DR.
SUSAN
LOVE'S
BREAST
BOOK

DR. SUSAN LOVE'S BREAST BOOK

Seventh Edition

Susan M. Love, MD

WITH ELIZABETH LOVE

IN PARTNERSHIP WITH
DR. SUSAN LOVE FOUNDATION FOR BREAST CANCER RESEARCH

CONTRIBUTORS
STEPHANIE L. GRAFF, MD & LAUREN A. GREEN, MD

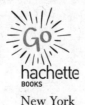

hachette
BOOKS

New York

Hachette Go, an imprint of Hachette Books
Hachette Book Group
1290 Avenue of the Americas
New York, NY 10104
HachetteGo.com
Facebook.com/HachetteGo
Instagram.com/HachetteGo

First Edition: October 2023

Published by Hachette Go, an imprint of Hachette Book Group, Inc. The Hachette Go name and logo is a trademark of the Hachette Book Group.

The Hachette Speakers Bureau provides a wide range of authors for speaking events. To find out more, go to hachettespeakersbureau.com or email HachetteSpeakers@hbgusa.com.

Hachette Go books may be purchased in bulk for business, educational, or promotional use. For information, please contact your local bookseller or Hachette Book Group Special Markets Department at special.markets@hbgusa.com.

The publisher is not responsible for websites (or their content) that are not owned by the publisher.

Print book interior design by Amy Quinn.

Library of Congress Cataloging-in-Publication Data
Names: Love, Susan M., author. | Lindsey, Karen, 1944– author. | Love, Elizabeth (Journalist), author.
Title: Dr. Susan Love's breast book / Susan M. Love, MD, with Karen Lindsey and Elizabeth Love.
Other titles: Breast book
Description: Seventh edition. | New York : Hachette Go, [2023] | Includes bibliographical references and index.
Identifiers: LCCN 2023010830 | ISBN 9780306833250 (paperback) | ISBN 9780306833267 (ebook)
Subjects: LCSH: Breast—Diseases—Popular works. | Breast—Cancer—Popular works.
Classification: LCC RG491 .L68 2023 | DDC 618.1/9—dc23/eng/20230530
LC record available at https://lccn.loc.gov/2023010830

ISBNs: 978-0-306-83325-0 (trade paperback); 978-0-306-83326-7 (ebook)

Printed in the United States of America

LSC-C

Printing 1, 2023

To all those dealing with breast cancer, with the hope that in the near future a cure will relegate this book to history.

Dr. Susan Love passed away from a recurrence of leukemia on July 2, 2023, three days after the last edits were sent in for the seventh edition.

Contents

Acknowledgments

Since 1990, I'd sit down every five years to completely revamp the Breast Book. This edition is a couple of years late and I got help from a team as I struggled with "chemo brain" after a relapse of acute myeloid leukemia. I am deeply grateful for the help of colleagues, especially Dr. Stephanie Graff and Dr. Lauren Green, who provided essential feedback, explanations, and anecdotes that brought material to life. They represent the new generation at the Dr. Susan Love Foundation for Breast Cancer Research. I also appreciate the input of Dr. Ana Lilia Aldrete in Guadalajara, Mexico, who is ready to assist with the new Spanish edition in the future. And, as always, I am also deeply grateful to all the support from family, colleagues, and friends, both online and off.

With continuing research, the diagnosis and treatment of breast cancer has become increasingly complex. It has become critically important to follow ongoing studies and touch base with friends and acquaintances who are in the thick of research and patient care. Their generous support is what makes this book valuable. Over the years, dozens of highly qualified experts have read, commented on, and enhanced new editions. For them we will always be grateful.

The other experts to whom I owe a debt of gratitude are the people who have shared their experiences with me. This includes not only the survivors I have met and talked to over the past years but also my Facebook friends, who always responded right away when I would post an urgent request for real-life stories to illustrate a point. I promised anonymity, but you know who you are.

Then there are the people in my life who facilitate the work and pitch in when needed. The team at the Dr. Susan Love Foundation for Breast Cancer Research has been terrific. Our CEO, Christopher Clinton Conway, is a steady and enthusiastic hand at the helm. The continual support of our wonderful board of directors is also critical to our mission. And keeping us all on track is Ileana Mendoza, our indefatigable director of business operations. Also hugely helpful in keeping us on track is Hilary Lentini, our project manager.

My terrific sister, Elizabeth Love, pitched in to help with research and writing, having already translated the fifth and sixth editions into Spanish. Sadly, Merloyd Lawrence, my wonderful and patient editor for decades, passed away recently. She was gifted at her job and always made sure everything fell together and made sense. We also lost our agent, Jill Kneerim, whose soft-spoken enthusiasm and continual support will be missed. Fortunately her talented protégé Sarah Khalil has taken over as my agent, for which I am grateful.

This book and these acknowledgments have tracked my life over the past three decades. The first edition was conceived before my daughter, who nonetheless beat it to being born. She is now married and living and working in Massachusetts. And my dear wife, Helen, has put up with "Dr. Susan Love's GD Breast Book" over the more than forty years of our lives together. To her I owe all my love and gratitude. You are the wind beneath my sails. And to all the people with breast cancer who share their stories with me online and in person, it is for you that I continue to do this work!

Introduction to the Seventh Edition

I did not expect to be writing an introduction to the seventh edition of my book, especially having written that the sixth was likely to be my last. This new edition came to light through the efforts of a supportive and energetic team. Just the kind of team you want to have by your side when confronting a serious and scary disease like breast cancer.

So much has happened in the three decades since the first book was published. Over the years we have witnessed a slow revolution in the way breast cancer is approached and how scientific research and medicine evolve.

In my first edition I explained what was then a new paradigm—that the most lethal part of breast cancer was the cells that may have spread into other parts of the body before diagnosis. At that time the addition of hormone therapy and then chemotherapy to the initial treatment of the disease was an exciting result of the new way of thinking. It also established the limitations of excessive surgery as the sole approach. The result has been a definite improvement in overall survival for many people with breast cancer.

But our belief that all breast cancers were the same and should be treated the same was wrong, as was the idea that more aggressive tumors required more aggressive treatments. At the time this had led to a high-dose chemotherapy and then stem cell rescue in an effort to kill every cancer cell—whether it was hiding somewhere or not. But ultimately this more aggressive approach proved no better than regular-dose chemotherapy.

Later observations suggested that cancer cells might be influenced by their surroundings. In the clinics, doctors noticed that some cancers were sensitive to hormones, whereas others weren't, and that some cancers had different molecular patterns that seemed to define their behavior.

Now we know that there are several different molecular subtypes of breast cancer, and each probably develops from a different step in the evolution of a tumor. That alone leads to the need to determine which subtype of cancer a person has at any particular time, then to personalize the treatment to match. We also have become aware that cancer cells do not function in isolation—the local and systemic environment plays an important role in goading them on.

Our sixth edition explored new findings on molecular markers and how cancer evades the immune system. We found that many cancers are made up of a variety of cancer cells as identified by molecular markers, leading to the possibility that a metastatic tumor may not match the original. We have tended to identify the dominant subtype and focus our treatments on it. Sometimes that works, but other times it allows less dominant molecular types to emerge. This means that we need to keep checking what type of cells we are dealing with but also that we may need a more systemic approach. That is where all the latest research and excitement with the immune system come into play—it is the security system that has the ability to adapt to the different types of cancer cells and destroy them when possible.

We now know that cancer cells do not function in isolation—you need more than a mutated cell to get actual cancer. You need it to be in a local environment, a sort of neighborhood that eggs it on. A bad cell in a good neighborhood will stay dormant most of the time, but if the neighborhood changes, there is likely to be trouble. This gives us a new way to think about risk factors, screening, and treatment. Without abandoning the goal to kill as many cancer cells as possible, we can also try to improve the neighborhood with healthy lifestyle changes.

In the past decade I have had my own experience with cancer, although it was leukemia (AML) rather than breast cancer. This taught me a lot about what it feels like to be a patient with no expertise, dependent on a good medical team, family, and friends to get you through. My experience taught me that even successful treatments come with a significant cost—the collateral damage—that we tend not to talk about. The chapter on "After Breast Cancer Treatment" reflects not only growing research on this damage but also ways to deal with it.

As this last edition is wrapped up, I am enrolled in a clinical trial to treat a recurrence of leukemia after nine cancer-free years. New breakthroughs in immunotherapy are particularly pertinent to me as I undergo a similar process as that used for metastatic breast cancer to jump-start my own immune cells.

Since the last edition, we have seen new drugs, new treatment combinations, and an increased understanding of how cancer subverts the immune system. There are more than a dozen new drugs being tested to alter and degrade estrogen receptors on cancer cells and several targeted immunotherapy drugs for specific subsets of cancer. There are also additional options for metastatic cancer, with new drugs and treatment options. In the first edition I did not even include metastatic disease because people died so quickly and there was so little we could do. Thank God this has changed a lot in thirty-two years. The treatments are much better, although still not good enough, and many people have been living with metastatic disease for ten years and more. In fact, not only are there advocacy groups for people with metastatic disease: there are numerous ones. If we could understand how to keep cancer cells dormant or put them back to sleep, metastatic disease could well become chronic rather than acute. This is certainly an important goal.

I truly believe we can be the generation that ends breast cancer. And we have to do it! We owe it to all the wonderful people who have died of this disease to make sure it ends with us. That is a fight I will not give up! I hope you will join me.

PART ONE

The Healthy Breast and Common Problems

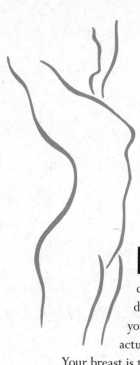

CHAPTER 1

The Breast

If you're reading this book, it's probably because you've come to think of the breast in terms of breast cancer: either it has the disease, or you're worried the disease may develop. But I think it is important to start your reading with a quick review of just what the breast actually is and does.

Your breast is the only organ in your body that you are not born with. You come into the world with a nipple and lots of potential: some cells behind the nipple that, given the right hormonal stimulation, will grow and become a breast. These are called stem cells. I like to think these stem cells are like those capsules you had as a kid that held collapsed sponge animals. When you added water, a sponge animal appeared. In the breast, what is added to the cells are certain hormones. These hormones cause your nipple to grow, and then a whole breast. When you get pregnant, the hormones take the breast tissue to the next level, making it ready to turn blood into milk to nurse a baby. The breast milk not only nourishes, it also passes on immunity to friendly bacteria and viruses needed to colonize the child's gut. Once that job is over, the breast cleans up all the milk-making cells and ducts and then makes new ones—to prepare for the next pregnancy. This continues for decades. When menopause comes along, this remarkable organ goes into retirement and just hangs out, literally and figuratively. Men's breasts develop similarly, but without that crucial role in pregnancy. Finally, despite all their marvels, it's important to know that you can live without breasts. People do it all the time. Still, breasts are pretty great and deserve some praise beyond their outward beauty!

Understanding a bit about anatomy will make much of the rest of the book clearer. The breast itself is usually tear-shaped (Figures 1.1 and 1.2). There's breast tissue from the collarbone all the way down to

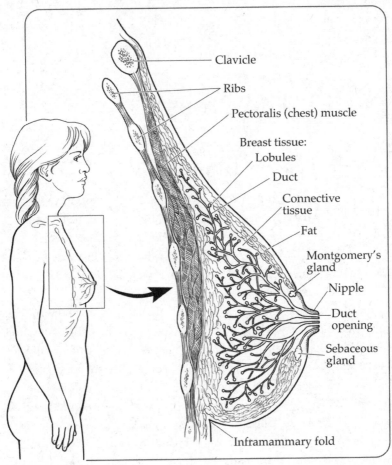

Clavicle

Ribs

Pectoralis (chest) muscle

Breast tissue:
    Lobules

Duct

Connective
tissue

Fat

Montgomery's
gland

Nipple

Duct
opening

Sebaceous
gland

Inframammary fold

Figure 1.1

the last few ribs, and from the breastbone in the middle of the chest to the back of the armpit. This becomes most obvious when you are pregnant and the tissue responds to the call to action. You suddenly notice parts of the breast you did not know you had. This, however, is also why it is impossible to tell a person with cancer that you removed all their breast. Unfortunately, breast tissue does not come in a different color or consistency than the surrounding flesh.

Luckily, removing most of the tissue is sufficient most of the time for people seeking prevention or treatment of breast cancer.

Often there's a ridge of fat at the bottom of the breast—the inframammary ridge (Figure 1.3). This ridge is perfectly normal, the result of

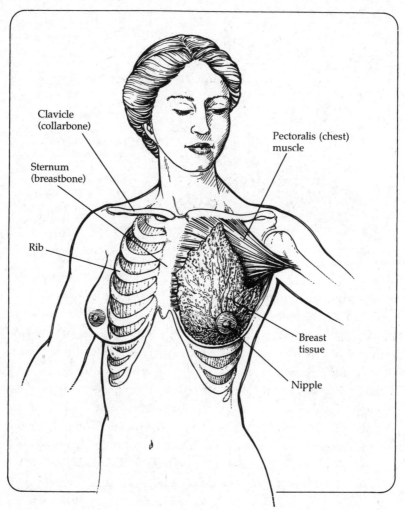

Figure 1.2

that fact that we walk upright and our breasts fold over themselves. Plastic surgeons take great care to reproduce this ridge when reconstructing a breast so that it will actually hang normally.

The areola is the darker area of the skin surrounding the nipple (Figure 1.4). Its size and shape varies from person to person, and its color varies according to complexion. In most people it gets darker after the first pregnancy. There are hair follicles around the nipple, so most people have at least some nipple hair. It's perfectly natural, and you can ignore it. If you don't like it, you can shave it off, pluck it out, use electrolysis,

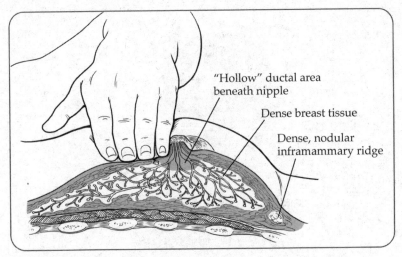

"Hollow" ductal area
beneath nipple

Dense breast tissue

Dense, nodular
inframammary ridge

Figure 1.3

or get rid of it any sensible way you want—it's just like leg or armpit hair except softer. You may also notice little bumps around the areola that look like goose pimples. These are the little glands known as Montgomery's glands. The nipple also has sebaceous glands, which I'll talk about later on in this chapter.

Sometimes nipples are "shy": when they're stimulated, instead of becoming erect they retreat into themselves and become temporarily inverted. This is nothing to worry about; it has no effect on milk supply, breastfeeding, sexual pleasure, or anything else. It is different when nipples suddenly become permanently inverted (see Chapter 2).

Inside, the breast tissue is sandwiched between layers of fat, behind which is the chest muscle. The fat has some give to it, which is why we bounce. The breast tissue is firm and rubbery. One of my patients told me while I was operating on her that she thought the breast was constructed like a woman—soft and pliant on the outside, and tough underneath. The breast also has its share of the connective tissue that holds the entire body together. This tissue has a solid structure—like gelatin—within which other kinds of tissues are loosely set. Sometimes called the stroma, it is getting more attention as recent studies show its importance in breast cancer.

Like the rest of the body, the breast has arteries, veins, and nerves. There is another, almost parallel, network called the lymphatic system, which consists of lymph vessels and lymph nodes. These recycle and filter lymph to help the body fight infection. The job of the lymphatic network

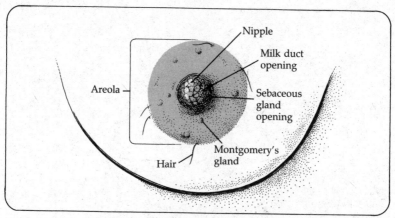

Figure 1.4

is to collect the debris from the cells and strain it through the lymph nodes found scattered in nests throughout the body; it then sends the filtered fluid back into the bloodstream to be reused (Figure 1.5). This system does more than just recycle, however. In the process of filtering the unnecessary fluid, the lymph nodes record what is in it. If there is anything threatening—a bacterial cell, a bit of material foreign to the body, or a virus—they hold on to it and use it to develop an immune response (see Chapter 3). They send cells to identify the invader and make antibodies to fight it. The lymph nodes are important when we talk about the way breast cancer spreads later in the book. It is crucial to identify which lymph vessels and which lymph nodes drain a particular area of the breast so that these nodes can be removed and examined for signs of cancer.

THE BREAST: AN INTERACTIVE COMMUNITY

During most of my career the critical component of the breast has been thought to be the system of milk ducts, with everything else just along for the ride. Yet there has been little research on the actual anatomy of the breast ducts. So I have devoted much of my own research to the subject.

Over the years my studies[1] have confirmed the findings of other researchers.[2] When we try to insert a tube (called a cannula) into the openings of the milk duct on the surface of the nipple, we find that there are between five and eight openings[3] (Figure 1.6). But this may be deceiving. When we examine a breast that has been removed and cut horizontally

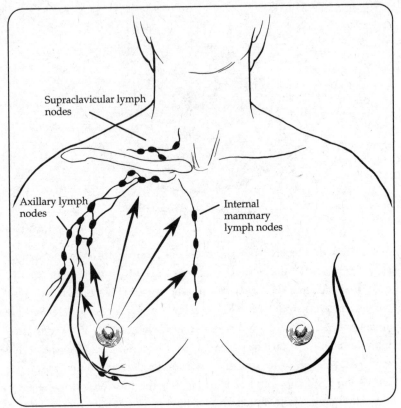

Figure 1.5

across the nipple, more ducts appear to exist—between fifteen and twenty-two ductlike structures.[4] This puzzle has still not been completely resolved, but recent work suggests that some of the ducts meet together inside the breast before they exit the nipple, thus sharing an opening, while others exit the nipple separately. In addition, some of what appear to be ducts may be something else: little glands that make a sebaceous material—a white, oily substance—and join with the milk duct. These sebaceous glands are found all over the body. We don't know what they're for, or why there are so many around the nipple. My own theory is that they provide a coating that protects the skin—sort of your own little skin-care system. The nipple, designed to be sucked on, is especially vulnerable to getting chapped and sore, so having a lot of these glands makes sense.

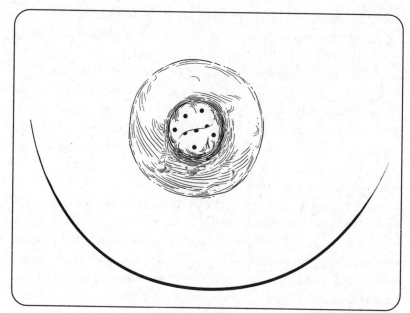

Figure 1.6

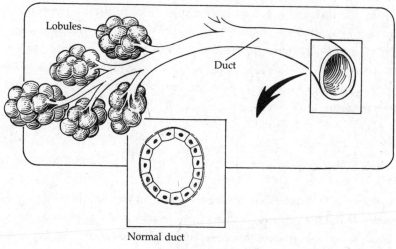

Normal duct

Figure 1.7

My colleagues and I studied the anatomy of the breast beyond the nipple, using both autopsies and breasts removed by mastectomy (with the patients' permission). We learned that the duct opening in the nipple leads into the breast in a straight line for a very short distance—only about a centimeter (less than one half inch). There's a little sphincter muscle here that prevents milk from squirting out when a breastfeeding parent is not nursing their baby. Behind that is a little antechamber called the lactiferous sinus. From there, the ductal system, like a tree, breaks up into little branches that go to the back of the breast. These branches are the ducts. Leafing out at the end of each branch are the lobules, which make the breast milk and then send it through the ducts to the nipple (Figure 1.7). Each ductal system is independent of all the others; each creates milk separately. They coexist, but they don't connect with one another. Each ductal system is completely lined or "tiled" by a single layer of small cells that completely coat the inside of the whole structure from the nipple to the very last branch closest to the chest wall. Breast cancer was thought to arise from changes in these lining cells, as we will see later. Initially we believed if we could selectively remove these lining cells from the inside of the ductal system when it is no longer needed for breastfeeding, we would be able to eliminate breast cancer. But recent studies have since shown that it isn't quite so simple. It turns out that the cells living around the ducts and lobules—fat cells, fibrous cells, and white blood cells—are as specialized and important as the cells lining the inside of the ducts and lobules. The cells all influence one another in a complex community that creates the breast's versatility, allowing it to go from the resting state to pregnancy and milk production and back to the resting state (Figure 1.8). What we do know is that when this interaction goes awry, it probably produces the environment that promotes cancer development and growth (see Chapter 3).

Supporting Cast

Besides the breast itself, there are two other organs that play an important role in breast cancer. These are the ovaries and the adrenal glands. These produce hormones that come into play in our current understanding of breast cancer and its treatment.

The Role of the Ovary

The Menstruating Years. From puberty on, the ovary produces the key hormones—estrogen and progesterone—needed to prepare for a pregnancy each month (Figure 1.9). This monthly process includes the breast.

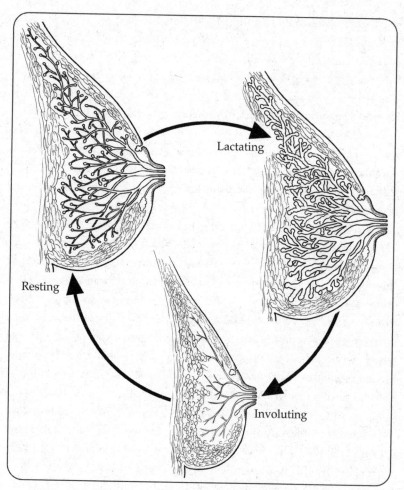

Figure 1.8

As the hormones stimulate the breast, we experience a familiar cyclical pattern of swelling, lumpiness, pain, and tenderness. This pattern, which involves over forty years of our reproductive lives, gives ample opportunity for minor changes in the breast to occur, resulting in many of the benign problems that people frequently experience (see Chapter 2).

Menopause. We used to assume that after menopause, when it is no longer capable of making eggs, the ovary shrivels up, dries out, and becomes completely useless. This resulted in part from the fact that we could not detect estrogen levels in the blood. Now we understand that with menopause, the ovary shifts from production of hormones to making the precursors of hormones and letting the organs themselves produce the final product. This is done by the stroma, or background tissue, in which eggs are embedded. In youth you have more eggs and less stroma. As time goes on, you have fewer and fewer eggs and more and more stroma. The stroma gives up the cyclical rhythm of the menstruating years and produces testosterone, and androstenedione—which are then converted into estrogen and progesterone in the breasts as well as in the bones, liver, and brain. This is why no estrogen was found in the blood—it is only the precursors of estrogen that circulate after menopause.[5] The hormonal dance doesn't end; the band just strikes up a different tune (see Figure 1.10).

Testosterone, of course, is a male hormone. But don't worry: you're not going to grow a beard, though you may find a few hairs on your chin. Much of a woman's testosterone and androstenedione is converted throughout the body to estrone, a form of estrogen, by an enzyme called aromatase. This continued production of hormones varies somewhat from one person to the next and may well explain some of the individual differences in symptoms after menopause. It also explains why people who have both ovaries removed surgically, thus losing all these hormones, often have worse symptoms of menopause and increased vulnerability to cardiovascular disease and osteoporosis.[6]

What all this means is that the ovaries have more than one function. Reproduction is their most dramatic task, but it isn't the only one. These organs have as much to do with the maintenance of the person's own life as they do with that person's role in bringing other lives into the world. A former medical colleague of mine, Bill Parker, confirmed the important role of the ovary postmenopausally when he demonstrated that people who had their ovaries removed preventively during hysterectomy had an overall increase in mortality compared to people who kept their ovaries. This was even though they had less breast and ovarian cancer.[7] The menopausal ovary is neither failing nor useless. It's simply beginning to shift from a reproductive function to a maintenance one. It's doing in midlife exactly what many people do—changing careers.

And what about the breasts? Clearly menopause is the ultimate involution—the breasts get the message that they will not be called into active duty again and can finally rest. But nothing is ever that simple. Different people have different levels of hormones after menopause,

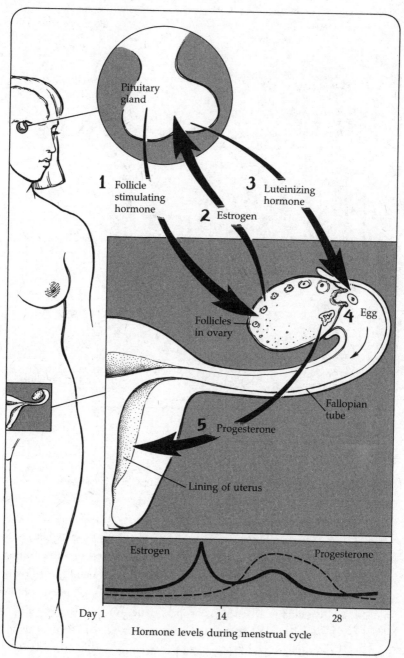

Figure 1.9

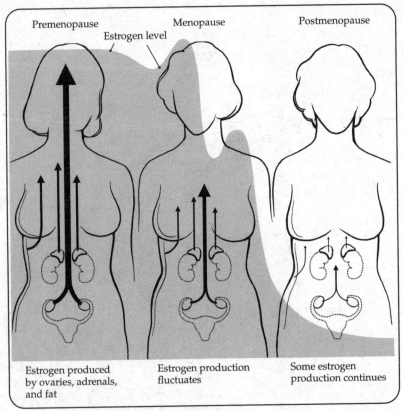

Figure 1.10

depending on several factors. If a person has reached menopause through surgery such as hysterectomy, or through chemotherapy, their hormone levels will change more dramatically than if they go through it naturally. Even in the latter case, however, some people naturally have higher levels of estrogen or testosterone, which will cause higher rates of vulnerability to breast cancer. We have observed, for example, that people with osteoporosis have 60 percent less breast cancer than those with normal bone density, and we believe that this is probably due to natural estrogen levels. If you have relatively high levels of estrogen in your body postmenopausally, you will have good bones and bad breasts; on the other hand, if your estrogen levels are lower, you will have good breasts and bad bones.

These differences in residual hormonal stimulation may be seen on a mammogram. A person's hormone levels may make the stroma appear denser than that of someone whose breasts have totally gone into retirement and become mostly ducts suspended in fat.

Synthetic Hormones

Giving people hormones (estrogen and usually progestins) can result in hormone-sensitive breast tumors (see Chapter 6). Also, people on postmenopausal hormones often, but not always, experience an increase in breast density, known to be a risk factor for breast cancer (see Chapter 5). Yet not every person who takes postmenopausal hormones gets breast cancer. It is likely that some people are more sensitive to postmenopausal hormones than others. Which ones and why remains a subject of much research. Recent studies suggest that mammographic breast density (see Chapter 7) may give us a hint. Karla Kerlikowske showed that postmenopausal people who still had dense breasts on a mammogram had a higher risk of cancer than those with fatty breasts.[8]

In addition, recent studies have shown that breast tissue itself has the enzyme aromatase, as noted earlier, which can convert testosterone and androstenedione into estrogen. This means that estrogen levels in the breast may indeed be higher than those in the rest of the body after menopause and may explain the estrogen-sensitive cancers that can occur at this age. Our increasing understanding of the postmenopausal breast's response to hormones will give us further insight into the cause of breast cancer after menopause.

Getting Acquainted

All this information can be intriguing and may lead you to a desire to get acquainted with your own breasts. This is a good idea, whether you are newly diagnosed or just worried. Those newly diagnosed may want to pay attention to how their breasts look and what is important to them as they try to figure out what surgical treatments are best for them. Those who have not been diagnosed will want to get to know what is normal for them so that they will recognize a change. And those who have had breast cancer will need to become acquainted with their new normal.

To start this process, look at your breasts. Stand in front of a mirror and look at yourself. See how your breasts hang and get a sense of how they project. If you're young they'll tend to stick out; if you're older they'll tend to be droopier. Feel the inframammary ridge, where the breast folds over itself, and the underlying muscles, the pectorals. Look at your nipple—what color is it? Does it have hairs or little bumps on it? If so, that's perfectly normal. You may want to swing your arms around and watch how your breasts move, or don't move, with the motion. Put your hands on your hips; flex your muscles; stretch your arms up. How do your breasts look with each change of position?

It's important to do this without judging your appearance. You're not trying out for a *Playboy* centerfold; you're learning about your body. Forget everything you've learned about what breasts are supposed to look like. These are your breasts, and they look fine.

The next step is to feel your breasts. It's best to do this soaped up in the shower or bath so your hands can slip very easily over your skin. Put the hand of the side you want to explore behind your head. This shifts the breast tissue that's beneath your armpit to over your chest wall. Since the tissue is sandwiched between your skin and your chest bones, you have good access to it. If you're very large breasted you may want to do it lying down, in the bathtub, or even in bed. You can then roll on one side and then the other to shift the breast closer to your chest wall so you can get a better feel for it.

Breast tissue generally has a texture that is finely nodular or granular, like large seeds. A lot of this more or less bumpy feeling is caused by the normal fat that intermingles with the breast tissue. Lumpy breasts have inspired some of the most unfortunate misconceptions about our bodies. Often this lumpiness gets confused with actual breast lumps, as discussed in Chapter 2. But lumpiness itself often gets bad press. People have been told their lumpy breasts are symptoms of "fibrocystic disease" (see Chapter 2) and have suffered from needless anxiety, fear, and even disfiguring surgery.

Lumpy breasts are caused by the way the breast tissue forms itself. In some people the breast tissue is fairly fine and thus not perceived as "lumpy." Others clearly have lumpy breasts, which can feel somewhat like cobblestone paving. Still others are somewhere between the extremes— just a bit nodular. There's nothing unusual about this—breasts vary as much as any other part of the body. Just as some people are tall and some short and some are fair-skinned and some dark, some have lumpier breasts and some have smoother breasts. There can even be differences within the same person's breasts. Your breasts may be a little more nodular near your armpit or at the top, for example, and the pattern may be the same in both breasts or may occur only in one. You'll find if you explore your breasts that there's a general, fairly consistent pattern. It's important to get a sense of what your pattern is.

Variations in Breast Development

Healthy breasts come in many different shapes and sizes. There's nothing "abnormal" about large, small, or asymmetrical breasts, or about extra nipples (Figure 1.11).

Common variations in breast development fall into one of two categories: those that are obvious from birth and those that don't show themselves until puberty. The latter are far more frequent.

(There are also variations due to accident or illness, the surgical remedies for which are essentially the same as those used for genetic variations.)

Variations Apparent at Birth. The most common variation to appear at birth is polymastia—an extra nipple or nipples. These can appear anywhere along the milk ridge (see Figure 1.12). Usually the milk ridge—a

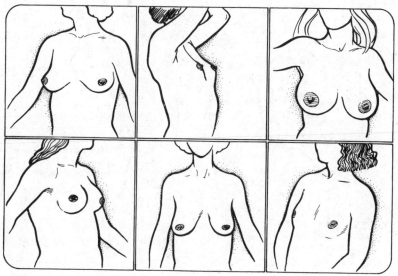

Figure 1.11

throwback to the days when we were animals with many nipples—regresses before birth, but in some people it remains throughout life. Between 1 and 5 percent of the population has extra nipples, usually inherited from their birth parent. Usually they're below the breast, and often people don't even know they're there, since they look like moles. When I would point out an extra nipple to a patient, it was usually the first time they had been aware of it.

Extra nipples cause no problems and usually don't appear cosmetically unattractive. One patient was actually fond of her extra nipple: she told me that her husband had one too, and that's how they knew they were meant for each other!

Extra nipples don't cause any problems, though they may lactate if you breastfeed. There's nothing wrong with this unless it causes you discomfort.

A variation of the extra nipple is extra breast tissue without a nipple, most often under the armpit. It may feel like hard, cystlike lumps that

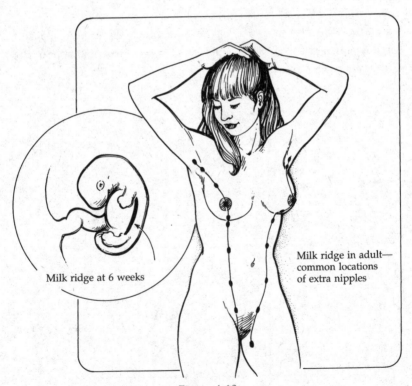

Milk ridge at 6 weeks

Milk ridge in adult—
common locations
of extra nipples

Figure 1.12

swell and hurt when you menstruate, the way your breasts do. Like extra nipples, this extra breast tissue is often unnoticed by doctor and patient. One of my patients had swelling under both armpits during her second pregnancy. It was probably caused by extra breast tissue, and it went down after she finished lactating. The extra tissue is subject to all the problems of normally situated tissue. I have had patients with cysts, fibroadenomas, or even cancers in such tissue.

Unless the extra nipple or breast tissue causes you extreme physical discomfort or psychological distress, there's no need to worry about it. If it does bother you, it's easy to get rid of surgically. The nipple can be removed under local anesthetic in your doctor's office, and the extra breast tissue can be removed under either local or general anesthetic.

A much rarer condition is *amastia*—being born with a breast that has breast tissue but no nipple. It's usually associated with problems in the development of the chest bone and muscles, like scoliosis and rib deformities. Aside from whatever medical procedures you may need because of the associated problems, you may want to have a fake nipple created by a plastic surgeon, in the same way a nipple is created during reconstruction after a mastectomy (see Chapter 13). The nipple can be created using skin from the breast, and the areola can be tattooed on or created using a skin graft, commonly from the inner thigh. Though this artificial nipple will look real, it won't feel completely like a real nipple. Its advantages are wholly cosmetic.

Some people have an underdeveloped breast on one side. This condition is sometimes called Poland syndrome, and it involves not just the breast but also the pectoralis muscle and the ribs, as well as, in some cases, abnormalities of the hand. A person with Poland syndrome may have a small but very deformed breast.

There is another condition in which people have permanently inverted nipples (they grow in instead of out)—a congenital condition that usually won't manifest until puberty.

Various injuries can affect breast development. This may happen surgically or with trauma. If the nipple and breast bud are seriously injured before puberty, the potential adult breast is destroyed as well. Sometimes injuring the skin can limit future breast development. Most commonly this occurs as a result of a severe burn. The resulting scars are so tight that breast tissue cannot develop. In the past, some congenital conditions such as hemangiomas (birthmarks) were treated with radiation, which damaged the nipple and breast bud and prevented later growth. Any serious injury to the breast bud can cause such arrested development.

Variations Appearing at Puberty. Three basic variations appear when the breasts begin to develop: very large breasts, very small breasts, and asymmetrical breasts.

Very Large Breasts. Very large breasts can occur early in puberty—a condition known as *virginal hypertrophy*. After the breasts begin to grow, the shutoff mechanism, whatever it is, forgets to do its job and the breasts keep on growing, becoming huge and greatly out of proportion to the rest of the body. Sometimes the condition runs in families. In very rare instances, virginal hypertrophy occurs in one breast and not the other. "Large" is both subjective and variable. A five-foot-tall person with a C cup is very large breasted; a five-foot-eight person with a C cup may not feel especially uncomfortable with their size. A five-foot-eight person with a DD cup is likely to be very uncomfortable.

Large breasts have been a problem for a number of my patients. "I almost never wear a bathing suit," one patient told me, "because people stare at my breasts." Another, at age 71, still "hunches over" when she walks to avoid having her breasts stared at.

Huge breasts can be especially distressful to a teenage girl. She faces ridicule from her schoolmates, and—unlike the small-breasted girl—extreme physical discomfort as well. She may be unable to participate in sports, and she may have severe backache all the time. She usually needs a bra to hold the breasts in, but the bra, pulled down by the weight of the breasts, can dig painful ridges into her shoulders.

If the breasts cause this much discomfort, the girl may want to have reduction surgery done while she's still in her teens. However, the surgical trauma involved in breast reduction can interfere with the ability to breastfeed. For this reason, some parents refuse to let their daughters have reduction surgery, urging them to wait until they've had children. Both parent and daughter must weigh the physical and emotional damage the girl may go through. If she decides to have children, pregnancy may worsen her problem. When the breasts become engorged with milk, they become even larger and, in a woman with huge breasts, more uncomfortable. Though it's unfortunate that someone so young is faced with a decision that affects her whole life, it's important to realize that not having the surgery will also affect her life. Many girls of fifteen or sixteen are mature enough to make their own decisions if all the facts are carefully explained to them, including the possibility of bottle-feeding. In any case, the losses and gains of either choice are the girl's, and she should be given the right and the time to decide for herself what to do. She should be encouraged to talk to doctors, mothers of young children, and very large-breasted women; to read all the material she can find about the pros and cons of the procedure and of breastfeeding; and to make her decision only when she feels she is fully informed.

Not all problems with huge breasts appear right after puberty. Some comfortably large-breasted individuals find that their breasts have expanded considerably after pregnancy; others become uncomfortable after their breast size has increased with an overall weight gain or after menopause. Many surgeons are reluctant to operate when the increase came with weight gain, preferring to wait until the patient has lost weight because of the increased risk of wound-healing complications. However, I've known people who were so depressed by their huge breasts that they compensated by overeating, thus intensifying both problems. In such cases, the pleasing appearance of their breasts created by reduction surgery can be a spur to continue their self-improvement.

In any case, the individual must make the decision; she's the one who lives with the problem and she's the one who can best judge its impact on her life. Some women with very large breasts don't mind them. One patient, who admits they cause her discomfort, says that she nonetheless enjoys their size because, she says, "they feel feminine and sexy."

Very Small Breasts. The opposite problem is extreme flat chestedness. Like "large breasted," the notion of "small breasted" is subjective and relative, and culturally determined. Some women, however, have breasts so small as to be almost nonexistent. This causes no physical or medical problems but can make a woman feel unattractive and sexless.

Because very small breasts can both feed babies and respond sexually, they don't bother some women. Simply wearing "falsies" or padded bras satisfies others. Some want to have the breasts altered surgically.

Asymmetrical Breasts. In most individuals breasts develop unevenly to some degree, but in some they develop quite differently, resulting in severe asymmetry. For someone who is bothered by this, plastic surgery can help achieve a reasonable match. Either the larger breast can be reduced or the smaller one augmented—or a combination of both can be done. It's important for the surgeon to discuss these options. Often we assume that a woman will want her small breast made larger and neglect to suggest the possibility of reducing the larger breast. What the patient decides will depend on the size of both breasts, the degree of asymmetry, and above all her own aesthetic goals.

It's fortunate that plastic surgery techniques exist for people who want them. But don't assume that because you have atypical-looking breasts, you have to get them altered. Many women are quite pleased with how their breasts look.

Thinking About Plastic Surgery

For a woman deeply unhappy with the way her breasts look, plastic surgery offers a solution that can make a major psychological difference in her life. No operation will make you look "perfect"—whatever that is—but these procedures can help you feel more normal and more comfortable in your body. Most of us have an emotional relationship with our breasts. Beyond size, consider issues like personal sense of style or breast sensation as it pertains to sexual intimacy and activities ranging from hugging a child to athletic performance. How much do symmetry and aesthetics matter to you and how might they affect sensation?

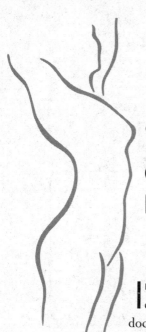

CHAPTER 2

Common Breast Problems

In the first edition of this book, I wrote about the common use of the term "fibrocystic disease," which doctors once used to describe a number of symptoms, often with no relation to one another, such as painful breasts, lumpy breasts, and breasts that got swollen and firm before a person's period. It seemed to me that "fibrocystic disease" meant "we don't know what is wrong with you but it isn't cancer so we are not going to pay attention to it." The term had no real meaning even though the symptoms were very real. So I began to call it a "garbage" term that lumps everything not related to breast cancer into one bucket (Figure 2.1). Luckily for us, over the past twenty-five years, a few researchers have focused on benign (noncancerous) breast problems and found that many of these conditions are related to various processes of reproductive life, with a spectrum that ranges from normal to atypical and, occasionally, to disease. As the breasts develop, go through the changes of pregnancy and lactation, and finally wind down with menopause, the potential for variations in timing, coordination, and resolution are enormous. These variations form the basis for most conditions that some consider benign breast disease.

Unfortunately some doctors still tell patients they have fibrocystic disease, as I have discovered from the comments people have sent to me on Facebook. And some people, having been told this years ago, still believe they have it. This might be harmless, except that it keeps patients from knowing precisely what their real condition is and, thus, whether it needs to be treated. Further, most of the conditions called "fibrocystic

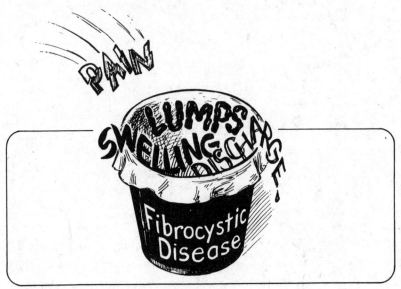

Figure 2.1

disease" are simply normal variations—they are not diseases, "fibrocys-tic" or otherwise.

In the following section I discuss the various kinds of benign breast problems people experience and try to give you a better understanding of what is really going on and how—or whether—it should be treated.

LUMPS AND LUMPINESS

Lumpiness, as I explained in Chapter 1, isn't the same as having one dom-inant lump. It's a general pattern of many little lumps in both breasts, and it is usually perfectly normal. The distinction between "lumps" and "lumpiness" is important; confusing the two can cause a person days and weeks of needless mental anguish. Doctors who don't usually work with breast cancer—family practitioners and gynecologists—often get ner-vous about lumpy breasts and fear that the lumps may be cancer. So your doctor may send you to a specialist—a surgeon or a breast specialist—to make sure you don't have a cancerous lump. If you or your doctor are uncertain about whether you've got a lump or just lumpy breasts, it's probably not a bad idea to check it out further. But understanding more about what a lump really feels like may make the trip to the specialist unnecessary.

Ellen Mahoney, a fellow breast surgeon, tells her patients to visualize what their breasts may be like inside—from butter to gravel to Bubble Wrap—and if it's the same all over, it's just the way they're made. The only area to be concerned about is one that is different from all the rest. The most important thing to know about dominant lumps—benign or malignant—is that they're almost never subtle. They're not like little BB pellets; they're usually at least a centimeter or two, almost an inch, or the size of a grape. The lump will stick out prominently in the midst of the smaller lumps that constitute normal lumpiness. You'll know it's something different. In fact, that's why most breast cancers are found by the person themself—the lumps are so clearly distinct from the rest of the breast tissue.

The obvious question here is: How do I know the BB-size thing isn't an early cancer? The answer is that you usually don't feel a malignant lump when it's small. The cancer has to grow to a large enough size for the body to begin to create a reaction to it—a fibrous, scarlike tissue forms around the cancer, and this, combined with the cancer itself, makes up a lump that you can feel, what we call *palpable*. The body won't create that reaction when the cancer is tiny, and you won't feel the cancerous lump until the reaction is formed. Although very large lumps and multiple lumps are rarely malignant, in this day and age it's easy enough to get an ultrasound test of the lump. Most breast surgeons have ultrasound in their offices and can check anything worrisome right there. Then if there is any question, they can have you get a diagnostic mammogram as well.

There are three main types of dominant lumps, two of which—cysts and fibroadenomas—are virtually harmless. It's the third type—the malignant lump—that you're worrying about when you have it examined by a health care provider. (I'll talk about cancerous lumps at length in Chapter 8.) It is important to remember that only about one in twelve palpable dominant lumps in premenopausal people are malignant. We often don't know the exact cause of any of the noncancerous lumps, though we do know they're somehow related to hormonal variations (see Chapter 1). Cysts and fibroadenomas form during a person's menstruating years and are probably variations in the formation (fibroadenomas) and shrinking (cysts) that occur in the breast tissue at different times.

CYSTS

Doctors tend to describe all nonmalignant lumps as cysts. They're not. A cyst is a distinct kind of lump. Typically it occurs in people in their thirties, forties, and early fifties and is most common in people approaching menopause. It rarely occurs in a younger person or in one who is past menopause. However, I've had patients in both categories, including a teenager and a woman who'd finished with her menopause long ago and wasn't on artificial hormones. (A person taking estrogen to combat menopausal symptoms fools their body into thinking it's still premenopausal.)

A gross cyst (*gross* meaning "large," not "disgusting") is a fluid-filled sac, like a large blister, that grows in breast tissue. It's smooth on the outside and *ballotable*—squishy—on the inside, so that if you push on it, you can feel that it contains fluid inside. This, however, can be deceptive. Cysts feel like cysts only when they're close to the surface (Figure 2.2). Cysts that are deeply embedded in breast tissue tend to stretch that tissue and push it forward, so that what you're feeling is the hard breast tissue, not the soft cyst. In these cases the cyst feels like a hard lump.

The classic cyst story goes something like this. A person in their forties comes to a specialist and says, "I went to the gynecologist six weeks ago and everything was fine. I had a mammogram, and that was fine too.

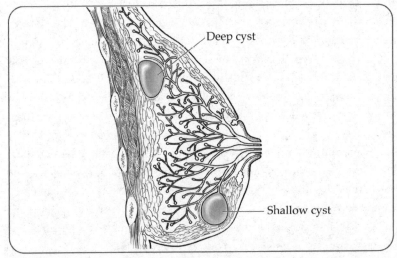

Figure 2.2

Then all of a sudden, in the shower last night, I found this lump in my breast, and I know it wasn't there before." So the doctor examines the patient and sure enough, there's a hard lump in their breast.

Because of its overnight appearance, the doctor is pretty sure it's a harmless cyst, but of course it's something the doctor—not to mention the patient—wants to be absolutely certain about: some cancers do seem to appear overnight. At this point the doctor has two options. If there's an ultrasound unit in the office, the lump can be imaged immediately to confirm the diagnosis. The ultrasound test works like radar or sonar. If you have a solid lump, the waves from the ultrasound will bounce back, showing a brighter spot with a dark shadow behind it. If it is a cyst, however, the sound waves will go right through it and there will be a black circle or oval without a shadow (see Chapter 7 to read about mammograms and ultrasound techniques). Once the cyst is diagnosed, the doctor can aspirate it right there. If there's no ultrasound in the office and the lump is easily palpable, it too can be immediately aspirated. To do this, the doctor takes a tiny needle, like the kind used for insulin injections, and anesthetizes the sensitive skin over the breast lump. Then a larger needle—like the kind used to draw blood—is attached to a syringe and inserted into the breast through the skin and into the cyst, where it draws out the fluid (Figure 2.3). The cyst collapses like a punctured blister, and that's that. Though the process sounds scary, it's usually almost painless.

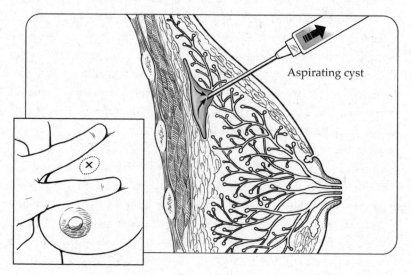

Aspirating cyst

Figure 2.3

Most of the nerves in the breast are in the skin, and that's been anesthetized. Some people with greater sensitivity to pain or especially sensitive breasts do find it painful, but most don't. The only possible complications from aspirating a cyst are bruising or bleeding into the cyst, neither of which is more than slightly uncomfortable. Another option is to order an ultrasound at an imaging center and if the area looks like a cyst, an aspiration can be done under ultrasound guidance.

The fluid looks disgusting, but it's harmless. It can be almost any color, but usually it's green, brown, or yellow. Sometimes the fluid can even be milk—a person who is breastfeeding can form a milk-filled cyst, called a galactocele, which is treated like any other cyst. There can be any amount of fluid—from a few drops to as much as a cup. One patient came to me with asymmetrical breasts; after I aspirated her cyst, her breasts were the same size.

Usually a person will get only one or two cysts in their entire life. But some get many, and often. A patient who has recurring, multiple cysts should be followed by a breast surgeon who has ultrasound and can monitor the cysts and aspirate them as needed. When a person has multiple cysts, chances are they'll go on getting them until menopause—only rarely are they a onetime occurrence.

If cysts are harmless, why do we bother to image and/or aspirate them? Mostly because we need to be sure it is a cyst. You can't be absolutely certain a lump in the breast isn't cancer until you find out what it really is. Once they know it's a cyst, doctor and patient can both rest easy.

There are other ways of finding out you have a cyst—it may show up as an area of density on a routine mammogram, and then you can have an ultrasound test done to see whether it's a cyst or a solid lump. If you've discovered a cyst through a mammogram and ultrasound and it doesn't worry you, don't bother having it aspirated—you already know it isn't cancer. Sometimes a cyst is painful, especially if it develops quickly. Aspirating it will usually relieve the pain.

Cysts are almost never malignant. There's a 1 percent incidence of cancer in cysts, and it's a seldom dangerous cancer called intracystic papillary carcinoma (Figure 2.4). It usually doesn't spread beyond the lining of the cyst, and unless there are specific signs that it may be present, it's not worth risking surgical removal. If there are signs that cancer may be present in the cyst, I'd operate on it—never otherwise, and only if the ultrasound looks suspicious.

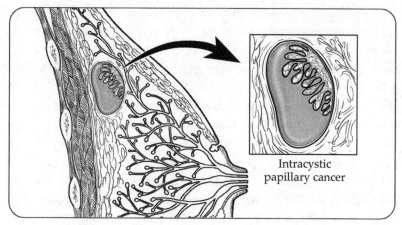

Intracystic
papillary cancer

Figure 2.4

Sometimes a doctor will aspirate a cyst and won't get any fluid. This isn't a cause for panic; it can happen for a number of reasons. The lump may not be a cyst after all, but a nonmalignant solid lump like those discussed shortly. Or the doctor may have missed the middle of the cyst. The doctor tries to get the cyst between their fingers and then puncture it, but it's easy to miss the middle, especially in a fairly small cyst. When this happened to me, I'd send the patient for ultrasound and let them aspirate it under direct vision. Operating on a cyst should be only a last resort.

Aspirating a cyst was once thought to be dangerous. If a person had an unknown breast cancer, doctors believed the process of aspiration would spread the cancer over the needle's track. We now know that's completely untrue.[1] It can be aspirated or left alone.

Cysts don't increase the risk of cancer. The real risk is mental rather than physical. A person with frequent cysts is likely to feel a lump and shrug it off as just another cyst—only to learn later that it was a malignant growth. Every lump should be checked out to be sure it isn't dangerous.

FIBROADENOMAS

Another common nonmalignant lump is the fibroadenoma. These lesions come from lobules that are particularly sensitive to estrogen stimulation.

They usually develop as the breasts are just getting used to hormonal cycling, during puberty and the teenage years. A fibroadenoma is a smooth, round lump that feels the way most people think a cyst should feel: it's smooth and hard, like a marble dropped into the breast tissue (Figure 2.5) where it can move around easily. It's often found near the nipple but can grow anywhere in the breast. It's also very distinct from the rest of the breast tissue. It can vary from a tiny five millimeters to a lemon-size five centimeters. The largest are called, logically, *giant fibroadenomas*. Generally fibroadenomas grow over a twelve-month period to a size of about two to three centimeters (from the size of a marble to that of a large grape), and then remain unchanged for several years. About 15 percent will go away on their own, while only 5 to 10 percent continue to grow. Studies in patients who were followed for up to twenty-nine years found that the fibroadenoma often shrank or disappeared. The researchers concluded that a fibroadenoma would probably disappear after five years in approximately 50 percent of cases and after fifteen years the rest of the time.[2]

A doctor can usually tell simply by feeling the lump that it's a fibroadenoma; if a needle aspiration is done and no fluid comes out, the doctor knows it isn't a cyst and is even more convinced it's a fibroadenoma. The diagnosis can always be confirmed by doing a core biopsy (see Chapter 8) and sending the tissue off to the lab just to make doubly sure.

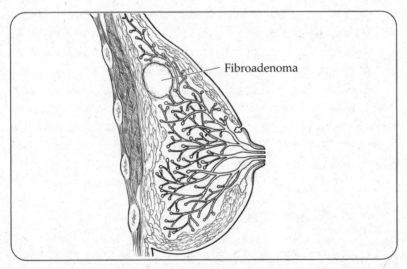

Fibroadenoma

Figure 2.5

Fibroadenomas are usually distinct on a mammogram or ultrasound test. They are harmless in themselves and don't need to be removed as long as we're sure they are fibroadenomas.

Because fibroadenomas develop at puberty, teenagers are more prone to have them and less likely to get breast cancer than are older people, so we may consider not removing them at all unless the patient desires it. In older patients we tend to do a core biopsy of all fibroadenomas, or simply remove them, to be sure they're not cancer.

If the doctor and the patient want the fibroadenoma removed, it can be easily done under local anesthetic. The surgeon simply makes a small incision, finds the lump, and takes it out (Figure 2.6). (Some surgeons prefer to make a small incision around the nipple and then tunnel their way to the lump, to minimize scarring. I don't think this is a great idea, and it's harder to find the lesion that way. If the doctor cuts over the fibroadenoma it's easier to find and the scarring doesn't usually remain noticeable in most patients.) If your core biopsy proves that this is a fibroadenoma, there is no need to have it removed unless you want to. Some patients remain nervous knowing there's a lump in their breast, in which case it's reasonable to have it removed for peace of mind. Another option has been developed that should appeal to many patients: a minimally invasive procedure in which the fibroadenoma is frozen in place under ultrasound guidance. It is almost painless because the cold is numbing, and it takes about a half hour in a doctor's office. Within about a year or two the fibroadenoma disappears.[3]

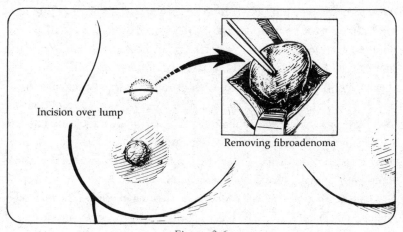

Figure 2.6

Usually a person has only one fibroadenoma; it's removed or treated, and they never get any more. But some people get several over a lifetime—and a few people get many of them. It's not uncommon to have three or four fibroadenomas in one breast, or for fibroadenomas to grow as large as four centimeters (one and a half inches) in diameter. One of my patients had a fibroadenoma in her left breast, and I removed it. She returned a couple of years later with another one on the exact same spot in her other breast—a kind of mirror image. Occasionally a person will have multiple fibroadenomas at once. After they are removed, more form. I had one patient with this problem, and I must admit it is a difficult one. Obviously a surgeon can't keep removing them, but equally obviously a person with this condition will be worried. One patient I talked to was told to have prophylactic mastectomies so the surgeon would not have to worry. This is pretty drastic for a benign condition that does not increase breast cancer risk. I'd generally recommend surgery only for the patient's—not the doctor's—peace of mind.

Fibroadenomas shouldn't be confused with fibroids, which by definition exist only in the uterus. There are similarities between the two conditions: in both cases one section of glandular tissue becomes autonomous, growing as a ball in the midst of the rest of the tissue. But there's no other correlation—having one doesn't mean you're likely to get the other. In fact, they usually occur at different stages of life: fibroids when you're heading toward menopause, fibroadenomas in your teens or early twenties.

However, fibroadenomas can occur at any age, up until menopause. As with cysts, you can get them after menopause if you're taking hormones that trick your body into thinking it's premenopausal. As we do more mammograms on a wider range of people, we find more and more fibroadenomas in people in their sixties and seventies. Probably they've had them since their teens and simply, in those premammography days, didn't know about them. There are some rare cancers that can look like fibroadenomas on a mammogram, so in postmenopausal people we usually do either a fine-needle aspiration, a core biopsy, or, if those don't give us the information, an excisional biopsy (removal of the whole lump), just to make sure it is a fibroadenoma.

There's also a rare cancer called cystosarcoma phyllodes, or phyllodes tumor (see Chapter 12), which is a cousin to a fibroadenoma. It is found about 1 percent of the time when a surgeon is removing what is thought to be a fibroadenoma. It's usually a big lump—lemon-size or larger. Generally this is a relatively harmless cancer that doesn't tend to spread to other parts of the body. Some doctors will insist on removing all fibroadenomas on the theory that this cancer may be present. It's not a very sensible attitude, especially if a core biopsy has proven that the lump is a fibroadenoma, because of both the rarity and the lack of danger.

Finally, fibroadenomas themselves never turn into cancer. Rarely, a cancer will arise in a fibroadenoma, but it won't be missed as long as you check the size at diagnosis and at six months. If all is stable, size doesn't have to be checked again until there is a suspicion of change.

What to Do If You Think You Have a Lump

If you have something that feels like it may be a lump, the first thing to do, obviously, is go to your doctor. If there is any question, they will do an ultrasound or send you to a specialist for one. If you are over thirty, you will have a mammogram to get additional information. The imaging may show evidence of a real lump. If the examination and imaging doesn't give the surgeon the necessary clarification, it's wise to do a needle biopsy to find out what it is. With the minimally invasive core biopsy, we can now easily get an answer without surgery. These core biopsies can be done by a surgeon if the lump can be felt or seen on ultrasound or, more often, by a radiologist, mammographer, or ultrasonographer. Find out who in your community has the most experience. In many places there are breast centers where you can have lumps evaluated by someone in the appropriate specialty.

It's important to stress one thing: if you're certain that something is wrong with your breast, get it biopsied, whatever the doctor's diagnosis. Often a person is sure they have a lump, the doctor is sure they don't, and a year or two later a lump shows up on their mammogram. The patient believes that the doctor was careless. Usually that's not the case. It's likely that the patient—who, after all, experiences their breast from both inside and outside, while the doctor can only experience the patient's breast from outside—has sensed something wrong and interpreted that in terms of the concept most familiar to them: a lump. I'm convinced that this is the basis of many of the malpractice suits that arise when a doctor "fails" to detect what later proves to be cancer. If you really feel something is wrong in your breast, insist on a biopsy. If you're wrong, you'll put your mind at rest—and if you're right, you may just save your own life. It's a minor procedure with low risks and potentially high gains.

BREAST PAIN

Another common breast symptom is pain—frequently called either mastalgia or mastodynia (one is Latin, the other Greek, and they both translate to "breast pain"). It can run the gamut of discomfort—from a minor irritation a couple of days a month to permanent, nearly disabling agony, and everything in between. A study of 1,171 healthy premenopausal American people revealed that 69 percent suffered from regular discomfort, 36 percent had seen a doctor about their pain, and 11 percent experienced moderate to severe breast pain.[4] A study in a clinic in Cardiff, Wales, documented three main categories of breast pain: cyclical (pain related to the menstrual cycle), noncyclical ("trigger zone" pain), and pain that does not originate in the breast. Of these, the most common by far is cyclical.[5]

The best way to determine which kind of pain you have is to keep a breast pain chart—a calendar where you mark every day whether your pain is severe, mild, or nonexistent.[6] In addition, you mark the days of your period. Looking at this, you can easily determine whether your pain is premenstrual or variable (cyclical or noncyclical).

Cyclical Pain

We know that cyclical mastalgia is related to hormonal variations. The breasts are sensitive right before menstruation, then less sensitive once the period begins. For some people, tenderness begins at the time of ovulation and continues until their period, leaving only a couple of pain-free weeks during their cycle. For some, it's barely noticeable; others are in such pain they can't wear a T-shirt, lie on their stomach, or tolerate a hug. Sometimes it's only in one breast, and other times it radiates into the armpit and even down to the elbows, causing its poor victim to think they've got cancer spreading to their lymph nodes.

Breast pain is annoying, but it usually isn't unbearable—what can be unbearable is the fear that it's cancer. The best treatment, therefore, is reassurance. The study in Cardiff suggests that 85 percent of people with breast pain worry much more about the possibility of cancer than about the pain itself. Most of them, after exams and imaging, can be reassured that their problem has no relation to cancer, leading to emotional relief and the feeling that they can live with their pain. This study was repeated in Brazil to see if it was only Welsh patients who responded to reassurance. Sure enough, Brazilian patients also responded to reassurance with a success rate of 70.2 percent. Only 10 to 15 percent of the patients had pain that was incapacitating and needed treatment.[7]

If you have breast pain, the first step is to get a good examination from a breast specialist or someone knowledgeable in the field who will take your symptoms and concerns seriously (this may take some searching). If you're over thirty, have a mammogram. Once you know you don't have cancer, you can decide whether you are able to live with your discomfort or want to further explore treatment. You may also want to look into Chinese herbs and acupuncture, which have been used for centuries in China. In some cases, herbs and acupuncture are used together; in others, the patient or practitioner prefers to use one or the other. They can also be used for noncyclical pain, discussed later in this chapter.

Another possibility is the use of meditation and visualization techniques, such as those discussed in Chapter 16. A number of studies have shown that these techniques can be effective in reducing pain, and they may well help relieve both cyclical and noncyclical breast pain.

If you are in your twenties and the pain is cyclical, you may want to try a birth control pill. Analgesics like aspirin, Tylenol, and ibuprofen can offer some relief, and wearing a firm bra will prevent bouncing breasts from increasing your discomfort. Nonsteroidal anti-inflammatory drugs (NSAIDs) can be applied directly to the breast in a gel, which can be beneficial.[8]

If these approaches do not work, then Nolvadex (tamoxifen), an estrogen blocker that has been used in treating and preventing breast cancer, can be helpful. Nolvadex is a selective estrogen receptor modulator (see Chapter 6). According to an English study, it's very good at relieving mastalgia (80 to 90 percent).[9] Side effects include hot flashes and menstrual irregularities. Luckily, it was shown to be just as effective at ten milligrams per day as at twenty milligrams, and three months of treatment were just as good as six. A group in Minnesota reports using ten milligrams for two months with good results and only a 30 percent recurrence rate.[10]

Noncyclical Pain

Noncyclical pain is far less common than cyclical pain. It also feels a lot different. To begin with, it doesn't vary with your menstrual cycle—it's there and it stays there. It's also known as "trigger zone" breast pain because it's almost always in one specific area: you can point exactly to where it hurts. It's anatomical rather than hormonal—something in the breast tissue is causing it (although we usually don't know what). Sometimes it can be a sign of cancer, so it's always worth checking out with your doctor, especially if you are over thirty.

One cause of noncyclical breast pain is trauma—a blow to the breast will obviously cause it to hurt, and a breast biopsy is likely to leave some pain (see Chapter 8). Many patients get slight shooting or stabbing pains up to two years or more after a biopsy. And you're never quite perfect after any surgery—just as after breaking a leg you can always tell when it will rain. This kind of pain is usually pretty obvious: it's on the spot where your scar is. It's unpleasant, but it's nothing to worry about.

Often doctors simply don't know what causes noncyclical breast pain; they'll operate and remove the area, have the tissue studied, and find nothing abnormal. Unfortunately this doesn't relieve the pain.

Treatment for this kind of breast pain is more difficult than for cyclical breast pain. Again, start with a good exam and, if you're over thirty, a mammogram. If there's an obvious abnormality, it can then be taken care of. For example, sometimes a gross cyst causing localized breast pain or tenderness can be cured by needle aspiration.

Because noncyclical pain is rarely caused by hormones, hormonal treatments are less likely to work. Some people, however, find relief with the kinds of treatments mentioned in the section on cyclical breast pain. Sometimes, though not invariably, having a biopsy relieves the pain—though you will experience pain for a while from the biopsy itself. A good test is for your doctor to inject some local anesthesia into the spot. If it gives relief, then surgery may work well; if not, then it probably isn't worth it.

Nonbreast-Origin Pain

This third category isn't really a form of breast pain, though that's what it feels like to the patient. It's usually in the middle of the chest and doesn't change with your period. Most frequently it is arthritic pain, in the place where the ribs and breastbone connect—an arthritis called costochondritis (Figure 2.7).[11] When men get costochondritis they think it's a heart attack; when women get it, they think it's breast cancer. You can tell it's arthritis by pushing down on your breastbone where your ribs are—if it hurts a lot more, that's probably what you've got. Similarly, if you take a deep breath and the middle part of your breast hurts, it's probably arthritis. If you take aspirin or Motrin and it relieves the pain, it's probably arthritis, as they're anti-inflammatory agents and thus work especially well on conditions like arthritis. Having your doctor inject the spot with local anesthetic and steroids will relieve 90 percent of chest wall pain.[12]

You can also get nonbreast-origin pain from arthritis in the neck (a pinched nerve).[13] This pain can radiate down into the breast the way lower-back arthritis goes into the legs. There's also a special kind of phlebitis (inflamed vein) that can occur in the breast, called Mondor's syndrome. It gives you a drawing sensation around the outer edge of your breast that extends down into your abdomen. Sometimes you can even feel a cord where it is most tender. None of these problems are serious. A

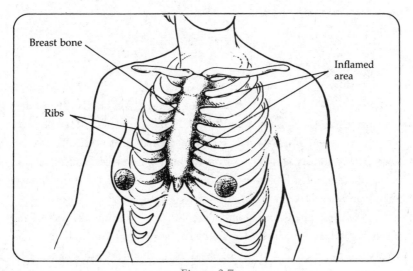

Figure 2.7

nonbreast condition that appears in the breast area is treated as it would be in any other part of the body. That usually means, for the conditions just mentioned, aspirin or another anti-inflammatory agent. These pains are usually self-limited and will go away in time.

Cancer Concerns

How likely is any breast pain to be cancer? Cyclical pain has no relation to cancer, so don't worry. Noncyclical pain is rarely a sign of cancer, but it can be, so it's worth checking out. One of my patients discovered while she was traveling in Europe that her breast hurt when she lay on her stomach. Though she couldn't feel any lump, she had it checked when she came home and discovered she did indeed have a tiny cancer on the spot. About 5 percent of all "target zone" breast pain is cancer. So it's worth having your doctor check it—if only for the relief of being sure you aren't in the 5 percent.

BREAST INFECTIONS

Breast infections and nipple discharge are fairly uncommon and usually are not much more than a nuisance, but they can cause great anxiety to people who experience them.

Lactational Mastitis

Lactational mastitis is the most common of these infections.[14] It occurs, as its name suggests, when a person is breastfeeding. The breast is filled with milk, a medium that encourages the growth of bacteria. You've got a baby biting and sucking on your breast on a regular basis, causing cracks in the skin and introducing bacteria—it's really amazing that more nursing parents don't get infections.

Probably it happens as seldom as it does because milk is always flowing through and flushing the bacteria out. However, sometimes when you're breastfeeding, a duct will get blocked up with thick milk that doesn't flow very well. Then bacteria become trapped in the breast, the milk feeds them, and suddenly you've got a reddened, hot, and very painful breast (Figure 2.8).

Your doctor will probably suggest that you try to unblock the duct with massage or warm soaks and other kinds of heat (which liquefies the milk for better flow). If the infection persists, an ultrasound should be done to determine whether there is an area of infection that needs to be treated with antibiotics or an abscess that needs to be drained. Don't worry about the antibiotics affecting your nursing child; your obstetrician will know which antibiotics are safe for children to ingest. Nor will the bacteria hurt the child, as they will be killed by the baby's stomach acid. It's actually good for you if the child goes on nursing. The sucking helps unblock the duct.

Antibiotics almost always get rid of infection, but in about 10 percent of cases an abscess forms, and antibiotics can't eliminate abscesses. An abscess, like a boil, is basically a collection of pus that the doctor has to drain. This is usually done through a needle while the patient is having an ultrasound, and it may need to be repeated more than once. The pus can be sent to the lab to identify the bacteria and what drugs they are sensitive to so that the infection will be treated with the best antibiotic. Surgery is rarely done anymore, and only as a last resort.

Breastfeeding can continue during the infection and its treatment.

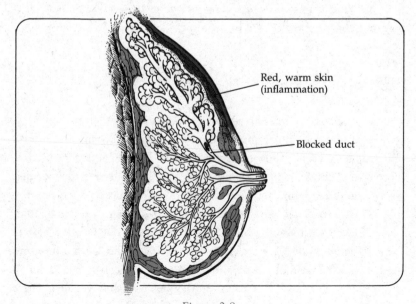

Red, warm skin
(inflammation)

Blocked duct

Figure 2.8

Nonlactational Mastitis

Mastitis can also occur in nonlactating people, especially in particular circumstances. For example, it may occur in people who have had lumpectomies followed by radiation, who have diabetes, or whose immune systems are otherwise depressed. Such people are prone to infections either because some of the lymph nodes, which help fight infection, have been removed or because their immune system is generally less strong than most people's. This type of infection will usually be a cellulitis (an infection of the skin) that is red, hot, and swollen all over rather than in one spot. It's generally accompanied by high fever and headache, both characteristics of a strep infection (staph infections, by contrast, are usually local). Your doctor will treat it with antibiotics, usually penicillin, and you may be briefly hospitalized.

Skin boils (or staph infections) can form on the breast, as they can on other parts of the body. If you're a carrier of staph and prone to infection as well—as in the case of people with diabetes—this is more likely to occur than in noncarriers or people who are less infection prone. It's also possible to get an abscess in the breast when you're not lactating and don't have any of the other risk factors, although this is unusual. Both cellulitis and these abscesses can mask cancer (as we'll discuss later), so, though such cancer is rare, if you've got one of these conditions it's important to have it checked out by a doctor.

Chronic Subareolar Abscess

The second most common breast infection—and it's rather infrequent—is the chronic subareolar (under the nipple) abscess, which we don't understand very well, though there is some evidence that it is more common in smokers. Two theories about its cause demonstrate the fact that we also don't really understand the anatomy of the breast ducts and the nipples. One theory states that this infection is caused by ducts that become blocked with keratin and then get infected.[15] But Dr. Bruce Derrick at Temple University and Dr. Otto Sartorius put forth a different view, which I find more compelling.[16] As you'll recall from earlier in this chapter, there are little glands on the nipple as well as ducts. These small, dead-ended glands can get infections, whether you're nursing or

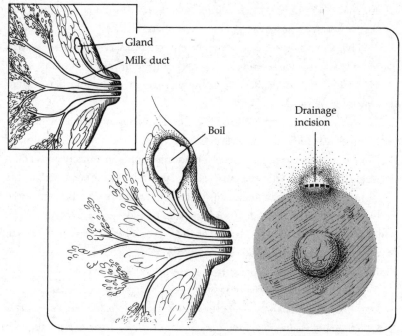

Figure 2.9

not. Bacteria from the skin or mouth of your child or sexual partner gets
into the gland; thickened secretions block it so it can't drain well, and an
infection forms. This is most common in people with inverted nipples,
because their glands have narrower openings.

Whether the culprit in this condition is the ducts or the glands doesn't
matter much to the patient. Either way, an abscess forms that can't drain
through the usual exit and therefore tries to drain through the weakest
part of the skin in the area—the border between the areola and the regular skin (Figure 2.9). The abscess is a red, hot, sore area—like a boil. It
looks and feels awful, and the frightened person often thinks they've got
breast cancer. They don't, and the infection doesn't affect their vulnerability to breast cancer.

If the infection is caught very early, before an abscess forms, it may be
helped by antibiotics and aspiration with a needle. But often it can't be
and needs to be incised and drained. I think it's best to make the incision
on the border of the areola, so that it doesn't show later. Once the pus
is drained, it's okay—for the time being. The trouble is that this type
of infection is apt to recur. The gland is a little dead-ended passage with

no internal opening, so it can reinfect itself and drain again at the same point. Eventually this leaves a permanent open tract.

I've had some luck reducing these recurrences by removing the entire gland or tract. To get the whole tract, the surgeon must excise a wedge of nipple. The method isn't perfect, but its success rate is a lot better than that of other methods.

We don't yet know the reason for the frequency of recurrence, even in the most skillfully done operations.[17] Perhaps there is a disease in more than one duct that makes it susceptible to infection. This has been termed duct ectasia or periductal mastitis. There are multiple descriptions of this condition, and there has been much hypothesizing about what causes it. Perhaps the infection spreads from one gland to another, or perhaps there's still lining left from the old gland that the surgeon isn't aware of. So if you have a chronic subareolar abscess, understand that you may have to keep dealing with it. About 40 percent of these infections do recur, sometimes as often as every few months—again especially if you are a smoker.

As so often happens, many doctors think surgery is called for, no matter how disfiguring it may be. One patient came to me after her doctor said he was fed up with these recurrences and wanted to remove both breasts. Fortunately she had the sense not to listen to him. A well-planned, non-mutilating operation solved her problem—but even if it hadn't, the most drastic procedure that would have made any sense at all would have been to remove the ducts behind her nipple, leaving the breast intact.

INFECTION AND CANCER

As I said earlier, breast infections do not lead to breast cancer. However, some breast cancers lead to infections or look like infections. As the cancer cells grow, noncancerous cells die off for lack of blood supply, and the necrotic (dead) tissue can get infected. So it's possible, though extremely unusual, for breast cancer to show up first as a breast abscess.

Inflammatory breast cancer can be mistaken for infection (see Chapter 12). This starts with redness of the skin, warmth, and swelling. There usually is no lump. What distinguishes it from infection is that it doesn't get better with antibiotics. Anyone with a breast infection that persists after ten days to two weeks of antibiotics should see a breast surgeon, who will probably want to do a biopsy.

If you get an infection, don't worry about it—but do see your doctor right away. The infection won't give you cancer, but it should be treated and gotten rid of, and you do want to make sure it is in fact an infection.

NIPPLE PROBLEMS

Cracked or Sore Nipples While Nursing

The nipple is an especially sensitive area and subject to a number of problems, such as the subareolar abscess discussed earlier. A new parent who is nursing sometimes develops a cracked or sore nipple, and it isn't a pleasant experience. The pain can be severe and the guilt from feeling unable to breastfeed adequately is hard to tolerate, especially because, at this time, the person's hormones are surging. Such pain occurs in as many as 17 percent of people in the first few weeks after giving birth. Typically there is a small erosion or crack on the nipple. Although it usually goes away on its own, if the baby is having trouble sucking or is sucking hard, the nipple may become painfully raw and progress to a larger crack in the nipple in about a week. It is often infected with bacteria. One study looked at four different strategies to treat a cracked nipple and found that oral antibiotics both provided the best relief and reduced the chance of developing mastitis.[18] This and good nipple hygiene are key to preventing this distressing condition.

Another source of pain in the nipple or breast while nursing is infection resulting from candida (a fungus that causes yeast infection). A study based on a microbiologic analysis of the parent's nipple, their milk, and the baby's mouth found that 19 percent of the parents had candida. The involved nipples were mildly inflamed and tender to the touch. It's easy to treat with a topical miconazole (antifungal) oral gel to the nipple and the baby's mouth, and oral nystatin to resolve this problem.

Discharge

The most common nipple problem—or rather concern, as it's not always a problem—is discharge. Most people do have some amount of discharge or fluid when their breasts are squeezed, and it's perfectly normal

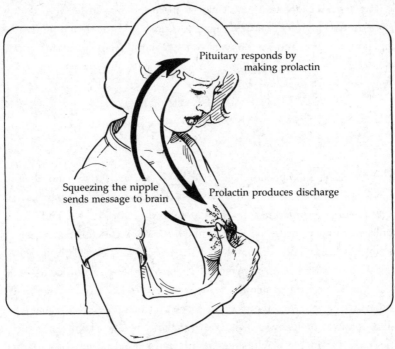

Pituitary responds by making prolactin

Squeezing the nipple sends message to brain

Prolactin produces discharge

Figure 2.10

(Figure 2.10). In a study at the old Boston Lying-in Hospital breast clinic, participants had little suction cups, like breast pumps, put on their nipples, and gentle suction was applied.[19] Eighty-three percent of these participants—old, young, parents, nonparents, previously pregnant, never pregnant—had some amount of fluid. As I will explain in Chapter 5, this fluid can be analyzed for precancerous cells.

The ducts of the nipple are pipelines; they're made to carry milk to the nipple, so a little fluid in the pipes shouldn't be surprising. (It can come in a number of colors—gray, green, and brown, as well as white.)

Sometimes people confuse nipple discharge with other problems—weepy sores, infections, abscesses (see the previous discussion). Inverted nipples (see Chapter 1) can sometimes get dirt and dried-up sweat trapped in them, and this can be confused with discharge.

Some individuals are more prone to lots of discharge than others: those who are on birth control pills, antihypertensives, or strong tranquilizers tend to notice more discharge, because these medications increase prolactin levels. This discharge may be aesthetically displeasing, but beyond that there's nothing to worry about.

There are also different life periods when you're more likely to get discharge than others: there's more discharge at puberty and at menopause than in the years between. And there's the milk sometimes briefly secreted by newborns. This makes sense, since the discharge is the result of hormonal processes.

When Should You Worry?

The time to worry about nipple discharge is when it's spontaneous, persistent, and only on one side. If it comes out by itself without squeezing, keeps on happening, is only from one nipple and usually one duct, and is either clear and sticky like an egg white or bloody, you should go to the doctor for evaluation of the discharge. There are several possible causes:

1. Intraductal papilloma. This is a little wartlike growth on the lining of the duct. It gets eroded and bleeds, creating a bloody discharge. It's benign; the surgeon removes it to make sure that's what it is.
2. Intraductal papillomatosis. Instead of one wart, you've got a lot of little warts.
3. Ductal carcinoma in situ (DCIS). This is a precancer that clogs up the duct like rust (discussed in detail in Chapter 9).
4. Cancer. Cancers are rarely the cause of discharge. Less than 10 percent of all spontaneous unilateral bloody discharges are cancerous. But it's important to have it checked.

Age is an important factor in predicting whether the discharge is related to cancer. Among patients with nipple discharges, only 3 percent who are younger than age 40, and 10 percent who are between ages 40 and 60, will have cancer, but the number jumps to 32 percent of those over age 60.[20]

Your clinician should first test for blood by taking a sample, putting it on a card, and adding a chemical (hemoccult test). If it turns blue, there's blood (which may not be visible to the eye because of the color of the discharge). The doctor may do a Pap smear, very like the Pap smear you get to test for cervical cancer. Discharge is put on a glass slide and sent to the lab for the cells to be examined. A recent study from Vermont showed this test to be quite accurate when it showed malignant cells but less accurate when it showed only apparently benign cells.[21] Next the doctor will try to figure out the "trigger zone" by going around the breast to find out which duct the discharge is coming from, though often the patient can give the doctor this information. An ultrasound evaluation can often identify an intraductal papilloma. If the patient is over thirty, they'll be sent for a mammogram to see if there's a tumor underneath the duct. If all these steps are negative for cancer, then surgery is not necessary.

If there is any question or if further investigation is warranted, many doctors will follow this with either ductoscopy or a ductogram. Ductoscopy is exactly what it sounds like: a very tiny endoscope (a long flexible tube used to check out an interior body part) is passed through a numbed-up nipple for the doctor to look around for any problems. This has been very useful in finding intraductal papillomas, and a German version of the scope even has the ability to remove the papilloma through the nipple.[22] Other tools for determining both the cause and location of ductal pathology include ultrasound and ductography, in which the radiologist takes a very fine plastic catheter and, with a magnifying glass, threads it into the duct, squirts dye into it, and takes an X-ray (Figure 2.11). This may sound ghastly, but it really isn't that bad—the duct is an open tube already, and the discharge has dilated it.

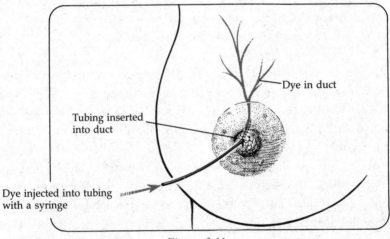

Figure 2.11

Two studies have documented that preoperative ductography increases the chance that if there is any abnormal tissue causing the pathology, it will be found.[23] So if your doctor does not recommend one of these techniques, you may want to look around for someone who does.

You may also have a simple operation under local anesthetic on an outpatient basis. A tiny incision is made at the edge of the areola; the areola is flipped up, and the blood-filled duct is located and removed (Figure 2.12). Sometimes the radiologist will cut a fine suture and pass it into the duct to the point to be removed, or blue dye can be injected into the duct to help identify it. Both of these techniques will help pinpoint the right area. Sometimes, if the ductogram has shown the lesion to be far from the nipple, the surgeon will localize the area with a wire, as described in Chapter 13.

Another form of problematic discharge is one that is spontaneous, bilateral (on both sides), and milky. If you're not breastfeeding and haven't been in the past year, this is probably a condition called galactorrhea—excessive or spontaneous milk flow. It occurs because something is increasing the prolactin levels. Rarely, the source turns out to be a small tumor in the brain, which can be detected on an MRI of the pituitary gland. This may not be as alarming as it sounds: often it's a tiny tumor that may not require surgery. A neurosurgeon and an endocrinologist

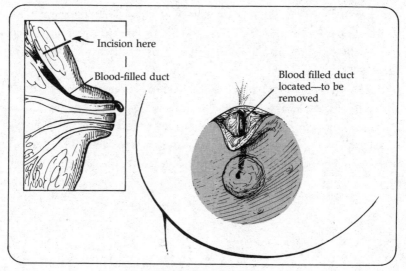

Figure 2.12

together need to check this out. You may be given a medication called bromocriptine to block the prolactin. Galactorrhea is often associated with amenorrhea—failure to get your period. It can also be caused by major tranquilizers, marijuana consumption, or high estrogen doses.

Galactorrhea is diagnosed only when the discharge is bilateral. Many doctors don't understand this and send patients with any discharge for prolactin-level tests. They shouldn't; the unilateral discharges are not associated with hormonal problems, and any money spent on prolactin tests is wasted.

Other Nipple Problems

There are a few other problems people can have with their nipples. Some patients complain of itchy nipples. Usually this doesn't indicate anything dangerous, especially if both nipples itch. You can get dry skin on your nipples as elsewhere. You may be allergic to your bra or to the detergent it's washed in. Pubescent young people with growing breasts often experience itching as the skin stretches. Otherwise, we don't know what causes itchy nipples. If they bother you, you can use calamine lotion or other anti-itch medication.

There is a form of cancer known as Paget's disease that doctors and patients often confuse with eczema of the nipple. It looks like an open sore area and it itches. If it's on only one nipple and doesn't go away with standard eczema treatments, check it out. A biopsy can be performed on a small section of the nipple. (Paget's disease is discussed at length in Chapter 12.)

If the rash is on both nipples and you tend to get eczema anyway, don't worry. The eczema has just decided to try a new place to show up.

Most of these infections and irritations are benign—they're more of a nuisance than anything else. If they appear, get them checked out, just to make sure they're what they appear to be and to get the relief available.

PART TWO

What Causes Breast Cancer and How Do We Prevent It?

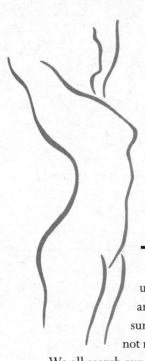

CHAPTER 3
Biology of Cancer

The first question asked by anyone diagnosed with cancer is "Am I going to die?" This fear is natural and understandable, but treatments for this disease are growing more effective every day and most people survive it. So my answer is "Eventually, yes, but probably not now." The next question is usually "How did I get this?" We all search our life experience for potential carcinogens. Could it have been the formaldehyde when I was taking anatomy in medical school, or the radiation from the airport screening? In reality, we rarely know exactly what caused any particular cancer, and it really doesn't matter much once you have been diagnosed. However, what we are learning about what cancer needs to develop and grow is giving us clues as to how to treat it and possibly even prevent it.

This chapter is for those of you who want a better understanding of the biology of breast cancer and immunology. It also provides the background for some of the treatments that we will discuss later. Some of you may want to skip ahead. No problem! But for those intrepid souls who want to understand as much as possible, here is my best effort.

In Chapter 1, I compared the breast to an interactive community in which the cells of the ducts and lobules interact and influence the surrounding fibrous tissue, blood vessels, immune cells, and even fat. This crosstalk and the elegant dance that results have begun to be studied in recent years, and what we have learned already is changing how we think about the causes of breast cancer.[1] It appears that at least two critical elements are necessary for any cancer to develop and flourish. The first is a cell that for some reason, either hereditary or environmental, has developed a mutation in a critical part of its DNA, and the mutation changes the cell's potential behavior. The second is a neighborhood that is egging this cell on.[2]

We get mutations all the time just by living on this earth. Imagine having one car your whole life. After a bit you start to collect dents (mutations), and the longer you own it, the more dents you have. Some of them are important dents that interfere with driving, while others are just cosmetic. Likewise, some of our mutations are more important than others. Figuring out all these many mutations and what part of the cell's activity they control is a huge part of current cancer research.[3] Radiation, environmental toxins, and even viruses can cause mutations.[4] Our bodies have anticipated this problem, and we have some built-in repair genes or mechanics to fix the dents. One of these is the gene known as BRCA (which stands for "breast cancer"), which is found in all the cells of the body.[5] BRCA is an important gene because it can repair damaged DNA. When one copy of BRCA has a hereditary mutation, the second backup copy from the other parent can still function. It's as if someone were born with one blind eye but can still see with the other. This is what occurs in people who inherit the gene (see Chapter 4). It is not enough to cause breast cancer.

However, if something happens in the breast to cause a mutation in the second copy (like losing the second eye), then the body can no longer repair damaged DNA, allowing it to propagate with errors and potentially leaving patches of mutated cells in the breast (Figure 3.1).

This alone is not enough to create cancer; here's where the second element comes in. The mutated cells are in a neighborhood of other cells—fat cells, immune cells, blood cells, and so on—known collectively as the *microenvironment*. If these cells are all well-behaved, they will have a good influence on the mutated cell, which will coexist peacefully with them, and no disease will occur. But if the neighborhood is not so "law-abiding" and stimulates or even tolerates bad behavior, there may be trouble. The combination of the mutated cells and the stimulating, or tolerant, neighborhood will create breast cancer (Figure 3.2).

I find this new way of thinking about cancer very exciting because it explains a lot and gives me a new way to think about the disease, its cause, and risk factors. We can figure out what causes mutations and how to prevent or fix them. We can also figure out what affects the community around the mutated cell. Because the community (microenvironment) is also composed of cells, they too can undergo mutations and alter

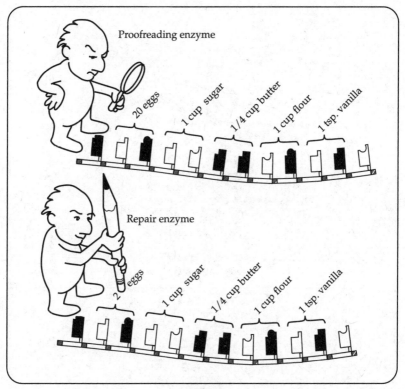

Figure 3.1

their behavior (Figure 3.3). Let's say the original nice neighborhood gets run-down and criminals begin to move in, or a factory gets built and pollutes the water, or a huge department store chain drives out all the small businesses. Each change in any part of the community can affect all its inhabitants, including the mutated ones.

So in this chapter we'll first explore the basic molecular biology needed to understand cancer and then describe the epithelial (ductal) cells and surrounding tissue or stroma—let's say we're introducing the town in which the crime drama will unfold. And we won't forget the law enforcement or immune system, which can help or hurt depending on whether it is efficient, overly aggressive, or lazy. In the next chapter we'll apply this information, looking at the known and suspected risk factors for breast cancer, as well as ways we might use lifestyle changes and the immune system to clean up the neighborhood.

To me, all this is both useful and immensely fascinating. It may be less so for some readers. If the thought of reading about biology is a drag, feel free to skip to the next chapter. You now have my version of the

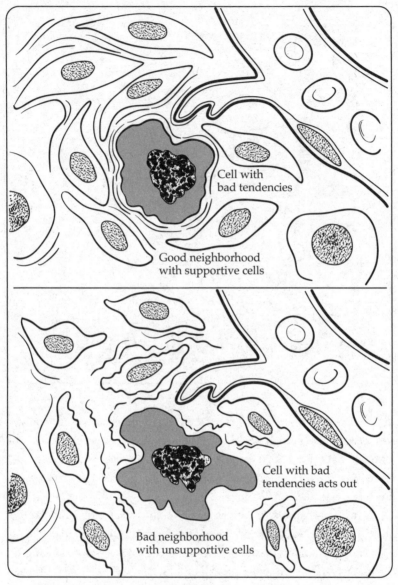

Cell with
bad tendencies

Good neighborhood
with supportive cells

Cell with bad
tendencies acts out

Bad neighborhood
with unsupportive cells

Figure 3.2

CliffsNotes. All you need to know is the metaphor of the mutated cell in its community and the immune system as our local and biological department of defense. But if you enjoy delving deeper into the why of things, then come along. I'll make it as easy as I can!

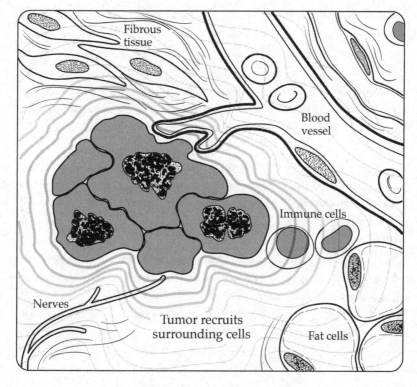

Figure 3.3

BACKGROUND

DNA

Because mutations occur in DNA, we have to start there. The way life works is through a magnificently elegant system. Every bacterium, every tree, every dog, every human being has its vital information coded into the DNA in the nucleus of its cells. This is responsible for transferring genetic characteristics. With a single system of four bases (like four letters), everything that's alive, including viruses and bacteria, is programmed. It's like realizing that with a single alphabet of twenty-six letters we have Shakespeare, *Mein Kampf*, and the Julia Child cookbooks.

These "letters" are called nucleotides, and they are the smallest unit of information in the body. How they combine to form DNA is crucial, because DNA codes all the information that your body contains. It determines the color of your eyes and your hair; it tells your lungs how to take in oxygen from the air and use it for energy. It's also complicated, so I'm going to use another metaphor for a while. I'm borrowing this metaphor from Mahlon Hoagland, Bert Dodson, and Judith Hauck's superb book *The Way Life Works*.[6] They depict DNA as a recipe. This recipe uses a definite code—four different nucleotides to which we have assigned letters (Figure 3.4). The nucleotides combine in pairs, known as "base pairs" because the pairs become the basis of whatever comes next. This pairing is very precise, like a tiny jigsaw puzzle. A and T fit together, as do G and C, and that can never vary.

Hoagland, Dodson, and Hauck use the analogy of the letters of the alphabet and the paragraphs the letters make, which as you can see I've borrowed, but I'm changing it slightly for my own use. These letters and paragraphs will all combine to create a "cookbook." The base pairs can be seen as two-letter combinations, and they come together in a chain to form a gene, which can thus be seen as a recipe made with those letters. The genes are arranged in a long row, side by side, to form a chromosome (a volume of the book). All the chromosomes together form the genome (or a set of volumes that contains all the recipes needed to make a full-scale banquet—a human being) (Figure 3.5). Here's a multivolume creation indeed!

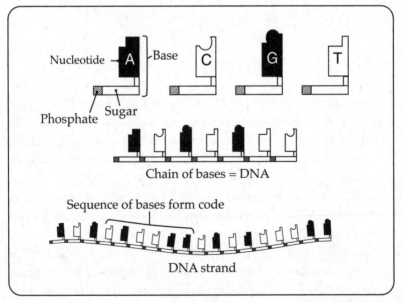

Figure 3.4

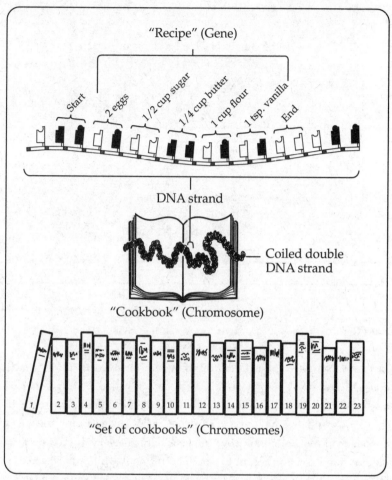

"Recipe" (Gene)

Start | 2 eggs | 1/2 cup sugar | 1/4 cup butter | 1 cup flour | 1 tsp. vanilla | End

DNA strand

Coiled double DNA strand

"Cookbook" (Chromosome)

"Set of cookbooks" (Chromosomes)

Figure 3.5

Why do the bases have to come in pairs? Each message is encoded in only one chromosome strand. But genes need to be able to replicate themselves or no growth takes place. So the strands come in pairs that are actually mirror images of each other. This is the famous double helix. When a cell needs to divide—as it will for any number of reasons, from healing a scratch on the body to creating a pregnancy—it can do so because there is a mirror image attached to the original strand. In order to replicate, the helix separates, and mirror images are made of each strand from other bases that are floating around in the cell (Figure 3.6). The two mirror images then reconnect, forming a new double helix—a nifty way to make sure the code is unaltered.

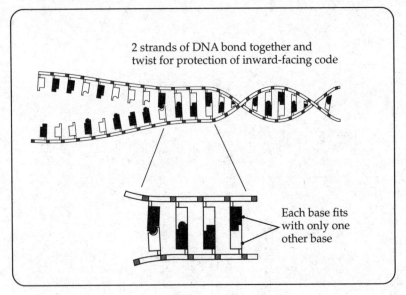

2 strands of DNA bond together and
twist for protection of inward-facing code

Each base fits
with only one
other base

Figure 3.6

RNA

In case DNA hasn't confused you enough, you need to know that it doesn't work alone. It's got a temporary partner, called RNA (ribonucleic acid). DNA, remember, is just a code—a code for creating proteins. By itself, it doesn't do anything. Let's use our recipe image again. You've got a wonderful recipe book in your kitchen, but it's a very rare, expensive, old book and you don't want to splatter stuff on it while you're cooking. What you'd like to do is have a copy of one page, which you can bring to the counter and use to make your soufflé. Well, the RNA provides that copy. It duplicates the gene that it needs at the moment. Then it takes the coding message to another part of the cell and translates that piece of code into a protein. When the copy is no longer used it disappears (you throw it into the trash bin).

The RNA copy can be produced frequently for certain genes (like your daily breakfast cereal) or it can be produced less frequently (like a holiday dinner). The production of RNA determines how much protein will be produced and therefore the levels of expression of a particular protein.

So the gene is like one recipe: it will make one thing. The DNA is the information that has gone into writing that recipe. The chromosome is one volume of the cookbook. And the RNA is the disposable copy of the recipe that keeps the whole cookbook from having to be carted around.

Proteins

Proteins are the body's building blocks, which are needed throughout our lives, making this recipe system vital. As Hoagland, Dodson, and Hauck write, proteins "do the daily business of living, giving cells their shapes and unique abilities." There are many kinds of proteins (just as there are many dishes)—enzymes, transporters, movers, and so on. There are

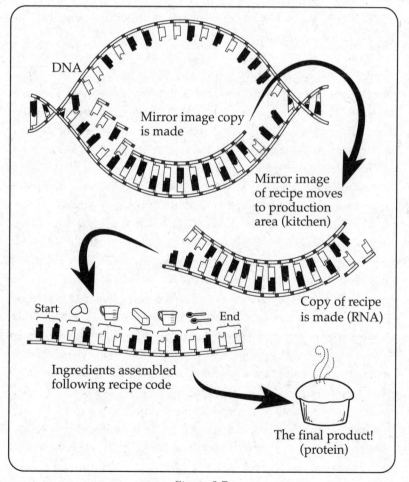

Figure 3.7

twenty-one amino acids (ingredients) that are hooked together as proteins, and the RNA is what directs how they're strung together. Proteins are the end product of a recipe—your delicious soufflé (Figure 3.7).

GENES AND BREAST CANCER

When you understand DNA, RNA, and protein, you can begin to comprehend what may happen with cancer. The process can break down at any of these levels. First it can happen at the DNA level. When human egg or sperm cells are made, the cells divide and only one DNA strand is put into each egg or sperm cell. So one parent gives the child half of that parent's DNA, the child's other parent gives half of their own DNA, and the combination makes a unique whole.

A mutation occurs when the wrong nucleotide gets inserted into the new strand as it is being made. Going back to our analogy, let's say there's a typo (mutation) in the recipe (Figure 3.8). These mutations can occur in either somatic cells (the ones that form the tissues of your body) or in germ cells (sperm and egg), which are passed onto your offspring. Both types of mutations are important: the first to the person who carries it, and the second to the next generation.

The mutations known as BRCA 1 or BRCA 2 germ cell mutations are found in some hereditary breast cancers. If one of your parents carries a mutation for BRCA 1 in one strand of DNA, there is a fifty-fifty chance that you have inherited it. Remember you only get half a DNA strand from each parent, so you could get the mutated one or the good one. If you inherit the mutation, it will almost always be matched with a good strand from the other parent in every cell in your body. This puts you closer to getting cancer because you need only to develop another mutation in your good strand of DNA in the breast or ovary to develop cancer. This is one reason that people who carry the mutation often get breast cancer at a young age: they start out halfway there. It is also why not every person with mutations in BRCA 1 or BRCA 2 gets breast cancer (see Chapter 4 for a full discussion of this situation).

Somatic—or acquired—mutations are more common. They happen with frequency over a person's lifetime because of exposure to carcinogens; radiation, electricity, infrared light, and dozens of other things can create a mutation. But most are no problem. If you have a typo in

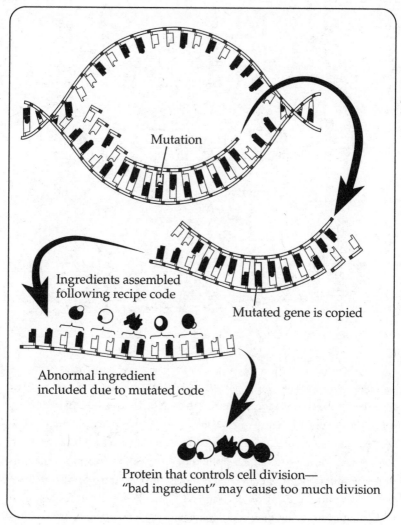

Figure 3.8

a recipe no one ever uses, and it never gets retyped, it doesn't matter. There are other mutations that don't matter either, because the "typo" doesn't obscure the meaning (Figure 3.9). If your recipe says "Add one cup of sigar," you may smile at it, but you know you need to add a cup of sugar. Once in a great while a mutation even creates an improvement. (If the recipe says to add a half cup of sugar, it may end up tasting just as good and being healthier.) In fact, there's an argument that civilization itself depends on mutations—the mutations that lead to evolution.

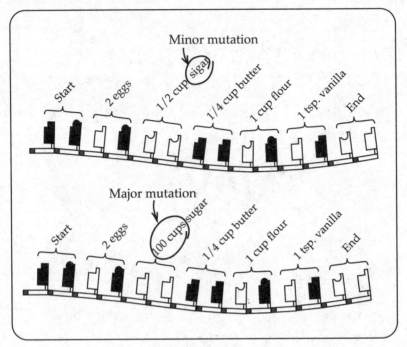

Figure 3.9

Then there are the cancer genes. These are genes that enable and regulate cell growth but that, if altered by mutation, can lead to cancer because they change DNA quality control, repair, or growth. Mutations in these cancer genes are usually caused by outside forces such as radiation, food toxins, or environmental pollutants. It usually takes more than one of these mutations for a cancer to develop, and of course it also requires the right community of other cells, all of which can also develop a somatic mutation. In other words, cancers are the result of multiple alterations in a number of genes.

BRCA 1 and BRCA 2 are genes involved in double-strand DNA repair. When women who carry a pathogenic variant (or mutation) in one of these get a second mutation in a breast cell, they can develop cancer because their bodies are less able to repair mutations that may arise (caused by radiation, for example). There is, however, a backup DNA repair system, based on poly (ADP-ribose) polymerase, which we call PARP, since "poly (ADP-ribose) polymerase" is ridiculously hard to say (Figure 3.10). The attempt to target this pathway is the basis of new drugs that we have been studying for more than a decade, and recent results are

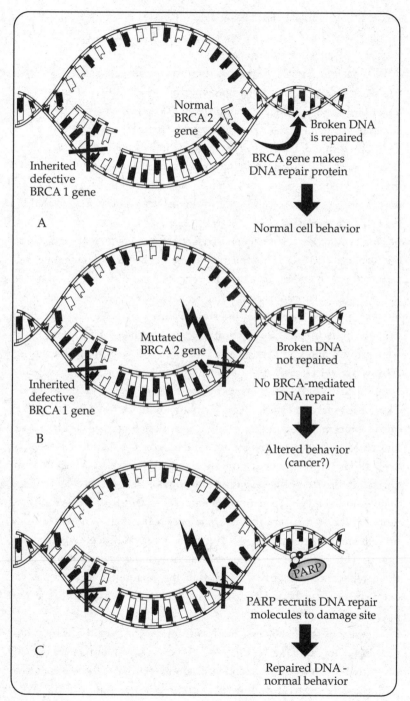

Figure 3.10

encouraging. Clinical trials have shown PARP inhibitors to be at least as effective as chemotherapy, and less toxic, in people with BRCA mutations and advanced breast cancers.[7]

For patients with high-risk early-stage breast cancer, either triple-negative or hormone-receptor-positive, and a BRCA 1 or BRCA 2 mutation, adding a PARP inhibitor for a year after surgery, chemotherapy, and/or radiation has been shown to decrease risk of recurrence.[8]

Another kind of cancer gene is involved in making cells divide. When they're normal, these are called proto-oncogenes; when they're mutated they're called oncogenes. Proto-oncogenes involved in breast cancer are mostly ones that cause more cell division—they contribute to making the cell cycle speed up.

One type of proto-oncogene is related to the epidermal growth factor receptor (EGFR). This receptor is on a cell; the epidermal growth factor comes in and attaches to the receptor and directs it to divide—so until the factor comes along, it's just a passive receptor (a lock without a key). These growth factors and receptors are necessary at certain times of your life, such as puberty, when big changes are going on in your growth and you need growth factors egging on the cells yelling, "Grow! Grow! Grow!" The epidermal growth factor finds a receptor, attaches to it, and signals the cell to replicate (grow) (Figure 3.11). There are different types of epidermal growth factors. An important one is epidermal growth factor 2. In the United States this is commonly known as HER2/neu (pronounced "her two new") and in Europe as erbB-2. The type of genetic alteration that HER2/neu has is called amplification. Instead of having only one copy of this gene, the cell makes many (ten to sixty) copies of this gene. When this happens the cell has more HER2/neu receptors than normal, which helps to create more protein and a louder message—like more powerful earphones for your laptop. This accelerates the growth of any cancer cells that may be in the neighborhood (Figure 3.11). Either the gene overexpression or the extra protein can be measured in a tumor by studying the tissue that has been removed.

Tempering the oncogenes and proto-oncogenes are the tumor suppression genes and the repair genes. These are the brakes and repair shop in the cell system—so that whereas you have some genes that push the cells to grow and divide, you have others there to say "Well, no, growing and dividing really isn't such a good idea." Or "Maybe we

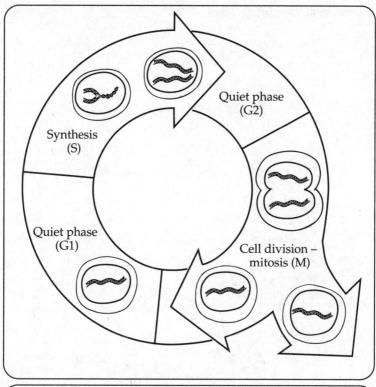

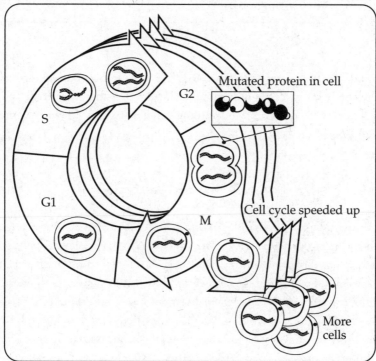

Figure 3.11

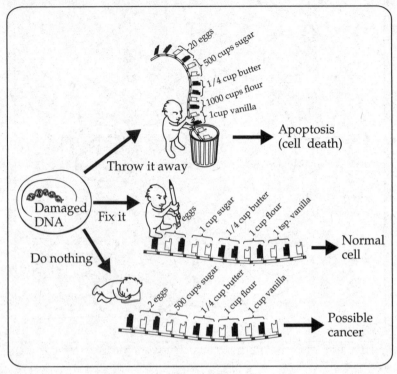

20 eggs
500 cups sugar
1/4 cup butter
1000 cups flour
1cup vanilla

Throw it away

Apoptosis
(cell death)

Damaged
DNA

Fix it

eggs
1 cup sugar
1/4 cup butter
1 cup flour
1 tsp. vanilla

Normal
cell

Do nothing

2 eggs
500 cups sugar
1/4 cup butter
1 cup flour
1 cup vanilla

Possible
cancer

Figure 3.12

should repair you first" (Figure 3.12). For example, one suppressor gene, p53, keeps cells with mutated DNA from dividing. If the p53 itself becomes compromised, nothing remains to slow down that mutated DNA.

TUMOR HETEROGENEITY

In the past we focused on identifying exactly what kind of breast cancer you had in order to match the treatment to the type. It was believed that each of the different kinds of cancer developed from different mutations and along different pathways. If we could target the mutation or the resulting growth factor or hormone, we could specifically treat the cancer. This was termed "precision medicine" and gained a lot of credibility when it was found that some mutations occurred in cancers in different organs. For example, HER-2 is sometimes overexpressed in stomach cancers as well as breast cancers. That suggests that a drug against this growth factor would work in both situations. Although these findings generated much excitement, hopes were soon dashed when scientists realized there were too many targets and not enough drugs.

Although this was a serious concern, the real problem soon became clear. Tumors are not homogeneous! That means that a tumor is a combination of cells with different mutations.[9] If you block the dominant mutation, then you allow or encourage smaller communities of mutations to rise up—if you knock out one gang in a troubled neighborhood, then the secondary gangs have the opportunity to dominate. This became more noticeable when genomic sequencing techniques were applied to cancer. Not only are there different mutations, but they can exist in different areas of the same cancer! (See Figure 3.13.) In addition, over time new mutations can occur. Mutations, or cancer cells, that have spread to other organs may not have the same characteristics as the primary cancer, a fact that is changing the treatment of metastatic disease. This ever-changing landscape of tumor mutations has made it clear that we are going to have to go beyond trying to kill every cancer cell with a targeted bullet and focus instead on changing the conditions that have allowed them to arise in the first place.[10] This is where we move from focusing on the cell to focusing on the tumor as a complex organism that depends on a variety of factors for its existence and propagation. It is not just the cell but the neighborhood it lives in that is critical.

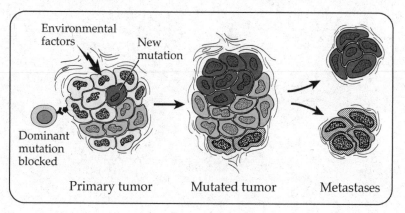

Figure 3.13

THE ENVIRONMENT OF THE CELL

We have considered the fact that a cell carrying a mutation requires the appropriate community for a cancer to develop. But can you really have mutated cells and no cancer? The answer, surprisingly, is yes. As we get older, we probably all walk around with mutated cells in our bodies. One study examined breasts that were removed at autopsy from people age 40 to 50 who had died of other causes. The researchers did not expect what they discovered—39 percent of the breasts had nests of cancer cells lying dormant inside them. Dr. Thea Tlsty of the University of California, San Francisco has been studying early mutations in breast cancer. At one point she was looking at tissue from reduction mammoplasties (when breasts are made smaller because they are too big). To her surprise, she found cells that had the same early cancer markers just sitting around doing nothing.[11] Mutated cells in a good neighborhood!

The proof comes from studies by my friend Dr. Mina Bissell, a biochemist in Berkeley, California, who has spent her career studying breast cancer cells within a breast tissue environment. She has taken cells that have the mutations of breast cancer and grown them in a culture of normal breast stroma. In that environment, the cancer cells behaved like normal cells—they made ducts and did the other things that healthy breast cells do.[12] The healthy influence of the surrounding cells caused the cancer cells, even though they were genetically altered, to behave

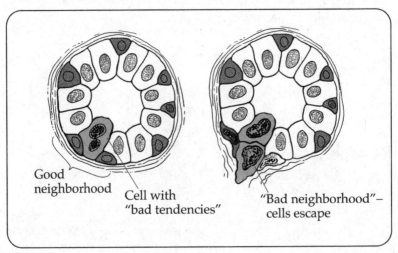

Good neighborhood

Cell with "bad tendencies"

"Bad neighborhood"– cells escape

Figure 3.14

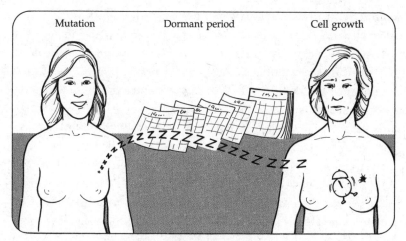

Figure 3.15

well. When Dr. Bissell and her associates put the same cells in a malignant environment, the cells went back to behaving like cancer (see Figure 3.14). This means that if we knew the right environment, the reverse would be possible as well: we may be able to keep the cancer cells from misbehaving. The ability to control or reverse cancer may also explain a phenomenon known as *tumor dormancy* (see Figure 3.15). This is thought to happen in patients who appear to be cured at the end of treatment but have a recurrence ten years later. What were the cells doing for ten years? They were asleep. What put them to sleep? What woke them up?

In summary, all cancer is probably caused by a combination of genes that are altered by carcinogens and stimulated by an environment conducive to growth and spread.

THE IMMUNE SYSTEM: OUR BIOLOGICAL DEPARTMENT OF DEFENSE

In the past, we considered the immune system to be just another part of the environment, but studies have shown that it plays a critical role in the development of cancer. First of all, the term "immune system" covers a lot of territory, including different kinds of cells, antibodies, and proteins. I think of it as the security system of the body, encompassing the local neighborhood watch; private security companies like ADT; specialized systems like police, fire, and emergency medical services; and, ultimately, the National Guard and military. After all, this is our personal Department of Defense. As I started researching the immune system in relation to breast cancer, I was both fascinated and overwhelmed. It seemed that every time I thought I understood things, a new study would come out and prove it all wrong! Nonetheless, we cannot ignore the immune system, as it probably holds the key to both why we get breast cancer and why it does or does not come back. With that in mind, I am going to give you a brief description so you will at least recognize the players later in the book when we discuss vaccines, immunotherapy, and checkpoint blockades.

In general, there are two components to the immune system: the innate immune system is nonspecific and local, and the adaptive immune system is more specific and systemic. First, let's go local. The *innate*, or *nonspecific*, *immune system* is composed of cells that are responsible for our "secure borders." These are cells that hang out at places where our body interacts with the outside world: think skin, mouth, gastrointestinal (GI) tract (we are, in fact, donuts with a hole down the middle), lungs, vagina, urethra, and liver. If there is a threat, such as a splinter, they immediately leap into action, checking out the intruder and sounding the alarm. They literally serve as the neighborhood watch, figuring out what the problem is and calling for help. Special white blood cells are mostly involved here, in the form of neutrophils and macrophages, although the

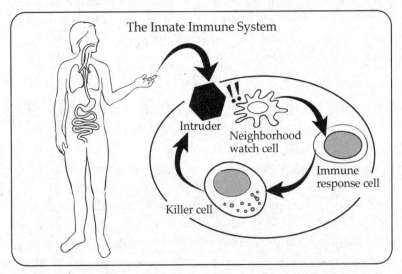

Figure 3.16

more we study this initial response, the more complicated it gets. The next line of defense comes in the form of increased blood supply to the problem area. This is the equivalent of the private security team. What you then see is redness, swelling, and pain in the area around the splinter and, ultimately, pus (neutrophils that died in the line of duty). If you are lucky, the local defenses will do the job, the splinter will be removed, and the wound will quickly heal (Figure 3.16).

But for the sake of argument, what if it doesn't? This is where the *adaptive immune system* kicks in (see Figure 3.17). The local neighborhood watch calls the local security patrol, which figures out what kind of problem it is and calls the appropriate experts: fire department, police department, or emergency medical department, depending on the situation. The antigen-presenting cells, called dendritic cells and macrophages, do this for us by taking a cell phone picture of the problem (this is getting to be a very loose analogy) and bringing it to the center of town where the

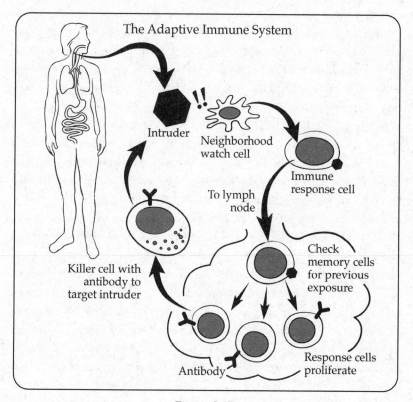

Figure 3.17

emergency services hang out, in this case a lymph node. Some of you may have had an experience where you started out with a local infection in your finger, foot, or even throat and then your lymph nodes swelled up. They are the second line of defense and they are where the more specific memory T cells hang out. These are the ones that check their database. If they recognize the picture as one they have seen before, they head out to do battle with the appropriate specific antibodies or killer T cells. This is how a vaccine works. The first time, you are given just a part of the virus, for instance, polio, but enough for your immune system to develop a file on it. In biological terms, this file would be kept by memory T cells and B cells. Then if you get exposed to the virus again, they recognize it and go right to work killing it, without the delay of the first encounter.

Or say a virus gets into your throat, making it red and sore and sparking a fever with lots of mucus as a result of the battle. Then your swollen glands, the adaptive immune system or next line of defense, get called in to banish the intruder.

This innate immune system (nonspecific neighborhood watch), and its interaction with the adaptive immune system in the lymph nodes, is critical in dealing with infections. (This is why people on chemotherapy, which kills all dividing cells including white blood cells, are more susceptible to infections.)

While all this is fascinating, the real question is: How does it relate to breast cancer? Why doesn't the immune system recognize cancer cells as bad and kill them before they kill you? It is sort of like asking how the 9/11 terrorists managed to get into the country and eventually take down the World Trade Center and attack the Pentagon.

The relationship between cancer cells and the immune system is complicated. I have come to think of cancer cells as terrorists. People are not born terrorists, but they become so because of their environment, traumatic experiences, armed conflicts, politics, and so on. This is also true of cancer cells. Remember that cancer cells originally came from normal cells that developed mutations. And like terrorists, they have ways of escaping recognition by the adaptive immune system—just as they sometimes get through the airport's Transportation Security Administration (TSA). This escape is achieved through a number of mechanisms, which include both direct interference with the cells of the adaptive immune response and indirectly the tumor microenvironment, or neighborhood.

The cancer cells that survive are the ones that have learned how to avoid, or block, the immune surveillance.

Can we harness the immune system or turn it around to help get rid of the cancer? As long ago as 1891, William Cooley[13] injected cancer patients with bacteria to ignite an immune response. This strategy is being used again in an attempt to use the immune system to treat cancer. Specific breast cancer immunotherapies will be discussed in Chapter 15. Here, however, I will try to give you the background to understand the current approaches and enough about the immune system and cancer to get a hint of what may well be coming down the road.

Checkpoint Inhibition

The immune system must have a way to recognize normal cells and leave them alone. It does this by responding to special codes that turn it off when it is not needed. If we go back to our security system analogy, these checkpoints are the equivalent of the code you punch in when you arrive, or the ID you show the TSA at the airport. When this fail-safe system doesn't work in the body, people develop autoimmune diseases in which the immune system starts to attack normal organs and cause disease. Examples include inflammatory bowel disease, rheumatoid arthritis and some kinds of thyroid disease, and skin diseases.

These checkpoints usually work but can be blocked, tricked, or over-ridden just like any security system. That is exactly what the cancers do. They suppress or block the immune system so that the cancer cells can divide and grow with impunity. One of the first examples of a blocker of immune response, CTLA-4, was discovered in the 1980s on the surface of T cells by French scientists who were not thinking about cancer. Immunologist James Allison, now at the MD Anderson Cancer Center, found that CTLA-4 is like a brake on T cells, preventing them from launching a full-out response (see Figure 3.18). He tried blocking it and, in 1996, showed that he could erase tumors in mice. This led to a new treatment for metastatic melanoma and opened up the field of immunologic therapy.

One example of changing the immune response to treat breast cancer (see Chapter 11) focuses on the receptor on T cells, PD-1, that must link with the tumor in order to cause an immune response. Tumors can

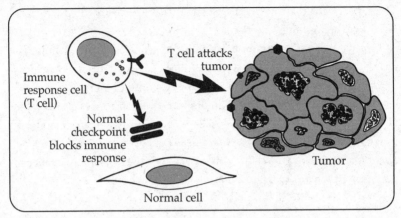

Figure 3.18

secrete a signaling protein, PD-L1, that links to the PD-1 receptor and tells the immune system not to bother (see Figure 3.19). Checkpoint inhibitors block either PD-L1 or PD-1 from this subversion of the surveillance and alert the immune system that the cancer cells are actually terrorists. One checkpoint inhibitor, Keytruda (pembrolizumab), has been approved for use in both early-stage and metastatic triple-negative breast cancer (see Chapter 11). These drugs block either PD-L1 or PD-1 from this subversion of the surveillance and alert the immune system that the cancer cells are a real threat.

Vaccines

Another approach to cancer involving the immune system is to vaccinate you against your own cancer cells. This has had some early success in preventing recurrence (see Chapter 11). Vaccines are tailored to target antigens found on the cancer cells such as HER2/neu and then given to patients after their initial treatment in an attempt to prevent recurrence. Another effort at a vaccine uses mammaglobin, which is a protein found on breast cancer cells. And yet another targets a protein that is produced in breastfeeding and is present in most triple-negative breast cancers. All these efforts are promising but still under study. Finally, there is the possibility that you could prevent the cancer in the first place by vaccinating against the cause of the mutation. This is what the human papillomavirus (HPV) vaccine is all about. Cervical, mouth, and anal

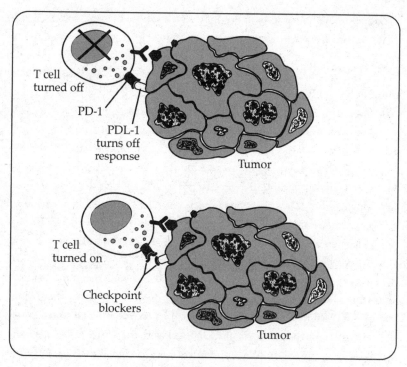

Figure 3.19

cancers are all caused by HPV. If a person is vaccinated against HPV, the immune system attacks the virus whenever it shows up. This is the ideal way to prevent cancer.

CHANGING THE NEIGHBORHOOD

In thinking about the environment of cancer cells, there is a question whether it is the local community of cells or the larger environment of the whole body. My guess is that it can be either or both. For example, we all know of people who go through a lot of acute stress in their lives and then get cancer. Did the stress cause the cancer? Probably not, but it certainly may have changed the body's hormones, as well as the immune system, thus cultivating an environment that may allow or encourage some dormant cells to grow. If we carry on with my terrorism/cancer analogy, there are factors in a country or the world that may encourage or support terrorism activity. At a different time, under different circumstances the same people might not have become terrorists. Does infection or chronic inflammation cause cancer? Or does it set up an environment in which the immune system is so busy that it lets the odd cancer cell get through? These are just analogies, but they illustrate how complicated it all is.

If you think about a "bad neighborhood" with gangs, drug pushers, abandoned buildings, and litter-strewn streets, you would not be surprised to learn it has a high crime rate. Cleaning up the vacant lots; encouraging socially acceptable groups like sports teams, scout troops, or bands; and giving kids legal ways to make money can decrease arrests and improve the safety of the neighborhood. Cancer is much the same.

We acquire mutated cells as we go through life. In fact, as I mentioned earlier, most of us walk around with cancer cells. Eighty percent of 80-year-old men have cancer cells in their prostates. And these are just the cancer cells we know about. We all probably walk around with dormant cancer cells. And as long as we get through life without them waking up and causing problems, we don't really care whether they are there.

So what keeps them asleep and what wakes them up? That is where the neighborhood comes in. We can control a lot of those cells by cleaning up the neighborhood, in this case by exercising, maintaining a healthy weight, and reducing stress. There will always be some cancer cells, like some people, who will be bad no matter what the neighborhood, but under the right conditions most cancer cells will behave.

We are starting to get evidence for this. When you look at breast cancers under the microscope, the ones with more blood vessels, suggesting an enabling environment, are more aggressive. On the other hand, the ones with a lot of associated white blood cells or tumor-infiltrating lymphocytes (TILs), suggesting a strong immune response, have a better prognosis. The immune system—or neighborhood watch, or police to mix up all my metaphors at once—has noticed shady activity in the neighborhood and has increased its surveillance!

Tumor as Organism

I once had the opportunity to hear a great scientist, Joan Brugge, give a talk about how we have to think of a tumor not as a few bad cells but as an organism (living creature) (see Figure 3.3, page 55) all its own. The tumor is composed of an enormous variety of cancer cells, as well as a large cast of supporting cells and tissues such as blood cells, nerves, lymphatics, immune cells, fibrous tissue, and fat cells. In other words, it's not just one large group of similar cells. This means that the cells removed on a tumor biopsy may—or may not—be the same as other cells that make up the tumor. Tumors are ever-changing organisms that continually develop new mutations. And they convert the supporting cells to their own use. They co-opt whatever resources are available to help them invade the body.

From a treatment perspective, we need to examine how to use chemotherapy and targeted therapies against an ever-mutating tumor. Will we need to customize therapies for primary and recurrent, metastatic cancers based on specific genetic alterations that are present in the tumor at each point in time? And even if these were feasible, we also have to account for the fact that the cancer cells can switch their phenotype—how they appear—depending on the microenvironment or neighborhood they are in. This is also an important element in predicting how the cells will behave.

We need to understand the entire ecosystem of the tumor so that we can eliminate it and prevent the development of resistant cells—while causing minimal harm to normal cells. Although the tumor ecosystem is robust and able to adapt to new therapies and environments, there also is a limit to the number of insults that it can withstand. This means we need to develop treatments that push the ecosystem beyond its ability to adapt; otherwise, it will become resistant. To do this, we need to stop trying to kill individual cells and target the whole tumor ecosystem. We need to identify the most effective immunotherapies for different classes of breast cancer, establish how to integrate them with current and emerging surgical and systemic therapies, and simultaneously target multiple places where the cells are vulnerable to prevent adaptation. In other words, if we could find the right tools to undermine the whole tumor as an organism, cancer may be reversible or at least controllable, and we wouldn't have to try to kill every last cancer cell. Or we could destroy the nests of mutated cells and prevent them from developing in the first place. This is much more complicated than the standard message of "early detection is the best prevention," but in my mind it is much more exciting because it tells us there are many routes to eradicating this disease.

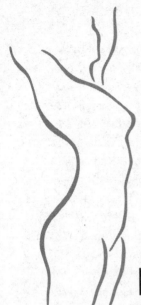

CHAPTER 4

Hereditary Breast Cancer

In the last chapter we discussed biological factors needed for breast cancer to develop. These factors are important to researchers trying to figure out the causes of the disease. But they are less helpful to you, individually, with the questions you may have at this particular point in your life. In this chapter and the next, however, we are going to consider tests that examine individuals to determine which ones have something in their genes or in their breasts that indicates a higher risk of getting the disease.

I often hear from a patient newly diagnosed with breast cancer that they fear their child is doomed—and that it is they, the parent, who has doomed the child. But it's unlikely that the child is fated to replicate their parent's experience, and, of course, the parent's guilt is wholly irrational. Although having first-degree relatives with a history of breast cancer increases a person's risk of the disease, most will never develop it. In countries where breast cancer is common, the lifetime increased incidence of breast cancer is 5.5 percent for women with one affected first-degree relative and 13.3 percent for women with two.[1]

Breast cancer in family members can be the result not of genes but of exposure to similar external risk factors. I have a friend who is one of five sisters who got breast cancer. The sisters were all tested for BRCA 1 and BRCA 2 and were surprised to discover they didn't have it. When all the cancer is in one generation, as in these sisters' case, it's possible that they were all exposed to an environment that caused the cancer with a temporary or permanent genetic mutation.

I am starting out with the genes because we know the most about them, and then I'll move to ways doctors can examine the breast itself for prediction. Remember in Chapter 3 we talked about cancer needing both a mutation and the right environment in order to grow. Some people start out with an inherited mutation that either is key for the development of breast cancer or makes them more likely to get that key mutation because of an inability to fix errors that occur in cell division. Since the last edition of the book, seventy-two previously unknown mutations linked to higher breast cancer risk have been found. In a large international study, a team of 550 researchers studied blood samples from 275,000 women, of whom 146,000 had breast cancer. They then compared the DNA from the healthy women to their counterparts, identifying common mutations in the latter group. Sixty-five of the new mutations are for breast cancer in general while seven are specific to hormone-receptor-negative cancers. Although this may seem ominous, the mutations increase a woman's risk by only 2 or 5 percent, but they are cumulative. So if a woman has two or more of these common mutations, her risk would increase accordingly. It is just one more factor to quantify risk and determine the best individualized screening approach.[2]

In case you are glumly thinking the list of mutations will never stop growing, a more heartening study recently revealed that several genetic mutations previously linked to breast cancer were found not to increase the risk of disease after all. According to the CARRIERS study of more than 64,000 participants, only twelve of the twenty-eight mutations included on genetic tests showed clear evidence of associated cancer risk. The study also debunked the commonly cited statistic that 7 to 10 percent of women carry mutations linked to higher risk. That specific statistic comes from studies of high-risk women with family histories, or cancer, at a young age—so it doesn't apply to all women. Results from the CARRIER study place risk in the general population of women closer to 5 percent.[3]

Most breast cancers are what we call sporadic—people have no family history of it and are therefore unlikely to have inherited their risk. Only 5 to 10 percent of women with breast cancer have hereditary breast cancer; in other words, they possess a dominant cancer gene that is passed on to succeeding generations from either parent. Not everyone with the gene will develop breast cancer, but those who inherit it will have a higher risk. Much larger is the group of people whose cancer is polygenic. This means there is a family history of breast cancer that isn't directly passed on through each generation in one dominant gene—some members of the family get it and others don't. This category includes the possibility that the cancer is actually genetic—there may be a dominant gene that we haven't discovered and thus don't know how to test for. People in this category are at greater risk for cancer than the general public, though less so than people with identifiably hereditary cancer. There are many possible genes that may make someone more prone to breast cancer. A person may, for example, inherit a gene that causes them to begin menstruating at an early age, a factor that has been linked to a higher incidence of breast cancer. Other family members, inheriting the same gene, are also more likely to get breast cancer. Or a person may inherit a mutation in a gene that is responsible for DNA repair after damage and before cell division (see Figure 3.10, page 63). The mutation would not cause breast cancer specifically, but it could make cancers more likely in organs where there is ongoing cell division for renewal, such as the colon, lung, and breast, and no alternative path for repair such as PARP in the breast.

BRCA 1 AND BRCA 2

Approximately 50 to 90 percent of hereditary breast cancer cases are caused by mutations in the BRCA 1 and BRCA 2 genes or, more accurately, 90 percent of cases from families with hereditary breast and/or ovarian cancer and 50 percent of cases from families with hereditary breast cancer. (Remember that the actual BRCA genes aren't bad: we all have them; it's the mutations they sometimes undergo that we need to worry about.) We have learned a lot about these genes since they were discovered in the early 1990s. For one thing, in addition to breast cancer, they also predict higher rates of ovarian and pancreatic cancers (the latter, however, is a much smaller risk). Mutations in the two genes are equally common and men can carry both of them.

According to studies, 1 in 300 women have BRCA 1 mutations, 1 in 800 have BRCA 2 mutations, and 1 in 40 have the Ashkenazi Jewish mutation.[4] The Affordable Care Act requires most private insurers to cover, at no cost to the patient, genetic testing for people at high risk of having BRCA 1 and BRCA 2 and with specific personal and/or family cancer history. Unfortunately, insurers are not required to cover any of the follow-up care for those confirmed to have the mutations.

The risk that women who have mutations in BRCA 1 or BRCA 2 will develop breast cancer is somewhere between 50 and 80 percent. At first researchers believed that anyone with the BRCA 1 gene had an 80 percent lifetime risk of getting breast cancer, based on studies of families with a lot of breast and ovarian cancer.[5] Additional studies were then done on women who, though they had the gene, had only one or two relatives with breast cancer. The studies found, predictably, that the risk was commensurately lower in this group—more like a 37 to 60 percent chance.[6]

Men who carry mutations in BRCA 1 or BRCA 2 are also susceptible to cancer; however, their risks are less understood. Male BRCA 1 carriers are at increased risk for cancer of the breast. In women BRCA 1 mutations carry the greatest risk; in men it is BRCA 2. The relative risk of developing cancer for male BRCA 2 mutation carriers is high before age 65, mostly due to breast, prostate, and pancreatic cancer. And of course both BRCA 1 and BRCA 2 carriers can also pass the mutated gene on to their children.[7]

But why aren't all the carriers getting breast cancer, and why does the risk increase over the years? The word we use to describe this variability is "penetrance," which means the lifetime (usually defined as up to age 70) risk of developing breast cancer. Whether the mutation in the gene results in cancer depends on whether that mutation has an effect. We don't know what causes this difference in penetrance, but some carriers probably won't get cancer unless there is an additional key genetic alteration or they may have inherited other genes that protect them as we said in the last chapter. Several mutations in sequence are probably needed to cause breast cancer (see Chapter 3). For example, suppose a person carrying a BRCA mutation is exposed to radiation and gets breast cancer. They pass the mutation on to their child, who needs only to acquire a second to get breast cancer. If the second mutation was for something that could be avoided (such as exposure to radiation), it would hypothetically be possible for the child to avoid exposure and thus escape breast cancer. Or the mutated cells could exist but the neighborhood they live in (see Chapter 3) is one that suppresses their growth. In fact, studies have shown that the risk of getting cancer has increased in recent generations, implying that nongenetic factors may modify the inherited risk. Not surprisingly, the factors that appear to modify the risk most strongly include reproductive histories and hormones (see Chapter 5). Oral contraceptives are associated with a profound reduction in the risk of ovarian cancer with little or no increase in the risk of breast cancer. Other factors include how old you are at your first period, whether you have been pregnant, whether you have breastfed your child, and whether you have had your ovaries removed. These factors can have different effects depending on which gene is mutated. Having more than one pregnancy appears to be protective in BRCA 1 carriers but is associated with an increased risk in BRCA 2 carriers.[8]

All that being said, penetrance for breast cancer is about 80 percent for both BRCA 1 and BRCA 2; for ovarian cancer it is about 40 percent for carriers of BRCA 1 and 20 percent for carriers of BRCA 2.[9] The risk of ovarian cancer rises steeply after age 40 in both BRCA 1 and BRCA 2 carriers, with an average age of 51.2 years at diagnosis.[10]

Men who carry BRCA 1 or BRCA 2 mutations have a 5.8 percent cumulative lifetime risk of breast cancer versus 0.1 percent for nonmutation carriers.[11]

Founder's Mutations

There are over seven hundred possible mutations in each of the BRCA genes, just as the same word can be mistyped in a number of different ways. Three of these mutations are found consistently in women of Ashkenazi (Eastern European Jewish) descent, like a word always mistyped in one of the same three ways. The mutations are 185delAG, 5382InsC, and 6174delT. These are often called *founder mutations* because they're more common in small, tightly knit populations. The founder is the first person who got the mutated gene, inadvertently "founding" it and then passing it down to their descendants. Intermarriage perpetuates the gene through many generations. Because one or another of the three founder mutations is present in 2.5 percent of Ashkenazi Jews, this group has been studied extensively.

Of course, such an effect isn't exclusive to Ashkenazi Jews. When researchers started looking at other populations, they found similar situations. In Iceland, where there's a lot of intermarriage, there is also a predominant mutation of BRCA 2. Only 9 percent of people in Iceland with a mutated BRCA gene have a BRCA 1 mutation, while 54 percent have a BRCA 2 mutation.[12] This is the reverse of the case in most other

Western countries, in which BRCA 1 mutations are far more common than BRCA 2 mutations. In Norway it's even more specific. Though Norwegians may have either a BRCA 1 or BRCA 2 mutation, which mutation a person gets depends on which fjord they live on.[13] One fjord has one mutation, while another has one of the others.

It is not always so simple, however. In a study of Hispanic women living in Los Angeles, Dr. Jeff Weitzel found that six mutations were responsible for 47 percent of the positive genetic tests, with four of the six seeming to be almost exclusively in families with Latin American/Caribbean or Spanish ancestry. Even more interesting was that another of the six mutations was the same as one of the three Ashkenazi Jewish founder mutations, suggesting that it dates back to the Jews who remained in Spain during the Inquisition, assimilated into Spanish culture, and immigrated to the Americas in the late fifteenth century.[14] And they also found a new BRCA 1 mutation in women from Spain or South America that had not been seen before. This mutation was estimated to have arisen 1,480 years ago, predating Spanish colonization, and represents 10 to 12 percent of BRCA 1 mutations in women who reported Mexican ancestry.[15]

At the time of writing this edition of the book, a specific founder's mutation had yet to be identified for Black women with African ancestry, who tend to get more aggressive breast cancer with higher mortality rates. A Nigerian study of the RNA of ninety-seven breast cancers identified a unique genomic subtype, but research in this area is still lagging.[16]

Returning to the typo metaphor, there are thousands of possible typos with the BRCA 1 or BRCA 2 genes. It's as though all Ashkenazi Jews used the same Hebrew keyboard with an *e* that didn't work. Icelanders used a different keyboard, on which the *t* didn't work. And the Native Americans in Mexico had yet another letter awry.

All this is important when it comes to testing. If you're from an Ashkenazi family and have breast or ovarian cancer, instead of looking for any of the thousands of possible mutations, doctors focus on the three mutations that are most common in this population—and the gene is much easier to test. Investigators have shown that if a Jewish woman does not carry one of those three founder mutations, it is highly unlikely that a different mutation will be found. In other populations, testing for a mutation means studying the whole paragraph to find the typo: it's more time-consuming, and thus more expensive, to test.

Further Questions About BRCA 1 and BRCA 2

What do these genes do? Why does a mutation in BRCA 1, which exists in every cell of your body, cause breast and ovarian cancer and not, say, kidney cancer? BRCA 1 and BRCA 2 are thought to be involved in checkpoint, or quality control, of the DNA. Before a cell can divide and replicate, its DNA has to be checked out to make sure there are no mutations. As part of their quality control job, BRCA 1 and BRCA 2 are involved in tagging badly damaged DNA for degradation. Both BRCA 1 and BRCA 2 are also involved in DNA repair. When a carcinogen like radiation causes a mutation in the DNA, these genes are critical to the machinery that repairs it. Sometimes there are backup repair genes like PARP in the breast, but they are not as good as the originals (Figure 3.10, page 63). When the genes themselves are mutated and can't be repaired, damaged genes accumulate. But this still does not explain why the cancers occur in the breast and ovary specifically. One theory is that the absence of functioning BRCA 1 and BRCA 2 can exacerbate the action of tissue-specific promoters like estrogen and progestin. As I was researching this chapter, I thought for a minute about this theory and then said, "Hmm. I thought BRCA 1 caused cancers that aren't sensitive to estrogen. Why would BRCA care about estrogen?" This sent me back to the books, only to find a new hypothesis: the breast cancer stem cells that seem to develop into BRCA 1 cancers are indeed estrogen-receptor-negative (ER-negative). But the cells right next door are not. Could it be that these surrounding cells may respond to estrogen and send pro-survival signals to the ER-negative cancer stem cells? I'll discuss this later when I review the options for mutation carriers. For now, I simply want to note that most of the treatments that reduce estrogen also reduce the ER-negative tumors of BRCA 1. Obviously we have far ways to go to understand how these mutations work, but research is moving rapidly and I am sure the answers are not far off.

Needless to say, both breasts have the mutations, so if a woman has a first cancer there is a higher risk, about 40 to 65 percent, of a second cancer. Interestingly, as we test more people for BRCA 1 and BRCA 2 mutations we find they also have an increased risk for other cancers. It is well-known that people with BRCA 1 also have an increased risk of ovarian cancer, but less publicized is the fact that carriers of BRCA 2 have an increased risk of pancreatic cancer, male breast cancer, prostate cancer, melanoma, and lung cancer.[17]

OTHER KNOWN MUTATIONS

As we have become more sophisticated in our ability to test for mutated genes, we have expanded beyond the common BRCA 1 and BRCA 2. Other moderate-risk (50 to 80 percent) breast cancer susceptibility genes include TP53, PTEN, STK11, and CDH1. TP53, which sometimes goes under the name Li-Fraumeni syndrome after the scientists who discovered it, causes significant problems, including childhood malignancies, sarcomas, brain tumors, leukemia, adrenocortical tumors, and colon cancer. PTEN, which is also called Cowden syndrome, can show up in childhood with head enlargement, skin findings, benign thyroid and uterine findings, and developmental delay. If this were not enough, these people have a higher risk of breast cancer, endometrial cancer, thyroid cancer, kidney cancer, colon cancer, and melanoma. Families with a lot of different cancers, including breast cancer, may be more likely to have a syndrome like this. Another syndrome, often called Peutz-Jeghers syndrome (STK11), sometimes manifests with lip freckling and indicates an increased risk for breast cancer, colorectal cancer, small bowel cancer, pancreatic cancer, and ovarian cancers. Finally, hereditary diffuse gastric cancer (HDGC) or CDH1 manifests in the breast as lobular cancers and also causes cancer of the stomach.

Many other moderate-penetrance genes have also been identified, such as CHEK2, ATM, BARD, and PALB2. Two of these are now considered to have more risk than we initially thought.

CHEK2 mutation is found in people of Northern and Eastern European descent. It is also involved in DNA repair, and women who carry the mutation have a two- to threefold increased risk of developing breast cancer and one and a half times increased risk of dying of the disease (if the average woman has a 30 percent chance of dying, they have a 45 percent chance) and three and a half times as high a chance of getting breast cancer in the other breast.[18] This means if the average risk is 1 percent per year, theirs is 3.5 percent per year. This gene has also been found mutated in women with hormone-positive breast cancer and is associated with PALB2.

PALB2, which stands for "partner and localizer of BRCA 2," was initially thought to be a moderate-risk mutation, but a study in 2014 found the lifetime risk to be equivalent to that of BRCA 2, with a risk of breast cancer by age 70 of 35 percent. The risk was highest among those younger than forty.[19] Men who are carriers of PALB2 have 8.3 times the risk of the general male population, which, you will remember, is pretty low.

TESTING

Over time, the world of genetic testing has undergone a huge shift. Almost two decades ago in the United States there was one company, Myriad Genetics, that had patented the BRCA 1 and BRCA 2 genes and their mutations. This made their facilities the only place that the test could be legally done. This monopoly was challenged in a lawsuit brought by the American Civil Liberties Union (ACLU). In 2013 the Supreme Court decided that genes cannot be patented, opening up the testing world to other techniques, companies and, most importantly, research.

This, together with next-generation sequencing technology, opened up the marketplace for genetic screening. There are now several commercial panels (genetic sequencing methods) that can test for a variety of low- to moderate-penetrance genes at once. In addition to genetic screening, panels that test for low-penetrance single nucleotide polymorphisms (SNPs) are also commercially available. These are common DNA sequence variants. The cost of mapping your whole genome is dropping fast as well. All this information far exceeds our ability to interpret it. This makes it more crucial than ever to seek the guidance of an expert if you are considering any genetic testing. It is essential for the results to be interpreted by someone knowledgeable, such as an oncologist who specializes in genetic risk or a genetic counselor. Commercial testers tend to check for only a handful of the most common genetic markers linked to breast cancer risk, so a negative result means only that you don't have these most frequent mutations, not that you are without risk. They also lack essential context like family history or environmental factors that may increase risk. A genetic counselor can help you determine whether the test should be done, identify which test should be done, and interpret the results. Furthermore, as new findings emerge that may relate to you, they will recontact you. To find such a counselor, you can check with a nearby medical school. The National Society of Genetic Counselors has a searchable directory of over 3,300 experts in the United States and Canada. A U.S. government website that also lists genetic cancer counselors geographically is www.cancer.gov/search/geneticsservices. For more context on hereditary cancer, the organization Facing Our Risk of Cancer Empowered (FORCE) has a website with up-to-date, expert-reviewed information (www.facingourrisk.org).

In an interesting article for the *Annals of Surgery*, J. D. Igelhart looked into the responses of people who were considering getting tested for BRCA genes and who sought counseling at the testing center.[20] Even after they had talked it over with counselors who explained the test's limitations, many people still believed that if they tested negative they wouldn't ever get breast cancer. When you desperately want something to be true, you often mentally edit what you hear to transform it into what you want it to be.

Whatever the limits of counseling, however, it's much more of a concern when people go into testing without it. And for the most part, they do. As Dr. Iglehart noted, "Physicians without genetic training are more likely to provide testing and least likely to provide counseling." And in fact few doctors have genetic training.

In the Iglehart study, high-risk participants likely to be positive because of their family history were asked before testing to estimate their risk of having the gene. The participants far overestimated their risk, thinking they had a 100 percent risk. The doctors not specializing in inherited risk thought most people had zero risk. They thought a few had a 10 percent risk, and a few had a 20 percent risk.

Who Should Be Tested

Some people have asked why the test for the breast cancer gene is being offered only to women at high risk for the disease. Why isn't it being suggested for all women with breast cancer, or even all women in the United States? Part of the reason is that the chance of having the gene is so low for most people that testing wouldn't be worthwhile. A study by Dr. Beth Newman, reported in the *Journal of the American Medical Association*, looked at a general group of women between ages 20 and 74 with breast cancer to see how many had the mutation.[21] Only 3 percent had the BRCA 1 gene. Another reason to avoid widespread testing is that the options for prevention at the moment mostly involve surgically removing normal body parts to prevent a disease.

However, the question of screening for breast cancer genes is subject to debate. As I was working on this book, Mary Claire King, who discovered the BRCA mutations, suggested that we should be doing population screening. She cited a study she had done in the Ashkenazi Jewish population in Israel.[22] They tested men first and, if they were positive, offered testing to their female relatives for the three common foundation mutations found in the Ashkenazi Jewish population. She points out that 50 percent of families found to harbor BRCA 1 or BRCA 2 mutations were from families that had none of the history of breast or ovarian cancer that would have triggered testing in the United States. This she attributed to smaller families, which then produced fewer people who had inherited mutations and, as a consequence, resulted in fewer cancers. Because tests can also turn up variants of unknown significance (VUS), which are DNA changes that lack enough information to classify, she suggests screening only for unambiguous loss-of-function genes. In the case of BRCA 1 and BRCA 2, these would be genes that have lost some of their DNA-repairing abilities. Finally, she points out that population-based screening enables mutation carriers to be identified independent of physician referral or family involvement (only 19 percent of U.S. primary care physicians accurately assessed family history for BRCA 1/BRCA 2 testing).[23] I thought readers should be aware of these two points of view, an example of differences of opinion in medicine.

In any case, it is important to stop and put the risk of genetic breast cancer into context. J. Peto and his group did a study in the United Kingdom in the summer of 1999, looking at women with hereditary breast cancer.[24] They divided them into age groups and looked at the correlation between hereditary cancer and the BRCA genes. In the group most likely to have the gene, women who had gotten cancer before they reached age 36, only 3.5 percent had BRCA 1 and 2.4 percent had BRCA 2. In women between ages 36 and 45, 1.9 percent had BRCA 1 and 2.2 percent had BRCA 2. So it's a very small percentage, even among young women. However, among women diagnosed with breast cancer before age 35 or women with a history of early breast cancer and a close relative with ovarian cancer, the risk of having the mutation can be greater than 30 percent.

If you think your family may be at risk for hereditary breast cancer and you don't have breast cancer, the best approach is for the relative who has had either breast or ovarian cancer to be tested first. If your mother has breast cancer, is tested, and discovers that she doesn't have a genetic alteration, there's no need for you to get tested. If the test finds that she has a mutation in the BRCA 1 gene, then you can be tested for that specific mutation and save money and time. And if you don't carry her mutation, then you know you didn't get it. This is called a true negative. Again, that's no guarantee you won't get breast cancer, but the risk is much reduced and is the same as that of anyone whose parents did not carry the genetic mutation.

One of my friends of Ashkenazi Jewish descent was diagnosed with breast cancer and was found to carry a mutation in the BRCA 1 gene. This led her sister and brother to be tested. Both her siblings were found to be carriers. Within a few months, her sister was also diagnosed with breast cancer. The good news came when her 25-year-old daughter decided to be tested after reviewing her options with a hereditary breast cancer specialist in Washington. Everyone breathed a sigh of relief when she was found to be negative for the mutation carried by her mother, her aunt, and her uncle.

A more complicated situation occurs when there is a lot of breast cancer in your family (two or more breast cancers under age 50 or three or more breast cancers in relatives at any age) and yet you test negative for BRCA 1 and BRCA 2. This is called a noninformative test because, though the test did not detect anything amiss, this does not guarantee that there is no increased risk. It doesn't mean you don't have any breast cancer gene; it just means you don't have a mutation in BRCA 1 or BRCA 2. You could have a gene we haven't yet discovered. Because only 25 percent of families with only breast cancer (no ovarian cancer) carry a mutation, this is a large group. For those families, a genetic counselor may suggest a panel to look for some of the other hereditary syndromes mentioned. One analysis by Steven Narod's group in Canada calculated that such families still had approximately a fourfold increased risk of breast cancer compared to the general population and still should be screened and maybe even consider chemoprevention (see Chapter 6).[25] A Facebook friend reported that she was the ninth person in her family to get breast cancer. All the computer modeling and genetic consultations predicted a 98 percent chance that she would be a carrier of BRCA 1 or BRCA 2, and yet she tested negative. Nevertheless she almost certainly was at increased risk. She probably has a gene/mutation/condition we just don't know how to test for yet.

A lot of other gene mutations linked to breast cancer risk are being identified as research gains momentum in that area. If you think you may have a mutated gene in your family, you should talk with a genetic counselor or specialist in this area.

The Risks and Benefits of Getting Tested

What precisely are the risks? As I noted, one is financial. The testing can be expensive, costing from $300 to $5,000 depending on whether you are testing for a specific mutation known to be in your family or doing an extensive screen. You can first be tested for the most common BRCA 1 and BRCA 2 mutations and PALB2 with several commercial laboratories, which should cost less, or do a more extensive screen. This again points out the benefit of knowing what you are looking for, such as a mutation that has already been found in the family as opposed to a more expensive fishing trip. If a particular mutation is identified, then other family members can get tested for less. That's because the really hard work is searching for a possible mutation. It's like proofreading an entire manuscript to find the typo; once you know the location, finding it in other copies is fairly easy.

Some insurers will pay for the test, but that is not always the case. Initially there was fear that insurance companies would discriminate against people who had been tested. The 2008 Genetic Information Nondiscrimination Act protects against discrimination based on an individual's genetic information or disability by health plans but not life insurance plans. The confidentiality of genetic information is protected under the HIPAA Privacy Rule as health information. You can also be tested under a code number or an assumed name. Still, it would be smart to check the laws in your state and the policy of your insurance company before proceeding.

Keep in mind that it isn't only you who will need to deal with the consequences of your decision. It becomes a family issue. If I get tested and I'm positive, this will have implications for my siblings—who may or may not want to get tested. It also has implications for my children. If you choose to be tested and learn you have a mutated gene, you will then need to decide what to do with the information.

When you already have breast cancer, the emotional conflict over gene testing intensifies. You tend to think that you must have the bad gene. Further, your own psychological issues almost inevitably get mixed into your perceptions. Were you mean to your parent when they had breast cancer, so now you're being punished by inheriting a killer gene? Even highly sophisticated people are to some extent trapped by unconscious expectations.

One benefit of being tested is the reduction in uncertainty. If the result is positive, the knowledge can allow you to make a plan for risk reduction (see Chapter 6). My Ashkenazi Jewish friend mentioned earlier told me she highly recommended that the daughters of people who carry BRCA 1 be tested. It was an enormous relief for her and her daughter to know that her daughter was negative, and she suspects that it would also be helpful to know if one's child is a carrier. Not knowing can cause anxiety.

A Facebook friend wrote that she had herself tested because there was ovarian and breast cancer on her father's side of the family, and her oldest sister had ovarian cancer. Ideally her sister would have been tested, but she refused because she did not want to know. However, my friend wanted to know for her own sake and her daughter's.

If you decide to be tested, there are several possible results. Most satisfying are the true positives and true negatives. In a true positive, the test finds that there is a clear mutation. In a true negative, the patient tests negative but another family member has an identified mutation. In this case you know you did not inherit the family gene. More complex is the situation in which the test identifies no known mutation, and no one else in the family has been found to have a specific mutation. Then you do not know whether there is a mutated gene that is not one of the ones we know how to look for, or if there is no genetic alteration. Also, abnormal genetic alterations of unknown clinical significance can be found that have not been linked to breast cancer. In both of these situations you are left with as many questions as answers.

The test that looks for any kind of sequence change may find that there is only one nucleotide off (see Chapter 3), and it may or may not be important. As I mentioned, it could be a variant of uncertain significance (VUS). This can be very frustrating for the doctor and the family. Between 10 and 15 percent of people undergoing genetic testing for BRCA 1 and BRCA 2 mutations will be found to have a VUS.[26] They are even more common in nonwhite populations, with frequencies as high as 14 percent among Americans of African descent.[27] Sometimes genetic detective work can help sort them out, but frequently a person is left not knowing whether to consider themself at risk.[28] In these situations it is important to be followed in a high-risk setting (such as a clinic or university medical center) where research is going on all the time. Ask about registries of these variants, so that you will become aware of any new information as soon as it becomes available. Again, as research continues, we'll learn more and more about this, but we don't have all the answers now. In addition to variants, there can be mutations that manifest through large rearrangements in a gene that go undetected by standard testing. These large rearrangements (not a single typo but a phrase in the wrong place in the sentence) account for about 10 percent of mutations identified and are more common in people of Latin American/Caribbean ancestry than in other ethnicities.[29] New tests for the BRCA 1 and BRCA 2 genes are more sensitive and can pick up such rearrangements.

Recommendations for Genetic Testing for Breast Cancer Risk

Guidelines for genetic testing for breast cancer are becoming broader as new mutations are discovered. Although hereditary cancer is still uncommon, this kind of testing can also help in making treatment decisions. The most detailed guideline for genetic testing is put out by the National Comprehensive Cancer Network (NCCN), a nonprofit alliance of thirty-one cancer centers. Their recommendations[30] are as follows.

You should get genetic testing if you have a personal history of breast cancer:

- At or before age 45
- At age 45 to 50 with any unknown or limited family history of breast cancer (first- or second-degree relative)
- At age 45 to 50 with multiple primary breast cancers
- At age 45 to 50 with one or more close blood relatives on the same side of the family tree with breast, ovarian, pancreatic, or prostate cancer at any age, on either parent's side of the family

- At or over age 51 with one or more close blood relatives with breast cancer before or at age 50, or with male breast cancer at any age
- At or over age 51 with one or more close blood relatives with ovarian, pancreatic, or metastatic prostate cancer at any age, on either parent's side of the family
- At or over age 51 with three or more total diagnoses of breast cancer for you and/or any close blood relatives
- At any age to aid in systemic treatment decisions using PARP inhibitors for breast cancer in the metastatic setting
- At any age to aid in adjuvant treatment decisions with olaparib for high-risk HER2-negative breast cancer
- At any age with triple-negative breast cancer
- At any age with lobular breast cancer with personal or family history of diffuse gastric cancer
- At any age with male breast cancer or one or more close relatives with male breast cancer on either parent's side of the family
- Personal history of breast cancer and Ashkenazi Jewish ancestry

Understandably, the NCCN guidelines have been criticized for being unnecessarily complex. A recent study has also demonstrated that their detailed parameters on testing inadvertently excluded patients who, when checked, did indeed have genetic mutations.[31]

The American Society of Breast Surgeons instead suggests that genetic testing be made available to all patients with a personal history of breast cancer. For those newly diagnosed, the identification of a mutation may impact local treatment recommendations. Furthermore, with the approval of PARP inhibitors for both early-stage and metastatic breast cancer, testing may be appropriate to expand treatment options for some patients independent of family history and should be discussed. Patients who were tested before 2014 may benefit from an updated test with a broader array of potentially relevant genes.[32]

There are several reasons for people with breast cancer to consider getting tested. They may want to know if others in their family are likely to get cancer. Or they may be thinking about having children, and the possibility of passing on a breast cancer gene could play a role in their decision making. People with cancer in one breast are more likely to get it in the other, and they may want to consider having a double mastectomy if they know they have the gene. In women without the mutated gene, the risk of a second primary cancer (unrelated to the first and thus not considered a recurrence) is between 0.5 and 1 percent a year, and 15 to 25 percent over their lifetime. For someone with the gene, it's probably between 1 and 2 percent a year, 30 to 50 percent over their lifetime. A person with BRCA 1 or BRCA 2 may want to have their ovaries removed, which reduces breast cancer risk by 53 percent.

I don't think it makes sense for every person with breast cancer to be tested, since hereditary breast cancer is so rare. Still, there are some profiles showing the likelihood of carrying a genetic alteration. If you are a Jewish woman younger than age 40 with breast cancer, there is about a 33 percent chance that you are a carrier. If you are not Ashkenazi Jewish and have breast cancer before age 30, you have a 12 percent chance of having a mutation. If you develop bilateral breast cancer between ages 40 and 50 and have a first- or second-degree relative with breast or ovarian cancer before age 50, there is a 42 percent chance that you carry a mutation. If you are over age 50 when you get breast cancer, your risk of having a mutation is lower. Furthermore, if you have two relatives who had breast cancer after age 50, your chances of having the breast cancer mutation are only 2 percent.[33]

CHOICES

If you test positive for the BRCA 1 or BRCA 2 gene, what next? First, getting a positive test result is not an emergency. It just confirms what you undoubtedly suspected: that you are at high risk for breast cancer. The question is, what are you comfortable doing about it? The choices range from ignoring it (probably not too wise) to close monitoring[34] and through chemoprevention or surgical prevention[35] (examined in Chapter 6).

In any case, you want to be seen by a clinic that specializes in high-risk individuals and those with genetic risk. They will review your options with you and consider your particular situation. Many factors have to be taken into consideration, from whether you still want to conceive children (which would preclude having your ovaries removed immediately) to whether you are claustrophobic and cannot tolerate an MRI. You need to discuss and digest all these matters before you launch into a plan that will work for you and your life.

Surveillance

The kinds of monitoring for people who carry a mutation has been evolving. Usually it involves having an exam every six months, beginning around age 25 to 35, as well as yearly mammography and breast MRIs (alternating every six months). Mammography is controversial because, as we will discuss in Chapter 6, it doesn't work as well in young people with dense breasts. In fact, it detects less than half the breast cancers in mutation carriers.[36] Still, it can find microcalcifications and sometimes a cancer. An alternative in the early years may be the addition of WBUS (whole-breast ultrasound; see Chapter 7), which is being used more frequently for screening high-risk people with dense breasts. At the moment, MRI with mammography and ultrasound, starting at age 25 to 30, seems to be the best approach to surveillance. But you must make sure you are getting the best breast MRI available, in a high-quality breast imaging center, particularly an American College of Radiology–accredited Breast Imaging Center of Excellence. Images are only as good as the person taking and reading the pictures.

Of course, the risk of having cancer as a result of carrying one of the BRCA mutations is not limited to the breast. You will also need to be monitored for ovarian cancer. In many ways, as I noted earlier, ovarian cancer is more deadly than breast cancer, although it's much less common. When found on screening, breast cancer is often more treatable, whereas ovarian cancer is less often found at an early stage. It is a very sneaky cancer: there are no symptoms until it's far developed. Pelvic exams rarely show signs of ovarian cancer. A blood test called CA125 is good for monitoring metastatic ovarian cancer, but it works only about 50 percent of the time when the cancer is in an early stage. It's particularly tricky in premenopausal people. There are a lot of false positives, leaving the patient terrified that they have an incurable disease and leading to unnecessary surgery. Transvaginal ultrasound is a more recent technique. An ultrasound tool is placed in the vagina and the technician can look around the ovarian area. The process has a very high resolution, but most of what it finds is benign. It may be a good idea for very high-risk people, but if used for screening, suspicious signs would be found in about fifty out of a thousand people, all of whom would undergo major surgery and only one of whom would turn out to have cancer.

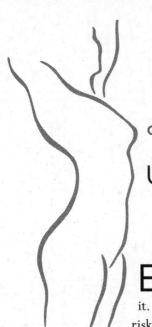

CHAPTER 5

Understanding Risk

Everyone wants to know what their chances are of getting breast cancer and what they can do about it. In this chapter we will discuss biological tests for risk, and in the following one we will go over prevention or risk reduction. I wish there were a simple way to calculate that risk, but it changes with exposures to carcinogens, with reproductive events, and over time. Three kinds of risk are commonly referred to in connection with breast cancer: absolute risk, relative risk, and attributable risk (Figure 5.1). Although the rest of this section will be less complex, I do think understanding relative risk is important when you are making choices about the benefits of prevention as well as of the treatments. So take your time and I will try to explain the kinds of risk and what they mean. If this is more than you want to know, skip to Chapter 6, where we discuss the evidence we have for certain links between behaviors, exposures, and breast cancer risk.

HOW WE RESEARCH CAUSE AND PREVENTION

We saw in Chapter 3 how molecular biology has helped us understand how abnormal cells develop. However, molecular biology is slow when it comes to finding causes or ways to prevent malignancy. Here we may have to move to a bigger picture: What causes the cell to mutate in the first place, and what influences the neighborhood? To learn this, we need to look at big groups of people in whom we can find the commonalities as well as differences. This is where epidemiology comes in. Many of the studies you hear about in popular media are of this kind. They suggest

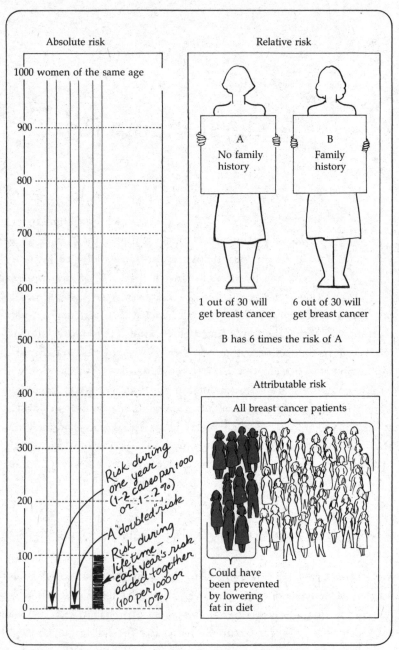

Figure 5.1

that food X increases the risk of getting breast cancer, or activity Y prevents the disease. Typically, these are big studies that compare groups of people. Although this type of study can give us clues, it can't prove cause and effect. It provides, at most, circumstantial evidence. For example, if you studied the lives of people with drug addiction, you would probably find that most of them drank milk as children. But you wouldn't conclude that drinking milk causes drug addiction. To find a connection, you'd need to compare both people who have addiction and people who do not, calling for a much larger, more complicated study.

There are many ways to conduct studies of diseases and the possible ways to control, treat, or prevent them. Unfortunately, a completely accurate, comprehensive study is impossible to achieve. There are too many variables in even the simplest area of research. But some studies are better than others. To understand how accurate a study is, you need to look at how it was designed. It may be weak in one area, strong in another, and excellent in a third.

Few people understand study design. Doctors are as predisposed to self-deception as anyone else: we all tend to believe the studies that feed our biases rather than the ones that don't. This same tendency is reflected by the media. Reporters often don't understand the nuances of a study, and their sound-bite reports usually fail to address any limitations in the study's design. In addition, they often exaggerate the study's implications. Data that form only one small part of the puzzle are presented as if they gave the whole situation. It's no wonder nonscientists are confused about what a study's results mean in real life.

Observational Studies

There are two basic categories of study, each with its own benefits and limitations. The *observational study* looks at, without intervention, people doing what they would normally do. The *clinical trial*, or *intervention study*, tests a certain treatment on a group of people who are assigned to use it in certain ways over a certain period of time. We will examine this category later when we talk about treatments (see Chapter 11). Here we will review observational studies, which are more relevant to risk and prevention.

Observational studies are great for generating a hypothesis. The researchers observe a phenomenon and then try to think of an explanation. For example, a study done in Boston observed that women with breast cancer were more likely to get their clothing dry-cleaned. The hypothesis was that the fumes may lead to breast cancer. This is an interesting idea but far from proven. The next step may be to do a study in mice and see if dry cleaning fluid increases cancers. We could also study people who work at dry cleaners to see if they had more cancer. If these studies still seemed to show a relationship, we could then go on to a controlled study in which people were randomized to use dry cleaners or not, and then see how many developed breast cancer. This last study, of course, would be difficult to do, but it would be essential to give us the final proof. In this particular case, the women who worked at dry cleaners did not have an increased risk of breast cancer. It turned out that people at higher socioeconomic levels are at higher risk in general and also use dry cleaners more often. Although both of these statements are true, they are unrelated. Observational studies are useful but far from definitive. Media headlines often use the word "may" to indicate these limitations, as in: Dry cleaning *may* increase breast cancer risk. This is okay as long as they then discuss the limitations of the study.

These limitations do not mean such studies are useless. They are great at telling us what to study in greater depth. Observational studies take the form of cross-sectional studies, case control studies, and cohort studies. These are increasingly more complex and expensive to do. For that reason we usually start with the easiest approach and do the most complicated and expensive study only if warranted. (See the Epilogue for more information on the HOW study in the Love Research Army, formerly known as the Army of Women.)

TYPES OF RISK

Absolute risk is the rate at which cancer, or mortality from cancer, occurs in a general population. It can be expressed either as the number of cases per a specified population (such as 50 cases per 100,000 annually) or as a cumulative risk up to a particular age. This cumulative risk is the source of the familiar 1 in 8 for non-Hispanic white women. (Other racial and ethnic groups may actually have a lower risk; see Figure 5.2.) Note that

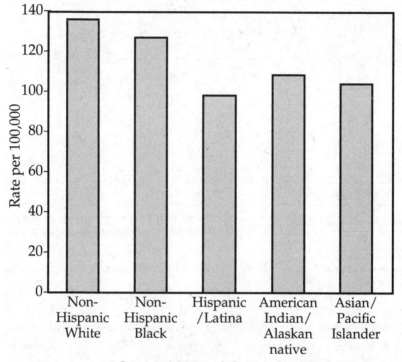

Female Breast Cancer Incidence by Race and Ethnicity
2015-2019 US

Source: National Cancer Institute

Figure 5.2

what it cannot do is tell *you* what *your* particular risk is as that changes all the time depending on life events, exposures to carcinogens, and drugs. For example, future risk at any one time depends to a great extent on your age. At age 20 the risk over the next ten years is 1 in 1,479 (0.1 percent), while the risk over the next ten years for a 50-year-old is 1 in 42 (2.4 percent) (see Table 5.1).

The second kind of risk we talk about is *relative risk*. This is the comparison of the incidence of breast cancer, or deaths from breast cancer, among people with a particular risk factor to that of people without that factor, or a *reference population*. This type of measurement is more useful to an individual because they can determine their risk factors and thus calculate how those factors will affect their chances of getting the disease. Even here you have to be very careful. For comparison, if you are a non-Hispanic white woman, you can't use the 1 in 8, or 12 percent,

Table 5.1 Age-Specific Probabilities of Developing Invasive Female Breast Cancer

If your current age is:	The probability of developing breast cancer in the next ten years is:	or 1 in:
20	0.1%	1,479
30	0.5%	209
40	1.5%	65
50	2.4%	42
60	3.5%	28
70	4.1%	25
80	3.0%	33
Lifetime risk:	12.8%	

Note: Probability is among those who have not been previously diagnosed with cancer. Percentages and "1 in" numbers may not be numerically equivalent due to rounding.

Source: American Cancer Society. *Breast Cancer Facts and Figures 2019–2020.* Atlanta: American Cancer Society, Inc., 2019.

figure generated in the absolute risk equation mentioned earlier, because that is based on all such women regardless of risk factors; rather, you need a number that will reflect your risk without the factors being considered. For a woman with no clear risk factors at all (no previous cancers, no family history, menarche (first period) after age 11, first pregnancy before age 30, menopause before age 52), this is 1 in 30, or 3.3 percent, significantly lower than the "average" risk of 12 percent.[1]

If you call the risk of the woman without any particular risk factors 1.0, you can report the risk of those with a particular risk factor in relation to this. This is how relative risk is derived. A woman whose mother had breast cancer in both breasts before age 40, for example, has a relative risk of 2.7 over her lifetime—in other words, 2.7 times that of the woman with no family history; not, as it may appear, 2.7 times the 12 percent mentioned earlier (see Table 5.2).

When you read a study or see one reported in the media, it is important to check the basis for the relative risk numbers. Most authors compare people with a specific risk factor to people without it. They assume that all the other risk factors are equal in both groups so that only their risk in terms of the risk factor of interest is being compared.

**Table 5.2 Factors That Increase the Relative Risk
for Invasive Breast Cancer in Women**

Relative Risk	Factor
>4.0	• Age (65+ versus <65 years, although risk increases across all ages until age 80) • Atypical hyperplasia • Lobular carcinoma in situ • Pathogenic genetic variations (e.g., BRCA1, BRCA2, PALB2, TP53)
2.1–4.0	• Ductal Carcinoma in situ • High endogenous hormone levels (postmenopausal) • High-dose radiation to chest (e.g., Hodgkin lymphoma treatment) • Mammographically dense breasts • Two or more first-degree relatives with breast cancer
1.1–2.0	• Alcohol consumption • Early menarche (<11 years) • Excess body weight • High endogenous estrogen or testosterone levels (premenopausal) • Late age at first-term pregnancy (>30 years) • Late menopause (≥ 55 years) • Never breastfed a child • No full-term pregnancies • One first-degree relative with breast cancer • Obesity (postmenopausal) • Personal history of ovarian or endometrial cancer • Physical inactivity • Proliferative breast disease without atypia (usual ductal hyperplasia, fibroadenoma) • Recent and long-term use of menopausal hormone therapy containing estrogen and progestin • Recent hormonal contraceptive use • Weight gain in adulthood • Tall height

Note: Relative risks for some factors vary by breast cancer molecular subtype.

Source: American Cancer Society. *Breast Cancer Facts and Figures 2019–2020.* Atlanta: American Cancer Society, Inc., 2019.

Relative risk is also used to give results regarding treatments for breast cancer. Women who took a particular drug had a 30 percent decrease in the chance of dying within five years compared to women who did not. Although this sounds hopeful, it is important to know what the risk of dying was. It could be that one group had a 9 percent chance of dying and the other 6 percent—or one-third less. You may not be willing to take a drug to reduce your risk by 3 percent.

Finally, we must consider *attributable risk*. This concept relates more to public policy than personal health. It looks at the amount of disease in the population that could be prevented by reducing risk factors. For example, a risk factor could convey a very large relative risk but be restricted to a few individuals, so changing it would benefit only these individuals. Dr. Anthony B. Miller has hypothesized that if every person in the world capable of giving birth were to have a baby before age 25, then 17 percent of the world's breast cancer would be eliminated.[2] If you were looking at this from a public health policy perspective, you'd have to weigh the possible advantages of pushing early pregnancy against the problems of young and possibly immature parents and the dangers of increased population growth.

To understand any of this, we need to understand what is meant by the term "risk factor." What do we mean by risk factors and how are they determined? "Risk factor" is a term referring to identifiable factors that make some people more susceptible than others to a particular disease; for example, smoking is a risk factor in lung cancer, and high cholesterol is a risk factor in heart disease. Medical researchers attempt to identify risk factors in order to discover who is most likely to get a particular disease, and also to get clues as to the disease's cause, and thus to the possible prevention and/or cure. A risk factor is usually determined by an observational study. For example, it was first noted that a risk factor for cancer of the cervix was more common in people who were sexually active and had multiple sexual partners.[3] This led to the suspicion that the cause may be sexually transmitted and ultimately to figuring out that it was HPV.

In breast cancer, we have come up with some risk factors—such as radiation exposure—that we'll look at in the next chapter. But so far, there is nothing comparable to the connections found between sexual activity and cancer of the cervix. With breast cancer, the sad reality is that we can't say, as with cancer of the cervix, "you're safe because you don't have the virus." In fact, 70 percent of breast cancer patients have none of the classical risk factors in their history.[4] It's important to understand this, for two reasons. Overestimating the importance of risk factors can cause needless mental anguish if you have one of them in your background. However, you may harbor a false sense of security if you don't have them. I can't count the number of times a patient has come to me with a suspicious lump that turns out to be malignant and, stunned, says, "I don't know how this happened! No one in my family ever had breast cancer!" I tell her she's in good company—most breast cancer patients don't have a family history of breast cancer. By virtue of being women, we are at risk for breast cancer.

Risk factors don't necessarily increase in a simple arithmetical fashion. If one risk factor gives you a 20 percent risk of getting breast cancer and another gives you a 10 percent chance, it doesn't always mean that now you're up to 30 percent. The interaction of risk factors is a tricky and complicated process. One interesting example concerns studies on alcohol and breast cancer (which we'll consider in the next chapter), showing that women with other risk factors who also drank alcohol didn't increase their risk very much, while women with no other risk factors who drank raised their risk dramatically.[5]

It reminds me of the old story of the blind men and the elephant. Each man carefully described one section of the elephant's anatomy, but no one got the whole picture. Our descriptions of risk are still fragmentary, and there is often the sense that we are missing something big that would tie it all together and enable us to say "This causes breast cancer so don't do it!" But breast cancer is complex and has many factors that interact with one another in ways we don't understand yet. It is looking likely that the four or five different types of breast cancer (see Chapter 10) may each have their own risk factors with little overlap. We may well be talking about several different diseases, all of which happen to occur in the breast, rather than different flavors of the same disease.

So read on, not to calculate your exact risk or that of your child or to learn how to live your life risk-free, but to understand what you read in the media and to explore the mystery that is breast cancer. And if you want to play your own role in sorting it out, join the Love Research Army and be part of the research to end breast cancer once and for all.

RISK FACTORS

Returning to the metaphor of the mutated cell in a community of supporting cells (Chapter 3), it makes sense to distinguish between the potential causes of breast cancer that create mutations and those that affect the community. However, readers who braved the previous chapter will know that nothing is that simple. For one thing, there is some evidence that postmenopausal estrogen can cause mutations in cells,[6] and there is plenty of evidence that it can also quickly change the environment that serves as fertilizer for mutated cells. And we know of other factors that can modify the potential cancer cell and/or its community.

As we saw in the last chapter, most people do not carry a gene for breast cancer, and yet many may still be at higher risk because of other biological factors beyond their control, such as hormones or the type of breast tissue they inherited. What the majority of people want to know is what are the risk factors, and how can we avoid them? What we really want to know is, what is the cause of nonhereditary breast cancer, and how can we avoid it? And for that matter, why doesn't everyone with a mutated BRCA gene get breast cancer? If I knew those answers I'd be sitting here with the Nobel Prize, instead of working on another edition of the book. That being said, there are definitely hints that we can get from studying what increases breast cancer risk and even the variability of risk in different countries and different ethnic groups. In 2014, researcher William Anderson[7] and others came out with a different hypothesis on breast cancer. They suggested there could be two or more causes of breast cancer just as there seem to be several types of breast cancer: for instance, there could be one for the basal-like hormone-negative cancers and another for the hormone-positive cancers (see Chapter 10). This is very intriguing and could be true. Certainly we see different patterns of breast cancer in Asian and African countries and even in different ethnic groups in the United States. It is complicated to sort out, however. The rates in Black, Hispanic,[8] and Malaysian women all seem to suggest that tumors not sensitive to hormones are more prevalent and appear at a younger age. Is this due to biology, ethnicity, socioeconomic status, or lifestyle? In general, ER-negative tumors have an earlier age of onset, increase rapidly, and then decrease after menopause, while hormone-positive tumors increase at a slower rate and peak at age 70. Could one kind of cancer come from one cell type and the other from a different one? I find this fascinating as a new way to think of breast cancer. Stay tuned—there is obviously a lot more to come that may help in both prevention and treatment.

Our Own Hormones

When you think about hormones and breast cancer, you tend to think in terms of hormone pills. Much attention (and much needed attention) has been paid to the relationship between cancer and use of oral contraceptives, menopausal hormone therapy, and fertility drugs. Less consideration has been paid to our bodies' own hormonal levels (see Chapter 1). How our own hormones exert their influence on breast cancer is not clear. They are also almost certain to be a factor that makes the neighborhood more welcoming to cancer cells. If they are not a cause, they most definitely are a major influence on breast cancer.

Prenatal Hormones

Some of the most intriguing data on the influence of hormones suggest that prenatal influences may also affect breast cancer risk. In studies, fetal mice were exposed to the estrogen-like bisphenol A (a substance used in making plastics). This resulted in long-lasting effects in the mice's mammary glands that showed up as precancerous changes during puberty.[9] These effects may apply in human females as well. This was tragically demonstrated during the 1950s and 1960s; a synthetic estrogen, diethylstilbestrol (DES), was widely prescribed to pregnant people to prevent miscarriages. Many years later we discovered that DES increased the risk of vaginal and cervical cancer in those patients' children. A recent follow-up study suggested—but did not prove—a slightly increased risk of breast cancer in their children under age 40 and a definite increase in risk in those over age 40.[10] Although far from definitive, these studies lead us to believe that there may be influences in the womb that set the stage for later disease.

Another way of viewing these influences is to look at hormone levels at birth. Data are pretty consistent that high birth weight (which gives us clues about estrogen levels in the womb) correlates with later breast cancer risk.[11] However, preeclampsia, a condition associated with low estrogen levels, decreases the child's subsequent breast cancer risk.[12] Other factors indicate that good nutrition during childhood also correlates with breast cancer risk. One hypothesis is that early stimulants for growth (internal and external factors that encourage growth, the way rain, sun, and fertilizer encourage a plant's growth) also increase the number of breast stem cells that are available to undergo mutations.[13] These mutations can be inherited or acquired by exposure to carcinogens. Another theory is that the early hormones cause temporary changes to the DNA (changes that have the potential to revert, though such reversion is not inevitable).

Adult Hormones

There is no question that exposure to hormones affects our risk throughout life. For example, the younger a person is at their first period and the older they are when they go into menopause (that is, the longer they have reproductive levels of hormones), the more likely they are to get breast cancer than is a person with a shorter reproductive period (Table 5.2). People who menstruate for more than forty years seem to have a particularly high risk. A person whose ovaries are removed early and who doesn't take hormone therapy has a greatly reduced risk of breast cancer.[14] But there may be costs. One recent study has suggested that ovarian removal increases mortality overall: although protecting you from breast cancer, it increases your vulnerability to other conditions such as heart disease.[15] If you've had a hysterectomy, it may or may not influence your risk of breast cancer, depending on whether your ovaries were removed. If you still have ovaries, your body continues to go through hormonal cycles, even though you have no periods; these cycles continue until the time you would normally go into menopause.

Pregnancy appears to affect breast cancer risk in two ways. During a pregnancy and for the ten years following it, a person has a greater risk of developing breast cancer, presumably because the hormones of pregnancy have caused more cell division and therefore more opportunities for mutations to occur.[16] This is particularly true for people who do not breastfeed. A recent hypothesis suggests that involution (resetting of the breast after weaning) could also set the stage for more cancer.[17] However, people who are able to give birth but who have never been pregnant seem to be more at risk than people who have a child before age 35. The-oretically the hormones of a pregnancy carried to term mature the breast tissue, making it less susceptible to carcinogens. People who have their first pregnancy after age 35 have a greater risk than people who have never been pregnant at all. Although it has been hypothesized that ther-apeutic abortion or miscarriage may increase breast cancer risk, large studies have shown no association.[18] Breastfeeding is protective against breast cancer, the relative risk decreasing 4.3 percent for every twelve months of nursing, in addition to a decrease of 7 percent for each birth. This could explain some of the discrepancy between more developed and less developed countries, as there tends to be more and longer breast-feeding in poorer countries.[19]

Although we have known of a link between hormonal levels in the blood and postmenopausal breast cancer, a study showed this is true in premenopausal people as well.[20] After menopause most estrogen comes from converting androgens—hormones from the adrenal glands—into estradiol. Most of this conversion is done by fat tissue. Thus estradiol levels tend to increase with body weight.[21] In contrast, body weight is not a risk factor for breast cancer before menopause because premenopausal estrogen comes from the ovaries (see Chapter 1).

We also know that in at least some people the breast tissue is also capable of making its own estrogen locally through the enzymes aro-matase and sulfatase.[22] The tissue around the tumor has been shown to have higher estrogen levels than the tissue far from it.[23] It should come as no surprise, then, that blocking estrogen reduces breast cancer risk and treats estrogen-sensitive cancers (see the discussion of prevention in Chapter 15). Cumulatively, research data suggest that there is a role for prolactin and testosterone in causing breast cancer as well.[24]

What about testosterone? (As I mentioned in Chapter 1, women have testosterone, though in much smaller amounts than men do.) Studies have shown that circulating estrogens and testosterone are associated with an increased risk of breast cancer in premenopausal people as well as postmenopausal people.[25] Interestingly, obesity was associated with much higher levels of hormones than those in lean women, as was smok-ing and alcohol consumption compared to those who did not smoke or drink. The effect of these hormone levels was apart from classic risk fac-tors such as age at first period, number of pregnancies, age at first preg-nancy, or family history of breast cancer.

Transgender individuals may have a slightly higher risk of breast cancer due to their own unique hormonal, and sometimes surgical, histories. Individuals who are lesbian, gay, bisexual, transgender, or queer are also less likely to seek cancer screening. Because of hormonal use, transgender women have a greater risk than people who do not undergo such types of hormone treatment, according to the American Society of Radiology and the Society of Breast Imaging. Transgender men and nonbinary people who do not undergo mastectomy remain at their previous risk for breast cancer.[26] Lastly, screening may still be necessary for transgender men and nonbinary people who have undergone double mastectomies, depending on family history. This is because there is usually some residual breast tissue left behind, and it could be a concern if there are any inherited mutations. In these cases, the general rule is "screen now, screen regularly, and screen what you have."[27]

Breast Density

Another condition suspected of posing a biological risk is breast density as seen on a mammogram[28] (see Chapter 8). Breast tissue, which is dense, shows up white on the mammogram, while the more transparent fat tissue shows up gray. Although some researchers have attributed this to an increase in breast cells, the evidence suggests it is the stroma, or local neighborhood, that is responsible. Some epidemiological data suggest that breast density may have two different effects. One is that dense tissue makes it more difficult to see lumps on the mammogram. The other is that the stroma in the breast tissue is being stimulated. When I was first told this, I thought it was foolish—the dense breast tissue that shows on the mammogram isn't what gets cancer; the cells within the ducts do. But now that we're learning that there is constant "crosstalk" between cells and their neighbors (see Chapter 3), the effect isn't quite so easy to dismiss.

Dense breast tissue seems to represent an activated breast tissue more prone to cancer. People whose mammograms show very dense tissue are at significantly higher risk of breast cancer than those whose mammograms are less dense, and this applies to people of any age. In fact, a recent overview of forty-two studies of mammographic density indicates that the relative risk of breast cancer for people who had 70 percent or more density was 4.64 times that of people with less than 5 percent density.[29]

Young people have dense breasts (remember when they stood straight up?). As we age, this density decreases, and we begin to sag. Some studies show that the rate of decline in breast density is slower in some people. Although we would like to think they are lucky not to sag, they actually have a higher chance of getting breast cancer.[30]

There are increasing data to support this theory. Studies regarding hormone replacement therapy (HRT) have suggested that people whose breasts become denser while taking these hormones have increased risk. A third of people taking them show increased breast density on mammograms, which starts as soon as the person begins taking the medication. Observational studies have suggested that progestin added to estrogen increases the density, resulting in more risk than that of estrogen alone. We have also seen that tamoxifen reduces breast density almost immediately.

Breast density is getting more and more attention. I will discuss alternatives to mammography that are being used or offered to people with dense breasts in Chapter 7; suffice it to say that breast density is one of many markers of risk that can be monitored.

Precancer in Breast Tissue

Hormones in the blood are one thing, but what you really want to know is what is happening in the breast. Specifically, you want to know whether you have cells that look like they are on the way to becoming cancerous. Although we have some ways to get a glimpse of this, they are not as reliable as we would like.

To understand the conditions we call precancer, we need to back up a minute and return to the breast's biology. As I noted in Chapter 1, the breast is a kind of milk factory. It has two parts—lobules that make the milk, and ducts, like hollow branches, that carry it to the nipples (see Figure 1.7, page 9).

Over the years, you can get a few extra cells lining the duct—sort of like rust in a pipe. This is called *intraductal hyperplasia*, which simply translates to "too many cells in the duct." We call these proliferative or dividing cells. In themselves they aren't a problem. Sometimes the cells become a bit strange-looking, and this condition is called *intraductal*

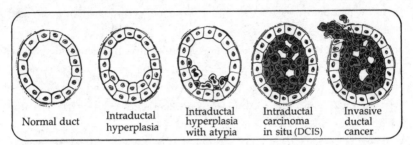

Normal duct	Intraductal hyperplasia	Intraductal hyperplasia with atypia	Intraductal carcinoma in situ (DCIS)	Invasive ductal cancer

Figure 5.3

hyperplasia with atypia (also known as *atypical ductal hyperplasia*, or ADH). If they keep on looking odd and multiply within the duct, clogging it, they get another name—*ductal carcinoma in situ* (meaning "in place"; DCIS) or *intraductal carcinoma* (Figure 5.3). You might imagine that this means there is a big difference between these two steps. After all, that frightening word "carcinoma" has been inserted into the phrase. But in fact, the only difference between ADH and low-grade DCIS is that DCIS requires two adjacent ductal structures to be filled with cells and ADH does not—a fairly arbitrary definition. We think that these DCIS cells represent the "seeds" of a potential cancer and that they can revert to ordinary cells if the neighborhood changes. It isn't until the cells are let out of the ducts and into the surrounding fibrous tissue or fat that they are called invasive or infiltrating ductal cancer.

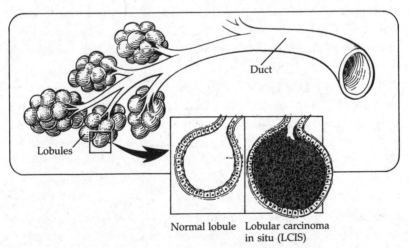

Duct

Lobules

Normal lobule   Lobular carcinoma in situ (LCIS)

Figure 5.4

The same stages can be seen in the lobules with *lobular hyperplasia*, *atypical lobular hyperplasia* (ALH), and *lobular carcinoma in situ* (LCIS) (Figure 5.4). And sometimes you see a mixture of ductal and lobular cells. This is not surprising since the first changes that lead to cancer are thought to start at the junction of the duct and the lobule.

Of course, we are making these distinctions based on how the cells look under the microscope. We need to analyze this further with genetic tests. It would not be surprising if they represented different types of DNA damage or mutations. Studies are now being done to try to figure this out.

The proliferation (hyperplasia and atypia) takes place inside the duct or lobule, so you can't feel it by examining your breast. In the past it was found only incidentally (2 to 4 percent of the time) during a surgical biopsy, not in the lump itself but next to the lump in the rim of apparently "normal" tissue, and the pathologist came across it by accident. A review by the Mayo Clinic[31] followed all patients who had benign biopsy findings between 1967 and 2001. Of these they followed a total of 698 patients with atypical hyperplasia for a mean of 12.5 years. Overall, 143 developed breast cancer, or 20 percent. The risk was twice as high in the breast with the atypia as in the other breast, especially in the first five years. The cancers were usually ductal (see Chapter 10). I will talk more about treating ADH and ALH in the following pages; however, this new data based on modern screening and pathology suggests that this is indeed a very early form of precancer. With mammographic screening we are finding that 12 to 17 percent of the microcalcifications biopsied are associated with ADH or ALH.[32] In addition to increased detection by mammography, a French study showed that people on postmenopausal hormones had double the risk of ADH compared to those who did not take hormones.[33] It will be interesting to see if the recent decrease in postmenopausal hormone use will result in less apparent ADH. I say "apparent" because autopsy findings on women who have died of causes other than breast cancer reveal that 30 percent or so had some degree of either hyperplasia or atypical hyperplasia.[34] This is not uncommon. One study[35] compared the incidence of hyperplasia with or without atypia in normal breast tissue donors (3.3 percent), reduction mammoplasties (17 percent), and benign breast samples (34.9 percent). So probably a lot of us are walking around with these conditions, and we don't know it because we have no reason to have biopsies, they don't show on mammograms, and the cells are dormant.

As you see, many questions still remain. For a person diagnosed with ADH or ALH, the most vital question is, what does it mean? The first step is to look at how it was diagnosed. If atypical hyperplasia shows up on a core biopsy, there is a consensus that an open surgical biopsy is indicated. This is because of a 20 to 25 percent risk that the hyperplasia is the tip of the iceberg—that next to it there may be an in situ or invasive cancer.[36]

But if it was found during a larger surgical biopsy, we can be more confident that the whole area has been removed. Most surgeons would agree that the best program in that case is close follow-up, so that any in situ carcinoma or invasive cancer is found. This would include a physical exam by a doctor every six months and yearly mammograms.

For people who have been diagnosed with ADH or ALH there is an alternative to surgery as studies have shown that people with ADH who took tamoxifen for five years had 86 percent fewer subsequent breast cancers than those who had no treatment.[37] Later studies showed that the benefits persist long after the five-year course is over. The risks and benefits of this approach are certainly worth considering (see Chapter 6). Some people may even consider a more drastic approach and have preventive mastectomies.

Lobular Involution

Another recent finding on biopsy that may give information about breast cancer risk is whether there is *lobular involution*. As mentioned earlier, involution refers to what happens when the tissue regresses or retires. You will remember from Chapter 1 that the breast develops lobules at puberty, and it develops even more with pregnancy when they're needed to produce milk. After you've finished breastfeeding the child, the lobules all undergo cell suicide. But don't feel sorry for the lobules; they've lived a good life—and new ones form to replace them and prepare your body for its next pregnancy. That is one form of involution.

As we age and especially after menopause, our lobules are no longer stimulated by hormones and become permanently involuted. These changes can be seen on a breast biopsy. Dr. Lynn Hartmann at the Mayo Clinic looked at a large series of benign breast biopsies from the past in people who had later developed cancer. She found that people who had experienced lobular involution had a significantly reduced risk of breast cancer. For example, people over age 55 who didn't appear to have involution had a threefold increase in breast cancer risk. This permanent involution occurs around menopause, with only 5 percent of people under age 50 showing it but is present in 20 percent of people between ages 50 and 59.[38]

This is a relatively new area of research, and the Susan G. Komen Tissue Bank has been key. In one study of normal samples from the bank, researchers looked at terminal duct lobular units (TDLUs), which can be likened to the end of the branches and attached leaves (lobules) of the breast ducts. Breast cancer is thought to start at the junction of the duct and the lobule, so if hormones make you produce more of them, the active breast has more places for breast cancer to grow. Researchers were able to show that all measures of TDLUs started declining when study participants were in their thirties and were lower in postmenopausal individuals. People capable of giving birth who had never been pregnant also had lower levels, but the age-related decline was faster among people who had given birth, perhaps explaining their lower breast cancer risk.[39] Researchers looked at how hormone levels correlated with the extent of lobular involution in the specimens. In premenopausal people, higher prolactin levels were associated with higher TDLUs—they had less involution—but higher progesterone showed lower levels. In postmenopausal people, higher levels of estradiol and testosterone were associated with higher TDLU counts. This suggests that hormones are at least one factor in keeping the breast active and at risk. This is an area of much interest and may well give us further insight not only on the risks for breast cancer but also how to prevent it.

TESTS FOR RISK

It is all well and good to find precancerous changes on a biopsy, but it would be much more helpful if there were an easy way to identify abnormal or precancerous cells. There are three current approaches to sampling cells: nipple aspirate fluid (NAF) collection, ductal lavage, and random periareolar fine-needle aspiration (RPFNA). They all depend on cytology (the study of cells), which involves looking at isolated cells under the microscope and determining by their appearance whether they are precancerous. Although the use of these three methods is still only for research, they are teaching us a lot about who is at risk.

Nipple Aspirate Fluid (NAF) Collection

As I said in Chapter 3, all breast cancer starts in the milk ducts. The idea of studying the ducts and their fluid was first mentioned in 1946 when a Uruguayan doctor, Raul Leborgne,[40] described a way to pass a small catheter into a breast duct and squirt saline in, take the catheter out, and collect the fluid as it dripped out. He termed his procedure a "ductal rinse." Then in 1958, American physician George Papanicolaou, the inventor of the cervical Pap smear, described applying suction to the nipple to obtain small drops of fluid from the milk ducts (Figure 5.5). He termed it a "breast Pap smear."[41] (As I explained in Chapter 2, it's not unusual to be able to obtain fluid from a breast.) The timing was not right, however, and the technique languished for years. This was probably because no one knew at the time how the information could be used to help people. But curiosity remained, and in the 1970s, several researchers reevaluated Papanicolaou's approach. Three major series of studies took place, each advancing our understanding in a slightly different way: one by Gertrude Buehring, another by Otto Sartorius, and the third by Eileen King and Nicholas Petrakis.[42] In all of them, researchers were able to obtain breast fluid from about 80 percent of premenopausal individuals and 50 percent of postmenopausal individuals by using a suction cup on the nipple.

King and Petrakis took the long view. Between 1973 and 1980 they collected fluid and then analyzed it. After twenty-one years of follow-up, 285 of the 3,633 women studied developed breast cancer. The researchers compared the outcome with their initial evaluation of the fluid they'd taken twenty-one years earlier. Not surprisingly, they discovered that the participants who'd had no fluid had the lowest incidence of breast cancer (4.7 percent). Those with fluid but with normal cells had a slightly higher incidence (8.2 percent) than those without fluid. Those with hyperplasia showed a bit higher (10.8 percent) incidence, and those with atypical cells had the highest incidence (13.8 percent). The researchers took into account differences in the individuals' ages and the years they entered the study. Those with atypical cells had nearly three times the amount of breast cancer of those with no fluid at all.

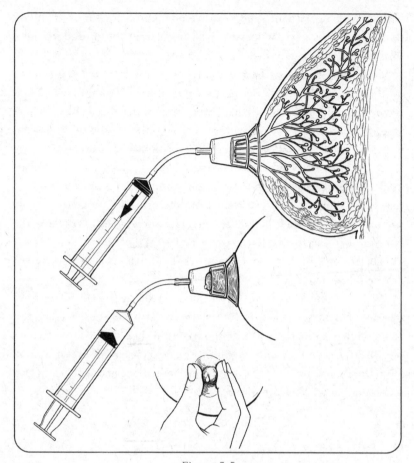

Figure 5.5

This study also led King and Petrakis to conclude that women with atypical cells and a first-degree relative with breast cancer were nearly twice as likely to develop the disease as those who had atypical cells but no first-degree relatives with breast cancer. This suggests that if you have both atypical cells and a family history of breast cancer, you have a fairly high risk of getting the disease. Virologist Gertrude Buehring completed a twenty-five-year follow-up of her series of NAF volunteers and confirmed a higher risk of cancer in those who had both NAF and abnormal cells.[43] Kim Baltzell has now completed the follow-up of the Sartorius series of 946 women and found that those with abnormal epithelial cells in NAF have a greater risk of breast cancer than those without fluid. Even women with normal cells in their NAF had a higher risk than those without cells or without fluid.[44] So we now know how most of the six thousand or so study participants who underwent the procedure more than twenty years ago have fared.

In addition to cells, there are also proteins, hormones, and even carcinogens in the fluid. Because cells require a cytologist to look at them, it would be better if there were something that could serve as an easier *marker* of what was going on biologically in the duct—a protein secreted by precancerous cells, for example. Ed Sauter, a surgeon from the University of Texas Health Science Center in Tyler, Texas, improved the suction technique of obtaining nipple aspirate fluid so that he was able to retrieve fluid from close to 100 percent of study participants.[45] He then looked for prostate-specific antigen (PSA; the same marker that is used for prostate cancer) and other markers. As yet the perfect one marker—one that can predict who is at risk for breast cancer—has eluded us.

We have been doing research on this approach at the Dr. Susan Love Research Foundation and are working on an easy, inexpensive home test based on finding markers like immune cells in the fluid or even bacteria or viruses. Could they offer a glimmer as to the cause of breast cancer? Does the fluid represent a low-grade inflammation, and if so, does that inflammation set the stage for breast cancer?[46]

Ductal Lavage

The problem we came up against with nipple aspirate fluid was that not all ducts had it. I found this surprising; the common belief among doctors, when they gave it any thought at all, was that it was always there. So I thought it would be important to look at cells and fluid from every duct. I developed a tiny catheter that could be used to thread through the nipple into a milk duct for a distance of about 0.5 inch (1 cm) (Figure 5.6). Using this catheter, we washed each duct with salt water and then retrieved cells from deep in each ductal tree. The fluid was then sent to be examined for cells, as we had done with NAF. In an early study we compared these cells to those in the fluid obtained by suction alone. We found that lavage, as we called the process, collected more cells than NAF and was better able to detect abnormalities.[47]

Although the procedure was approved for high-risk people, the question remained: How do we know that these cells are precancerous? We

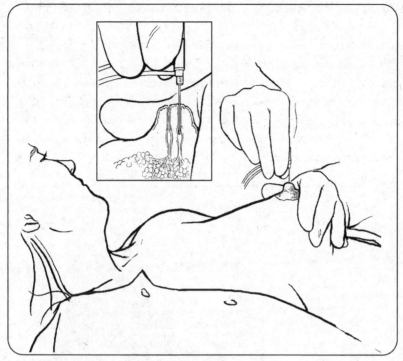

Figure 5.6

found that there were limits to our procedure as far as answering the question. First of all, not all ducts with cancer gave fluid that contained any cells, let alone cancer cells. In addition, when we repeated lavage in the same duct six months later, we found that most of the time the atypical cells had gone away on their own, much as they often do when the doctor repeats a Pap smear. One of my colleagues, Dr. Bonnie King, looked not just at the cells themselves but the DNA inside them. This turned out to be more accurate.[48] Research is continuing and expanding. As I mentioned, some researchers are looking for substances in the fluid that can identify who has cancer or is at risk: patterns of proteins, for example, or hormone levels. Although lavage is still a research tool, I am confident that we will find a good marker of risk in the fluid, and when this happens it will become a useful test on a wider level.

Another aspect of this approach is ductoscopy. This involves threading a very small scope through the nipple and down a milk duct and biopsy-ing the lining. Although many surgeons have identified known cancers through this technique, it is not clear whether it will be a good diagnostic test for precancerous lesions.[49]

Random Periareolar Fine-Needle Aspiration (RPFNA)

In a different approach to the problem of identifying people with high-risk changes in the breast, Dr. Carol Fabian in Kansas explored the use of fine-needle aspiration—sticking small needles into both breasts on both sides of the nipple and then suctioning out some cells (Figure 5.7).[50] Although this technique has found more atypical changes in the tissue of high-risk individuals than in those of normal risk, it also has its limitations. Placed at random, the needles can detect only the changes that

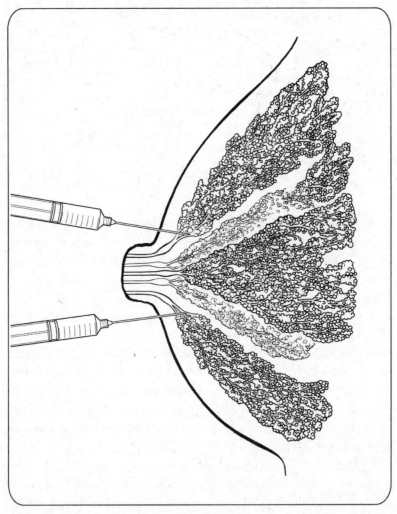

Figure 5.7

are going on somewhere in the breast. If typical cells are identified, it is more difficult to ascertain which duct they are in and get back to the precise spot six months later. Nonetheless this approach has proved useful in testing new drugs to see whether they have any effects on the breasts of high-risk individuals. First RPFNA is done and then the person takes a new drug for six months, at which time the needle biopsies are repeated, looking for changes in markers of hyperplasia and atypia.

STATISTICAL RISK

In this chapter we have focused on concrete ways to determine your risk based on either your genes or changes in your tissue. Sometimes we resort to calculating a statistical risk based on some of the family history and lifestyle risk factors. In an attempt to do this, several statistical models have been developed based on risks across a population and then applied to individuals. These are usually based on various combinations of family history, age, reproductive history, race/ethnicity, hormonal factors, and benign breast disease. The one most commonly used in the United States is the National Cancer Institute (NCI) breast cancer risk assessment model based on the Gail model (www.cancer.gov /bcrisktool/). It has been validated for use in most women age 35 or older and provides estimates for an individual's five-year and lifetime risk for developing breast cancer on the basis of five to six questions. The Women's Contraceptive and Reproductive Experience (CARE) model has allowed them to update it for Black women.[51] Another aimed at that same underserved population is the Black Women's Health Study (BWHS) to estimate an individual's risk of developing invasive breast cancer over the next five years. It was derived and tested solely using data from Black women in the United States.[52] A model from Dr. Jeffrey Tice of the University of California, San Francisco incorporates breast density into its calculations and has been shown to be a good tool in a multiethnic population.[53] The inclusion of breast density in traditional risk models for breast cancer has resulted in an increase in accuracy, according to recent studies and reviews.[54]

A model based on the Women's Health Initiative study predicts the risk of ER-positive cancers in postmenopausal people. None of these models work well in those with a strong family history, however, and so the Claus model or the Tyrer-Cuzick (https://ibis-risk-calculator .magview.com)[55] model (both of which include detailed family history) is used in these situations. Finally, a model known as BRCAPRO[56] is frequently used to estimate how likely an individual is to carry a mutation in BRCA 1 or BRCA 2 and whether testing is worthwhile. These last three are most often used in high-risk or genetic clinics.

Risk models that do well in predicting the proportion of women in a population who develop cancer have only a modest ability to discriminate whether an individual will develop breast cancer. It is like predicting that people who graduate from college and live on the East Coast are more likely to go to Europe at some point in their lives versus predicting that *you*, who live on the East Coast, will go to Europe. Most people who are identified as being at increased risk for breast cancer will never develop the disease, and most who develop breast cancer have no known risk factors and would not be identified ahead of time using any of these models. But if these models are so limited, why do we even use them? We use them, for instance, to figure out whom to include in studies of chemoprevention so that we know we are comparing similar people. That way we can say that if, based on this model, you have this risk, then you may be a candidate for this type of prevention. As of yet we do not have the perfect test, statistical or otherwise, to identify those who are most strongly at risk.

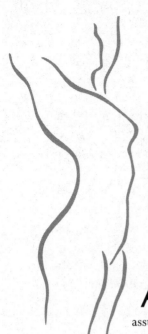

CHAPTER 6

Prevention and Risk Reduction

As we continue to research the biology of breast cancer, new revelations prompt us to revisit past assumptions. In the past decade a lot of new information came to light on what this disease requires to thrive. As we explained in Chapter 3, for cancer to develop you need mutated cells (inherited, acquired, or both) as well as a local and systemic (whole-body) neighborhood egging them on. The mutations can be caused by radiation, carcinogens (environmental and viral), and age. At this time we don't know enough about the relationship between environmental carcinogens and breast cancer to make a data-based recommendation. For now, risk reduction means limiting radiation exposure (especially medical), uncalled-for hormonal exposures (hormone replacement therapy, whether bioidentical or pharmacological), and other known carcinogens when possible (especially occupational). Medical radiation is an important risk that is often overlooked. We have become used to getting an X-ray or an even stronger CT scan every time we have a symptom needing diagnosis. Although this can be satisfying to the doctor and patient, it is done more often because physicians think the patient expects it rather than because it is necessary. Every time an X-ray is recommended, we need to get into the habit of asking whether it will change the treatment. If the answer is no, then politely decline. It is not worth the extra radiation.

Beyond avoiding mutations, we can try to change the local and systemic neighborhood that our cells live in. This becomes increasingly important as the limits of "precision medicine," or finding a single mutation and fixing it, become clear. For now the cell's neighborhood—hormonal, immunological, and metabolic—is a better starting point for prevention strategies. Some things that improve the cell community are lifestyle changes, such as reducing obesity, exercising regularly, and following a healthy diet. Other changes can come from drugs that can alter the hormonal, inflammatory, or metabolic milieu. Finally, as a last resort in breast cancer prevention, we have the option of removing the organ itself.

A woman with average risk is most likely fine with lifestyle changes, whereas one whose parent has had breast cancer may want to consider chemoprevention as well. The drastic option of preventive surgery may be weighed by a carrier of the BRCA 1 or BRCA 2 mutation. In this chapter I'll review all these options and the data supporting them. I will also highlight some other new prevention research that looks promising—including vaccines to prevent breast cancer.

LIFESTYLE

The bad news is that there is no new magic! Weight loss, exercise, and healthy eating still appear to be the best ways to reduce your risk of breast cancer. The American Institute for Cancer Research released a review of all the studies examining lifestyle changes that could prevent breast cancer. Their conclusion was that more than seventy thousand breast cancer cases a year—40 percent of all cases—could be prevented with lifestyle measures such as maintaining a healthy weight, breastfeeding, eating well, exercising, and limiting alcohol consumption. Of these measures, the biggest single thing a person can do to lower their risk, especially after menopause, is exercise and maintain a healthy weight. There is a growing body of evidence indicating that being overweight as we get older increases estrogen and also affects insulin and other growth factors in ways that give cancers a more stimulating neighborhood in which to grow and, at the same time, make it more difficult for the body to eliminate emerging abnormal cells. A 2012 study from Seattle showed that weight loss in postmenopausal people lowered serum estrogens and free testosterone, giving a biological rationale for why weight loss may lower breast cancer risk.[1]

A lifestyle issue that is not discussed much is age at first pregnancy. The data are clear that early first pregnancy is protective and that getting pregnant for the first time after age 35 increases the risk more than never being pregnant at all. The full reason for this finding is not clear. Breast-feeding also has been shown to decrease breast cancer risk, especially in people with a family history of the disease. The longer in total months that a person has breastfed, the greater the risk reduction.[2]

It is hard not to notice that all these lifestyle changes relate to estrogen levels. Later period, early pregnancy, breastfeeding, early menopause, and even weight loss are all associated with less estrogen stimulation. If you combined them all, the risk would go down significantly.

Epidemiologist Graham Colditz, who has been studying this his whole life, reported that "women can slash their breast cancer risk by avoiding alcohol or drinking very moderately; maintaining a healthy weight; being physically active; eating plenty of fruits, vegetables and whole grains; and, if they have children, breastfeeding them."[3]

Diet

The connection between diet and breast cancer is proving to be more complex than we initially thought. Researchers continue to explore this link, finding different effects depending on a person's age and the kind of tumor examined. The role of fruits and vegetables as a means of pre-venting breast cancer received a blow in 2005 with the report from the European Prospective Investigation into Cancer and Nutrition (EPIC). An amazing 285,526 women between ages 25 and 70 completed a di-etary questionnaire and were then followed prospectively for a median of 5.4 years. Although 3,659 breast cancers were reported, the study found no association between the consumption of fruits and vegetables and the risk of developing breast cancer.[4] However, the question is prob-ably more complicated. A 2013 study pooled several cohort studies and looked at 993,466 women who were followed for eleven to twenty years with ER-negative tumors.[5] What they found was that total fruit and veg-etable intake caused a statistically significant decrease in these hormone insensitive tumors but not in the hormone-positive ones. As was men-tioned in Chapter 5, these may well be two different kinds of breast can-cer with different risk factors and causes, and we obviously need to take that into account when we evaluate studies. This is clear in the results of the randomized controlled study by the Women's Health Initiative on low-fat diets, which included postmenopausal people. This study began in 1992 and randomized participants between ages 50 and 79 into two groups, one given a diet with less than 20 percent of calories from fat, at least five daily servings of vegetables and fruit, and at least six servings of grains, and the other group on their usual diet. Between 1993 and 1998, the researchers studied 48,835 participants, and they found no effect on breast cancer overall. Because postmenopausal people are more likely to have hormone-positive cancers, this is not surprising.[6]

At this point I think it is wise, for many reasons, for all of us to eat a diet low in animal fat and high in fruits and vegetables. Reducing the risk of the more aggressive ER-negative tumors is worth it.

Soy, Flaxseed, and Green Tea

Soy as a food has had a mixed reputation regarding breast cancer prevention. It has often mistakenly been termed a phytoestrogen (literally, plant estrogen). Although it does contain phytoestrogens, it has a much more complex hormonal composition, acting more like tamoxifen than estrogen. Studies in Western populations have shown no association between high soy intake and breast cancer prevention.[7] However, a large study from Shanghai found that adult soy food consumption was associated with a lowered risk of premenopausal breast cancer.[8] Again, timing matters, as it was the high intake of soy foods during adolescence that appears to be the most important. The weak plant estrogens in soy may enhance early differentiation and maturation of the breast tissue, which in turn may protect a person from developing breast cancer.[9] A U.S. study of Asian American women confirmed that soy intake during childhood, adolescence, and adult life was associated with decreased breast cancer risk, in this case with the strongest and most consistent effect from childhood intake.[10] This is encouraging, and you may want to try to coax your adolescent into eating more tofu. But we can't be totally certain it will help: the possibility remains that these children and adults had other elements in their lifestyle that were also or even exclusively protective. We get a hint of this in the study: when adjustments were made for aspects of a Western lifestyle, the investigators found reduced benefits of soy intake among adolescents and adults.

Regarding soy supplements, it's probably a good idea to play it safe and stay away from them as they may not have the same effects as soy in real foods. Although you would think the label would tell you the dose, supplements are not compelled to either control or report this information the way drugs are. They could have no soy in them at all or a lot, as they are not regulated.

Flaxseed, sesame, and several other oily seeds and edible fibrous plants contain high amounts of lignans (complex elements in a plant cell's walls that give the plant rigidity and strength), which have some weak estrogenic and antiestrogenic properties distinct from soy. Flaxseed is currently advocated by professional gynecologic associations in Canada as a treatment for cyclic breast pain,[11] and a small placebo-controlled trial in early breast cancer has also shown that it can reduce growth of cancer cells.[12] A more recent trial, however, found that flaxseed did not make a notable difference compared to a placebo.[13]

Another substance being studied is green tea, which, like soy, is often part of an Asian diet. A study of Chinese women in Singapore found that daily intake of green tea had a strong effect on decreasing mammographic density.[14] Black tea, much more common in the West, had no such effect. I must say this finding brought a smile to my face as I sipped my evening mug of green tea!

Vitamins and Minerals

Changing one's diet is never easy, and researchers have tried to figure out the key ingredients in vegetables, fruits, and fats so they can put them in a pill. This can be a tricky business. I am always reminded of the study done on vitamins and lung cancer. Initial work had shown that people who ate a lot of carrots had less lung cancer. Researchers postulated that it was the beta-carotene and decided to test it. They gave smokers beta-carotene capsules and were shocked when they found more cancers in the smokers taking the pills than those in the control group.[15] The answer is probably that vitamins and minerals are meant to be eaten together in a healthy diet. Beta-carotene needs to be eaten with all the other vitamins and minerals in the carrot, not in isolation.

Still, a lot of research continues to focus on specific vitamins, hoping that one will be the holy grail. More recently, it was vitamin D, which also is thought to help maintain healthy bone, muscle, immune system, and probably other tissues as well. We make most of our vitamin D in the skin as a result of sun exposure. Our current indoor lifestyles and increased use of sunscreen limit this route for many people. As a result there are a lot of people, including some people with breast cancer, who have low blood levels of vitamin D. This has led some researchers to question whether vitamin D can prevent breast cancer. Epidemiologic studies comparing women in areas of high versus low sun exposure, animal studies, and some case control studies, particularly in young women, suggest that it can, especially if higher blood levels are achieved than we usually see with conventional doses of supplements. However, these investigations are only first steps. Women who have lower body fat from diet and exercise are also likely to have higher levels of vitamin D.[16] We are not sure of the ideal blood level of vitamin D or the age at which vitamin D supplementation would need to start to prevent breast cancer. Further, overly high levels of vitamin D can result in side effects such as kidney stones.

Studies to evaluate cancer incidence in women randomized to placebo or calcium plus vitamin D have been inconclusive. A small study in postmenopausal people in which the vitamin D dose was 1,100 IU suggested a benefit in reducing all types of cancers, including breast cancer, but the numbers of each specific cancer that developed were too small to single out a single kind.[17] The Women's Health Initiative randomized postmenopausal individuals to take calcium and 400 IU of a specific form of vitamin D, or a placebo. Study participants in both the placebo and treatment arms were allowed to take up to 1,000 IU of nonstudy vitamin D because the study actually focused on whether calcium prevented fractures. No reduction in risk of breast cancer in the treatment arm compared to the placebo one was observed, nor were baseline blood levels of vitamin D correlated with breast cancer risk.[18] However, these baseline levels were rarely in the range associated with substantial risk reduction in other studies.[19] The researchers did find that baseline levels correlated with weight and exercise.[20] So one possible explanation of the previous studies may be that the participants with higher vitamin D levels were more likely to be thinner and also to exercise. Because both of these factors can also reduce breast cancer risk, it is hard to know which is more relevant. A more recent randomized controlled trial to study vitamin D and omega-3 concluded that supplements of the vitamins did not result in a lower incidence of invasive cancer or cardiovascular events.[21] Still, vitamin D's more modest benefits are worth exploiting. Younger people in particular may consider taking a supplement or spending fifteen minutes a day in the sun without sunblock unless you are very fair or have a personal or family history of skin cancer. Many vitamin D experts recommend taking a supplement of 1,000 IU daily for general health.[22]

Studies of vitamin A supplements have also been equivocal, with some suggesting a benefit and some not.[23] However, in studies that measure vitamin A compounds in the blood, low levels of the vitamin correlated with an increased risk of breast cancer.[24] Recent reviews of epidemiological data suggest that vitamin E in foods may provide some protection against breast cancer, whereas vitamin E supplements appear not to.[25]

Finally, the Women's Health Initiative looked at whether taking a multivitamin would reduce the risk of getting cancer. This observational study[26] found that taking a multivitamin had little or no influence on the risk of common cancers, cardiovascular disease, or total mortality in postmenopausal individuals.

Overall the data are not strong enough to talk about a "breast cancer prevention diet," but in general a diet low in animal fat and high in whole grains, fruits, and vegetables is most likely to keep you healthy and help you maintain a good weight. It also makes sense to drink alcohol only in moderation, since regular consumption of alcohol may affect your vulnerability to breast cancer.

Exercise

Exercise is important for cardiovascular health and for preventing osteoporosis, heart disease, and breast cancer. A 1994 study by my friend and colleague Leslie Bernstein at the City of Hope Medical Center demonstrated that women who participated in four or more hours of exercise a week during their reproductive years have a 58 percent decrease in breast cancer risk.[27] Exercise is one of the first lifestyle changes shown to decrease risk. Bernstein has recently updated this finding in a prospective study of retired and active California teachers and other public school professionals followed for ten years.[28] She found that strenuous long-term exercise can indeed protect against invasive and in situ breast cancer, with a 20 percent greater risk reduction in women who exercised more than five hours a week compared to those who exercised minimally or not at all. Interestingly, participation in moderate to strenuous activity also reduced the risk of

ER-negative breast cancer by about half. More than fifty studies have shown that women who are physically active have a lower risk of invasive breast cancer. Several have shown that the same is true for in situ breast cancer. This suggests that physical activity affects early phases of breast cancer development. What causes this to happen is not clear, and the benefits may differ at different times of life. In young people the mechanism is thought to be hormonal as exercise results in alterations in menstrual cycle patterns and less frequent ovulation, both of which are correlated with lower risk (Figure 6.1).[29] A study of estrogen metabolism in premenopausal people randomized either to thirty minutes of moderate to vigorous aerobic exercise five times a week for about sixteen weeks or to no exercise program showed changes in premenopausal metabolism of estrogen compared to the sedentary group. This is thought to be one mechanism for the effect.[30] Even though delaying the onset of the menstrual cycle seemingly should prevent hormonal tumors, it is also possible that the effect is on the interactive

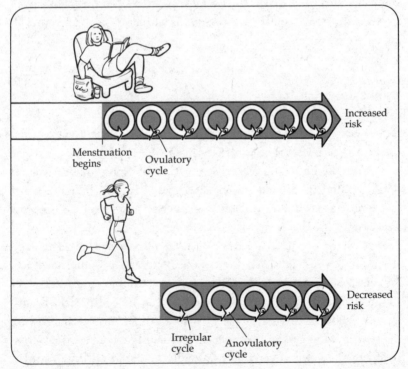

Figure 6.1

community of cells (neighborhood) that support ER-negative tumors. Another possibility is that exercise has an anti-inflammatory effect, which reduces the incidence of all kinds of cancers. Finally, there is the fact that it helps maintain a healthy weight, which reduces risk in postmenopausal people.

A long-term prevention approach thus may be to get girls into the habit of exercising early on. The late Dr. Rose Frisch of Harvard Medical School and Harvard School of Public Health showed that women who were involved in athletics during high school and college have a decreased risk of breast cancer.[31]

A delightful proposal has been put forth: increase funding for girls' high school athletics. Expanded participation in athletics would likely decrease breast cancer, strengthen bones, and prevent future osteo-porosis; it would also help prevent heart disease and type 2 diabetes. However, physical activity doesn't have to be athletics. My daughter joined the folk dancing club in college and got a great workout that way. And it is never too late to begin! I am a born-again exerciser, hav-ing started running at age 50. I learned to enjoy the stress reduction from my regular slow run, as well as the sense of moral superiority I felt for the rest of the day.

Lifestyle changes are interesting from a public health standpoint and probably are worthwhile to consider on an individual basis, but they may or may not be applicable to any particular person, and I don't advise using them as the sole influence in decision making. For example, I had my first child at age 40 and do not regret it. The advantages to me far out-weighed the slight potentially increased risk for breast cancer. Would I have been wiser to have had a child in my twenties, when I wasn't ready for it? Or, since having no children is actually less of a risk than having a first child later in life, should I have deprived myself of the joy Katie has brought me? For me, there was no question. However, I do exercise reg-ularly and eat a good diet high in fruits and vegetables and low in animal fat. My weight is finally at a healthy place. The occasional twinge I feel at the sight of a juicy hamburger or wedge of Brie is a reasonable price to pay for the possibility that I may be decreasing my breast cancer risk and improving my overall health. Another person in my position may decide to adopt rather than become pregnant, or they may decide that the plea-sure they get from fatty foods isn't worth abandoning. These are very personal decisions.

CHEMOPREVENTION

Hormones

Because hormones are heavily implicated in the development of breast cancer, and the more menstruating years you experience, the higher your risk of breast cancer, one proposed approach has been to put people into temporary menopause.[32] This approach, which could combine birth control and breast cancer prevention, has been shown to reduce mammographic density,[33] but so far no long-term studies have been done to demonstrate its safety and effectiveness for breast cancer prevention.

Another approach is based on the recognition that the younger you are when you have your first child, the lower your risk. This has led to the idea of inducing a hormonal "pregnancy," in which a teenager would be given pregnancy hormones for nine months to mature the breast tissue and thus mimic the protective effect of early pregnancy. To my knowledge, this has been tried only in rats, but it's an interesting possibility. One ingenious study took advantage of the fact that human chorionic gonadotropin (HCG, a pregnancy hormone) was once used in weight loss clinics allegedly to help women lose weight (it has no such effect, but many women took these shots). Professor Leslie Bernstein was the only one ever to collect such data, and she showed that it does reduce breast cancer risk in premenopausal individuals, just as the animal studies would have predicted, with the strongest effect seen in those who had never been pregnant and therefore had not had a chance to be exposed to their own pregnancy-induced HCG.[34] There are several small studies looking at whether HCG could be used for prevention.

Another use of drugs to prevent breast cancer is based on the idea of blocking the estrogen receptor to keep estrogen from having its usual effect. This is the theory behind efforts to avert the disease by giving women tamoxifen, raloxifene, or an aromatase inhibitor.

The first two drugs are actually not estrogen blockers but rather selective estrogen receptor modulators, or SERMs. They have some estrogenic effects (Nolvadex/tamoxifen can increase bone density) and some estrogen-blocking effects (hot flashes). Evista (raloxifene) was originally developed as an osteoporosis drug and found to also reduce breast cancer. In several large clinical trials it has been found to reduce the risk of bone fractures in postmenopausal individuals but not heart disease. Like

Nolvadex, Evista is associated with an increase in blood clots, hot flashes, and vaginal bleeding. The good news is that it acts like estrogen in the bone and blocks it in the breast, so it is a good chemoprevention drug. Two newer, third-generation SERMs, Fablyn (lasofoxifene) and arzoxifene, have similar effects with slightly different profiles.

A meta-analysis of all the studies of SERMs combined published by Jack Cuzick and his colleagues[35] concluded that SERMs significantly reduce the risk of all breast cancer in high-risk and average-risk women without the disease. (Only Nolvadex [tamoxifen] has been studied in premenopausal people.) The reduction is largely in hormone-positive disease, with no effect on ER-negative tumors. Again, this harks back to the discussion in Chapter 5 about the two different causes for the two types of breast cancer (hormone-positive versus hormone-negative). Interestingly, the benefits of the SERMs persist during the five years after treatment. The new drug Fablyn (lasofoxifene) was particularly promising for prevention because it not only had a large effect on breast cancer but also decreased strokes, cardiac events, and fractures with no increase in uterine cancer.

Aromatase inhibitors are being widely used to prevent recurrence in women with breast cancer. They decreased not only recurrence but also cancer in the other breast. This has prompted prevention trials in women with DCIS and women at high risk. Initial results of the NCIC-MAP.3 trial[36] demonstrated that Aromasin (exemestane) reduces the incidence of invasive breast cancer by 65 percent and ER-positive cancer by 73 percent. The study reported no significant impact on quality of life or serious toxicities. However, follow-up studies over the years revealed many of the participants who took aromatase inhibitors for longer periods of time experienced musculoskeletal problems such as bone loss and fractures in addition to more manageable side effects like arthritis and hot flashes.[37] Initial results from the IBIS-II study of anastrozole for prevention in high-risk postmenopausal individuals showed that the risk of breast cancer with five years of treatment was 2 percent compared to the control group, whose risk was 4 percent.[38] While this sounds small, it does mean that the drug reduced the risk by half. A long-term follow-up to the IBIS-II study noted that the reduction in breast cancer incidence was maintained for up to twelve years, although a side effect during the active treatment period was an 11 percent excess of fractures.[39]

In 2019 the American Society of Clinical Oncology (ASCO) updated recommendations for hormone therapy, such as chemoprevention, to include pre- and postmenopausal individuals over age 35 with a five-year projected risk of at least 3 percent, or with a ten-year risk of at least 5 percent, or a diagnosis of atypical ductal or lobular hyperplasia, or lobular carcinoma in situ (LCIS).[40]

Chemoprevention should not be used in women with a prior history of deep vein thrombosis, pulmonary embolus, or stroke or transient ischemic attack (TIA), or in combination with hormone replacement therapy (HRT). The only exception is the drug Fablyn (lasofoxifene), which has proved effective in reducing strokes. And finally, gynecological exams should be done before starting treatment and yearly thereafter to monitor for uterine cancer. Evista (raloxifene) is recommended only for postmenopausal individuals and has the same warnings as other hormonal chemoprevention regarding thrombosis, pulmonary embolus, and stroke and TIA. The main difference is that the recommendations allow for longer use in individuals with osteoporosis as it is a good drug for preventing fractures. If you have low bone density and are not at high risk for blood clots, then it is a good drug for you. However, if you are at risk for these problems, you shouldn't take it.

Soon after issuing updated guidelines on hormone therapy, ASCO revised them to include Arimidex (anastrozole) based on IBIS trial results.[41] In postmenopausal individuals at increased risk, options for hormone therapy now include Arimidex (anastrozole) (1 mg/day) in addition to Aromasin (exemestane) (25 mg/day), Evista (raloxifene) (60 mg/day), or Nolvadex (tamoxifen) (20 mg/day). The choice of therapy should consider age, other ailments, and any adverse reactions to treatment. Premenopausal individuals should not be prescribed Arimidex, Aromasin, or Evista for breast cancer risk reduction. Nolvadex (20 mg/day for five years) is still considered the standard of care for risk reduction in premenopausal individuals who are at least 35 years old and have completed childbearing.

Other Drugs

Anti-inflammatory Drugs: Aspirin and NSAIDs

Many of the drugs in our medicine cabinets have also been shown to have some value in cancer prevention. There is a lot of interest in aspirin as a chemopreventive, as well as other nonsteroidal anti-inflammatory drugs (NSAIDs). In epidemiological studies there are signs of a reduced risk of breast cancer in women who take it. In some but not all studies,[42] regular aspirin use has been associated with up to a 25 percent reduction in the incidence of postmenopausal hormone-receptor-positive breast cancer. It does not seem to change estrogen levels in postmenopausal individuals,[43] but it may work by blocking inflammation (changing the neighborhood). Although some researchers think it is too soon to identify aspirin as a chemopreventive,[44] others are publicly advocating it.[45] Certainly those of you who are taking aspirin or another NSAID regularly for arthritis or heart disease prevention may be getting an added benefit.

Fortamet/Metformin

Fortamet (metformin) is a drug that has been used for type 2 diabetes, and some studies have found that women who take it have a lower chance of getting breast cancer than those on other drugs used to treat diabetes.[46] The problem with these studies was that they were largely done with people who had diabetes and were often obese, which in itself has a risk of breast cancer. In 2014 a careful review[47] and analysis of these studies focused on metformin, cancer risk, and mortality. It did show that Fortamet (metformin) may reduce cancer incidence and mortality in patients with diabetes, but it was hard to say whether it was cause and effect or resulted from the benefits of diabetes control and weight loss. Furthermore, the reduction was modest and did not affect everyone. The authors of the review suggested prospective clinical trials to test the effect of this drug further. If you take Fortamet (metformin) for your diabetes, there may be an additional benefit regarding breast cancer risk, but it is too soon to recommend it for chemoprevention.

HER2/EGFR Inhibitors

There has been a lot of interest in ways to prevent the more deadly hormone insensitive tumors, but less success. Research is being done in the use of HER2/neu blockers commonly used in therapy for chemoprevention. Initial studies are not as encouraging as one would like, but in a few cases there has been enough of a response for researchers to continue the search for the right approach.[48]

VACCINES

One exciting area of prevention research is in vaccines. Most of the current work is focused on preventing recurrence in established invasive cancers, but as we saw with the hormonal therapies, this can often lead to use in prevention down the line. Here vaccines are made against proteins that are uniquely found on tumors and not in the normal breast. Several vaccines against HER2 have been developed and are being tested to decrease recurrence in women with HER2-positive breast cancer. Brian Czerniecki of the University of Pennsylvania has been working on a HER2 vaccine for ductal carcinoma in situ (DCIS),[49] and William E. Gillanders of the Washington University School of Medicine in St. Louis has interesting preliminary data on his mammaglobin—a DNA vaccine.[50] The National Breast Cancer Coalition's Artemis Project, which had hoped to end breast cancer by 2020—or at least gain the knowledge of how to eventually eliminate breast cancer—focuses on a vaccine. They are currently discussing a phase 2 clinical trial focusing on women previously treated for DCIS.

Another vaccine is targeting a protein produced in breastfeeding that is present in more than two-thirds of triple-negative breast cancer. This α-lactalbumin vaccine is still undergoing testing for safety and dosage. The majority of these early breast cancer vaccines will be tested in clinical trials over the next decade. Of all the pathways, I think this is the most promising.

PREVENTIVE SURGERY

Most people assume that the foolproof way to prevent breast cancer is to remove the breasts. If you don't have breasts, the reasoning goes, you won't get breast cancer. There are two problems here. For one thing, it's a drastic solution. Most cisgender women like their breasts for aesthetic and erotic reasons, even if they're not planning to use them for breastfeeding. Yet some individuals are so terrified of the possibility of breast cancer that preventive mastectomy seems to be a good idea.

Most of the studies on preventive mastectomy have followed individuals who are at high genetic risk because of mutations in BRCA 1 or BRCA 2, and they show that preventive mastectomy reduces the risk of

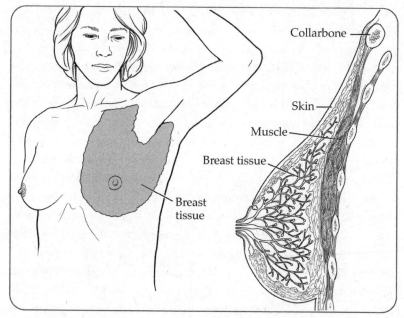

Figure 6.2

subsequent breast cancer by 90 percent. That's the other issue. It's a large reduction, but not a total one. No mastectomy can be guaranteed to remove all the breast tissue, which extends from the collarbone to below the rib cage, from the breastbone around to the back. Further, it doesn't separate itself out from the surrounding tissue in any obvious way (Figure 6.2). The most brilliant surgeon in the world couldn't be certain of digging all the breast tissue out of your body. When we do a mastectomy we do our best to get out as much as possible.[51]

The Society of Surgical Oncology currently recommends risk-reducing surgery for individuals with:

1. Mutations in BRCA 1 or BRCA 2 or other genetic susceptibility genes
2. Strong family history with no demonstrable mutation
3. Histological risk factors (LCIS, ADH)
4. Difficult surveillance

Although I concur with the first three, I think the fourth is the one most subject to interpretation. People who either have been diagnosed with breast cancer or are at risk often tell me that they need to have pro-phylactic mastectomies because their breasts are dense and mammograms are not valuable. As you will see in Chapter 7, there are many ways to monitor the breasts beyond mammography, and MRI has proved to be a great way to find early cancers in people with BRCA mutations. Finally, there is the fact that breasts don't stay the same your whole life. After menopause and/or post-treatment hormones (see Chapter 15), the density decreases and turns to fat in many individuals. This may unfortunately make you droop more, but it ensures a more accurate mammogram.

Without discounting anyone's right to make such a choice, I have to say that prophylactic or preventive mastectomies make me a bit uneasy.

Interestingly, part of the growing popularity of these mastectomies seems to be driven by the increased use of preoperative and sensitive MRIs noted earlier. This test (see Chapter 8) finds lots of "things" that may not be cancer but need to be investigated. It often scares people so much that they want to just get rid of both breasts once and for all.[52] In fact, how-ever, the risk of cancer developing in the second (contralateral) breast is not high, about 10 percent over a lifetime. Most people will not have fur-ther problems—particularly if they are taking or have taken a hormonal treatment that has been shown to decrease the risk of contralateral breast cancer. Often the risk of recurrence of the first cancer is higher than the risk of a new cancer in the other breast. This is relevant because having a bilateral mastectomy with immediate reconstruction and the subsequent recovery time often leads to a delay in starting chemotherapy or other sys-temic treatment (see Chapter 11) for the first cancer.

I think part of the problem is that surgeons are rushed and often don't take the time to explain to patients the risks and benefits of either mas-tectomy or double mastectomy. But then I may be a bit biased. We fought so hard in the 1980s to give patients the option of lumpectomy, which conserved the breast and equaled the effectiveness of mastectomy, that I find it hard to see public opinion shifting the other way without data to support the shift.

Some individuals who are newly diagnosed or consider themselves high risk but without a known mutation wonder about having their ovaries removed. Although this will reduce the risk of breast cancer and ovar-ian cancer, there is a significant downside. Recent studies have shown that preventive removal of the ovaries increases the risk of early death from other diseases, including lung cancer and heart disease, which over-rides any benefit from decreasing breast or ovarian cancer in the average person.[53] (Note that the person with BRCA will have a different balance of risk and benefit.) And removing the ovaries after menopause has been shown to have no effect on breast cancer risk. Further, because ovarian tissue, like breast tissue, still remains in the area surrounding the organs, removal of the ovaries isn't a guarantee against getting the disease (see the following section).

PREVENTION IN BRCA 1 AND BRCA 2 MUTATION CARRIERS

In women who are carriers of a genetic mutation in BRCA 1 or BRCA 2, the situation is a bit different. Their risk of developing cancer is 65 to 80 percent over their lifetime, and in the absence of other alternatives, they may well decide that it makes sense to choose preventive surgery. In a multicenter study of 483 mutation carriers from the Prevention and Observation of Surgical Endpoints study group (PROSE), the women were monitored for an average of 6.4 years. Two of 105 carriers (1.9 percent) who had preventive mastectomy developed breast cancer as opposed to 184 out of 378 (48.7 percent) people in the control group. When they looked only at the participants who still had their ovaries, prophylactic mastectomies led to a 90 percent reduction in risk.[54] The Rotterdam Family Cancer Clinic updated its experience with risk-reducing mastectomies in 358 women who had known mutations. The participants underwent skin-sparing mastectomies (see Chapter 13), often followed by immediate reconstruction. In 4.5 years there was only one case of metastatic breast cancer in a previously unaffected woman. The mastectomy specimens were carefully examined for the presence of cancers, which were found in 10 out of 358 women, or 2.8 percent.[55]

If you are a mutation carrier, having your ovaries removed before age 50 reduces the risk of ovarian cancer by 96 percent and decreases the risk of breast cancer by 47 to 61 percent.[56] It doesn't reduce the risk of ovarian cancer 100 percent because, as I said, there can be specks of ovarian tissue in the peritoneal lining of the abdomen (this is the smooth, glistening lining of the inside of your belly, something like the inside of your mouth), which can still become cancerous. In a large follow-up study of people at high risk for ovarian cancer at the Gilda Radner Familial Ovarian Cancer Registry, 6 of the 324 participants (2 percent) who underwent prophylactic oophorectomy developed peritoneal carcinomas.[57]

This occurs because the cells that are at risk are found in all the tissue that developed from the same embryologic root. That means it not only includes the tubes and ovaries but also the lining tissue of the abdominal cavity (peritoneum). Although surgeons look at the peritoneum (the lining of the whole abdominal cavity) when the ovaries and fallopian tubes are removed, they cannot remove all.

And finally, in people over age 50, the risk reduction was 89 percent for ovarian cancer and 48 percent for breast cancer.[58] Interestingly, in at least one study, taking estrogen after oophorectomy did not seem to affect this lowered risk, probably because the hormones are given at a lower dose than premenopausal people are likely to have naturally.

And what if you do both? Have your ovaries and breasts removed? We are unlikely to get this information because the number of mutation carriers who have had this surgery is not large enough to do the kind of randomized controlled study that would be needed. When actress Angelina Jolie, who carries a mutation, picked this path in 2014, experts thought it to be a reasonable choice for her.

If all this seems overwhelming, remember that you don't have to do everything at once. One of my Facebook friends had a strong paternal history of breast cancer (great-grandmother, grandmother, father, two cousins, and three aunts), and they all tested positive for BRCA 2. Initially she opted for close surveillance and then, after many years, had bilateral oophorectomy. Five years later she decided to reduce her risk further with bilateral preventive mastectomy. Now, two years later, she is very happy with her decision, saying, "My husband and I talk about it every once in a while, satisfied with the knowledge that we can grow old together without the huge threat of cancer for me."

Having a genetic risk of breast cancer is not an emergency, and you do not have to rush. Take your time to decide what is appropriate for you, and don't be afraid to change your mind over time.

Not all individuals who are carriers of the BRCA genes and thus face a very high risk of breast cancer choose to undergo preventive surgery. They still have options. One choice, as mentioned in the last chapter, is close monitoring, which, though not prevention, aims to find a cancer as soon as it becomes detectable. This approach, however, has not yet shown a reduction in breast cancer mortality.

The National Comprehensive Cancer Network (NCCN), an alliance of thirty-one leading cancer centers, issues guidelines for screening high-risk patients and those with a family history of breast cancer. Screening with mammography should begin ten years prior to the age the youngest family member was diagnosed with breast cancer, but not before age 30, or should begin at age 40 (whichever comes first).

According to the NCCN, annual breast MRIs for high-risk patients should also begin ten years prior to when the youngest family member was diagnosed with breast cancer, but not before age 25, or should begin at age 40 (whichever comes first).

Those who qualify but cannot undergo MRIs should consider contrast-enhanced mammography or whole-breast ultrasound. This would apply to individuals who may have a reaction to the gadolinium contrast material or to the scanner itself because of embedded metal such as shrapnel or a device like a pacemaker.

One interesting analysis modeled the benefits of screening versus preventive surgery for 25-year-old BRCA 1 and BRCA 2 carriers. The researchers found that preventive mastectomy at age 25 plus preventive oophorectomy at age 40 maximizes the probability of survival. However, mammography plus MRI screening starting at age 25 with preventive oophorectomy at age 40 is about the same.[59] But the downsides to oophorectomy prior to age 40, mentioned earlier—such as increased heart disease—must be taken into account.

Beyond surveillance, there are lifestyle changes that may have some impact. As noted earlier, modulating estrogen appears to be relevant; for example, oral contraceptives decrease ovarian cancer. So does breastfeeding.[60]

There are several interesting new approaches on the horizon. An animal study at Johns Hopkins found that giving low-dose chemotherapy into the ducts results in the equivalent of a chemical mastectomy.[61] It removes the ductal cells but not the others. My research has involved safety studies in which we put chemotherapy into the ducts of individuals scheduled for mastectomies to see if it has any side effects. The original studies have not shown negative effects, and we are now looking at the effects of this approach in patients with DCIS. My hope is that one day it will allow people to prevent breast cancer without removing the breast.

Another possibility would be a drug specific to the BRCA defect that could prevent cancer from developing. This class of drugs (PARP 2 inhibitors, which we considered in Chapter 3 and will examine at length in Chapter 15) has been developed and tested in individuals with metastatic disease and has had very promising results. Whether these drugs will be useful for prevention has yet to be determined, but it is certainly a possibility. Because so much research is going on, mutation carriers who want to take measures to prevent the disease should go to a high-risk center that specializes in women with genetic breast cancer, where they will get the very latest and best advice available.

PUTTING IT TOGETHER

So, once again, what can most people do? There are some steps that the average person can take to reduce their risk.

1. Exercise for at least thirty minutes a day, preferably four to five hours a week (enough to break a sweat).
2. Maintain a normal weight, especially if you are postmenopausal.
3. Have your children before age 35 if you can.
4. Breastfeed your children for as long as possible.
5. Avoid unnecessary X-rays, including CT scans.
6. Drink alcohol only in moderation.
7. Avoid taking noncontraceptive hormones (HRT, fertility drugs) unless necessary.
8. Have a doctor evaluate any breast symptoms or changes that develop.
9. Have a mammogram when appropriate (see Chapter 7 on screening).
10. Join the Love Research Army (https://drsusanloveresearch.org /love-research-army/) to participate in studies to find causes and ways to prevent breast cancer.

If you have a family history of breast cancer or think you are at risk, you can be evaluated at a high-risk center to see where you stand. Those who are at increased risk may consider taking Evista (raloxifene) or Nolvadex (tamoxifen) for five years. If you fit the criteria for genetic testing (see Chapter 4), you should see a genetic counselor to consider your options. Those who are mutation carriers will want to consider prophylactic surgery and close surveillance. Finally, you can get involved in the research yourself (see the Epilogue).

PART THREE

Finding Breast Cancer

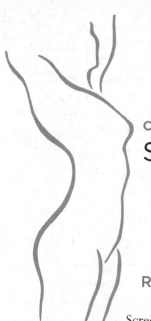

CHAPTER 7

Screening

RISKS AND BENEFITS OF SCREENING

Screening means looking for a cancer before it produces a lump or other symptom. It is used for a number of cancers, such as colon, prostate, and, recently, lung, but breast cancer screening has engendered the most controversy.[1] This stems not from lack of data, which are pretty clear at this point, but from differing views about risk and benefit and our limited understanding of the biology of the disease (see Chapter 3). When screening was first introduced, the understanding was that cancers grow at a certain steady rate and at some point get out into the rest of the body. Thus, we concluded, if we could just find the cancers before this happened, we could prevent people dying from breast cancer.

This rather simplistic notion of cancer was appealing to doctors and the public because it was easy to understand and suggested that there was something we could do to mitigate one's chances of dying from the disease. The problem, as we have discussed in Chapter 3, is that nothing is so simple. Some cancers are so slow growing or even dormant that they will never cause you a problem; we don't need to find those. Others will slowly grow and eventually spread and kill you if not found "early." And some grow so quickly that by the time they are detectable on exam or imaging, they have already spread and early detection will not be early enough. Screening guidelines are now focusing more on the degree of risk a person may have of getting breast cancer in the near future.

Overlooked and underserved populations are particularly vulnerable to faster-growing breast cancers, according to the American College of

Radiology (ACR) and Society of Breast Imaging (SBI). "Minority women are 72 percent more likely to be diagnosed with breast cancer before age 50, are 58 percent more likely to be diagnosed with advanced stage disease prior to age 50, and are 127 percent more likely to die of breast cancer before age 50 compared to white women," said Dr. Debra Monticciolo, author of screening guidelines for the ACR and SBI.[2] A key recommendation is for women to get a risk assessment at age 30 to see if screening prior to age 40 is needed.

Screening, however, is not a perfect process despite increasingly sophisticated equipment; but it can be worth it when an early diagnosis translates to less aggressive treatments. To find potential terrorists, the TSA screens for certain characteristics at the airport. But they pull over many people who are perfectly innocent (false positives) and, as we know all too well, sometimes miss the person who is planning trouble (false negatives) while thwarting many attempted terrorist attacks in the process (true positives).

In breast cancer screening a false positive is when a breast mass on a mammogram is identified as suspicious for cancer, requires further workup to find out, sometimes including a biopsy, and the biopsy turns out to be benign. Whew! But in spite of the relief for the individual, false positives are one downside of screening. They can be expected 7 percent of the time in people between ages 40 and 50 who are screened each year for ten years by mammography.[3] They add a cost to the health care system—not to mention the cost to your psychological health during those days to weeks of worry. Is it worth it? Most people think it is. In one study, 90 percent of participants who had experienced a false-positive test still regarded mammography as having no downside.[4]

Being called back for additional testing after screening mammography is very common, and usually there is nothing of concern, so don't lose sleep over it. Out of a thousand patients who have a screening mammogram, about a hundred will be told to return for additional mammographic views or ultrasound or both. About sixty-five of those recalled will be told there is nothing of concern; the original finding was due to overlapping normal tissue or a cyst or other benign (noncancerous) finding. About twenty of the patients recalled will be recommended to have short-interval follow-up imaging, usually in six months, for a "probably benign" finding (BI-RADS 3). BI-RADS 3 findings are specific findings that have been well studied and have less than 2 percent chance of being cancer; it has been shown to be safe to watch such findings even in the rare instance when the abnormality is cancerous, and this approach avoids unnecessary biopsy for the 98 percent of patients who do not have cancer. Only about fifteen of the hundred patients recalled for additional testing will be recommended to have a biopsy, and only two to five of those who have a biopsy will be found to have cancer. Even when there is cancer, if it is found because of screening, it is usually small and easily treated.

Then there is the problem of overdiagnosis. This is when you are diagnosed with a tumor that was actually dormant and would not have harmed you if it had not been found. Unfortunately, we cannot predict who will develop the harmless tumor. Because we are unable to be sure it is dormant, we treat it as if it were not, and you get some combination of surgery, radiation, and hormone therapy you didn't need—each treatment produces its own collateral damage. Though this situation is estimated to happen about 22 to 31 percent[5] of the time, these figures are not widely known. We tend to see these as breast cancer survivors rather than as people who have been overdiagnosed, having "survived" a disease that would never have developed. As mentioned in Chapter 3, there is much research devoted to identifying these harmless tumors.

False negatives are more dangerous. This is when you have been dutifully screened and nothing showed up, but later a lump or other symptom is found, indicating a cancer that the screening missed. People with dense breasts are more likely to get a false negative. Their breasts have less fat, which is translucent on the mammogram, and more glandular and fibrous tissue, which makes it harder for radiologists to see through. The technology is not perfect as the statistics about false positives and false negatives show. We all wish the accuracy of breast self-examination (BSE), doctor's exams, and mammography were better and the results were not so hard to interpret.

But numbers are important and, as you can see in Figure 7.1, the benefits may be less or more than you thought.

MAMMOGRAPHY SCREENING

A mammogram is an X-ray of the breast—*mammo* means "breast" and *gram* means "picture." It isn't the same as a chest X-ray, which looks through the breast and photographs the lungs. Mammograms look at the

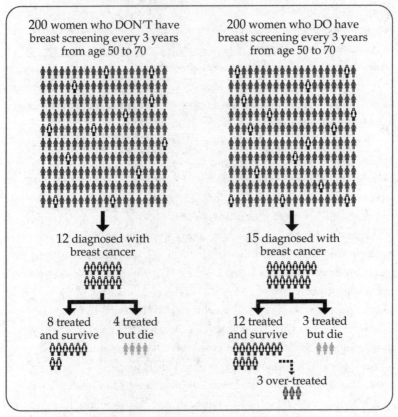

Figure 7.1

breast itself and take pictures of the soft tissue, allowing the radiologist to see anything unusual or suspicious. Mammography can pick up very small lesions—about 0.2 inch (0.5 cm), whereas you usually can't feel a lump until it's at least 0.4 inch (1 cm), unless it is deep. Findings on mammograms can be benign or malignant. In addition, mammograms can sometimes pick up noninvasive cancers (see Chapter 12).

Mammography has its limits, though. The mammogram can photograph only the part of the breast that sticks out—the plates are put underneath the breast or on the sides of the breast—so it's easier to get an accurate picture of a large breast than of a small one. The periphery of the breast does not fully get into the picture (see Figure 8.1, page 170). In addition, if your breasts are dense, with less fat and more glandular and fibrous tissue, masses may not be visible through the tissue. So a mammogram isn't perfect. Physical exams, ultrasounds, and mammograms complement one another. You can see some lumps on a mammogram that you can't feel, and you can feel some lumps (palpation) and see them on ultrasound even though you can't see them on a mammogram.

The U.S. Preventive Services Task Force (USPSTF) recently made a huge shift in its updated guidelines, pushing back the age to begin getting regular mammograms from 50 to 40 years. The draft guidelines recommend that all cisgender women and people assigned female at birth get screened every other year starting at age 40. This shift reflects the increasing importance of early screening in catching the more aggressive cancers that strike younger individuals and populations of color. Some medical professionals consider the suggested interval of every other year to be inadequate in diagnosing the more aggressive cancers. Although the USPSTF guidelines must still undergo a review before becoming official, it is important to remember that all guidelines like these depend on a goal. If the goal of a national screening program is to reduce mortality in the most efficient and cost-effective manner, then programs that screen every other year from ages 50 to 84 demonstrate the most benefits per screening examination.[6] However, if the goal is to minimize deaths from breast cancer, then annual screening mammography beginning at age 40 would be most appropriate. Guidelines for different levels of risk are also issued by the American Cancer Society, the National Comprehensive Cancer Network (NCCN), and the American College of Radiology (ACR).

The goal for individuals may differ and may depend on their risk of developing breast cancer and their tolerance for false alarms.

To put things into perspective, a recent analysis estimated that among ten thousand women aged 40 years undergoing annual mammography for ten years, thirty-one deaths would occur despite screening (young women tend to have more aggressive cancers that are less amenable to screening), and five deaths would be prevented because of screening. Among 50-year-olds screened for ten years, sixty-two deaths would occur despite screening; ten would be averted. And among 60-year-olds screened for the same length of time, eighty-eight deaths would occur despite screening, and forty-two would be averted.[7] It is clear that screening is more effective in older people probably because the cancers in this age group are often less fast-growing and their breasts are less dense. This is a much more complex message than can fit on a T-shirt, however; if you were one of the fifty-seven people out of thirty thousand whose life was saved because of screening mammography, you would certainly be glad it was done.

The study did not mention the risk from having radiation every year. Several studies have estimated that the risk is real, although very low compared to the potential lifesaving benefit.[8] One modeling study concluded that of 100,000 women screened at age 40 to 74, radiation induces 125 breast cancers leading to 16 deaths. But in the same group, 968 breast cancer deaths are averted through early detection.[9] And the radiation risk is not the same for everyone. People with large breasts require extra views, and thus more radiation and risk. People who received high-dose radiation therapy during childhood as a treatment for Hodgkin lymphoma when their breasts were still developing will have much higher risk. Partly due to low numbers of people with breast cancer before age 40, partly due to the radiation risk, and partly due to the increased breast density in this population, mammography is not routinely performed for screening before age 40. The exception is high-risk patients such as BRCA carriers, for whom the NCCN recommends screening mammograms after age 30.

When viewing the screening recommendations of different health organizations, it is important to remember that mammography has been proved to decrease deaths from breast cancer.[10] The arguments regarding screening refer to the value of recommending frequent mammography as a public policy. Only you and your doctor can decide on what is the best approach for you. But bear in mind that screening can catch aggressive cancers early, allow time for more treatment options, and increase the chance of survival.

SCREENING DURING A PANDEMIC

Since it looks like COVID-type viruses and their many variations may be around for a while, I thought I'd add a brief section on the unique challenges posed by a pandemic. In addition to the obvious suspension of mammograms during lockdowns, in some people the COVID vaccine itself caused swollen lymph nodes in their armpit. This side effect, called axillary adenopathy, is a reaction by your immune system to the vaccine and is a good thing, although feeling a lump under your arm can be disconcerting. This condition can last as long as forty-three weeks, so you shouldn't delay a mammography if you have it. Axillary adenopathy usually appears within fourteen days of the first vaccination and has been seen with all brands of the COVID shots, although it appears more often with the Moderna version.[11] Radiologists will assume the condition is benign in patients with no breast cancer history or suspicious findings on their mammogram.

Understandably, at the peak of the pandemic there was a big drop in mammogram screening as health care centers prioritized urgent needs to reduce the risk of spread. Communities hit hard by the virus stayed away as well, as people struggled with competing priorities and limited access.[12] But as these conditions ease, it is important to get back on track and re-schedule any delayed tests. Most of our coping strategies during lockdowns haven't always been healthy. In a 2021 poll on pandemic stress, the American Psychological Association found that 42 percent of respondents gained more weight than they intended (an average of 29 pounds) while 23 percent reported drinking more alcohol. A change in physical activity was also noted.[13] Taken together, weight gain, drinking, and lack of exercise can lead to an increase in breast cancer risk.

Those of you already being treated for breast cancer may have a weaker immune system and thus are at higher risk of infection, so it is important to mask up in public. Get your vaccines and boosters, follow the science, and keep up with screenings and follow-up appointments.

SPECIAL SITUATIONS

As I alluded to earlier, there are situations where screening recommendations may be different from those for the general population. These include people who carry a genetic risk of developing breast cancer, those who received radiation as a child or teenager, or those who are calculated to have a risk over 20 to 25 percent by one of the current risk models. They are advised to get MRI screening in addition to mammography (see the following discussion).

People who have dense breasts are also at higher risk of developing breast cancer. First of all, breast density makes it harder to see cancers because the dense tissue and cancer cells or small lesions blend together. It is like looking for a polar bear in the snow! In addition, the density itself may represent an environment more conducive to developing breast cancer (see Chapter 5). This is particularly true in people whose breasts remain dense after menopause. In 2019 the U.S. Congress passed national breast density legislation to ensure that all mammography reports included information on breast density, so patients would know their status. You should ask whether your breasts are dense, but that information should also be on the mammogram report sent to you and your doctor.

People with dense breasts may need additional screening techniques, including tomosynthesis and/or whole-breast ultrasound, both of which are described shortly. In some situations MRI may be added.

Trans men who have had top surgery to remove their breasts sometimes assume they no longer need screening for breast cancer. This is wrong. There will always be some breast tissue left behind in these operations, and that tissue can still get breast cancer (see Chapter 12, page 293).

OTHER SCREENING TECHNIQUES

Tomosynthesis

Tomosynthesis is a fancy name for 3D mammography. The problem with the standard mammogram is that it shows the breast from two vantage points: top down (CC) and from the side (lateral). If you have a very fatty breast, this is probably fine; however, if you have dense breasts they may hide a lump. It is like looking at a solid red ball sitting in a round glass bowl. If the glass of the bowl is clear, you will easily see the ball within it; however, if the glass is tinted red you may not be able to recognize the ball even if you look at the bowl from several different angles. To solve this problem, tomosynthesis takes pictures of your breast in slices at different intervals and then uses computer software to combine them into a 3D image. The middle slice will show the ball within the bowl, whereas the one in the front or back might have missed it. Likewise, this technique can find more cancers in dense breasts. Two studies[14] have confirmed that adding tomosynthesis to digital mammography increases the number of cancers found and also decreases the number of patients who are called back for further imaging. In screening to detect recurrence in people with a history of breast cancer, it was found to decrease the rate of false positives but did not lead to an improvement in detection when compared to digital mammography. Many mammography units have added tomosynthesis to the machine, and it is quickly becoming the new standard.

MRI

As discussed in Chapter 8, MRI is significantly more complicated than mammography or ultrasound. You usually need to schedule it during the first half of the menstrual cycle (the first day of your period begins the cycle), although newer "abbreviated" techniques don't require it. Some claustrophobic people require sedation, which may or may not be offered. And finally, it is important that you have a radiologist who is experienced in breast MRI and capable of doing a biopsy under MRI if indicated. Although it currently takes about forty-five minutes, newer "fast" MRI[15] techniques are being evaluated and may well become the norm during the life of this edition. It requires you to have a contrast agent, a metal salt, injected intravenously.

Screening studies using MRI have been limited to high-risk patients but have demonstrated improved survival.[16] If a patient with a genetic mutation is under age 30, MRIs alone are used in screening. But after age 30, MRIs combined with mammograms have proved effective in those at greater risk.[17] For the general population with average breast cancer risk, MRIs sometimes find abnormalities that are not cancer but, once found, must be ruled out. Most studies so far have demonstrated that MRI has a higher sensitivity to breast cancer than does mammography, ultrasound, or both. In other words, it finds more cancers. The largest study (1,909 participants) was done in the Netherlands. It compared three screening methods and found that the sensitivity (cancers found) of clinical breast exam was 17.9 percent, whereas for mammography it was 40 percent, and for MRI it was 71 percent. The specificity (how many abnormalities were really cancer) was 98 percent for clinical breast examination, 95 percent for mammography, and 89 percent for MRI. In other words, it finds more benign lesions as well as cancers. The authors noted that screening with MRI led to twice as many unneeded additional examinations (420 versus 207) and three times as many unneeded biopsies (24 versus 7) as did mammographic screening.[18]

At present, the chance of a false positive and greater expense of MRI means it is not a good screening test for the majority of people. Currently it is recommended only for people with a very high risk of breast cancer, where it has been shown to reduce the number of patients who progress to late-stage disease[19] and the false-negative cancers (those that show up between screenings).[20] In a large study of people of intermediate risk and dense breasts, adding MRI resulted in a higher breast cancer detection rate, albeit at the cost of an increase in false positives.[21] A study of 3,002 high-risk women that compared mammography alone to mammography plus breast MRI found that the overall cancer detection rate was significantly higher in the combined screening group. Furthermore, of the eleven recurrences and five deaths found on long-term follow-up, all the deaths were in the mammography-alone group. Combined screening in individuals with elevated risk significantly improved overall survival.[22]

An interesting study back in 2010, however, showed that women are not as eager to have MRIs as was once thought. In a study of screening techniques, participants were invited to participate in an MRI substudy. Of the 1,215 women eligible, 42.1 percent declined to participate.[23] Reasons included claustrophobia (18.2 percent), time constraints (12.1 percent), financial concerns (9.2 percent), a decision either by themselves or their doctors that it was unnecessary (7.8 percent), objection to getting an intravenous injection (5.3 percent), concern because they were leery of biopsies or extra procedures that may be needed afterward (4.1 percent), and a handful of other reasons.

The ultimate role of MRI in screening is evolving as we try to determine the best approach for young people, mutation carriers, and those with dense breasts on mammogram.

Whole-Breast Ultrasound

Ultrasound is another technology with an expanding role. It has always been a useful tool for investigating palpable lumps and masses seen on a mammogram, suggesting that it might be used for screening as well. A multicenter study[24] looked at physician-performed ultrasound screening in people with dense breasts in addition to mammography and MRI. Of the 110 participants who had cancer, 33 were detected by mammography only, 32 by ultrasound only, 26 by both, and 9 by MRI after mammography plus ultrasound. Finally, there were 11 that were not detected by any imaging. An Italian study also supported adding ultrasound.[25] In multiple studies, whole-breast ultrasound has been shown to be a good adjunct to mammography, with the final assessment made at the time in 99 percent of the cases.[26] The lack of enough trained technicians has precluded its widespread use in screening. But a relatively common alternative is the use of automated whole-breast ultrasound that uses a computer to control the probe. An early study showed that 13 percent of patients had to come back for targeted ultrasound first and then either a six-month follow-up or biopsy.[27] Obviously this is not as good as human diagnosis but may play a role in areas where trained personnel are not available. In fact, this method is even used in facilities with trained personnel. Some radiologists prefer it as it is more standardized and less operator dependent than handheld ultrasound.

Breast Self-Exam

Breast self-exam has always seemed to be the easiest and most obvious way to find breast cancers. But just finding cancers does not mean that you are making a difference in their outcome. Before I start explaining the data, I want to be clear about my definitions. Health care professionals or researchers who talk about "breast self-exam" usually mean a formal procedure you do in four positions, covering the whole breast in a certain pattern and taking a half hour to perform. These are the ones you see on the shower card or video version. When a person talks about breast self-exam, they are often talking about poking around either because it is "that time in the month" or because a pain or twinge has brought their attention to their breast. The question is not whether people can find their own cancers—they can. But do they find them while doing a formal regimen every month, like a religious ritual, or simply in the normal poking around that we all do?

To answer that question, a randomized controlled study of formal breast self-exam was done in Shanghai and reported in 1997.[28] In the study, 267,040 women from 520 factories were randomly divided between a self-exam instruction group and a control group. Then they were studied for over five years. (The study was done in China because the Chinese did not have screening mammography or doctors doing physical exams at that time to complicate things, so the only way for a person to be diagnosed with breast cancer was to find it themself.) The participants in the instruction group were given intensive training in breast self-examination. The others, those in the control group, were not. All participants were followed up for the development of breast diseases and for death from breast cancer. Approximately equal numbers of breast cancers were detected in the two groups (331 in the instruction group and 322 in the control group). The breast cancers detected in the instruction group were not diagnosed at a significantly earlier stage or smaller size than those in the control group. The death rates from breast cancer in the two groups were also virtually equal. What is clear from this is the fact that the participants in the control group found their own cancers. They found them while showering or lovemaking or moving their arms or any of the other ways we tend to touch our bodies without even thinking about it. They just did not find the cancers by doing a formal breast self-exam.

Our radiology advisor Dr. Lauren Green tells her patients they are their own best advocates, and it is their duty to be familiar with their own bodies. "If something does not feel right or seems different and you are unsure about it, you have to talk to your health care provider. I've had a number of patients or their partners find their breast cancer that way," she notes.

Interestingly, in the Chinese study cited earlier there was even a downside to formal BSE. The participants in the instruction group detected more benign lesions requiring biopsy (1,457 versus 623) than did those in the control group. This means that formal BSE not only failed to benefit those in the instruction group by finding cancers earlier but led them to be subjected to more biopsies than were participants in the control group.

In 2009 the USPSTF guidelines recommended that doctors stop teaching formal breast self-exam.[29] This was misconstrued to mean that people should not do it, or indeed should not even explore their breasts. What it really meant was that because formal breast self-exam was no better than people's normal acquaintance with their breasts, it was not worth having health care professionals spend their limited time teaching it. So get to know your breasts and check in on them regularly, but don't feel guilty if you don't follow the shower card exactly!

Breast Physical Exam

What about the exams done by health care professionals during yearly checkups? This process (known as clinical breast exam) has not been studied as much in terms of its usefulness in detecting cancer. I've always wondered about that, since it's so ubiquitous. If its value is negligible, we could then save time and energy for busy medical professionals, as well as sparing patients the mild discomfort and embarrassment involved.

A recent nine-year study from Israel assessed the contribution of clinical breast exam to cancer diagnosis in women participating in a modern breast screening program. The exams, performed by surgeons, resulted in a high number of abnormal findings regardless of age and rarely contributed to early diagnosis of cancer. As breast cancer screening becomes more personalized in the future, the role of clinical breast exam in specific subgroups, particularly younger people, will need to be evaluated.[30]

One problem is that most doctors haven't been trained to do clinical breast exam. The breast has always been considered the property of the general surgeon, so hardly any gynecologists and primary care doctors have formal training in the breast. Yet most women with breast problems go to their gynecologists or primary care doctors rather than surgeons. A colleague of mine, Dr. William Goodson, reported on an interesting study. Researchers developed a form for primary care doctors to document their findings after they did a clinical breast exam.[31] Just adding this reminder not only increased the number of exams done but also increased the number of lumps found. With all the available imaging, there has been a tendency to stop paying attention to physical examinations. Nonetheless, many cancers that are not detectable on imaging will be picked up this way. So we need primary care doctors to be well trained in breast examination. Then every patient will have access to a good clinical breast exam as part of their yearly checkup. It's a very helpful, low-tech tool.

SCREENING RECOMMENDATIONS

Many countries have government-sponsored mammography screening programs that start inviting people to screening when they turn 49 or

50. In the United States, we do not have organized screening, but many of the top medical organizations recommend annual screening as of age 40 for women of average risk. After age 50, some organizations recommend screening every other year for those with average risk factors.[32]

If you're very young, you should begin getting acquainted with your breasts, not in a rigid breast examination but in comfortable awareness of how your breasts look and feel. Have your doctor examine your breasts during your regular checkups; after age 40, make sure to have this done at least once a year. Discuss with your doctor whether you should get a mammogram between ages 40 and 50. After age 50, make sure you have a mammogram at least every two years. (See Chapter 8 for discussion of the procedure.)

Many doctors stress the importance of a "baseline" mammogram. Your first mammogram, whenever it is, could be called your baseline, and usually is not recommended before age 40 unless you are at high risk or have had breast cancer or breast symptoms (such as a lump, bloody nipple discharge, or skin retraction). What's more important is that you have serial mammograms once you're in your fifties, several a year or two apart so that we can compare each mammogram against the previous one. Often that's how we catch a cancer—this year's mammogram has something that wasn't there last year or the year before. There are people who believe they can get one mammogram and that's it. However, as much as I oppose overdoing mammography, underdoing it is just as bad.

It's important to point out that this discussion of mammograms has focused on screening for people who have no symptoms but want to get checked out. Before age 40, get to know your breasts, have physical exams during your yearly checkups, and discuss with your doctor whether you need breast imaging.

As noted earlier, the USPSTF has updated its guidelines, lowering the age of screening from 50 to 40 years, every other year. They note that Black women are 40 percent more likely to die of breast cancer than white women and too often get aggressive cancers at young ages. They also stressed the need to address screening disparities among minority populations. It is essential that you discuss your screening options with your health provider taking into account your level of risk and breast density. There seems to be a growing push for more individualized screening, tailored for each persons level of risk. MRI is appropriate for screening people at high risk;[33] many options can be considered for supplemental screening of people with dense breasts (see https://densebreast-info.org for more information), and further studies are ongoing.

What mammography can do is important—detect some cancers earlier than they would be detected otherwise, thus reducing the chances of dying from breast cancer. A large Swedish study found that participants who regularly got mammograms had up to a 49 percent lower risk of breast cancer mortality.[34] For now, it's what we have, and it makes sense to use it.

So although I agree with the current guidelines and get my own mammogram every couple of years as a woman over age 70 who doesn't have dense breasts, I cannot fault those of you who choose to get yearly mammograms. The problem, as aptly pointed out by Lisa Rosenbaum, MD, is that "we do not think risk, we feel it."[35]

Meanwhile, the ultimate goal has to be preventing the disease in the first place, which would make all this discussion become moot.

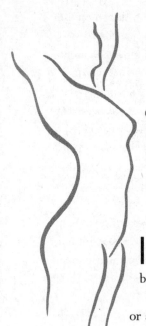

CHAPTER 8

Diagnosis

In this chapter we will review the many different imaging and biopsy techniques and how to read your biopsy report.

Once you or your primary care doctor notice a lump or abnormality in your breast, then what? First you need time to let the initial panic subside. Of the lumps detected on breast self-exam in a large study of people under age 40, only 53 percent, or half, were actually lumps that needed evaluation.[1] Even among the lumps identified as significant by surgeons, 28 percent were benign.[2] In people past menopause, the potential for a palpable lump to be cancer is higher because there are no more hormonal changes to cause benign lumps.

When I started in practice, the first stop for a patient with a breast lump or abnormality was with the surgeon, who then determined whether it was worthy of imaging and/or biopsy. Things have changed remarkably since then, with the addition of better imaging and imaging-directed biopsies. Now the first stop after the primary care doctor is to radiology, where an ultrasound with or without a mammogram will be done. This is a very good way to identify lesions needing biopsy as well as a good way to guide the biopsy. If the lump is a cyst or a fibroadenoma (see Chapter 2), it will usually be left alone. A patient may also be given the option of aspiration if the cyst is large and painful, and removal of the fluid can relieve discomfort. Ultrasound is nearly 100 percent accurate in identifying benign cysts.[3] If there is a question whether a new mass is a cyst or a solid mass, the cyst may be biopsied or aspirated to confirm that it is a benign cyst. Besides cysts, the other most common noncancerous lump is a fibroadenoma, and another benign possibility is *fibrocystic disease* or normal lumpy breast tissue (see Chapter 2). These types of masses can usually be distinguished on ultrasound and mammography, if indicated, and usually do not need treatment.

MAMMOGRAMS

If you're over age 30 and you find a lump or have another breast complaint, you'll get a diagnostic mammogram (as opposed to a screening mammogram) in addition to the ultrasound. If on the mammogram a lump looks jagged rather than smooth, it's a sign that further investigation may be needed. If you've got a lump your doctor thinks may be cancerous, a mammogram can help determine if there are other lumps that should be biopsied at the same time; it can also document the location and size of the lump.

A mammogram, like any other X-ray, presents a two-dimensional view of a three-dimensional structure. Denser areas appear bright. Glandular breast tissue, for example, is dense and shows up white on the mammogram. Fat, which is not very dense at all, shows up gray (see the images below).

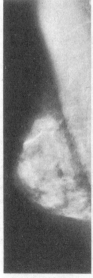 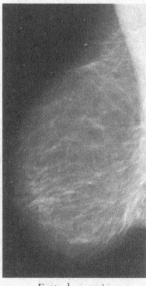 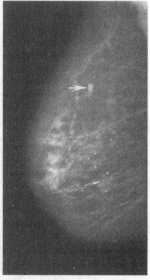

Dense breast in young woman

Fatty breast in older woman

Small cancer in fatty breast (arrow) and benign calcifications

As you'll recall from Chapter 1, when you're young—in your teens and early twenties—your breasts are made up mostly of glandular breast tissue (where the milk is produced) and are usually very dense. As you grow older, the breast ages, much as your skin does, and there's less glandular breast tissue and more fat. However, people vary in the proportion of glandular tissue remaining after menopause.

Beyond assessing breast density, mammography allows a radiologist to find lesions or abnormalities. If you have felt a lump, the radiologist will look particularly in that area to decide how suspicious it may be and will almost always do an ultrasound too. Generally, when noncancerous lesions expand, they push the normal breast tissue away and create smooth edges (like blowing up a balloon), whereas cancers expand by growing between the normal cells—*infiltrating*—and this leads to indistinct or jagged, irregular edges (like a mold expanding into a cheese). Thus, when mammograms show something round and smooth, it's likely to be a cyst or a fibroadenoma. The mammogram can't distinguish between them; you follow up with an ultrasound (discussed later in this chapter) to see if it's a cyst. If a mammogram shows a mass with jagged (*spiculated*) or indistinct edges, with radiating strands pulling inward (*distortion*, like pulling a thread in a piece of fabric), it's more likely to be cancer. But until it is biopsied, we can't tell for sure; several benign conditions can mimic cancer on a mammogram. Scarring or fat necrosis (dead fat) can look very suspicious. A noncancerous entity—a radial scar—is caused by an increase in local fibrous tissue (see Chapter 2) trapping some of the glands in a way that can look suspicious; it can be confusing even under the microscope and often requires an expert breast pathologist to rule out cancer.

A mammogram may also show intramammary (in the breast) lymph nodes. In fact, until the mammogram came along, we didn't even know there were lymph nodes in the breast. We now know that 5.4 percent of women have them. Sometimes you'll hear about a "normal" mammogram. But there's really no one normal pattern—there is only normal for you.

A standardized reporting system for mammography was developed to indicate how suspicious a particular finding may be. It is now used by most radiologists who interpret mammograms. This is called the Breast Imaging Reporting and Data System (BI-RADS; see Table 8.1). It is important that the radiologist who interprets your mammogram uses BI-RADS for the report so the findings won't confuse your doctor. (BI-RADS is also used to categorize breast ultrasound and breast MRI.)

Table 8.1 What Do the BI-RADS Categories Mean?

CATEGORY: 0

Definition: Incomplete. Additional imaging evaluation and/or comparison to prior mammograms (or other imaging tests) is needed.

What it means: This means the radiologist may have seen a possible abnormality, but it was not clear and you will need more tests, such as another mammogram with the use of spot compression (applying compression to a smaller area when doing the mammogram), magnified views, special mammogram views, and/or ultrasound. This may also suggest that the radiologist wants to compare your new mammogram with older ones to see if there have been changes in the area over time.

CATEGORY: 1

Definition: Negative

What it means: This is a normal test result. Your breasts look the same (they are symmetrical) with no masses (lumps), distorted structures, or suspicious calcifications. In this case, negative means nothing new or abnormal was found.

CATEGORY: 2

Definition: Benign (non-cancerous finding)

What it means: This is also a negative test result (there is no sign of cancer), but the radiologist chooses to describe a finding that is not cancer, such as benign calcifications, masses, or lymph nodes in the breast. This can also be used to describe changes from a prior procedure (such as a biopsy) in the breast. This ensures that others who look at the mammogram in the future will not misinterpret the benign findings as suspicious.

CATEGORY: 3

Definition: Probably benign finding—Follow-up in a short time frame is suggested.

What it means: A finding in this category has a very low (no more than 2%) chance of being cancer. It is not expected to change over time. But since it's not proven to be benign, it's helpful to be extra safe and see if the area in question does change over time. You will likely need follow-up with repeat imaging in 6 to 12 months and regularly after that until the finding is known to be stable (usually at least two years). This approach helps avoid unnecessary biopsies, but if the area does change over time, it still allows for early diagnosis.

(continues)

(continued)

CATEGORY: 4

Definition: Suspicious abnormality. Biopsy should be considered.

What it means: These findings do not definitely look like cancer but could be cancer. The radiologist is concerned enough to recommend a biopsy. The findings in this category can have a wide range of suspicion levels. For this reason, the category is often divided further:

4A: Finding with a low likelihood of being cancer
(more than 2% but no more than 10%)
4B: Finding with a moderate likelihood of being cancer
(more than 10% but no more than 50%)
4C: Finding with a high likelihood of being cancer (more than 50% but less than 95%), but not as high as Category 5.

CATEGORY: 5

Definition: Highly suggestive of malignancy—Appropriate action should be taken.

What it means: The findings look like cancer and have a high chance (at least 95%) of being cancer. Biopsy is very strongly recommended.

CATEGORY: 6

Definition: Known biopsy-proven malignancy—Appropriate action should be taken.

What it means: This category is only used for findings on a mammogram (or ultrasound or MRI) that have already been shown to be cancer by a previous biopsy. Imaging may be used in this way to see how well the cancer is responding to treatment.

BREAST DENSITY

Your mammogram report will also include an assessment of your breast density, which is a description of how much fibrous and glandular tissue is in your breasts, as compared to fatty tissue. The denser your breasts, the harder it can be to see abnormal areas on mammograms. (Having dense breasts also slightly raises your risk of getting breast cancer.)

Mammogram reports usually mention the breast density. Approximately 80 percent of women will have scattered density (40 percent) or heterogeneously (mixed) dense breast tissue (40 percent), and only 10 percent will have extremely dense or fatty breasts.[4] Although increased breast density is correlated with increased risk of developing breast cancer and increased risk of cancer being hidden on a mammogram, breast density has not been shown to cause breast cancer. Many states now require mammography centers to inform you if your breasts are dense. Your doctor may then recommend that you consider supplemental screening with ultrasound or even MRI if you have a strong family history or otherwise meet defined risk criteria. Our radiology advisor Dr. Lauren Green recalls a patient who had been receiving notifications of dense breasts with annual mammograms and requested supplemental screening. Her doctor refused, saying it was unnecessary. Years passed and one day while vacationing abroad, she noticed her breast swelling, getting red and feeling painful with thickened skin. A local doctor diagnosed her with inflammatory breast cancer. On returning home it was clear when comparing mammograms that cancer had likely been present for some time, but it was difficult to discern due to density. She would have greatly benefited from supplemental screening with ultrasound, which would have found the cancer at an earlier stage. Sadly, she died of treatment complications in her forties, leaving behind two young children.

The main reason to know how dense your breasts are is that this affects how sensitive the mammogram may be to showing cancer if it is present. If your breasts are extremely dense, the sensitivity is only about 69 percent.[5] If your breasts are mostly fatty, you can be more assured that when a mammogram shows that there is nothing suspicious in your breast, there probably isn't. But it is also important to point out, as we mentioned in Chapter 6, that our breasts don't stay at a given density: they normally become less dense after menopause. Having dense breasts after menopause indicates an increased risk for cancer.

Calcifications

One of the more important discoveries that has come from the study of mammograms is that breast cancer is often associated with very fine specks of calcium that appear on the picture; they look a bit like tiny specks of dust or salt on a film.

We discovered that these microcalcifications, as we call them, are sometimes an indication of cancer or DCIS (noninvasive cancer) (see Chapter 12). At least a few calcifications can be found on nearly every mammogram, though, so the radiologist needs to try to distinguish the few mammograms with calcifications that merit further evaluation and possibly biopsy from all the rest. But it's nothing to panic about—even among calcifications biopsied, 80 percent have nothing to do with cancer; they're probably just the result of normal wear and tear on your breast.[6] Ironically, when you age, calcium leaves your bones, where it's needed, and shows up in other places, where it's not. It can show up in arteries, causing them to harden, and in joints, causing arthritis. The microcalcifications in your breast won't cause any problems if they're not indications of cancer or noninvasive cancer. (The appearance of this calcium in your body has no relation to how much calcium you eat or drink, by the way.)

How do we distinguish between the bad calcifications and the harmless kinds? We look at the shape, the size, and how many there are. If they're tiny and tightly clustered, and there aren't a whole lot of them elsewhere in either breast, they're more likely to indicate noninvasive cancer. If they're bigger and/or scattered all over the place in both breasts, they're more likely to be benign.

Noninvasive cancer occurs in the duct or lobule, which is very small. For the calcifications to fit in a duct, they have to be very small and they tend to assume the linear shape of the duct in rather a dash-dot pattern. The big chunks of calcium we sometimes see on the mammogram couldn't possibly fit in the ductal system, so we know they're benign. They're usually old fibroadenomas that you had as a teenager, which have faded and become soft and less dense and now are calcifying. Sometimes they're calcifications in a scar or in a blood vessel that's getting older and harder.

There's a middle type of calcifications that is less easy to characterize. They may be new, but there are just a few of them and possibly they are associated with a scar, or some of them may "layer" on the side-view mammogram because they are floating in tiny cysts. In that situation, we'll recommend a follow-up mammogram in six months and consider it BI-RADS 3, probably benign. If it's noninvasive cancer, we may see more calcifications, or a change in the shape or size, whereas if there's no worrisome change, it's more likely to be benign. Patients get nervous about that; if it's cancer and we wait six months, won't it grow and kill you? But in fact, if we wait six months it's because we don't think it's cancer. And even in the worst-case scenario, it's usually noninvasive cancer, and noninvasive cancer takes years to develop into cancer. So six months won't make any difference, and the wait prevents needless biopsies.

Some calcifications associated with noninvasive cancers don't grow or change, so they don't get picked up on the second mammogram. But that's because they aren't growing and, thus, we don't expect there to be any associated invasive cancer.

Any time doctors are worried about calcifications, they can proceed to a biopsy. This is usually done as a core biopsy (described at the end of this chapter). If we want to prove an area benign just by imaging, usually we need to do a mammogram every six, twelve, and twenty-four months.[7] In the days of wire-localized excisional biopsies, this was acceptable and proved safe. But the more modern invention of the core biopsy has proved less invasive and can resolve the issue sooner.

Types of Mammograms

Though early mammography in the 1950s produced a fair amount of radiation, over the years X-ray techniques have been refined so that very little radiation is actually used. Most mammography now is digital. Like a digital camera, digital mammography is a way of computerizing the image so it can be viewed on a computer monitor screen. Because it's a computerized rather than a photographic technique, the radiologist can magnify different areas to focus on what they want to see. Digital technique allows the images to be stored more efficiently and transmitted more easily, as with the photos taken with a digital camera. Though this technique has definite advantages, it is only slightly better than the older film-screen mammogram, and only better in people with dense breasts. What it has allowed is computerized *marking* of mammograms (computer-aided detection, or CAD). A computer prescreens mammograms and points out potentially worrisome areas so that the interpreting radiologist can examine them more carefully. This was intended to make reading more accurate as computers don't get distracted or blink at the wrong moment. In many studies, it has been shown to help find more cancers; unfortunately, this benefit does not seem to translate as well to the real world when tested in a large clinical practice because there are too many marks (think of the boy who cried wolf); only about one in one thousand marks is useful, so radiologists must ignore most of the marks even when they may help.[8]

Tomosynthesis (3D Mammography)

As mentioned in Chapter 7, a newer technology called a 3D mammogram (also known as tomosynthesis) is often performed in addition to or instead of a standard 2D mammogram in both screening and diagnosis. Tomosynthesis uses X-rays that produce about the same radiation exposure to the breasts as a standard mammogram: if you have both 2D and 3D, your breasts will receive nearly twice the amount of radiation as from a standard mammogram, though the combined dose is still within standard safety limits.

A 2D mammogram finds about two to seven cancers for every one thousand patients who have a mammogram. Another one to two cancers will be found per one thousand patients when tomosynthesis is added to a standard mammogram. Tomosynthesis also makes it easier to identify normal tissue (versus an area that might have needed more follow-up based on a 2D mammogram) and therefore reduces the chance of being called back for additional views or an ultrasound.

Contrast-Enhanced Mammography (CEM)

Contrast-enhanced mammography (CEM), a hybrid type of mammogram, is gaining traction because it can obtain similar information as breast MRI but in less time and at a lower cost. Approved by the U.S. Food and Drug Administration (FDA) for clinical use in 2011, CEM uses iodinated contrast to detect tumors with an abundance of blood vessels—which are a sign of cancer. Preliminary studies have shown that the images, while looking very different, are as sensitive to cancer as MRIs.[9] A major study called the Contrast-Enhanced Mammography Imaging Screening Trial (CMIST), led by the Breast Cancer Research Foundation, is now comparing CEM with other breast imaging techniques. CEM works by taking an initial image of the breasts before contrast is injected. After the contrast is administered, more images are taken, and then the plain, precontrast image is subtracted from the postcontrast ones, removing unneeded background and featuring only highlighted suspicious areas.

Quality of Mammograms

Today all mammography units must be certified as meeting FDA standards and must prominently display the certificate issued by the agency. The initial quality standards for mammography facilities to meet FDA certification went into effect in December 1994. They include the following: radiologic technologists who perform mammography, physicians who interpret mammograms, and medical physicists who survey equipment must all have adequate training and experience, and each facility must have a system for following up on mammograms that reveal problems and for obtaining biopsy results. In 1996, the FDA along with the National Mammography Quality Assurance Advisory Committee developed additional and more comprehensive final standards, including (1) a consumer complaint mechanism to provide patients with a process for addressing their concerns about mammography facilities, (2) special techniques and personnel qualifications related to mammography of people with breast implants, (3) communication of mammography results to referring physicians and *all examinees (that means you)* in writing, and (4) additional clinical image review and examinee notification requirements when a facility's images are determined to be substandard. In addition, the BI-RADS system provides standardized terminology for reporting mammogram results whereby all of them are classified according to one of seven categories (see Table 8.1) that must be used.

The radiation used in mammography is low risk, according to the American Cancer Society; two views of each breast generates the same amount a person would get from their natural surroundings over seven weeks (0.4 millisieverts). Mammography is one area where we really do have quality control—something we have little of in the rest of breast care, and indeed in much of medicine.

It should come as a comfort that a growing number of facilities have additional accreditations that require meeting high quality standards for not only mammography but other types of imaging and breast care. The American College of Radiology, for example, offers a Breast Imaging Center of Excellence status to facilities that meet high standards in mammography, breast ultrasound, MRI, ultrasound-guided biopsy, and stereotactic biopsy. The National Accreditation Program for Breast Centers (NAPBC) requires high standards in all areas of breast care, principally surgery, radiology, pathology, radiation oncology, genetics, plastic surgery, and physical therapy.

Procedure

When you go to a new doctor or screening center, it is important that they receive copies of your X-rays from your previous provider. The new site will then be able to do a comparison and possibly save you extra radiation spent trying to figure out something that has been there for years!

The atmosphere you face when you get there will vary from one mammography facility to another. Some are cold and clinical, whereas others provide a warm ambience and reassuring, friendly personnel. But the actual procedure is pretty standard. You have to undress from the waist up, and you're usually given some kind of hospital gown. You'll probably be X-rayed standing up. The technologist will have you lean over a plastic plate and help you place your breast on the plate (Figure 8.1). This can feel a bit uncomfortable, especially when the plates press your breast together. Two pictures of each breast are usually taken, one from the

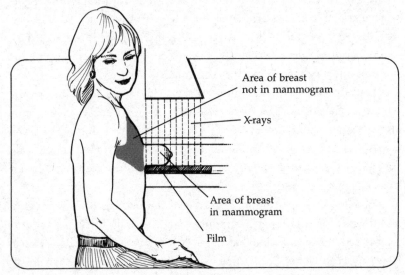

Figure 8.1

side, the other from the top. In addition, the way the technologist takes the X-rays is important. The tighter your breasts are squeezed, the more accurate the picture is and the less radiation is necessary to penetrate the tissue. It is very important to hold still during the exposure.

The process really isn't all that painful. It has been shown that breasts are less tender and less dense in the second half of the menstrual cycle (about a week after your period ends), so you may want to schedule around your period. For people who do find mammograms uncomfortable, taking aspirin, ibuprofen, or naproxen half an hour before the exam can make all the difference.

People with disabilities may have difficulty getting a clear mammogram, particularly if they're unable to stand up. Fortunately a good technologist can do a mammogram while a patient sits for the procedure, provided the patient can cooperate with positioning and hold still during the exposure. If you're told this can't be done, you should insist on it or go to another facility.

The whole process lasts only a few minutes. With digital mammograms, the technologist can check the mammograms on a computer screen a few seconds after they are taken. If you are having a diagnostic mammogram, the radiologist will review the images while you wait, and you will receive the results immediately following the examination. In some places, the radiologist will also come out and tell you what the screening mammogram shows. In other high-volume settings, the radiologists will read the screening mammograms later in the day when they can focus and not be interrupted. Then the results are sent by mail and you have to wait several days to a week to get them. Studies have shown that centers that do a high volume of mammograms and read them later usually provide more accurate interpretations, so this is worth the trade-off of having to wait for a result.

Please don't ask your technologist to interpret the mammogram for you. Technologists aren't doctors; their job is taking the pictures, not reading them.

Limitations of Mammography

Frustration with the limitations of mammography has led to a search for other ways of looking at the breast. Mammography uses radiation, which carries some risk, and it is limited in its ability to see through dense breast tissue and determine clearly whether a lump is benign or malignant. For people age 30 and over, ultrasound should be used in addition to mammography to evaluate a breast symptom, such as a lump that is felt. These issues are especially important for young, high-risk people. Ultrasound is one alternative used to assess lumps, nipple discharge, other symptoms, and mammographic abnormalities and can be used in addition to mammography to screen people with dense breasts. MRI is recommended for screening people at high risk (see Chapter 7) and is occasionally used for problem-solving when ultrasound and mammography both remain unclear.

ULTRASOUND

In the ultrasound method, high-frequency sound waves are sent off in little pulses, like radar, toward the breast. A gel is put on the breast to make it slippery, and a small transducer (a device that both sends out and picks up sound waves) is slid along the skin, sending waves through it. When something gets in the way of the waves, they bounce back again, and if nothing gets in the way, they pass through the breast. Ultrasound is appealing because it doesn't use radiation and works well in dense breasts where mammography is limited. It has more limitations in large breasts, however.

We use ultrasound mostly for looking at a specific area. If we know a lump is there, we can get more information about it. It can help determine whether a lump is fluid-filled or solid—if it's fluid-filled, like a cyst, the sound waves go through it very well, and if it's solid, like a fibroadenoma, they are partially blocked. If a lump shows up on a mammogram that we can't feel in a physical examination, and we want to determine whether it's a cyst or a solid lump, ultrasound can give us the answer.

Ultrasound can also help us interpret findings seen on a mammogram. If the doctor feels a lump and the mammogram shows just dense breast tissue, the ultrasound can still show a lump within the dense breast tissue. Mammography will show a mass in dense tissue only as overlapping areas of brightness, but ultrasound can distinguish masses because the sound waves travel differently through masses than through normal tissue. Ultrasound adds another dimension to the imaging possible with mammography. Therefore, if there is a suspicious area other than calcifications on a mammogram, most breast imaging centers will also do an ultrasound. Many breast surgeons have an ultrasound machine in their office so that they can immediately check on a lump that you or they may have felt.

Because, as far as we know, sound waves are harmless, ultrasound is often the best tool for studying benign problems at length, particularly in people under age 30 or in people who are pregnant or breastfeeding. If a doctor has a younger patient with a lump and wants to determine if it's likely to be a fibroadenoma or a possible cancer, ultrasound in that area can differentiate between a distinct lesion with smooth edges or an irregular area with infiltrating borders.

A limitation of ultrasound is that it depends, more than mammography does, on the experience of the person operating the equipment. Unlike mammography, which shows the whole breast on each picture, each ultrasound picture shows only a small section of the breast—so it can be harder to figure out where that section is in the breast as a whole. Therefore the technologist or physician who operates the ultrasound equipment must be able first to find the abnormality and then demonstrate it well on the pictures. The technologist or physician holds the transducer directly over the suspicious area, and the angle at which it is held changes the image. Looking at the photograph of the image at another time can be difficult. The ultrasonographer is standing at the patient's side, looking at the screen while performing the examination and taking the pictures. It may be hard for the physician to pick up an ultrasound picture after the fact and then interpret it accurately.

We can also use ultrasound in much the same way we use mammograms to guide core biopsies.[10] Often ultrasound guides us into a mass more effectively than mammography does. Physicians experienced in breast ultrasound can approach the mass from different directions, which may make it easier to biopsy hard-to-reach areas in the breast, and many find the ultrasound method faster and more comfortable for the patient. It is the way most radiologists and surgeons prefer to do an image-guided core biopsy as it is the most comfortable for the patient, who is lying face up. For the same reason, sometimes radiologists and surgeons find it easier to use ultrasound in surgical planning as the patient is in the same face up position that they will assume in the operating room.

Automated Whole-Breast Ultrasound

Automated whole-breast ultrasound is a technique that was developed to overcome the variability issues with regular handheld ultrasound. The device is put over the breast and pictures are taken in an organized way so that they can be reconstructed in 3D. A large study reported that it was able to increase not only the number of clinically important cancers detected but also the number of false positives or lesions that looked like they could be cancer but weren't.[11] These lesions are then confirmed by handheld ultrasound and of course biopsy if indicated.

MRI

Magnetic resonance imaging (MRI) takes advantage of the magnetic qualities of the hydrogen nucleus. Hydrogen is part of water, and water is a large part of our bodies. MRI uses a huge magnet. You are put in the middle of the magnet, which turns on and off. The way the hydrogen realigns within the magnetic field allows the MRI machine to make an image of the tissues.

This test was initially used in the brain and has been very accurate in diagnosing brain tumors. It is also now recognized as the most sensitive and specific way to evaluate whether a silicone breast implant has leaked.

MRI is finally taking its place in breast cancer diagnosis. MRIs are significantly more complicated than mammography or ultrasound. For one thing, if you are premenopausal and having the MRI for screening, it is best to schedule your MRI during days seven to ten of the menstrual cycle (day one being the first day of your period) to reduce the normal hormonal changes that can affect the interpretation.[12] When MRI is performed on a patient with known breast cancer, we do not worry about the timing in the menstrual cycle as we do not want to delay care. On the day of your exam, leave your jewelry and other metal items (pins, hairpins, metal slippers, removable dental work, pens, eyeglasses, body piercing jewelry) at home or in the locker provided as they can distort the images. Watches, credit cards, cell phones, and hearing aids also interfere and can be damaged by the machine. The strength of the magnet can also cause metallic objects to become projectiles or heat up to dangerously high temperatures. Let your MRI technologist know if you have a pacemaker (some of the new ones are MRI compatible), cochlear (ear) implant, or clips used on brain aneurysms, as well as metal pins, screws, plates, or stents. Most joint replacements are okay, but it is always good to let the technologist know in advance. MRI tables are usually restricted to 350-pound weight limits, and some people who weigh less but are broad and stout also won't fit in the machine.

Traditional breast MRI currently involves a movable examination table that slides into a circular magnet. Some newer machines are open at the sides but may not be appropriate for your exam. At the moment, open MRI is not ideal for breast exams. If you are worried about feeling claustrophobic, ask which machine will be used. About one in twenty women will need a sedative to help them relax prior to the exam, so don't be afraid to ask your doctor if you want one. Contrast material is going to be used in the exam to highlight abnormalities (unless the study is being done only to evaluate breast implants), so a nurse or technologist will insert an intravenous (IV) line into a vein in your hand or arm. A saline solution will be dripped through it to keep the vein open during the procedure.

The MRI exam is done with you lying facedown on a table with your breasts hanging into cushioned coils and your arms over your head (see Figure 8.2). Once you are positioned on the table, the technologist will leave the room. He or she can see and hear you, however, so speak up if you need to. First an exam is done without contrast material to get a baseline. You will be told what to expect but it is good to anticipate that there will be a lot of humming and tapping noises, not unlike a low-level jackhammer. You can request earplugs if you want. Once the first images have been obtained, the contrast is injected into the intravenous line. This usually causes no side effects, although occasionally it produces a warm feeling and discomfort near the breast bone. To get good results, you will be asked to stay still during the exam. It can be helpful to try relaxation techniques (see Chapter 16) or imagine yourself somewhere else that you find comforting. The exam itself takes between thirty and sixty minutes. Although the procedure may seem scary, there are no known risks from the magnet, and the only side effect is a potential allergy to the contrast material, called gadolinium. There is a low risk of complications for people with kidney disease or damage. There are now faster, abbreviated MRIs (AB-MRIs) that use fewer images to obtain the same information and speed up the procedure, with a sensitivity comparable to the conventional exam, but their use is not yet widespread.

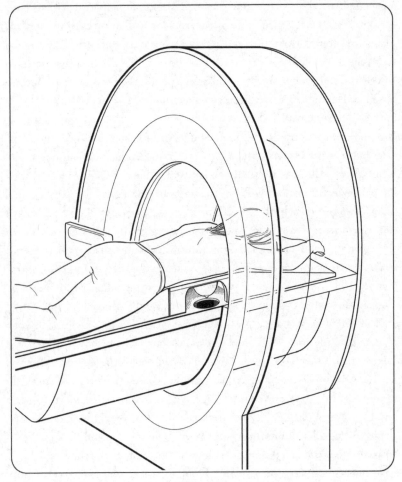

Figure 8.2

The downside of MRI is the fact that, like ultrasound, it finds all kinds of abnormalities, most of them benign. At first you may think this is a good thing, but actually it means lots of patients are getting unnecessary biopsies in an effort to track down every finding on the MRI. If an MRI finds a suspicious lesion that cannot be seen on mammography or ultrasound and is to be used to guide the biopsy, the biopsy must be done with special nonmagnetic equipment, adding yet another level of difficulty.

Breast MRI is best done by a dedicated team that does breast MRI regularly. To determine how experienced the team is, ask if they are able to do

MRI-guided biopsies and if they are certified by the American College of Radiology. Good diagnostic centers should be able to do the whole workup.

MRI, like ultrasound, is useful in conjunction with mammography, not as a replacement for it, though for high-risk patients between ages 25 and 30, sometimes a screening MRI is performed without mammography to avoid radiation to young breast tissue. Occasionally MRI is used to further distinguish an abnormality found on mammography and ultrasound. It can also be used to follow the results of chemotherapy in large cancers treated systemically prior to surgery (see Chapter 11) or instances in which there is cancer in a lymph node but no cancer has been found in the breast (see Chapter 12). Finally, as noted in Chapter 4, it is used to screen very high-risk people such as those who carry the mutation for breast cancer.[13]

The American College of Radiology suggests supplemental MRI screening if a woman has higher-than-average risk,[14] such as the following:

- Genetics-based increased risk with a lifetime risk of 20 percent or more
- A history of chest, neck, or armpit radiation during childhood/adolescence (once given for Hodgkin lymphoma)
- Personal history of cancer and dense tissue
- A diagnosis of breast cancer by age 50

A common practice is to do an MRI preoperatively for a person diagnosed with breast cancer to make sure that they are a candidate for breast conservation. Some argue that this has not been shown to be worthwhile in most cases and can potentially increase the cost of care and slightly delay treatment of the cancer (see Chapter 11). Some studies show that preoperative MRI decreases the rate of positive margins and the need for reexcision of lumpectomies. But other studies conclude that preoperative MRIs make little difference. One disease where it has proved highly useful is invasive lobular cancer, which can be particularly difficult to adequately assess on mammography or even ultrasound: MRI changes the surgical management in about half of patients with invasive lobular cancer. MRI should *not* be used to characterize suspicious lesions (BI-RADS 4 or 5) that already need to be biopsied. It is better just to have the core biopsy, since it is more accurate, more definitive, and cheaper than an MRI.

PET SCANNING

No, this doesn't mean we scan your hamster. Positron emission tomography (PET) is another detection technique that has received a lot of press. PET is a completely different way of imaging breast tissue; we don't look at the structure itself but at the activity going on in it. All tissues need glucose (a sugar) as fuel to survive. Cancers are rapidly growing and turning over, so they use more glucose than normal tissue. PET scanning looks at how much glucose is being used by a tissue. Like MRI, PET was first developed to study the brain, and it has been very useful for that. It is routinely used in locally advanced breast cancers to identify distant metastases. It is not ideal for evaluating the primary cancer within the breast at this time.

To do this scan we inject the patient with a small amount of radioactively labeled glucose molecules, which the tissue takes up and metabolizes. You have to fast before the study and wait an hour after the tracer has been injected to allow it to be distributed throughout the body. The scanner can then demonstrate where and how much glucose the tissues take up.

Specific PET scanners for the breast have been developed and show greater detail and accuracy in imaging breast cancer than whole-body PET or PET-CT, where it is combined with computed tomography (CT) in an effort to produce more detailed images than either alone.[15] The question remains regarding how they fit into the detection and treatment of breast cancer. The radiation dose is higher for PET scanning than for molecular breast imaging, which uses a radioactive tracer and gamma cameras to "light up" any areas of cancer inside the breast. PET scanners extend to the whole body, so it is not appropriate for screening. However, it is perfect for patients who are receiving neoadjuvant chemotherapy (see Chapter 11) to shrink their tumor prior to surgery. Whole-body PET-CT and dedicated breast PET with the same dose can thus reveal any metastases as well as the size of the breast tumor.

OTHER IMAGING

There is no doubt that standard breast cancer screening will continue to evolve at a rapid pace in the coming years. Current approaches are effective but imperfect and are constantly being tweaked. The use of artificial

intelligence is becoming increasingly common as machine-learning al-
gorithms improve quality and interpretation. Several new screening
approaches are in various states of clinical development as this is being
written. If there is a kind of screening you haven't heard of, or you are
unsure of its safety or effectiveness, check the FDA website (www.fda
.gov), as they are the government entity in charge of regulating medical
devices used for breast cancer screening. If something is not up to standard, they will say so. An example of this is a statement they issued on
thermography, which measures temperature differences on the surface
of the breasts based on the theory that fast-growing cancer cells radiate more heat. "The FDA is not aware of any scientific evidence to support these claims," they noted. "Thermography has not been shown to
be effective as a stand-alone test for either breast cancer screening or
diagnosis in detecting early stage breast cancer."[16] So if your health care
provider suggests a new screening technique that you haven't heard of or
that makes you uneasy, don't be afraid to do a little research.

BIOPSY

When the doctor says you need a biopsy, it usually means a needle or core
biopsy. Although the two types of biopsies are done with needles, in the
United States, core biopsies are the procedure of choice because they obtain more tissue and are easier for pathologists to interpret (Figure 8.3).
A fine-needle (like the kind used to draw blood) biopsy takes only a few
cells out of the lump; a large-needle biopsy, called a core biopsy, cuts a
small piece out of the lump. These can be done in a doctor's office but
more often are done under imaging guidance in a breast imaging suite
on lumps that are palpable or on lesions identified only on imaging. As I
mentioned at the start of this chapter, it is very unusual these days for a
surgeon to perform an operation to make a diagnosis on a breast lump or
abnormal mammogram. If that is being suggested for you, it is important
you find out why and then consider getting a second opinion.

The term "biopsy," by the way, refers to the procedure itself, not the
process of studying the lump in the laboratory, which the pathologist
or cytologist does later. Anything that we cut out of the body should be
sent for analysis, and the connection between the two procedures causes
people to confuse them with each other. The basic rule with any biopsy

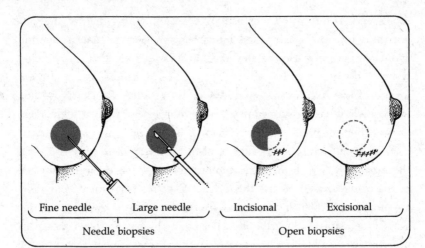

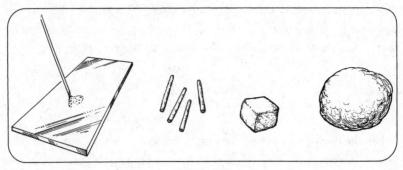

Figure 8.3

is that three elements should be in agreement in order to determine that the lesion is benign or malignant.[17] If I think on examination that it's a fibroadenoma, if it looks like one on the ultrasound, and if it also looks like one to the cytologist or pathologist under the microscope after a needle aspiration, then I feel certain that's what it is. But if one of those elements is different—if it seems like a cancer to me, even though the mammogram and core biopsy suggest it is benign, another biopsy may be needed.

Core Biopsy

Core biopsy should be the first choice for patients with a suspicious palpable lesion and/or one that is judged to be BI-RADS 4 or 5 on imaging (see Table 8.1). Core biopsies are done by a radiologist or, in some centers, a surgeon. Your doctor will get the results and refer you for further treatments. If the core biopsy shows cancer, you can then have the treatment you need, which may be chemotherapy first or surgery. If the core biopsy report is benign, you are done.

If the lesion can be felt, a core biopsy can be done without imaging, although an improved diagnosis results when ultrasound is used to direct the core into the lesion. This is by far the most comfortable for the patient, who lies on their back while the procedure takes place under local anesthesia. The ultrasound approach is also preferred because it does not require equipment such as X-ray machines and does not expose the patient to radiation. If the lesion is only seen on a mammogram, then a stereotactic core biopsy (see the following discussion) is done under X-ray guidance. This requires the patient to lie still on their stomach for about thirty minutes. For lesions seen only on MRI, a core biopsy can also be done in the MRI machine. This is the most complicated procedure, as it involves contrast material as well as special nonmagnetic needles and has you lying on your stomach for forty-five minutes. This eliminates anyone with significant claustrophobia (unless it can be controlled with medication), with arthritis in the neck or back, with chronic cough, with severe kyphosis (a condition that causes the person to hunch over), or anything else that prevents absolute immobility for forty-five minutes. Newer stereotactic/tomosynthesis biopsy devices allow for the patient to be seated upright, and the equipment attaches directly to the mammography machine. Patients tend to tolerate core biopsies quite well. Our radiology advisor Dr. Lauren Green, who is head of breast imaging at the University of Illinois Hospital, says that often fear and obsessive googling make anticipation of the procedure worse than the core biopsy itself. Usually the greatest discomfort comes from the injection of local anesthesia. After that, patients do not experience much pain, if any.

Core Biopsy with Ultrasound

In a core biopsy with ultrasound, the patient lies on their back on a table and the radiologist or surgeon identifies the lesion using a handheld ultrasound device. The patient is given local anesthesia and then the doctor makes a nick over the site where the biopsy needle will go in. The doctor passes a device through the incision and positions it for the biopsy (see

Figure 8.4). (This device was first called a "biopsy gun," an unfortunate name considering it is aimed at people's breasts. In the UCLA breast center, I persuaded doctors to use the less lethal-sounding "biopsy device.") When this device is used, the needle enters the lesion rapidly and cuts a core of tissue. Although this sounds scary, the function is similar to having your ears pierced with the tool used in jewelry outlets, although with local anesthesia, it should not feel that way. Most patients describe feeling pressure but not pain. Some devices use a vacuum or suction to pull

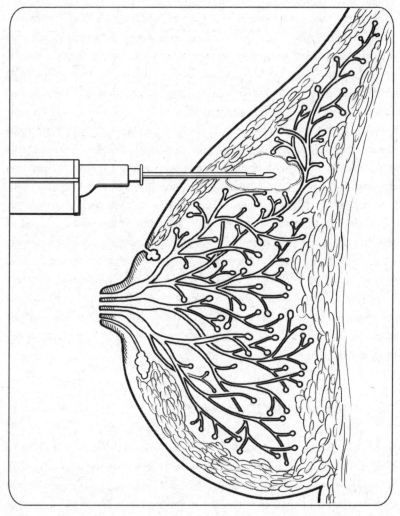

Figure 8.4

the tissue into the needle, then drill out a core. Others use a quick freeze to make the tissue more solid and therefore easier to cut. Which device is chosen depends on the situation and the experience of the doctor. Usually several passes are taken to make sure the lesion is well sampled. The size of the nick depends on how big the core biopsy needle is; usually a little, bandage-like covering called a Steri-Strip is enough to close it. Typically three cores are taken out for masses; for microcalcifications it may be six to ten or more. A vacuum-assisted device is more accurate when sampling calcifications, as we need to sample the tissue around the calcifications as well as the calcifications themselves.

After the core biopsy, it is standard to place a tiny metal clip to permanently mark the site of any biopsy, and a mammogram is usually obtained to show the clip position. The clip will not set off metal detectors in the airport, but it will show up on later breast imaging. It is important to have a clip placed to mark the spot that was biopsied in case the lesion cannot be seen any longer on imaging (or sometimes after chemotherapy) and it is cancer. Even if the biopsy does not show cancer, the clip helps show your doctors in the future that a particular area has already been biopsied and found to be benign, and this can avoid someone biopsying the same area all over again because they did not know. Radiologist Lauren Green likes to ask patients if they have a nickel allergy or are sensitive to costume jewelry prior to the biopsy. If so, she will place a nickel-free clip at the site of the biopsy. "I let my patients know they won't be able to see or feel the clip and that thousands of women have clips without any issues—many of whom don't even know they have one."

Pressure is applied to the breast for a few minutes after the biopsy until the breast stops bleeding. The afternoon and evening after the biopsy, you will be instructed to use an ice pack intermittently on your breast to reduce swelling. A tight-fitting wireless bra, like a sports bra, can also help.

Stereotactic Core Biopsy

A stereotactic core biopsy differs from core biopsy done with ultrasound, mainly in that it is done under mammographic guidance and usually uses a vacuum-assisted device. The patient lies down on the table with their breast suspended below them between two X-ray plates (Figure 8.5).

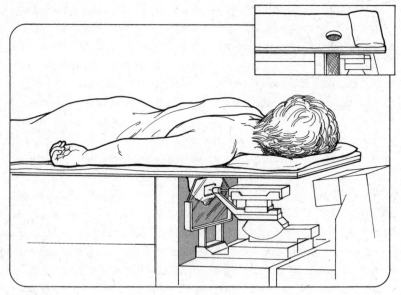

Figure 8.5

Some facilities now perform these in upright seated positioning. The radiologist marks the target on each of the pair of 2D images, and then the computer calculates the third dimension/depth to insert the needle and obtain the biopsy. When microcalcifications are biopsied, a mammographic image should be obtained of the specimens to ensure that they have been successfully sampled. Some centers put the individual pieces of tissue that contain calcifications in a separate container to help the pathologist find them.

There are few complications, whether done under X-ray or ultrasound. Rarely the doctor may miss the lesion. In 1 percent of patients there may be a hematoma (blood collection); up to 3 percent of patients have a hematoma when a vacuum-assisted device is used. Infection is extremely uncommon. You may have some minor bruising.

Tomosynthesis-Guided Biopsy

Taking all those images during a stereotactic biopsy can take time and sometimes can be complex; this can lead to additional discomfort for the patient, whose breast is compressed this entire time.

In tomosynthesis-guided biopsies, the images and artificial intelligence work to generate all three dimensions much more quickly. The initial shots are taken without having to manually reposition the X-ray machine. The radiologist then scrolls through that image set and marks the target lesion on a single image. Based on that, the computer calculates the rest and instantly generates all three of the coordinates. The procedure is far less time-intensive and there is less room for error—which is a huge benefit for the patient. This procedure is often performed with the patient in an upright seated position, which can help with patient comfort.

Fine-Needle Biopsy

If you have a lump that is easily felt, the surgeon will anesthetize your breast with a small amount of lidocaine and then use a needle and syringe to try to get a few cells (see Figure 8.3, page 180). The material is squirted onto a slide, which is examined under a microscope. This can often show whether it is benign or cancerous. However, because there's no tissue to look at, just individual cells, the procedure requires a good cytologist (a specialist in the field of looking at cells rather than tissue) who can identify cells out of context.

Fine-needle biopsies are usually not done on lesions that can be seen only on mammogram, as generally we use a core biopsy in that setting.

As I've mentioned before, things have changed a lot since the earlier editions of this book: some for the better and some not. Since you are now often sent directly to radiology for a biopsy by your gynecologist or primary care doctor, a radiologist may be the one to give you your results. You should ask when they think they will be calling so that you can have someone you trust with you. Sometimes it is the patient navigator who will be sharing the biopsy results with you. They are trained nurses whose job it is to help you navigate the different steps and doctors recommended for your situation. Biopsy results are usually available within forty-eight hours, although not on weekends. The biopsy report should reflect the findings on the mammogram, known as concordance. If they are not in agreement, the biopsied tissue sample may not have been enough. If you have cancer, hearing this news is shocking and scary. Unfortunately the person telling you may not be expert on your diagnosis and thus can't answer all your questions. The next step for many patients is to go on the Internet, which can be dangerous in itself. If you are lucky, you have a good friend who has been through it, or you have stumbled across this book. Take a deep breath!

If the biopsy is clearly benign (and this result agrees with the earlier imaging and clinical findings), you can relax and celebrate. However, you should still get and read your whole pathology report.

If your biopsy shows cancer, ideally you want to go somewhere that has a multidisciplinary breast program where you can be seen by a surgeon, oncologist, and radiation therapist. The latter should also receive the recommendations made by the radiologist who took your initial mammogram. They will be able to evaluate your biopsy and suggest a course of action. Breast cancer treatment has become more complicated. While we used to go first to surgery and then radiation and then chemotherapy and/or hormonal therapy, sometimes treatment now involves systemic therapy such as chemotherapy and/or hormonal therapy first, then surgery and radiation later. These decisions are based on factors like the type of tumor (see Chapter 10) or the size of tumor as well as your health in general. You have to take time for all this, and you have to have a doctor or team who will travel this road with you along with your local reputable breast cancer support organization. Progress has also occurred in the form of options for chemotherapy, or hormonal therapy, which are very complex, with results that are even better. A better result—less mutilation—is the upside. The downside is that it takes time and patience to wade through the pros and cons of all these options.

HOW TO READ YOUR BENIGN BIOPSY REPORT

Even when the doctor tells you that the lump was benign, it's important to find out exactly what it was—*benign* isn't enough. You should ask to see a copy of your pathology report. For help reading a biopsy report with findings of cancer, please see Chapter 10.

The report will have two parts. The first is the *gross description*. It describes what the doctor gave the pathologist—a slide with some cells on it, or a core, or a piece of tissue measuring, for example, three by five centimeters. If it's microcalcifications, the pathologist won't see these with the naked eye, and so they won't be described.

The second part describes what the tissue looks like under the microscope. Some reports will give you a detailed description—what the cells look like, what the surrounding tissue is like, and so on. Others cut to the chase and give just the final diagnosis. So it may read, "1. fibroadenoma." It almost always adds "2. fibrocystic change." That's because, as I said in Chapter 3, the fibrocystic change is the background that we see normally in breast tissue, so it's always there. The report may say "fibrocystic change" alone if it's just breast tissue. That may or may not be an adequate diagnosis, depending on the target of the biopsy. It is important to make sure that the correct tissue was biopsied.

In addition, if your biopsy was done for calcifications, you want to be sure that the pathologist saw calcifications under the microscope, so you can be sure that they are looking at the right tissue.

You should save the copy of the report; it may become relevant at some later time, and it's important for you to have it in your records. Ideally, you would also have a *concordance assessment* for your files, which integrates clinical examination, imaging, pathology, and surgical planning into the optimal interdisciplinary approach for your particular case. We're starting to realize that some of the changes in the basic molecular biology of the breast tissue (see Chapter 5) can be identified in earlier biopsy tissue. It may be important for you to be able to have the pathologist go back and look at the slides and determine what kind of fibroadenoma you actually had. Probably they won't keep the tissue, but if you at least keep a record of your biopsy, with the date and the hospital, you can go back and find the slides. That can be very important.

PART FOUR

Decisions

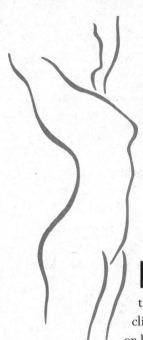

CHAPTER 9

Coping with a Breast Cancer Diagnosis

I n this chapter we will talk about the emotional fall-
out of your diagnosis, how to cope, and how to pick a
treatment team. We will also tackle the nuts and bolts of
clinical trials and the option of becoming part of a study
on breast cancer treatments.

FEELINGS

The first thing most people think when they're diagnosed with breast
cancer is "Will I die?" This is quickly followed by "Will I lose my breast?"
Or conversely, "I want both my breasts off now!" Clearly breast cancer
has a major psychological impact. Whenever you find a lump, get a mammogram, or have a biopsy, you rehearse the psychological work of having
breast cancer. Although most people don't die of breast cancer and most
do not have to lose their breasts, these fears remain.

How does a person react to this terrifying diagnosis? In my experience, people go through several psychological steps in dealing with it.

First there is shock. Particularly if you're relatively young and have
never had a life-threatening illness, it's difficult to believe you have something as serious as cancer. It's doubly hard to believe because, in most
cases, your body hasn't given you any warning. Unlike, say, appendici-
tis or a heart attack, there's no pain or fever or nausea—no symptom
that tells you something's going wrong inside. You or your doctor have
found a painless little lump, or your routine mammogram shows something peculiar—and the next thing you know you're being told you've
got breast cancer.

Many people find this to be the worst time. The initial shock can leave you feeling confused and unsure as to how to proceed. Your mind is seesawing between numb denial and terrified comprehension. But once you get the medical information you need to make decisions, things get better. Once those decisions have been made, things get better still.

You also feel anger—even fury—at your body, which has betrayed you in such a deceitful fashion. The thought of losing a breast is almost unbearable, and at the same time your anger can make you want a mastectomy. In spite of the horror you feel at the thought of losing your breast, often your first reaction is a desire to get rid of it: as one patient cried out to me: "Take the damned thing off and let me get on with my life!"

As an immediate emotional response, this makes perfect sense. As an active decision, it doesn't. Getting your breast cut off will not make things go back to normal; nothing can ever do that. Your life has been changed, and it will not be the same again. You need time to let this sink in, to face the implications cancer has for you, and to make a rational, informed decision about what treatment will be best for you both physically and emotionally.

Because patients are so vulnerable when they receive their diagnosis, in my surgical practice I didn't like to list all their options at the same time I told them they had cancer. I preferred to tell a patient they had cancer and that there were a number of treatment options to discuss the next day at my office.

If you were told about cancer by your primary care doctor or gynecologist, you may not have all the facts yet, much less a plan of action. This is a very scary time when you know you have something bad, but not how bad or what you will need to do about it. I remember all too well as I heard about my leukemia diagnosis on a Friday. I may know everything about breast cancer but I knew nothing about a blood cancer like leukemia. Of course I turned to the Internet, but, not unlike you, I did not know what information pertained to me and what did not. It is a frightening time and the best thing you can do is make an appointment as soon as possible to learn more. This can be done either by sitting down with the surgeon who did the biopsy or by finding a multidisciplinary clinic where you can be seen by a team including a medical oncologist, radiation oncologist, surgeon, and pathologist. You need to find out exactly what kind of cancer you have (see Chapter 10) and what the best plan is for your situation.

WEIGHING THE OPTIONS

Today there's much more emphasis on doctor and patient sharing the decision-making process, and there are more choices. There's also a lot more knowledge available—there are articles about breast cancer and survival rates in both the medical and the popular press and on the Internet; patients *know* they have no guarantee that everything will be fine once their doctor makes them better. All this is good, but it's also very stressful. In the long run, I'm convinced you're better off when you consciously choose your treatment than when it's imposed on you as a matter of course. In the short run it may be more difficult, but more anxiety ahead of time while you are trying to make decisions about your treatment may make for fewer regrets afterward.

Of course, different patients have different needs. Some people still want an "omniscient" doctor to tell them what to do. I was involved in a pilot study on how patients decide their treatments and what kinds of decision making had the best psychological results. I expected to find that patients coped better when they got a lot of information from their doctors and learned all they could about their disease, its prognosis, and the range of available treatments. But we found this wasn't always the case. Far more important was whether the doctor's style matched the patient's. Some patients preferred to deny their cancer as far as possible and have their doctor take care of it for them. They did better with old-fashioned paternalistic surgeons who told the patient what was best for them, giving them minimal information. Others liked to feel in control of their life and to know all they could about their illness and its ramifications. They did better with surgeons like me, who wanted to discuss everything with them. Still others wanted a great deal of information but deferred to the doctor for decision making. There is no right or wrong style, so don't feel guilty if your needs are not the same as those of your friend or neighbor. In choosing a doctor, you want someone whose style works best for you.

I experienced this when I was in practice. There was a well-respected breast surgeon in Boston when I was at the Faulkner Breast Center there. He was much more in the taciturn, old-fashioned mode, and he and I would lose patients to each other all the time; sometimes we referred patients to each other. It worked out very well, and we were both happy about it, since we were both able to help people while remaining true to our own styles and philosophies.

Sometimes I would get a patient who clearly preferred not to know a lot, and over the years I learned to recognize the signs and to respect them. I'd give such a patient enough information but not in as much detail as I usually did, and then try to hear what they were choosing and say something like "It seems to me that you're leaning toward mastectomy, and maybe that's the best decision for you." I still wouldn't tell her what to do, but I'd give a little more guidance than usual.

Although the style matters, so does the doctor's knowledge and experience. You may need to do some research to find the most knowledgeable medical team available. In many urban areas this will be a surgeon who specializes in breast cancer or, better yet, a team at a multidisciplinary breast center. Because the treatment of breast cancer involves a team (see Chapter 11), consulting with the nearest breast center or breast cancer advocacy organization will help you find the best care.

If the first stage is shock, the second is investigating your options. (Sometimes, however, it works in reverse, and these stages can vary in order and intensity.) How extensive this investigation is varies enormously among patients. Some of my patients simply went over what the doctor had told them with their families and friends. Others did research in medical libraries and on the Internet, and then went for multiple opinions. You can't take forever, but you don't want to hurry yourself either. In my experience, most patients are able to assimilate the information and make their decisions in a month, including any second opinions they may need.

When you're exploring the options, you should reflect seriously on what losing a breast would mean to you. Its importance varies from person to person, but there is no one for whom it doesn't have some significance. Although many people say, "I don't care about my breast," deep down this is probably not true for most of us. A mastectomy may be the best choice for you, but it will still have a powerful effect on how you feel about yourself. Often the loss of a breast creates feelings of inadequacy—the sense of no longer being "a real woman."

The fear of feeling this way may start long before the mastectomy—indeed, it plays a part in how the patient copes with their breast cancer from the first. In the early 1980s, Rose Kushner surveyed three thousand women with breast cancer and concluded that most patients "think first of saving their breasts, as a rule, and their lives are but second thoughts."[1]

My experience was different. The first reaction of most of my patients was "I don't care about my breast—just save my life." Later, when the first shock had worn off and they'd had time to think about it, their priorities remained the same, but they realized they did in fact care very much about their breast. Many patients feel robbed of their sexuality when they lose a breast. This can be true even with reconstruction, which leaves you with no sensation in your reconstructed breasts. Holly Peters-Golden points out the importance of distinguishing between the distress caused by mutilating surgery and the distress that comes from having a life-threatening disease.[2] Certainly in my experience with patients, the latter far outweighs the former. Still, the fear of losing a key body part can stress a relationship and affect one or both members sexually. It is also important to be clear what you want rather than try to please a spouse, partner, or even adult child. As I used to say in the early days of breast conservation, "Husbands may come and go but you are stuck with your body forever."

Sociologist Ann Kaspar studied twenty-nine women between ages 29 and 72, twenty of whom had mastectomies, and nine of whom had lumpectomies.[3] Although, as she hastens to explain, she had no illusions that twenty-nine women constituted a definitive study, her findings are interesting. Most of the women with mastectomies had been deeply concerned before surgery that the mastectomy would "violate their femininity." Yet, with only one exception, they reported that after the surgery it was much less traumatic than they'd anticipated, and that they'd realized that being female didn't mean having two breasts. "They got in touch with their identity as women, separate from social demands. Even the ones most determined to get reconstruction didn't feel that the plastic surgery would make them real women—they knew they already were real women," Kaspar says. She did find that anxiety was higher among the single women in her study, especially the single heterosexual women, who worried that "no man will ever want me." Those already in relationships usually found that their partners were still loving and sexual, and more concerned with the women's health than their appearance.

Although the experience of the young, single, heterosexual women in this study is consistent with my patients' experience, I've also had many other patients who had different reasons for wanting to keep their breasts. Middle-aged women approaching or just past menopause can have very strong feelings about their breasts. They've experienced the loss of their reproductive capacity with menopause; often their children are leaving home, and they are rediscovering their relationship with their spouse. This is no time for a woman to experience yet another loss around her womanhood. Beyond sexuality, the shape of breasts matter for things as ordinary as the fit of clothes, how we move during exercise, and how we express physical affection like hugging children or pets to our chest.

Many elderly women also want breast conservation. They're already experiencing loss and may not want to add the loss of their breasts, which have been a part of them for such a long time. Nothing makes me angrier than hearing of an elderly woman who has been told by her surgeon, "You don't need your breasts anymore; you may as well have a mastectomy." Different choices may make sense at different stages in a woman's life. Your choice should be based not only on the best medical information you can gather but also on what feels right to you. Don't let generalizations about age, gender identity, sexual orientation, or vanity get in your way.

Generally when a patient is given a choice or options, it's because these are reasonable choices in their situation. When a mastectomy is a better option, your surgeon will say that. However, in most cases both mastectomy and lumpectomy with radiation work equally well, and breast conservation can even be better as it treats more tissue (see Chapter 11). It is not as though if you choose wrong you'll die, and if you choose right you'll live.

Along with the fears and stages of recovery, a number of related issues also come up for people with cancer. One of these is the tendency to feel guilty for having cancer—a sense that you've somehow done something wrong. People have a way of blaming themselves for being ill anyway, and irrational though they know it to be, a person often feels that they have betrayed their once traditional function as the family caregiver by getting breast cancer.

In this connection, the holistic perspectives that I discuss in Chapter 16 can have their negative side. The mind-body connection is real, and its validation is important, but it's not the only force at work in any disease. Most of the studies on the relation between stress and cancer have been done on rats and are equivocal at that—some studies show that stress is a factor in cancer, others that it's a factor in *preventing* cancer. In my opinion it probably has little effect in most people. I wish there were some simple, clear cause of cancer so I could say, "Don't do this and you won't get breast cancer." Unfortunately it doesn't work that way. We don't have total control over our own bodies; we don't always, to use the popular New Age phrase, "create our own reality." You didn't give yourself breast cancer, and you won't help your healing by feeling guilty.

COPING: WHAT TO TELL YOUR CHILDREN

A particularly trying issue people face is the question of what to tell their children. Again, it's an individual decision, and there are no hard-and-fast rules. I do think, in general, it's wise to be honest with your kids and use the scary word "cancer." If they don't hear it from you now, they're bound to find out some other way—they'll overhear a conversation when you assume they're out of the room, or a friend or neighbor inadvertently says something. And when they hear it that way, in the form of a terrible secret they were never supposed to know, it will be a lot more horrifying for them. By talking about it openly with them, you can demystify it. In addition, if all goes well, your children learn about survival after cancer. Kids need to know they can trust you—you don't want to do anything to violate that trust. It's a two-way communication; remember to listen to their fears. If you find it difficult to bring up the subject, there are children's books that can help you begin.

How you tell them, of course, depends on the ages of the children and their emotional vulnerability. With a little child you can say, "I have cancer, but we were lucky and caught it early, and the doctors are going to help me get better soon." What younger kids need to know is that you're going to be there to take care of them, that you won't suddenly disappear. They also need to know that the changes in your life aren't their fault. All kids get angry at their parents, and they often say or think things like "I wish you were dead." When a parent suddenly has a serious illness, the child may well see it as a result of those hostile words or thoughts. They must be told very directly that they did not cause the cancer by any thoughts, words, anger, dreams, or wishes. Your children will also be affected in other ways. You may be gone for a few days in the hospital and will need to rest when you come home. You may be getting daily radiation treatments, which consume a lot of your time and leave you tired and lethargic. You may be having chemotherapy treatments that make you sick to your stomach. Your children need to know that the alteration in your behavior and your restricted accessibility to them aren't happening because you don't love them or because they've been bad and this is their punishment. In short, your children need honest, age-appropriate information and assurance that it is okay to talk—or not—about your breast cancer.

Some surgeons encourage their patients to bring young children to the examining room. I found that it could be very helpful for a daughter in particular to see me examining her mother. If you're being treated with radiation or chemotherapy in a center where your children are permitted to see the treatment areas, it's a good idea to bring them along once or twice. The environments aren't intimidating, and a child who doesn't know what's happening to you in the hospital can conjure up awful images of what "those people" are doing to Mommy.

It is also important to be careful about changes in your older children's roles at home. You don't want to lean too heavily on them to perform the tasks you are unable to do; on the other hand, you want to give kids things they can do that make them feel useful. Wendy Schain, a psychologist and breast cancer survivor, and David Wellisch, a psychologist I worked with at UCLA, did a study on daughters of women who had had breast cancer. They found that the daughters who had the most psychological problems in later life were the ones who had been in puberty when their mothers were diagnosed. This was in part because their own breasts were developing at a time when their mothers' breasts were a source of problems. But interestingly enough, that wasn't the major reason for their problems. Far more damaging was the fact that they were expected to perform many of the mother's traditional household tasks. They were physically capable of this work, but they were not psychologically able to cope with the responsibility and they felt guilty about their resentment.[4]

Hester Hill Schnipper, a clinical social worker, points out that it is important not to make promises that you may not be able to keep. It is a mistake to promise kids, for example, that the cancer won't kill their parent. Instead, if your child asks, "Will you die?" you can reply, "I expect to live for a very long time and die as an old person. The doctors are taking good care of me, and I am taking good care of myself, and I hope to live for years and years."

Judi Hirshfield-Bartek, a clinical nurse specialist in Boston, usually recommends to couples that the partner take the kids out for some special time together. This gives them a chance to ask questions they may be afraid to ask their parent with cancer and know they'll get honest answers. A close relative or friend can also do this.

Frightening as it can be for kids to know that their parent has a life-threatening illness, if you're honest and matter-of-fact with them, chances are it won't be too traumatizing. One of my patients decided when she learned about her breast cancer that she would demystify the process for her seven- and ten-year-old daughters by showing them a prosthesis (artificial breast) and explaining what it would be used for. The next day she came into my office for her appointment. When I asked her how her experiment worked, she started to giggle. "Well, they certainly weren't intimidated by it. They listened very carefully to my explanation—and then started playing Frisbee with it!"

Breast cancer has particularly complex ramifications for a mother and her daughter. Aside from the normal fears any child has to deal with, a daughter may worry about whether this will happen to her too. It's not a wholly unfounded fear. As I explained in Chapter 4, there is a genetic component to breast cancer. You need to reassure your daughter, explain to her that it isn't inevitable, but as she gets older she should learn about her breasts and, like everyone, have them checked.

Often teenage daughters of my patients came to talk with me about their mother's breast cancer and their fears for themselves. It can be very useful to a girl to have her mother's surgeon help her put the dangers she faces into perspective, and it may be worth asking your surgeon to meet with your daughter. This may also be useful years later if your daughter does develop problems—she's already built a relationship with a breast specialist, and she's more likely to seek treatment with confidence and a minimum of terror.

Often daughters find themselves feeling angry at their mothers, as though the mother created her own breast cancer and thus made her daughter vulnerable to it. Mothers often react the same way; their feeling that they caused their own cancer expands into guilt over their daughter's increased risk. Often patients would say to me, "What have I done to my daughter?" These feelings need to be faced and dealt with. Without openness, the cancer can become a scapegoat for all the other unresolved issues between the mother and daughter, putting the relationship at risk.[5]

It's a good idea to let the people at your child's school know about your illness. That way if the child begins acting out or showing other problems, the school knows what's going on.

COPING: MALE BREAST CANCER

Men diagnosed with breast cancer undergo much of the same psychological angst, tests, and procedures as women (see Chapter 12), but with the stigma of having what is considered a female disease. Because it is so rare—less than 1 percent of all breast cancers are male—society generally reacts with surprise at a man with the disease. "Even after my diagnosis and surgery, I called it 'chest cancer,'" said Michael Singer on the Cancer.net blog.[6] Receiving social support from family and friends is essential. Small published studies of men with the disease describe the anxiety and defensiveness they feel with terms like "defensive functioning" and "repressive coping."[7] Groups like the Male Breast Cancer Global Alliance (www.inspire.com/groups/male-breast -cancer/) can create a sense of community and solidarity online when cases are so rare.

COPING: YOUR LOVED ONE'S FEARS

Spouses, partners, or lovers of people with breast cancer also have feelings that need to be acknowledged. They worry that their loved one may die and about how best to show their concern. Should they initiate sex, or would that be seen as callous and insensitive? Should they refrain, or would that be seen as a loss of attraction to their partner sexually?

The cancer is affecting your whole family, not just you. While you're in treatment, you focus chiefly on yourself. But as soon as possible you need to deal with how it's affecting those closest to you. Sometimes couples therapy with your spouse, or family therapy with your spouse and children, can help. They too are feeling frightened, angry, depressed, maybe even rejected if all your attention is going to your illness, and they may not have as much support for their feelings as you do for yours. It's crucial to communicate with one another at this time, to work through the complex feelings you're all facing.

SEARCHING FOR INFORMATION

Because many patients these days want to know as much as possible, I've set up a website, www.drsusanloveresearchfoundation.org, where new information is posted as it emerges. The Internet is a wonderful source of information, but you need to be a savvy surfer. If you are searching there, make sure you follow a few guidelines.

1. Know the site's sponsor and whether it has anything to gain from the information given. For example, a site sponsored by a pharmaceutical company may have good information but may be biased toward its own drugs. Some of the sites pushing alternative therapies are also selling them.

2. Know who is answering questions or giving medical advice. Is it someone you have heard of? What are their credentials? Are they an expert in breast care? You can get good advice from other people with breast cancer on the bulletin boards, but you don't know if their experience is standard or if they have an axe to grind.

3. Check who wrote the information on the site and when it was last updated.

4. Look to see if the information is backed up by references in scientific journals.

5. If information that you get on a site disagrees with what your doctor says, print out the page and bring it to your doctor for discussion.

The same provisos can be applied to books and articles.

WHAT TO LOOK FOR IN A DOCTOR AND MEDICAL TEAM

When we are sick, we are largely socialized not to question authority. A good place to begin is to put together a questionnaire that will help you assess your potential doctor or medical team. This doesn't have to be an actual document, but if it helps keep your thoughts, questions, and needs organized and concise, there's nothing wrong with putting pen to paper.

What are some of the things you will want to include? The items may vary a bit from person to person, based on insurance coverage (or lack thereof), diagnosis, and so on. The following questions will give you a good start:

DO THEY LISTEN? We all know doctors are busy, pulled in many directions, and pressed for time. When you are dealing with people you may otherwise find intimidating, you may be a bit reluctant to make demands. But remember, they are people just like you, and you can bet they'd want someone to pay close attention if they were in your shoes. Never lose sight of this fact—and don't choose a doctor who has.

DO THEY SIT DOWN, LOOK YOU IN THE EYE, AND CONNECT WITH YOU? You should expect your doctors to hear you. As a way of showing they are listening and caring, it is not unusual for doctors to pull up a chair and sit face-to-face while discussing your diagnosis and treatment options. You need to feel that your doctor sees you as a person.

DO THEY SOLICIT AND ANSWER YOUR QUESTIONS? If only one of you is doing the talking, there's a problem. You will want to make certain that your doctor not only answers any questions you may have but also provides you with information that allows you to make decisions or shows you where to look for the answers.

DO THEY SHOW YOU YOUR X-RAYS AND TEST REPORTS AND EXPLAIN THEM IF YOU ASK? Each of us has a comfort level when it comes to facing what lies ahead in terms of surgery, adjuvant therapies, prognosis, and possibilities. You may want to know every detail. If this is the case, you should expect the doctor you select to explain tests and procedures you will be undergoing. However, you should decide in advance how much you really want to know. Some of us need the hard, fast facts; others just want a broad overview; still others want only the information needed to take their first step. One size does not fit all, so feel free to ask about anything that comes to mind.

DO THEY ALLOW YOU TO RECORD THE VISIT OR BRING SOMEONE CLOSE TO TAKE NOTES? Because you may be nervous or frightened— or simply because you may be asking questions that require lengthy or complicated answers—you may want to record conversations with your doctor. Don't be afraid to ask. But bear in mind that some health care practices have policies restricting it. An alternative is to bring a close friend or family member to take notes. It is a great way to make sure you aren't missing anything important. It provides you with the opportunity to review what you discussed, and also allows you to absorb what was said at your own pace, in your own time. See if there are portals that patients can access to view shared records and notes. If your doctor dismisses all these options up front, you should consider whether this is someone you feel safe and confident with, or if it's time to move on.

DO THEY ASK YOU ABOUT YOUR USE OF ALTERNATIVE AND COMPLEMENTARY THERAPIES? In this day and age, it is not uncommon for people with breast cancer to seek out therapies that may be considered outside the realm of Western medicine. A growing number of patients feel they need to approach the cancer on more than one level. You may try acupuncture, massage, Chinese herbs, Reiki therapy, vitamins, or many other therapies currently labeled alternative or complementary. Your doctor should want to know about them and may have useful advice about things such as combinations of herbs or vitamins and mainstream drugs that may be helpful or should be avoided. You want to pay close attention to reactions when you discuss any therapies you may be trying or want to try. If your doctor dismisses these therapies without evidence that they are harmful or ineffective, you may want to leave that doctor and find one who acknowledges that alternative treatments can help your physical and emotional well-being. Many women feel that having the option of an alternative therapy provides them with a sense of control when everything else seems to be out of their hands. However, always be skeptical of practitioners who promise a cure, ask for large amounts of money for treatment, or make statements that simply sound too good to be true (see Chapter 18).

DO THEY SUGGEST ADDITIONAL SOURCES OF EDUCATION AND SUPPORT? Ideally, your doctor will present you with brochures, pamphlets, and the names of books and other resources designed not only to assist you in making decisions about your treatment options but also to help you regain your equilibrium. You are going to need information that allows you to ask questions when you need to, talk to other people who have faced what you are going through, educate yourself about your specific type of breast cancer, and even have a shoulder to cry on once in a while. You should see a red flag if you are given a diagnosis, told you need surgery, and then sent home to prepare without any of the resources mentioned.

DO THEY SEEM TO FEEL THREATENED WHEN YOU BRING INFORMATION FROM THE MEDIA TO DISCUSS? Although not every bit of information you retrieve from the Internet, magazines, newspapers, and so on may be relevant, it's imperative that your doctor be willing to evaluate what you find, discuss it with you, and assist you in making decisions. Procedures, drugs, and information are changing so rapidly that you may stumble on an article, a web page, or even information in a chat room that could have a profound effect on your treatment—and that your doctor may not have heard about. A good doctor won't be threatened by this sort of information but will want to help you interpret it.

DO YOU FEEL THAT THEY ARE PARTNERS IN THIS PROCESS? Although no one else can travel the emotional, physical, or psychological path you will be following, it is important that your doctors convey a sincere aura of understanding, support, and partnering. You should feel that any decision you reach is one both of you can agree on, discuss honestly, and then act on in a spirit of hope and possibility.

DO THEY DISCUSS CLINICAL TRIALS? A clinical trial (sometimes called a protocol or study) is designed to decide whether a new drug or procedure is an effective treatment for a disease or has possible benefit to the patient. These trials give doctors and researchers an opportunity to gather information on the benefits, side effects, and potential applications for new drugs, as well as help them determine which doses and combinations of existing drugs are most effective.

DO THEY CLEARLY EXPLAIN HOW THEY, OR SOMEONE COVERING FOR THEM, CAN BE REACHED 24/7? DO THEY TELL YOU WHETHER THEY PREFER PHONE CALLS OR EMAILS AND APPROXIMATELY HOW LONG YOU MAY HAVE TO WAIT FOR A RESPONSE? You need to know how to reach them or their associates and not have to worry whether you are annoying them. Clearly establishing the best means of communication is critical to your care.

HOW DO THEY FEEL ABOUT SECOND OPINIONS? Exploring the options often means getting a second opinion. Some people assume this is just a confirmation of the treatment plan chosen. Often patients came to see me with their surgery scheduled for the next day and became upset if I disagreed with their doctor's plan. But that is the risk you take. As anyone reading this book knows, the treatment of breast cancer is far from straightforward. A second opinion may well be different from the first; having to think about what both doctors have said and make a decision can be extremely stressful. You feel very insecure because your life is on the line and no one seems to know what to do. But the truth is that there are choices. There are different ways to approach the problem and there is no one right answer. Although there may be more evidence at this point supporting one choice or another, it is still your decision. Even getting a third opinion may not prevent the uncertainty. We would all like to believe that there is some objective truth—one right way to treat diseases. But this is often not the case.

Sometimes patients are shy about seeking a second opinion, as though they're somehow insulting their doctor's professionalism. Never feel that way. You're not insulting us; you're simply seeking the most precise information possible in what may literally be a life-and-death situation. Most doctors won't be offended—and if you run into a doctor who does get miffed, don't be intimidated. Your life, and your peace of mind, are more important than your doctor's ego.

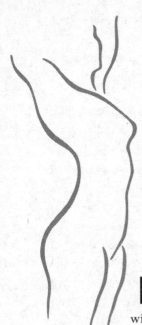

CHAPTER 10

What Kind of Breast Cancer Do I Have?

M ost of you who are reading this book are doing so because you or a loved one has been diagnosed with breast cancer. Face it—most people don't pick up this book out of idle curiosity or for a good beach read. You need to know what's going on with your cancer. I decided to put the chapter on diagnosis first, as that is the first thing that happens, and then the chapter on coping with it emotionally, and now this chapter on finding out what kind of cancer it is.

This chapter will help you sort out your pathology report and also discuss the key questions you'll want to ask your doctors so you can sort out the decisions you will need to make. Then in the next chapters we'll expand on the different situations and different kinds of cancers and their ramifications for treatment. A lot of new vocabulary will be coming at you—don't let that intimidate you. You'll only have to read what is relevant to your situation. My plan is that after reading the next several chapters you will be able to understand the nature of your cancer and, thus, the options available to you.

First ask your doctor for a copy of the pathology report from your needle/core biopsy, lumpectomy, or mastectomy for your records. If the doctor doesn't give it to you, call the pathology department in the hospital where you had the procedure and ask for a copy. Once you have it, sit down with the next section of this book; it will help you translate your report from medicalese into terms you can understand. If you haven't had your surgery yet, there will be a second pathology report once it is done (lumpectomy or mastectomy and sentinel node or node dissection).

It will be a variation on this same theme. It too will be worth obtaining and reading.

HOW TO INTERPRET A PATHOLOGY REPORT

First we will talk about the report from the diagnostic core biopsy that was used to diagnose your cancer. Most of the discussion is also applicable to the report from a lumpectomy or mastectomy as well. In the lumpectomy or mastectomy report, the pathologist has more than a small sample of the tumor to examine. And the lymph node report could be from a needle biopsy or a surgical removal. Regardless, the terminology and interpretations are pretty much the same.

The pathologist is a doctor who specializes in looking at tissue under the microscope. Your surgeon should select a pathologist who has had a lot of experience in diagnosing breast cancer. The language of a pathologist's report can be puzzling and intimidating, and for this reason you should always discuss the report with your surgeon or oncologist. The pathologist normally targets the report to the referring or treating physician and not directly to the patient. But if you still have questions, you can ask the pathologist to answer them. Don't be shy about this: addressing patients' questions is part of any doctor's job.

Some reports start with a summary (it should be labeled *Summary*), but most begin by describing what the pathologist received from the surgeon. It includes measurements and comments on the appearance of the tissue. We call this a *gross description*, in the sense of the word "gross" that means "obvious"—they need to see how the fresh tissue looks to the trained naked eye. The gross description is different from the *microscopic description*, which tells how the tissue looks magnified forty to four hundred times under the microscope after it has been chemically processed, sectioned, and placed on glass slides.

The pathologist looking at the tissue can usually tell whether breast cancer is present and, if it is, what kind of breast cancer you have. I say *usually* because sometimes a core biopsy gets only a small piece of the lesion. In this situation the pathologist can report only on what is there. It is important to remember this when reading a pathology report. The pathologist may say that the tumor is *widespread*, creating an alarming

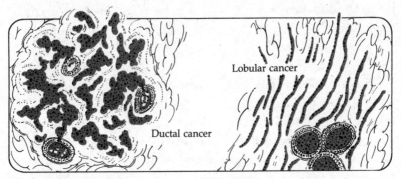

Figure 10.1

image of cancer all over your breast. But in fact, it just means the tumor is widespread *in the small piece of tissue* that's under the microscope, obtained by a needle. However, the pathologist may say that the tumor is small or *focal*; this reflects only what is in the tissue piece removed, which is usually, but not always, representative of what is in your breast.

Further, there are limitations in terms of the kind of cancer the pathologist sees in that one piece of tissue. Most breast cancers are *heterogeneous*—several different types of breast cancer can coexist. The cells are not all alike. It is possible for the biopsy to look like one type of cancer and the lumpectomy or mastectomy to show that other types are also present in the same tumor. When you read your pathology report, remember that a report based on a biopsy may not tell the whole story. Still, it can usually tell if you have cancer—and that is where we will start.

The report then offers a description of what the pathologist can see under the microscope. All breast cancer begins in the lining of the milk ducts. Some cancers originate from the duct cells themselves and others from the lobules that populate the ends of the ducts like leaves at the ends of tree branches. Thus, your cancer will probably be described as either ductal carcinoma or lobular carcinoma (Figure 10.1), indicating whether the cells look like they came from the duct or the lobule. Some cancers contain elements of both ducts and lobules and are considered mixed cancers. Next, the report will say whether the cancer is invasive. If the cancer is not invasive, it is called *intraductal carcinoma* or *ductal carcinoma in situ* or *lobular carcinoma in situ* or even *noninvasive carcinoma* (Figure 10.2). As we mentioned earlier, noninvasive means the cells are contained and have not grown outside the duct or lobule where the cancer started and into the surrounding tissue. Invasive, or infiltrating, means it has gotten out of the duct or lobule. In this case the report will read either *invasive ductal (or lobular) carcinoma* or *infiltrating ductal (lobular) carcinoma*. This can sound scary—has your cancer spread to the rest of your body? But that isn't what it means. The pathologist has only a piece of breast to look at and is describing only that small piece; they cannot tell whether something has spread beyond the breast. Sometimes both cancer and noninvasive material are present in one lump, and the report may read *infiltrating ductal carcinoma with an intraductal component*. It is important to remember that the initial biopsy may only show part of the cancer—for example, the in situ component—and it is not until the cancer is entirely removed that the pathologist can fully describe the whole tumor.

Oncologist Stephanie Graff, one of our medical advisors, tells patients that a needle biopsy is a little bit like putting a needle in a chocolate chip cookie. "You may get cookie, you may get chocolate chip, you may get pecan—but it doesn't mean it isn't a chocolate chip cookie. It simply means needles are small. If the needle were a little to the left or a little to the right, we might find the other part of the cookie. So until the final surgery, we can't tell what all the ingredients are."

Because lobules and ducts are kinds of glands and the medical term meaning "related to a gland" is "adeno," sometimes these cancers are called *adenocarcinomas*. People can be confused by this term, thinking it's a different kind of cancer. In reality, it's just a broader category—like calling someone from Los Angeles a Californian.

An infiltrating ductal cancer forms a hard, firm lump because the neighborhood or surrounding tissue will cause scar tissue (fibrosis) around the cells as well as some reaction. This scar tissue is called *desmoplasia*. Infiltrating lobular cancer, however, is sneaky. It sends individual

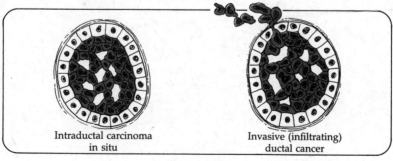

Intraductal carcinoma in situ	Invasive (infiltrating) ductal cancer

Figure 10.2

cells in little fingerlike projections (cells extending in a single-file line) out into the tissues without inciting a lot of desmoplastic reaction around them, and so you may feel it as a little thickening rather than a hard lump, or you may not feel it at all (Figure 10.3). For this reason it's harder for surgeons to tell whether they've got all the lobular cancer out: the little projections can't be felt as easily as a hard lump. Because lobular cancers elicit less scarring, they tend to grow to larger sizes (average five centimeters or almost two inches) than ductal carcinoma (average two centimeters or a little under an inch) before they are detected. The prognosis is based on size *and* type of cancer. Infiltrating lobular cancers are almost always sensitive to hormones (see the following discussion) and seem to be more common in people who have taken hormone replacement therapy. In addition, there's a slightly higher tendency for lobular cancer to occur in the other breast at a later time. Although an infiltrating ductal cancer has about a 15 percent chance of occurring in the other breast over your lifetime, a lobular cancer has about a 20 percent chance—an increase in risk but not an overwhelming one.[1]

Other names for cancers may also appear on the pathologist's report. For the most part they're variations on invasive ductal cancer, named by the pathologist according to the visual appearance of the cells under the microscope. *Tubular* cancer, in which the cancer cells look like little tubes, is very unusual—1 to 2 percent of breast cancers—and generally

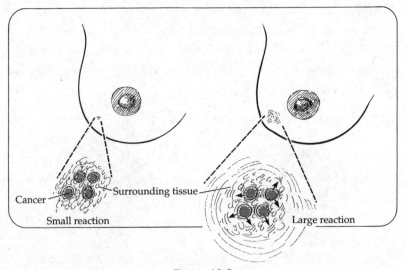

Figure 10.3

less aggressive. *Medullary carcinoma* resembles the color of brain tissue (the medulla), though it has nothing to do with the brain. *Mucinous* (or *colloid*) *carcinoma* is a form of infiltrating ductal cancer that makes a kind of gluey-looking material ("colloid" is the Greek word for "glue"). *Papillary carcinoma* has cells that stick out in little fronds (fingerlike projections). These special cancers tend to have a better prognosis than do typical invasive ductal or lobular cancers, but they are treated according to the same principles. Other types of cancer, such as inflammatory or cystosarcoma phyllodes, are a different matter. These we will discuss in Chapter 12.

After deciding what kind of cancer you have, the pathologist studies the appearance of the cells further to try to predict how aggressively the particular type of cancer will behave—like trying to pick out the criminal in a lineup by how they are dressed. Sometimes the lawbreaker is the guy in the three-piece suit rather than the scruffy-looking dude. Needless to say this isn't 100 percent accurate, which is why it is combined with an analysis of the molecular biology of the tumor—looking at the DNA of the suspects to be sure which one is the culprit.

The pathologist will describe any wild-looking (*poorly differentiated*) cells, which tend to behave more aggressively, whereas the cells that look more normal (*well differentiated*) are usually better behaved (see Figure 10.4). The cells in between are called *moderately differentiated*. But poorly differentiated cells aren't a sign of doom—the fact that they look wild doesn't guarantee that they will act that way or can't be treated. Most breast cancers are either moderately or poorly differentiated, and yet many patients who have these cells do fine.

Another thing the pathologist looks for is how many cells are dividing and how actively they're doing it; this is known as *mitotic rate* or activity. The most aggressive cancers tend to have a lot of cells dividing at the same time because they're growing rapidly. Less aggressive cancers tend to have fewer dividing cells. Another feature indirectly related to tumor growth and differentiation is the *nuclear grade*. The nucleus of the cell is the part that contains the DNA, so the grade gives you an idea of how abnormal the DNA looks. Pathologists usually grade on a scale of 1 to 3 or 1 to 4, with the higher number being worse (see Figure 10.4).

The pathologist will also look for cancer cells inside a blood vessel or lymphatic vessel. If there are any, it's called *vascular invasion*, *lymphatic invasion*, or *lymphovascular invasion*, and sometimes even *neural (nerve) invasion*. This too suggests that the cancer is potentially more dangerous.

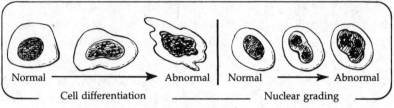

Figure 10.4

In addition, the pathologist sometimes counts the number of blood or lymph vessels associated with the tumor. This is because tumors secrete substances that cause blood vessels to grow, a process called *angiogenesis* or *lymphangiogenesis* (growth of new lymphatics). A lot of blood vessels may indicate that the tumor is growing rapidly and, thus, is more aggressive. I noticed that if I was operating on a lump I thought was benign and there was significantly more bleeding than I would have expected, it was often the tip-off that the lump was cancerous. Another sign we look for is *necrosis*, or dead cells. This usually can mean the cancer is growing so rapidly that it has outgrown its blood supply (Figure 10.5). The pathologist checks all these factors to get as much information as possible about the cancer. All are useful to help determine the nature of the cancer cells, but none are 100 percent perfect at predicting behavior. Usually all these observations are combined as a score. One commonly used scoring system is the Nottingham histologic score, otherwise known as the modified Bloom-Richardson score. (I know, it's hard enough to take in even one name, and then they have to go around and invent a second one. It reminds me of one of those medieval novels where there's a guy named Edgar, Duke of Buckingham, and you're never sure who he is because one moment they're talking about Edgar and on the next page they're talking about Buckingham and you have to stop and figure out who Buckingham is. Medicine is like that.) The score is based on three features: degree of tubule formation (well-formed tubules are better than poorly formed ones, as you might expect), nuclear grade (regularity in the size, shape, and staining character of the nuclei, with small being better than large), and mitotic activity or cell division (no or little mitosis is good, and much mitosis is not as good). Each of these gets a score of 1, 2, or 3, with the higher number reflecting poor tubules, large nuclei, and high mitotic rate. The scores are then added up: 3 to 5 is grade one, 6 to 7 is grade two, 8 to 9 is grade three. Grade 3 is the highest and supposedly the most

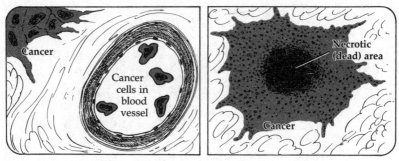

Figure 10.5

aggressive. (Be careful not to confuse grade with stage—grade describes the appearance of the cancerous cells, while stage focuses on tumor size and spread.) Unfortunately all these features are very subjective. A comparison of different pathologists' Nottingham or Bloom-Richardson scores on the same cancer showed that they agreed only 75 percent of the time. If you see a Nottingham or Bloom-Richardson score on your report, you will know what it is and you will also know that it is just a way to quantify how the tumor looked.

The pathologist's next job is to try to determine if the tumor has been completely removed. These days almost all cancers are diagnosed with a core biopsy, so it is understood that the tumor has not been completely removed. However, if you are reading the pathology report from your lumpectomy or mastectomy, this will be a key point. Margins are evaluated by a very imprecise technique. Ink is painted all around the outside of the sample before it is cut up and fixed, and slides are made. If the slides show cancer cells next to the ink, this means there's cancer on the outer border and presumably some left in the patient. If there are cancer cells only in the middle, away from the ink, there is a *clean margin* (Figure 10.6). So the report may say *The margins are uninvolved with tumor*, or *The margins are involved with tumor*, or *The margins are indeterminate*. If the lump has been taken out in more than one piece, we usually can't tell whether the margins are clean. Some surgeons remove the lump or area in question and then remove an extra rim of tissue at each edge as if the tumor were a cube. They send these additional pieces to the pathologist labeled as *superior* (toward the head), *inferior* (toward the feet), *medial* (toward the middle), *lateral* (toward the side), *anterior* (toward the skin), and *posterior* or *deep* (toward the chest wall). The pathologist comments on these sections separately in the report. The idea is that

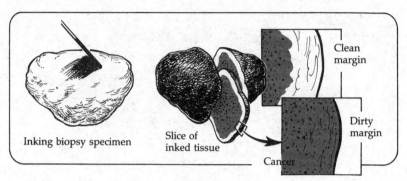

Inking biopsy specimen

Slice of
inked tissue

Cancer

Clean
margin

Dirty
margin

Figure 10.6

if a margin is involved, the surgeon knows where to go back and take more tissue. It is important to realize that there are enormous sampling problems with this approach. We can only do representative sections of the margin; to get them all, we'd have to make thousands of slides. So when we say the margins are clean, we're only making an educated guess—we can't be 100 percent sure. (See Chapter 12 for a discussion of margins and DCIS.)

Margins are often misunderstood as a black-and-white type of test rather than simply a predictor of the amount of cancer that may remain in the patient's breast. We ink the tumor's margins, but ink can sometimes run, and drawing on breast tissue is about as neat as drawing on a paper towel. A lumpectomy that shows just one spot of cancer at a margin suggests that there is not a lot of disease behind, while one with a lot of cancer throughout it and several "dirty" margins probably indicates that there is more disease left in the patient. Most guidelines[2] now agree that the definition of a clean margin is "no ink on tumor." In other words, as long as there are a few cells between the cancer cells and normal cells, it is okay. We know this based on a lot of clinical studies that have demonstrated that the additional treatment such as radiation, hormones, and chemotherapy are perfectly capable of taking care of a few cells that may be left behind, just not large clumps. So close margins are okay.

If the pathology report includes the sentinel node biopsy or axillary dissection, then it will describe how many nodes were removed as well as their size and shape. If there are cancer cells seen in a node, they will be described by size. If the pathologist is not sure whether the cells they are seeing are cancer, they may do special stains to see whether they can confirm it. This too will be described. Sometimes pathologists use the terms "metastatic focus" or "metastatic disease" in describing a lymph node. Don't panic if you see this. Strictly speaking, the word "metastatic" means that there are breast cancer cells outside their organ of origin. Clinicians, however, are more likely to use the term when the disease has spread outside its region—not in the adjacent lymph nodes or chest wall, but in the liver, lungs, or bones. But the pathologist sees only the bit of biopsied tissue, and none of the other parts of the body. Also, the mere presence of cancer cells in a lymph node is no cause for alarm. Lymph nodes that contain single isolated tumor cells or small clumps of tumor cells, so-called micrometastases, may not signify any worse behavior than if they are completely negative.[3]

The summary will also say how many nodes were positive for cancer and how many altogether were removed—for example, *one of two sentinel nodes removed showed cancer*.

Some of the things I've described aren't easy to see on the slides. Identification can be somewhat subjective: Are these cells bizarre-looking enough? Are they invading other structures? It's worth getting a second opinion. Often the pathologists themselves will ask other pathologists on the staff to look at the slides and give their opinions. If you live in a small town with a small hospital, you may want your slides sent to a big university center, where someone sees a lot of breast pathology. You can call the university hospital's pathology department and arrange to have them look at your slides, then call your hospital and have the slides sent. Make sure it is the slides themselves they send, since that's what the second pathologist needs to see, not just the first pathologist's written interpretation. And, yes, they still use physical slides. You need to get the best information possible to decide what course of treatment to pursue.

In the digital age, getting a second opinion can be facilitated by having your original slides scanned into "virtual" slides and sent anywhere in the world through the Internet. Centers are emerging with this capability.

Biomarkers

The pathologist's work doesn't end with these slides. The next step is studying and reporting on the molecular markers, also known as biomarkers. These tests often take longer to do than looking at the slides, and so they may come back later than the original report informing you that you have cancer. Although most of these markers are done only on invasive tumors, we are increasingly using them in the treatment of non-invasive tumors as well. The markers are classified into three categories: (1) ones that are used to help determine the prognosis of a particular cancer (how life-threatening it is), (2) ones that are used to predict whether a cancer will respond to a certain treatment, and (3) ones that do both. These markers can be used to classify tumors into the molecular subgroups that dictate both the kind of tumor and the best treatment for it, as we will discuss later in this chapter.

I'll discuss the biomarkers that are most frequently reported and used in all three categories. Remember, however, that these are just more ways of describing your tumor—and a snapshot of the tumor at that! But the tumor sits in a body—yours—and how it will behave is as much dependent on that neighborhood, from your immune system to your hormone levels and even some genetic factors we have yet to determine. There are days when I could be described as a disheveled older woman in jeans. That does not mean that I can't clean up and do an interview on CNN if needed. First impressions can be deceiving!

The most common analysis is one that explores the estrogen and progesterone receptors to find out whether the tumor is sensitive to these hormones (Figure 10.7). The report will tell you that the tumor is estrogen-receptor-positive or -negative (ER-positive or ER-negative) and progesterone-receptor-positive or -negative (PR-positive or PR-negative). More often than not, the report will include the percentage of positive

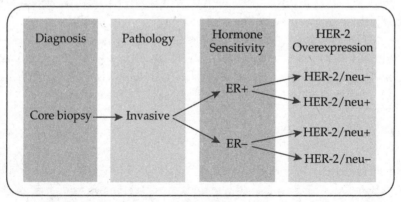

Figure 10.7

cells. Tumors lacking both estrogen and progesterone receptors are not sensitive to those hormones and are called ER- and/or PR-negative. This is not necessarily bad.

The implications of the hormone receptor tests are both prognostic and predictive. In general, tumors that are sensitive to hormones—that have receptors—are slightly slower growing and have a slightly better prognosis than tumors that aren't.[4] Generally postmenopausal people are more likely to be ER-positive, and premenopausal people are more likely to be ER-negative. Why premenopausal people who have a lot of estrogen get ER-negative tumors and why postmenopausal people and those who have reduced estrogen get ER-positive tumors is one of the great mysteries that remain unanswered. Further, the test tells whether the tumor can be treated with some kind of hormone-blocking therapy. As long as there are some positive cells, such therapy will have some response. If it's not sensitive to hormones, it rarely responds to hormone-blocking treatments (see Chapter 11) but still can be treated with chemotherapy and/or targeted therapies.

Another biomarker is overexpression (too many copies) of the HER2/neu oncogene, also known as erbB-2 (see Chapter 3, page 64). HER2/neu is one of the dominant oncogenes that contribute to cancer by telling cells to grow. Instead of being mutated, however, HER2/neu is frequently overexpressed and amplified: in other words, there are too many copies of the oncogene, so the intensity of the message telling the cells to grow is increased.[5] This occurs in about a fifth of invasive cancers. Having your tumor tested for the HER2/neu receptor is important because the test can function not only as a prognostic indicator (HER2/neu-positive tumors tend to be more aggressive) but also as an indicator of the best treatment. Several tests can be used for HER2/neu overexpression. One, *immunohistochemistry* (IHC), assesses whether there is more of the HER2 protein, whereas the other, *fluorescence in situ hybridization* (FISH), assesses whether there are too many copies of the actual gene. It is the difference between measuring the effect or the cause. Initially IHC was used, but later work indicated that FISH may be more precise in certain categories (2+ on IHC).[6] Generally tumors will first be tested by IHC as it is less expensive. If it is positive (3+), then the patient knows that their tumor is HER2/neu-positive. If the IHC test is negative or 1+ or 2+ out of a possible 3, it will usually be sent for FISH, which is more precise, to confirm that it is positive. If the FISH is negative (not amplified), then the cancer is considered negative for HER2, regardless of the IHC score.

As this edition was being updated, researchers have begun reframing this last group and considering a new category: HER2-low. This is when the IHC test comes back as 1+ or 2+, but the FISH is negative. Traditionally these cases were considered negative for HER2, although they still express HER2 to some degree. Now researchers are beginning to call them HER2-low and estimate that nearly 60 percent of patients have this kind of breast cancer.[7] Clinical trials focusing on HER2-low cancer have already produced positive results with a new drug combination called Enhertu (trastuzumab deruxtecan) in metastatic breast cancer.[8]

Herceptin (trastuzumab) alone is an effective drug that targets HER2/neu specifically. It is currently used in patients with HER2-positive cancers (see Chapter 11). Almost all DCIS is HER2/neu-positive, but this does not mean it should be treated with chemotherapy or Herceptin.[9] It is still precancer, growing only within the duct and not worth the risks of the drug (see Chapter 12).

Next, we try to figure out how rapidly the breast cancer cells are dividing (we call this being *proliferative*), based on the idea that the more they divide the more aggressive they must be.

More biomarkers are being discovered, but none were ready for prime time at the time we went to press.

When all these tests have been done, your tumor will be characterized in a description something like the following: *This is a stage II (T2): 2 centimeter, node-negative (N0), estrogen-receptor-positive (ER+), HER2/neu-amplified (HER2+) tumor* or *T2: N0, ER+, HER2+ or triple-positive.* (Note it is assumed that the tumor is progesterone-positive [PR+] if it is estrogen-positive [ER+].) Triple-negative is when the result is ER−, PR−, and HER2−; "triple-negative" is a poor choice of words but not one that necessarily means three times as bad (see Chapter 11). Other combinations are ER+, PR+, HER2−, and ER−, PR−, HER2+, which we will discuss at length in the next chapter.

MOLECULAR CLASSIFICATIONS

It is becoming clear that not all breast cancers are the same. Although we had suspected this for a long time, we had assumed that it all started with the same mutations and that the difference occurred over time when some tumors became more aggressive. We now know that there are at least five kinds of breast cancer that are different from the start, based on their specific mutations or molecular biology. There are probably more subgroups that await our discovery—and we're searching for them. Identifying these different kinds of cancer has allowed us to better determine the prognosis of each tumor and, even more importantly, to match the treatment to the type of tumor. This growing ability to personalize treatment means that it will both work better and limit the potential side effects to those that are absolutely unavoidable.

The most important tool in this regard has been the cDNA microarray analysis. This is done with a wonderful tool that new technology has enabled us to create. The *microarray* is a cDNA chip that gives researchers the astounding ability to look at the expression of hundreds of genes in hundreds of tumors at the same time. What we are actually looking at is the levels of messenger RNA (mRNA), the signal from the DNA to the protein that determines the expression levels of genes (see Chapter 3). When this tool is applied to the tumors of patients who participated in previous research, the patterns of gene expression can be associated with what we know has happened within the participant's body in the years since their study. The five main kinds of breast cancer identified by cDNA analysis correlate pretty well with the combinations of biomarkers noted in Table 10.1. These analyses are looking at *all* the cells in the tumor, which include both the cancer cells and the cells around it. Together they give us a picture of the conditions in which cancer has occurred.[10]

The most common types of breast cancer in Western countries are the luminal subtypes, so called because their genetic pattern is close to that of cells lining the lumen, the hollow center of the duct. The group is subdivided into luminal A and luminal B, and all are sensitive to estrogen. The rare occurrence of breast cancer in men (see Chapter 12) includes almost exclusively luminal A and luminal B.

Luminal A tumors generally have high levels of estrogen receptors, are HER2/neu-negative, and have little cell division. They comprise about 30 to 40 percent of breast tumors, and they generally have a good prognosis. Although we have not yet figured out the risk factors for the specific subtypes of breast cancer, it seems that most of the traditional hormonal risk factors (see Chapter 5) are predictors for the luminal A

Table 10.1 Luminal Subtypes

Molecular Markers	Hormone Receptors (ER/PR)	HER-2 Status	Tumor Grade
Luminal A	Positive	Not overexpressed	Low to intermediate (low recurrence score)
Luminal B	Positive	Not overexpressed	High (high recurrence score)
Triple positive	Positive	Overexpressed	Any
HER 2 neu type	Negative	Overexpressed	Any
Triple negative	Negative	Negative	Any

kind.[11] Luminal A cancers generally have a well-differentiated pathology. Many are the tubular cancers we described earlier in this chapter. These tumors are also more common in postmenopausal patients.

The luminal B tumors are less common, about 20 percent of breast cancers, and are still ER-positive, although less so than the luminal As. They also have more cell division and tend to be moderately or poorly differentiated.[12] Some classifications have designated a luminal C classification. These tumors correspond to infiltrating lobular carcinomas.

HER2/neu overexpressing tumors can be ER-positive or ER-negative, and they have their own groups. So you can be triple-positive (ER-positive, PR-positive, and HER2/neu-positive) or just HER2/neu-positive (HER2/neu-overexpressing but ER-negative and PR-negative). The HER2/neu-overexpressing ER-negative tumors have high rates of cell division and are more aggressive-looking. In the era before Herceptin was discovered, these tumors had a poor prognosis. Fortunately, targeted therapy using Herceptin has changed all that (see Chapter 11).

Another subtype is triple-negative breast cancer. I think this is an unfortunate designation because it sounds like these tumors are triply bad! In fact, *triple-negative* refers to the fact that the estrogen receptor, progesterone receptor, and HER2/neu are all negative. These

ER-negative breast cancers include but are not limited to the basal carcinomas.

Just to demonstrate how complicated this really is, in the mRNA analysis of these basal tumors we find a mixture of hormone-positive luminal genes and low levels of HER2/neu. They are dominated, however, by tumors with high levels of the proliferation genes that drive cell division. In addition, they have their own unique additional cluster of genes, which gives it its name, the basal cluster. Eighty percent of women who carry the mutation in BRCA 1 and develop breast cancer have the basal type of cancer.[13] However, most basal breast cancers are *not* in women with BRCA 1, which suggests that the BRCA pathway may be disrupted by acquired mutation rather than inherited. Interestingly, these tumors are more common among Black women of all ages and premenopausal people of all races. Though very aggressive, these tumors are also very sensitive to chemotherapy.[14] Generally the basal type of tumor is characterized by being triple-negative[15] (ER-negative, PR-negative, and HER2/neu-negative), but not all basal tumors are triple-negative. Their defining characteristic is that extra unique basal cluster of mutated genes. I should also point out that this key cluster is a research finding and is not routinely looked for in clinical practice because we don't have an easy way to do it. So don't expect to see it mentioned on your pathology report. Finally, there is the overlapping triple-negative group, 70 percent of which will not have the basal cluster. Both of these groups represent a therapeutic challenge because they do not offer specific molecular targets. Luckily they respond very well to chemotherapy.

Obviously this is not only complicated stuff but still a work in progress. I would not be surprised if there were several more groups or subgroups that are uncovered over the next few years. I spent some time delineating them because you will hear these terms and need to recognize where they come from. Not only are they helpful in estimating your prognosis, but, as you will see in the next chapter, they play a key role in predicting which treatment will be best for you. Once you have reviewed the three main markers (ER, PR, and HER2/neu) in your pathology report, you will have a pretty good idea of whether you have a HER2/neu overexpressing tumor, a triple-negative tumor, or a luminal one. Although this may sound hopelessly arcane to you now, it will help you sort out the decisions ahead of you.

COMMERCIAL TESTS

Another approach to identifying different types of tumors and matching the therapies has come from commercial tests of patterns of gene expression based on a limited sampling of genes, whereas the molecular classification discussed previously is based on an analysis of ten thousand genes. Although there are overlaps with the types of tumors, these tests have actually been validated and in some situations actually can predict the best therapy. The first such test to be clinically available, Oncotype DX, is from Genomic Health.[16] Scientists selected twenty-one genetic markers that held promise for both prognosis and prediction. They then developed a method to analyze these genes in fixed tissue (leftover tissue from a removed tumor that had already been used to make diagnostic slides). They first tested the genes on the tissue from a completed NSABP (National Surgical Adjuvant Breast and Bowel Project) study on women with ER-positive, node-negative tumors who were randomized between tamoxifen and placebo.[17] Because this study had been completed, they knew which participants had cancer that recurred within the ten-year follow-up. Their test was able to distinguish high-risk, low-risk, and intermediate-risk groups from supposedly good prognostic tumors. The high-risk group had a 30 percent chance of recurrence, whereas the low-risk group had a 6 percent chance. This recurrence score was more predictive of outcome than age or tumor size. In fact, they found some very small tumors that had a high chance of recurrence and some larger ones that did not. The value of the test has increased as it has been further applied to previous studies. By applying their test to women who had received chemotherapy in addition to tamoxifen, they showed that the high-risk group benefited significantly from chemotherapy, whereas the low-risk group did not. The benefit from tamoxifen was examined using this test in another retrospective study and showed that women with a low recurrence score and high estrogen receptor score got the biggest benefit from tamoxifen, whereas the women with a high recurrence score got none. More exciting are the data from node-positive, ER-positive women. The old "the worse the disease, the stronger the treatment needs to be" theory would suggest that these women all needed chemotherapy. However, when the Oncotype DX test was applied to these women, their prognosis looked just like the node-negative women's.[18] The ones with a lower recurrence score did better and responded very well to tamoxifen, whereas the ones with a high recurrence score had both a higher rate of recurrence and a better response to chemotherapy, suggesting that the biology of the tumor is more important at predicting prognosis and the best treatment than the stage of the cancer.

It reminds me of infections and antibiotics. Before we knew about bacteria, we would talk about tuberculosis and streptococcal pneumonia as if they were the same disease because they were both lung infections. In fact, they are very different, requiring different treatments and having different outcomes. We would not treat a really bad streptococci pneumonia with a higher dose of a tuberculosis drug and expect it to work. Similarly, if a breast cancer is one that has a low recurrence score that indicates that it's very sensitive to hormones, it makes no sense to give the patient chemotherapy, which it is not sensitive to. Some of you may wonder about the patients with an intermediate recurrence score. A large clinical trial called TAILORx concluded that most women in that group showed no benefit from receiving chemotherapy in addition to hormone therapy.[19] Furthermore, the current test does not address risk of recurrence in ER-negative cancers.

Oncotype DX is currently clinically available through Genomic Health. If you are interested, you have to ask your doctor to order it or your pathologist to send the fixed tissue or slides. Check in advance to see if your insurance will cover it.

An additional combination test from Europe (MammaPrint), based on the cDNA microarray discussed earlier, combined seventy genes to predict which women with stage I or stage II breast cancer who had not received chemotherapy developed metastases fourteen years later.[20] This test has been validated by a randomized controlled trial in Europe called MINDACT, which showed an excellent five-year metastasis-free survival rate in women with high clinical and low genomic risk who did not receive chemotherapy.[21] The advantage of this test is that there is no intermediate group, allowing the results to be more clear-cut. It has been approved by the U.S. Food and Drug Administration (FDA) for small to intermediate-size node-negative cancers regardless of hormonal status.

Both of these tests are available today, although you may have to ask your surgeon or oncologist to have the tissue sent for analysis. They can be very helpful in decision making. An older friend of mine called me to say that she had been diagnosed with ER-positive, node-positive breast cancer and was worried about getting chemotherapy as she had a history of heart disease. I was able to tell her to have her tumor tested for Oncotype DX. Her oncologist balked, saying that the test was only valid on patients with negative nodes. My friend was able to direct this oncologist to the latest study on node-positive patients and the test was done. It came back with a low recurrence score, indicating not only that she had a relatively low chance of recurrence but that chemotherapy would not help and hormone therapy was just fine. She was delighted. I think most patients with hormone-positive cancers should consider this test. Although it initially caused some controversy in the oncology community, the use of the Oncotype DX test is still growing a decade later as results provide valuable information for patient treatment and prognosis.[22] If the test comes out with a high recurrence score, then you can feel some reassurance that chemotherapy is worth it.

STAGING

The staging system is a bit of an anachronism. It is an attempt to categorize tumors in a way that helps predict the best approach to treatment and was developed before we had all the molecular markers to play with. It combines the microscopic aspects of the tumor that the pathology report addresses with clinical features of the tumor in a staging system. This classification system, known as the TNM (short for tumor, nodes, and metastasis), categorizes cases so that we can keep statistics and determine likely long-term survival rates that various treatments can create. The system is still used, but it is actually a holdover from the past. It doesn't fit very well with our current knowledge of biology because it is based only on the size of the tumor in the breast, the number of lymph nodes involved, and clinically detected spread to other organs. It is a static system based on a snapshot in time when we know that cancers are a dynamic disease in evolution. It is like looking at the students who cut classes in high school and predicting that they will grow up to be irresponsible in the workforce. Obviously other determinants of behavior (such as parenting, peer pressure, and health) also influence future performance. Similarly, other determinants of tumor behavior, such as the molecular biology of the tumor or its rate of growth—did it spread to the lymph nodes while small or after it had been around awhile?—are not reflected in the TNM classification system but are important in predicting prognosis and response to therapy. However, because the TNM system is still being used and you will probably be exposed to it, I'm including a summary of it here. Just keep its limitations in mind.

The system has been changed various times throughout the years. In an attempt to make it more relevant, a seventh version was introduced in 2010.[23] The major changes have to do with sentinel nodes and smaller tumors. I will provide a general overview of how it works and a look at the large classifications. In the appendix you'll find a check sheet to help you classify your own tumor.

In this system (Figure 10.8), the tumor size is first judged clinically, based on the surgeon's exam or an imaging modality such as mammography, ultrasound, CT scan, or MRI scan. If it's between zero and two centimeters, it's T1; between two and five centimeters, T2; above five centimeters, T3. Each of the T classifications can be further subdivided.

If it's ulcerating through the skin or stuck to the chest wall, it's T4. Again we have subgroups, with T4a when the tumor has spread to the chest wall; T4b when it has spread into the skin and the breast may be swollen; T4c when it has spread to both the skin and the chest wall and T4d when it is inflammatory breast cancer (see Chapter 12) and the overlying skin is red, swollen, and painful. Although the original tumor staging is based on the clinical estimate, it is further refined once the tumor has been removed surgically and examined pathologically so that the full extent of the cancer can be determined. This is called the pathological T stage and is based on the size of the invasive tumor only, without regard to its possible in situ component. If there is more than one tumor in the same breast, the largest of them is used for determining the T size. As we are diagnosing smaller and smaller tumors, subclassifications have been developed. *Tis* refers to in situ or noninvasive tumors as well as Paget's disease (see Chapter 12), while T1mic refers to micro-invasion 0.1 centimeter or smaller in the tumor's greatest dimension, T1a tumor between 0.1 centimeter and 0.5 centimeter, T1b tumor between 0.5 centimeter and 1 centimeter, and T1c tumor between 1 centimeter and 2 centimeters.

Then the lymph nodes are examined either by the surgeon or by an imaging test such as CT scan or ultrasound. If there are no palpable nodes, it's N0; if the surgeon feels nodes but thinks they're negative, it's N1a. If they're positive, it's N1b. If they're large and matted together, it's N2; if they're near the collarbone, it's N3. Nodes that cannot be

226

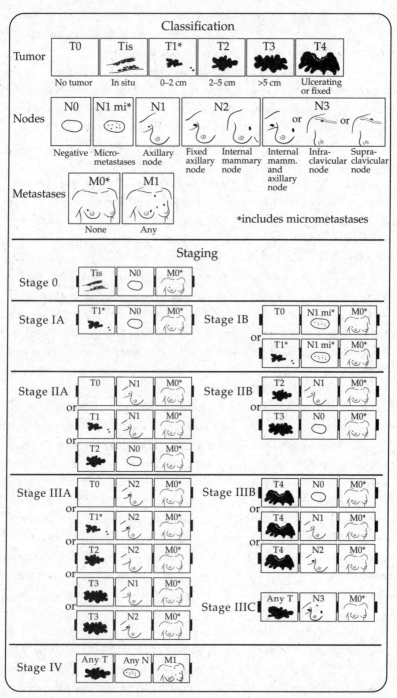

Figure 10.8

accurately accessed are termed Nx. Nodes are also reclassified once they are removed. With the increasing use of the sentinel node biopsy, this has been incorporated into the new staging system. For example, if only one or several clumps of cells of breast cancer are found in a lymph node based on IHC staining only (see Chapter 8) or RT-PCR (a technique to detect and quantify RNA) only, and they measure less than 0.2 milli-meter, they are considered isolated tumor cells and the nodes are still considered negative (pNi+). This is because we think a few cells may be dislodged during the procedure but that they have no long-term conse-quence; only cells that make it to the nodes on their own seem to count. But some researchers have been reexamining isolated tumor cells and are concluding that they may signal a poor disease outcome and should be considered when deciding on treatment.[24] Cancer deposits greater than 0.2 millimeter but less than 2 millimeters are considered micrometas-tasis and are termed pN1mi, whereas any bigger than 2 millimeters are considered pN1. The other change in the newer system is subdividing the nodes based on the number that are positive: pN1a for one to three positive nodes, pN1b for four to nine positive nodes, and pN1c for more than ten. These breakdowns are as much to help researchers collect data as they are to improve survival prognostications.

Finally, if an obvious metastasis has been discovered by any of the tests I'll describe shortly, it's M1; otherwise, it's M0. If we can't tell whether there is metastasis, we designate it Mx.

Then this information is combined into stage numbers. Stage I is a T1 tumor with no lymph nodes. Stage II is either a small tumor with positive lymph nodes or a tumor between two and five centimeters with nega-tive lymph nodes. (Sometimes this is designated as stage IIA.) Tumors between two and five centimeters with positive lymph nodes or tumors larger than five centimeters with negative lymph nodes are also stage II, but these latter types are designated stage IIB. Stage III is a large tumor with positive lymph nodes or a tumor with "grave signs." Stage IV is a tumor that has obvious metastasis.

The complexity of this system suggests that we still don't completely understand breast cancer. As we have seen in this chapter, the new tech-niques of DNA analysis are beginning to help us differentiate breast can-cers based on the specific mutations in each cancer and on which genes are either over- or underexpressed, and thus to determine more accu-rately both prognosis and treatment. We are still in a transition between molecular, biological, and traditional TNM classification. But in spite of its limitations, the TNM system gives us a conceptual framework for categorizing each case of breast cancer so that different treatments can be compared in the same types of patients.

Anatomical Staging

Before we had all these fancy molecular tests, we would stage breast cancer based on the anatomy. This was originally used to decide who was operable before the days of scans and circulating tumor cells (CTCs) that detach from a tumor and are detected in a patient's blood. Although anatomical staging is really less relevant today, we still use it in order to categorize the extent of disease.

The first level is based on how the cancer appears at diagnosis. Certain signs and symptoms statistically indicate a higher chance of microscopic cells being elsewhere. These have been incorporated into stage III (T4 lesions) of the TNM system. Dr. Cushman Haagensen first described what he called the "grave signs"—findings on a physical exam that indicated the likelihood that microscopic cells had spread to other areas of the body (Figure 10.9). His work was done in the 1940s before chemotherapy was used to treat early-diagnosis cancer. Haagensen's plan

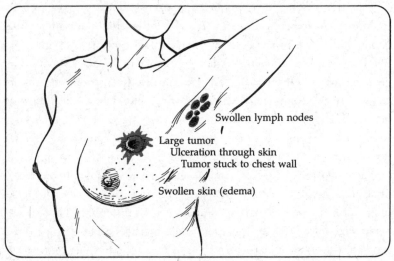

Figure 10.9

was to determine which patients would really benefit from a radical mastectomy. If there was no hope of saving a patient's life, he didn't want to cause needless suffering and destroy the quality of whatever life they had left. His system is still useful in a general way.

The question is no longer whether a cancer has spread but rather the likelihood of what has spread growing as a life-threatening metastasis. Evidence is emerging that large primary tumors have more of a stem cell component, suggesting that they have more potential to recur and metastasize.

Another danger sign is swelling of the skin (edema) in the tumor area. As the skin swells, ligaments that hold the breast tissue to the skin get pulled in, and it looks like you've got little dimples on the area. Because this can look like an orange peel, it's known as *peau d'orange* (Figure 10.10). If the tumor is ulcerating through the skin, it's ominous. If it's stuck to the muscles underneath so it doesn't move at all, that's also a bad sign. If there are lymph nodes you can feel above your collarbone (supraclavicular nodes) or walnut-size lymph nodes in your armpit, that's also dangerous. And if the skin around the lump appears red and infected, it can indicate inflammatory breast cancer (see Chapter 12), which is also likely to spread.

Any one of these signs suggests a high probability that microscopic cancer cells elsewhere in the body could grow and develop into metastases. In that setting, we plan a systemic treatment (see Chapter 11) as well as a local treatment for the cancer. These tumors are called *locally advanced* and are often treated with chemotherapy rather than surgery as a first step. (See Chapter 12.)

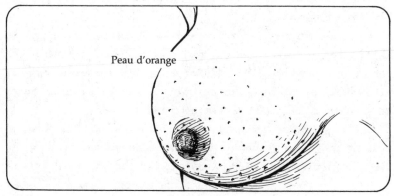

Peau d'orange

Figure 10.10

Most people don't have any of these grave signs, but we still need to figure out the likelihood of microscopic cancer cells existing and growing in other organs. The way we do this is to remove some axillary (armpit) lymph nodes. There are between thirty and sixty lymph nodes under the arm. We look at these lymph nodes because they are a good window for what is going in the rest of the body. If they reveal cancer cells, we assume there's a high probability that there are microscopic cancer cells in other parts of the body. If they don't show cancer, it means there is a lower probability. We do this by a procedure called a *sentinel node biopsy*, which involves finding the few nodes that are most likely to have cancer cells present, and if they do, examining them very thoroughly. (Sentinel node biopsy is discussed in detail in Chapters 11 and 13.)

The lymph node evaluation, however, doesn't give us a perfect answer either. Positive lymph nodes don't necessarily mean that there are microscopic cells elsewhere with the ability to grow. In fact, they don't in about 30 percent of cases. Conversely, even if the lymph nodes are negative, it does not mean that the cancer has not spread—20 to 30 percent of breast cancers with negative lymph nodes have spread elsewhere.

To a certain degree, though, the number of positive lymph nodes gives us a sense of the probability of having microscopic breast cancer cells elsewhere in the body. With one or two positive nodes, you're less likely to have the metastatic potential than with ten or fifteen, and this is reflected in the new TNM system, which separates N1 into a, b, and c categories based on the number of positive nodes. However, because with any positive lymph nodes there's a pretty high chance that there are cancer cells elsewhere capable of growing, we almost always treat patients with positive nodes with either hormone blockers or chemotherapy or both (see Chapter 15).

In patients with negative nodes, it's trickier. What we want is a way to identify the 20 to 30 percent who have microscopic cells elsewhere and not overtreat the other 70 percent. At present we don't have a direct way to do this. However, we do it indirectly by examining the primary tumor for the features described earlier in this chapter.

One obvious way to predict a poor prognosis is to find cancer cells in other organs. When the first edition of this book was written, all newly diagnosed patients would undergo tests to look for cancer cells in their liver, lungs, or bones. The problem with that approach, however, was that the imaging tests we had, and indeed still have, are useful only for finding chunks of cancer (one to two centimeters), not isolated cancer cells, and they often show other things that are probably not cancer but need to be checked out to be certain. So we don't do those tests now unless we have reason to think the cancer is likely to have spread because it is large or aggressive or you have worrisome symptoms such as a cough or weight loss. The exception to this is when we are going to give chemotherapy first and surgery second and you have symptoms (see the discussion of neoadjuvant chemotherapy in the next chapter). In order to see and document the amount of disease present, a CT scan of the chest, abdomen, and pelvis is done as well as a bone scan prior to starting treatment.

By the way, a cancer that starts out as a breast cancer remains a breast cancer, wherever it travels, and treatments used for the cancer are breast cancer treatments, not liver cancer or lung cancer treatments (very few cancers travel *to* the breast). Often you'll hear someone say "She had breast cancer, but now it's metastasized and it's liver cancer." But it isn't—it's breast cancer within the liver. It's a bit like what happens when a Californian moves to Paris. She's living in a new environment, but her language, her personality, her basic approach to life are still those of a Californian. She hasn't become a Parisian.

For those of you that are scheduled to have these tests, I will review what is involved. The rest of you can skip ahead!

Bone Scan

A technician injects a low level of radioactive particles into your vein, where the bones selectively pick them up. After the injection, you wait a few hours while the particles travel through the bloodstream; then you go back to the examination room, where you are put under a large machine that takes a picture of your skeleton (Figure 10.11). The machine whirs above you, reading the number of radioactive particles in your body. (The husband of one of my patients used to wear a Geiger counter, and right after her bone scan it started clicking whenever she came near it.) In the areas where the bone is actively metabolizing— doing something—the radioactive particles will show up much more strongly than in the more inert areas.

This doesn't necessarily mean that what the bone is doing has anything to do with cancer, however. It can mean there's arthritis (which most of

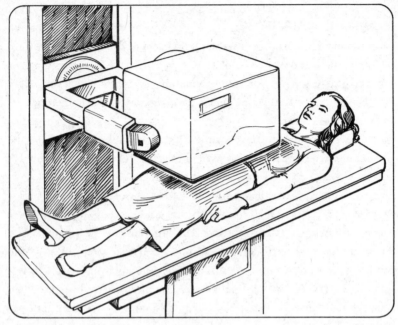

Figure 10.11

us have in small amounts anyway), a fracture that's in the process of healing, or some kind of infection. All the scan tells us is that something's going on. If the scan is positive, the next step is to X-ray the bone. This will help tell us what it is.

Markers

There are also some blood tests for patients with breast cancer—CEA, CA 15-3, CA 27.29. All these are nonspecific markers found in the blood. They can be followed over time and will often go up if metastases develop. It was initially hoped that these tests would detect the presence of a few cancer cells that had spread before they were visible on a scan; unfortunately, we've found that they're neither specific nor sensitive enough for that. But because they tend to go up in people with extensive metastases, they're useful in following patients with metastatic disease because they help us adjust treatment.

Remember that all tests have limits. A negative finding doesn't give you a clean bill of health; it simply tells you that there are no large chunks of cancer in those organs. Most people who are newly diagnosed don't have spread of this magnitude. So, as I mentioned, we no longer do these tests in the usual stage I or stage II breast cancers—in fact, they are actually discouraged. If you have stage III or locally advanced breast cancer, or if you have symptoms in any of the organs breast cancer typically spreads to—like low back pain that started right after you found your lump and hasn't gone away—we may do these tests. But we no longer do them routinely.

Most doctors' current recommendation is that all patients who are diagnosed with breast cancer undergo a history and physical exam, tests of liver function, and bilateral mammography.

In most patients without advanced disease (palpable matted lymph nodes in the armpit or above the collarbone, tumor in breast growing into the chest wall or skin, inflammatory breast cancer), there is no reason to do any additional staging until after surgery, if at all. Patients with stage tumors larger than five centimeters and positive nodes as well as those with tumors two to five centimeters and positive nodes with high-risk tumors or who are going to receive neoadjuvant chemotherapy may undergo bone scan, liver ultrasound, CT and chest X-ray, or CT alone.

Based on our current knowledge of breast cancer biology, we would expect a percentage of breast cancer patients to have micrometastases in

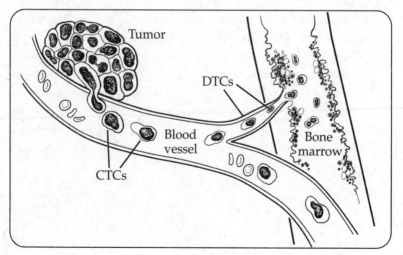

Figure 10.12

terms of either circulating tumor cells (CTCs) or disseminated tumor cells (DTCs) (Figure 10.12). The difference between them is that CTCs are cells that detach from a tumor and enter the bloodstream, while DTCs are the fraction of these that manage to reach distant sites like the bone marrow or an organ. The significance of DTCs is hotly debated.[25]

Although one may think looking for these cells would be the most accurate at finding cells that have "gotten out," the question is whether it has significance. For a cancer to spread, it needs not only to get out of the breast and into the bloodstream but to find a neighborhood in another organ that will take it in and support it (Figure 10.12). Packing up and getting into the car does not mean you will find a place to live at the other end. Many of the DTCs and CTCs, like a lot of travelers making a treacherous journey, die on the way (spontaneous cell death), have a run-in with the border patrol (immune system), or can't manage to successfully adapt to their new home (organ). Others may make it to another organ but not be able to survive there. Most patients with breast cancer are successfully treated initially. Some will get recurrences later on, and most will never get them. You really don't care whether a few cells got out and are retired (dormant) in your bone marrow if they stay dormant for the rest of your natural life.

A different kind of cell is now being examined for its potential to predict cancer recurrence through a blood test (also known as a *liquid biopsy*). Called circulating free DNA (cfDNA), these cells are degraded DNA fragments released into the blood plasma, and a portion of those are CTCs. Normally they are cleaned up by the body's immune system, but the overproduction of cells in cancer leaves some of them behind. Studies have concluded that measuring these cfDNA cells can be an effective and minimally invasive way to monitor cancer and predict treatment response. It would not only be quicker than imaging but also provide insight into the molecular evolution of the tumor.[26] Whether this approach will be incorporated into the arsenal of tools already in use against breast cancer remains to be seen.

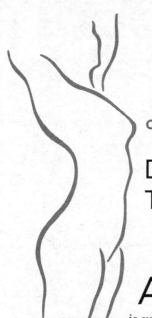

CHAPTER 11

Decisions About Treatment

Anyone receiving a cancer diagnosis may want to rush into treatment immediately. But if this is your reaction, don't follow through on it right away. Spend a day or two reflecting on the new reality you're facing. Obviously, if you've got cancer, you want it taken care of as soon as possible. But the week or so you give yourself won't kill you, and it will help you make the clearest decision possible. Whatever you choose, you'll have to live with your decision for the rest of your life—and that life won't be shortened by giving yourself a little time to think it over.

In the past it was common to make the decision—or rather, allow the doctor to make the decision for you—before the cancer was even diagnosed. You'd sign a consent form before your biopsy, agreeing to an immediate mastectomy if cancer was found. Fortunately that's much less common now, though it still sometimes happens. It's a terrible idea. No one should be put to sleep without knowing whether they will still have their breast when they wake up. If your doctor wants you to sign such a form, don't do it. What you think you'll want when you're not sure if you have cancer may or may not mirror what you really want when you have a definite diagnosis.

Part of the sense of urgency comes from the way we used to think about the disease before we had the numerous options we have today. Now you have choices. Any given procedure or combination of procedures may or may not be right for you, depending on the kind of cancer you have, the location of the cancer in your breast, its size, and, very importantly, your own thoughts and feelings. This chapter contains an overview of how different types of breast cancer relate to the different available treatments, and in the next chapter I'll explain how particular cancers are treated in particular situations. Finally, in Part 5 we'll consider each different treatment and what it entails.

GOALS OF TREATMENT: KILLING CELLS AND CHANGING THE ENVIRONMENT

Treatment for breast cancer involves removing cells, killing cells, and controlling cells by changing their neighborhood or environment. Surgery certainly removes all the cells, good and bad, from a defined location. Radiation therapy kills whatever dividing healthy and malignant cells are in its path. It takes advantage of the fact that most healthy cells are usually capable of recovering from the damage of radiation and/or grow back, leaving the irradiated breast intact. Chemotherapy kills cancer cells in many different ways, among them by causing fatal mutations in the cell's DNA. In general, the effects of chemotherapy are quite similar to those of radiation therapy—both interfere with the cancer cell's growth. But here too, the process harms healthy cells, changing the environment along the way. Surgery and radiation do this by causing the inflammatory reaction needed to heal the damage they wrought. Targeted therapy and chemotherapy interact with the immune system in ways that are only beginning to be discovered. Finally, the stress your body experiences in response to cancer and its treatment also influences your ability to fight it.

Hormone therapy, whether it is tamoxifen, an aromatase inhibitor, or even ovarian ablation (removing or blocking the ovaries), targets specific cancer cells, changing functions needed for the cells to survive or grow. At the same time, it also changes the environment. Thus, it causes a different hormonal milieu in the whole body, including the breast and the neighborhood directly around the tumor.

Nolvadex (tamoxifen) is a great example of how changing the neighborhood can have a lasting effect. It blocks the estrogen receptor in the cells and the neighborhood, preventing estrogen from reaching them. You would think that stopping Nolvadex (tamoxifen) would stop its effects. But the effect persists long after a person stops taking it. One Swedish study showed that taking Nolvadex for only two years provided benefits that lasted for at least fifteen years.[1] The longer a person takes it, for a period of up to ten years, the greater the benefit.

Undoubtedly it kills some cancer cells and also affects the stromal environment they live in. It may even put some of the cancer cells to sleep. The idea of living with cancer cells remaining in your body may seem alarming, but it shouldn't be. If you are feeling fine and ultimately die of a stroke at age 95, will you care that you had sleeping cancer cells in your body? Probably not.

The newer, targeted therapies also have mixed effects. Herceptin is an antibody that blocks HER2/neu, the growth factor receptor that spurs cancer cells on (see Chapter 10). Does it kill cells or change the environment? Probably both. It changes one of several key processes necessary for the cancer cell's survival and/or growth as well as enlisting the immune system in the fight. These processes exist in normal cells too but are much less prominent. The newer immune treatments change the response of the body's defense systems by removing the block some cancers have put on them, much like removing a roadblock to allow first responders through. This lets the immune system attack the cancer or make the neighborhood less conducive to its growth. Finally, there are all the complementary and lifestyle approaches. How do stress reduction, weight loss, or increased physical activity prevent recurrence? My bet is that they change the environment of the body, reduce inflammation, and thus maintain the cancer cells in a more dormant state.

So we can take advantage of all these approaches to help you achieve a long life. Most initial treatment plans, as we will see, reduce the amount of cancer through surgery and radiation (local therapy) and then add one or more systemic therapies (chemotherapy, hormone therapy, or targeted therapy) to kill or control any remaining cells. This is what the doctors do. You can add the lifestyle changes that are as key as anything else in keeping things under control (see Chapter 16).

STEP ONE: THE TEAM

The treatment of breast cancer is a team sport! Once you have received a diagnosis, it is important to assemble a team. Some specialized centers have multidisciplinary teams with all the appropriate specialists (breast surgeon, radiation therapist, medical oncologist, and possibly plastic surgeon) while hospitals often have de facto teams of people working on a common cause. Sometimes you'll have to assemble your own dream team. Don't be afraid to get a couple of opinions and combine specialists from different hospitals if it feels right for you. Most centers and doctors will allow you to refer yourself, so don't feel that you need to have a doctor call for you. Ask your local breast cancer support group members who they recommend. This is a time to engage your whole network.

In addition to the treating doctors, you will want to have a support team, including the clinical nurse specialists, physical therapy, palliative care (meaning symptom management, not end of life), and mental health. You may want to be the captain of your team and coordinate them all, or you may want your significant other, sibling, or best friend to take the reins. There is no right way to do this! Usually the professional leadership of the team shifts depending on the phase of treatment, with the surgeon leading on local therapy, and the oncologist on the use of drugs.

In the past, your surgeon gave you your diagnosis and then chose an intervention (lumpectomy, mastectomy, and so on) to prevent breast cancer from recurring. After that, you moved on to a radiation therapist and then an oncologist for some chemotherapy. Now this sequence is sometimes stood on its head. Sometimes the first step is chemotherapy or hormone therapy, followed by surgery and ending with radiation, depending on the kind of tumor you have (see Chapter 10) or whether you have chosen to participate in a clinical trial that gives the chemotherapy, hormone therapy, or targeted therapy first (see the discussion later in this chapter). So if you haven't read Chapter 10, read that first, as the next steps depend on the kind of cancer you have. You'll still have some decisions to make, but not nearly as many as those outlined in the earlier editions of the book. And you will still need a team.

FIRST DECISIONS

When you are newly diagnosed with breast cancer, there are generally three sets of decisions that need to be made, and the options and order will depend on your personal situation as well as the kind of cancer you have. The first is whether and what you are going to do to treat any cancer cells that may already be in the rest of your body. The first decision will involve chemotherapy, hormone therapy, and targeted therapies alone or in combination. The second decision is how to treat what we call the *local* area, which is the breast lump and lymph nodes under your arm.

Options for this are usually combinations of local therapies, including surgery and radiation. The third decision is how to prevent the cancer from coming back. The options here can include lifestyle changes such as losing weight, exercising, and reducing stress. These are not simple, cut-and-dried decisions.

The goal of these decisions is to give you the best shot at a cure of your disease—that is, to prevent it from recurring in the breast, the mastectomy scar, or the rest of the body. There is more than just one factor to consider. For example, we now know that a recurrence in the breast or lymph nodes is more than an inconvenience; it increases the chances of dying of cancer. We also know that tamoxifen and chemotherapy not only treat microscopic cells elsewhere in the body but also reduce local recurrences. So although doctors often separate the decisions, they are all part of a whole. While the local decisions are usually determined with a surgeon and radiation therapist, and the systemic ones are the province of the medical oncologist, there has to be coordination. In our current health care system you are the quarterback. Although this can be intimidating, it is important to remember that you are the patient and have to make the choices that work the best for you, not for your doctor or team. There is no right or wrong answer. If you feel uncomfortable or uneasy or just don't like the doctor, get a second opinion. You need to trust that the doctors who are treating you will work with you to get the best outcomes for you.

And remember that although this chapter focuses on the benefits of various treatments, there are also side effects from every approach. I encourage you to read through the entire treatment section and maybe even Chapter 18 on collateral damage, to ensure that you understand beforehand what you are getting into.

LOCAL TREATMENTS: SURGERY AND RADIATION

For years, most surgeons began any treatment course with mastectomy, assuming that this drastic procedure was the most effective way to save lives. But studies have proved them wrong. As we have seen again and again in breast cancer treatment, more is not necessarily better. The main goal of surgery to the breast is to prevent breast cancer from coming back in the specific area in which the cancer appeared. This can be done by taking out just the cancer with clear margins and the necessary lymph nodes, and letting radiation destroy any remaining cells: we call this breast-conserving therapy, as it does not remove the breast itself. (Less formally, it's called lumpectomy, wide excision, or even partial mastectomy—they all mean the same thing.) The cancer can also be removed by a mastectomy and excision of necessary lymph nodes, which in small tumors with little or no lymph node involvement usually takes out enough tissue to prevent local recurrence, eliminating the need for radiation. Finally, with very large tumors or significant lymph node involvement, we use both mastectomy and lymph node dissection to remove as much of the tumor as possible, and radiation therapy to take care of leftover cells. The best choice is generally dictated by not only the biology of the tumor but also by the patient's choice and the size of the tumor compared to the size of the breast.

Mastectomy Options

Many patients naturally conclude that the more drastic treatment will be better and that having a mastectomy will remove not only the breast but any possibility that cancer will return. But that isn't the case. Breast cancer can come back in the scar, chest wall, or axilla (armpits) after a mastectomy, just as it can after a lumpectomy. In fact, all things being equal, the local recurrence rates are the same for mastectomy without radiation (6 percent) and lumpectomy followed by radiation (6 percent).[2] The first patients treated with breast conservation compared to extended radical mastectomy showed no difference between the two treatments in terms of cancer in the other breast, distant metastases, or new cancers in the area of the same breast after twenty years.[3]

In June 1990 the National Cancer Institute Consensus Conference concluded: "Breast conservation treatment is an appropriate method of primary therapy for the *majority* of women with Stage I and II breast cancer and is *preferable* because it provides survival equivalent to total mastectomy while preserving the breast" (emphasis mine). What amazes me is that twenty-five years later we are still doing so many more mastectomies than breast conservation. Recently two studies revisited the benefits of breast conservation versus mastectomy with and without radiation therapy. Although the study was not randomized, it compared the ten-year breast cancer survival rate and found that 94 percent of the participants who underwent breast conservation had survived breast cancer, while those who had a mastectomy reached 90 percent and those who had a mastectomy and radiation 83 percent.[4] This was confirmed in a California study where again the participants who had breast conservation did better than those with mastectomy.[5] This despite the fact that more patients of higher socioeconomic status had mastectomies than breast conservation. The additional benefit of breast conservation was higher for patients over fifty with hormone-positive disease but still was there for younger patients with breast cancer of all subtypes. I can hypothesize that surgery or anesthesia perhaps sets up an inflammatory reaction that increases cancer spread, or explore the potential benefits of radiation, but the key is that *contrary to what we tend to believe, more surgery is not necessarily better and may well be worse.*

Still, it seems that more and more people are choosing mastectomy or even bilateral mastectomy. Part of this may be because, as breast conservation surgery became more common, surgeons started removing larger pieces of tissue to achieve clean margins, often at the expense of cosmetic results. It has been reported that 20 to 30 percent of patients who have lumpectomies have a poor cosmetic result.[6] Yet it needn't be that way. I wonder whether these patients are fully aware that the technique of reconstruction, so much associated with mastectomy, is nowadays also available for lumpectomies: you can achieve an excellent aesthetic result while, most importantly, conserving the sensation in your breast. If the potential cosmetic effect plays a large part in your choice of cancer surgery, you should be reassured by the increased availability of reconstruction for either path. If your surgeon doesn't mention this, you should ask about it and then do some research yourself. This is clearly better than having a cancer operation and being left with a dent or a widely unmatched set. And having sensation is significantly better than having bilateral mastectomies with numb reconstructions! My colleague Ben Anderson says that it is important to understand that reconstruction is a cosmetic procedure, not a functional one. It is worth spending the time asking around or looking online to find someone comfortable with this approach. Ask to see pictures and talk to people they have operated on. In the situation when chemotherapy can be done first, there is often plenty of time for this research and it will be well worth it.

Despite this option, in the past decade, higher proportions of patients who could have breast conservation underwent mastectomy and even bilateral mastectomy.[7] This may be due in part to the American tendency to think that more is always better in virtually any situation. If it hurts more or it's a bigger operation, it must be the best. It is almost magical thinking: "If I offer my breasts to the gods, I will get my life back in return!" I wish it were that easy. As you face many frightening choices it is important that you try to separate the feelings from the facts and make the best decision you can for yourself. You are the one who is going to have to live with the results for a long time to come.

Without question, some of the increase in people getting mastectomies is because of MRIs. When an MRI shows a separate "unidentified white spot"—even if that spot turns out to be benign—patients often panic, thinking "the cancer must be everywhere in my breast" and then elect to get a mastectomy. The thing to try to remember is that in the majority of cases of early breast cancer, the "cure" rates after lumpectomy and radiation are the same and often better than mastectomy—no matter how many "false positive" false alarms the MRI may show.

And in some cases, lumpectomy plus radiation is as important medically as it is cosmetically. If your cancer is right near the breastbone, the best mastectomy won't allow the surgeon to get a normal rim of tissue around the lump. But radiation will treat the surrounding tissue. And sometimes mastectomy is the best medical choice—for instance, if you have a large cancer in a small breast or extensive ductal carcinoma in situ (DCIS; a form of noninvasive cancer). More recently patients with large cancers have chemotherapy or hormone therapy before surgery to shrink the tumor and thus allow breast conservation. And radiation therapy is also given after mastectomy in certain situations.

If you decide on a mastectomy, breast reconstruction can be done either immediately at the time of mastectomy or later, when and if you want it. Commonly a surgeon will leave a large envelope of skin (skin sparing) for the plastic surgery to fill when reconstruction is planned. Nipple sparing is also sometimes used, although it is important to point out that the breast skin and spared nipple are usually numb. There is still some controversy about whether there is an increased risk of recurrence in the nipple, which has been difficult to assess based on evidence. In addition, the degree of ptosis (how much your breast droops) makes a big difference in the cosmetic outcome. If the patient has a very droopy breast, the nipple can end up in the wrong place.

Although the subtype of the cancer (see Chapter 10) affects the risk of recurrence, the data suggest that the type of local treatment you and your doctor choose is not the deciding factor.[8] It is still important to get out most of the tumor with surgery. That's *most of the tumor*—not every speck of cancer. Remember that what kills people with breast cancer is not what is in the breast but rather the microscopic cells that may already be elsewhere in the body. However, in some kinds of breast cancer (see Chapter 10) where there is a distinct lump with only short "tentacles," removing it with lumpectomy is enough. Sometimes the margin is just barely involved in one spot and is otherwise clear. This may still be acceptable for radiation therapy.[9] The key is determining the likelihood of cancer being left behind. In the usual type of cancer, the chance is low, and radiation therapy can get rid of whatever malignant cells may remain.

We determine whether we've removed the majority of the tumor by evaluating the margins of the tissue (see Figure 10.6, page 214). If they're free of tumor, breast conservation is fine. This can be affected by the tumor's pathology. Breast cancers have tentacle-like protrusions stretching out into the breast tissue from the original lump. Ductal carcinomas with lots of DCIS (also called *extensive intraductal component*, or EIC) associated with them can reach much farther out. When this occurs, the margins may not be clean on the first try (the surgeon can't see or feel the "tentacles") (see Figure 11.1). A re-excision, where some additional breast tissue is removed, will sometimes take care of it. But there are some cases in which even a re-excision won't get clean margins, and a mastectomy, the ultimate wide excision, is necessary to get it all out. Infiltrating lobular carcinomas are another kind of cancer that has a tendency to be stealthy and difficult for the surgeon to find (see Chapter 10). These too need a wider excision and clean margins if they are to be treated with breast conservation, and they may still end up requiring a mastectomy. These can be good cases for oncoplastic surgery (see Chapter 13). An additional option is to give chemotherapy (for triple-negative or HER2-positive tumors) before surgery or hormones such as aromatase inhibitors (especially for lobular tumors) to shrink the tumor. This can convert a tumor that is too big for a cosmetic resection to one that is easily removed. It is termed neoadjuvant therapy, which we will discuss later in this chapter. If you prefer breast conservation, you should ask your surgeon if they are skilled in oncoplastic techniques, and if not, find someone who is. Or if you are going to need chemotherapy or hormone therapy anyway, ask about having those first to give the tumor a chance to shrink to a more manageable size for removal.

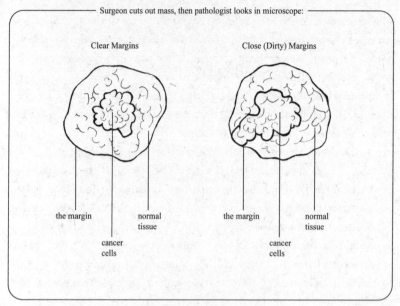

Figure 11.1

All this leads me to repeat my warning to patients against *routine* preoperative MRIs. Surgeons sometimes order these to determine whether a person is a candidate for breast conservation. In other words, they are looking for other suspicious lesions in addition to the cancer. We have always known that there will be other spots in the same breast.[10] That is why we treat the remaining breast tissue after a lumpectomy with radiation. Unfortunately, once an MRI is done and other potentially suspicious areas are noted,[11] they become hard to ignore, and many patients decide just to have a mastectomy as I discussed earlier. Some argue that they sometimes find cancers in the other breast with preoperative MRIs. Although this may be true, it is unclear whether it matters. It takes me back to the 1970s when Gerald Urban, a New York surgeon, was recommending "mirror image" biopsies of the other breast to find hidden cancers. They did find some, but the findings did not make a difference in the outcome. My colleague Ben Anderson has told his team that prior to ordering an MRI for preoperative evaluation, they have to state an explicit reason for the MRI (other than "because she hasn't had one") in which they describe how they anticipate it will change the treatment. The American Society of Breast Surgeons does not recommend diagnostic breast MRI until after clinical examination and conventional breast imaging. But it notes that MRIs can be effective in searching for a hidden breast cancer that has eluded conventional imaging, and in viewing extremely dense breast tissue where the extent of disease is hard to assess.[12]

In addition to unease at unexpected MRI findings, the other reason patients choose mastectomy is that the surgeon tells them that they can't remove the tumor and leave an "attractive" breast. In this situation it is important to get a second opinion from a surgeon who uses neoadjuvant therapy to decrease the size of the tumor first or is trained in oncoplastic techniques. As noted earlier, oncoplastic technique[13] means applying the techniques of a plastic surgeon to the removal of the lump and then, in some cases, reducing the opposite breast to match the first. The results can be both cosmetically and medically pleasing while maintaining the sensation in your breasts. With these options, it makes no sense to me to remove a breast and try to reconstruct it when it can usually be preserved in a cosmetically acceptable way with the same risk of recurrence and the same chance of cure and still retain normal sensation. Your doctor may recommend radiation after your procedure to kill any cancer cells that may remain. In short, there are both medical and cosmetic implications to whatever course you choose, and you should be fully informed about both.

Luminal A tumors (ER-positive, PR-positive, HER2-negative) do the best (1 percent recurrence) with breast conservation, and triple-negative tumors (ER-negative, PR-negative, HER2-negative) have the highest rate of local recurrence (10 percent). Before you conclude that people with this type of tumor should chose mastectomy, I need to point out that they also have about the same local recurrence rate (about 10 percent) after mastectomy.[14]

There are only three absolute reasons breast conservation can't be done:

1. The patient has a history of previous therapeutic radiation to the breast region (such as for Hodgkin lymphoma) that, combined with the proposed treatment, would result in an excessively high total radiation dosage. Still, even this may not be such a contra-indication after all, with the newer techniques of partial-breast radiation (brachytherapy).[15]
2. Widespread or multicentric disease that cannot be removed through one incision with clean margins and a satisfactory cosmetic result.
3. Diffuse, suspicious, malignant-appearing microcalcifications.

Relative contraindications include the following:

1. Specific, active autoimmune diseases, particularly scleroderma or lupus, which can result in severe short- and long-term complications in the presence of radiation
2. Focally positive margin (ink on tumor) without extensive DCIS

Sometimes a person will choose mastectomy without radiation over breast conservation because they have been told that if they have breast conservation and the cancer recurs later, the radiation will make it impossible to have reconstruction at that time. This is not entirely true. To begin with, only about 6 percent of patients develop a local recurrence (cancer coming back in the breast or lymph nodes) and require a mastectomy. Although it is harder to do reconstruction with an implant or expander (see Chapter 13) in this situation, studies have shown that patients who undergo reconstruction with a pure myocutaneous flap (skin and muscle taken from another part of the body) after postmastectomy radiation have the same outcome as those who have not had radiation therapy.[16] Of course, very thin women may not have enough to spare.

Radiation Options

Another issue that leads patients to choose mastectomy is the perceived inconvenience of receiving radiation for fifteen minutes every day for six weeks. This has been addressed with new, shorter schedules of hypofractionated radiation (*hypofractionated* means fewer fractions and therefore fewer visits) as well as intraoperative radiation and partial-breast radiation.

Accelerated or Partial-Breast Radiation

Accelerated or partial-breast radiation (they are the same thing) is considered an option for patients with early breast cancer (less than two centimeters, negative sentinel node and ER-positive), particularly if postmenopausal. It uses a higher dose over a shorter period and focuses only on the section of the breast where the tumor was, reducing treatment time and sparing healthy tissue. Two recent phase 3 trials comparing partial-breast radiation to whole-breast radiation concluded that the long-term difference in recurrence rates between the two techniques was minimal.[17] The larger of the two trials, conducted in 154 clinical centers in the United States, Canada, Ireland, and Israel, found an absolute difference of less than 1 percent in the ten-year incidence of ipsilateral (same side) breast tumor recurrence, in favor of whole-breast

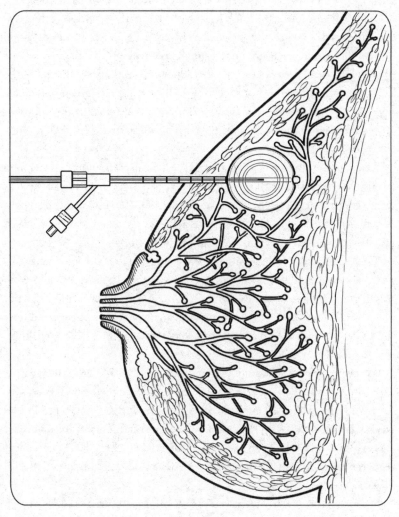

Figure 11.2

radiation. But a smaller Italian study found treatment-related toxicity to be greater in the whole-breast irradiation group.

Accelerated or partial-breast irradiation can be done with classical radiation machines, usually in five visits. Alternatively, another common approach is to place a balloon catheter in the lumpectomy site at the time of surgery to deliver radiation twice a day for about five days, and then remove the balloon (see Figure 11.2). These methods will be described in Chapter 14.

The American Society of Therapeutic and Radiation Oncology (ASTRO) recommends that this approach be used in patients over age 50 who have tumors that are less than or equal to two centimeters, are ER-positive, and show no visible invasion by cancer cells of blood or lymph vessels.[18] Patients over age 40 who meet all other standards of suitability can also receive it. Intraoperative radiation therapy is the most convenient method of receiving radiation, as it is given in a single dose at the time of surgery. However, it requires specialized equipment and is therefore offered only at particular centers or as part of a clinical trial.

After an important Canadian trial[19] demonstrating that sixteen to twenty-five treatments to the entire breast had an equivalent outcome as thirty treatments over the traditional six weeks for invasive breast cancer, many radiation oncologists have adopted accelerated whole-breast radiation (hypofractionation) for patients with node-negative breast cancer. If you are one of these patients and your doctor is offering the traditional six weeks instead of a shorter regimen, ask them to explain why. And if you have left-breast cancer (the same side as the heart), it is particularly important to ask to see your treatment plan and understand how the radiation doctor is planning to avoid treating your heart and lungs (see the following discussion).

An even shorter schedule of hypofractionation was effective against early breast cancer in another multicenter trial, named FAST-Forward. This study showed that for local tumor control, five treatments in one week were as effective as the standard fifteen treatments in three weeks, and in a five-year follow-up was as safe for normal tissue.[20] The low local recurrence rates are similar to those with standard treatments but with fewer side effects.

If you are considering breast conservation, make sure you meet with a radiation therapist to discuss all these options.

Postmastectomy Radiation

With mastectomy, we often don't do radiation because the tumor has been removed. But studies have shown that it may be worth it, even after a mastectomy. For some people there can be more than a 20 percent chance of the tumor recurring in the mastectomy scar, skin, or lymph nodes. These include people with four or more positive axillary lymph nodes and a tumor over five centimeters. Postmastectomy radiation therapy is also indicated for those with involvement of the skin overlying the breast or the chest wall, who are at highest risk.

Decisions on postmastectomy radiation should always take into account tumor size, number of positive lymph nodes, and, in early cancer, whether side effects may outweigh benefits. A guideline on postmastectomy radiotherapy issued by the American Societies for Clinical, Surgical, and Radiation Oncology[21] noted that radiation depends a great deal on clinical judgment and patient input in patients with tumors of two to five centimeters, one to three positive lymph nodes, and an axillary lymph node dissection. If the sentinel node is positive and there has been no lymph node dissection, postmastectomy radiation is recommended only if there is already sufficient information to justify it. Patients with stage I or II cancers who have received preoperative systemic therapy should get radiation only if the axillary nodes are still problematic.

Patients with an intermediate risk of local recurrence (10 to 20 percent) may consider postmastectomy radiation if they had less than clean margins (cancer cells at the edge of the mastectomy) and significant amounts of invasion of the lymphatic or blood vessels in the breast tissue (called lymphovascular invasion). Others who also may benefit are patients with triple-negative breast cancer, those younger than age 45, or those who have tumors with lymphovascular invasion.

Postmastectomy radiation reduces the risk of local recurrence substantially in all the situations just described, and the higher the chance of recurrence, the higher the chance the radiation will keep the recurrence from happening. If a patient with four or more positive nodes undergoes postmastectomy radiation therapy, their risk of regional recurrence is reduced by 19 percent, which would translate to a 9 percent reduction in breast cancer mortality, according to a meta-analysis by the Early Breast Cancer Trialists' Collaborative Group (EBCTCG).[22] Although patients with minimally involved lymph nodes could consider postmastectomy radiation therapy, the benefit would be relatively small.

Current recommendations are to evaluate individual risk, taking into account the stage and genomic profile of the cancer and any preoperative treatment.[23] Remember that systemic therapies have advanced considerably in the past decade, and radiation has its own risks. Studies show that people who had cancer on the left side and got radiation had an increase in heart disease, although this risk has decreased substantially as radiation techniques have improved[24] (see Chapter 14). Furthermore, recent studies have shown a doubling of the risk of lung cancer ten years after postmastectomy radiation therapy.[25] (This risk is related to smoking history as well as the amount of lung that has been treated and, interestingly, does not apply to radiation therapy after breast conservation.) This is because the breast protrudes out from the chest, allowing it to be treated from the side or in tangents. Fortunately the more modern, computer-planning-based techniques of radiotherapy are better at sparing the heart and lung when treating the chest wall and scar after mastectomy. It is important to ensure that your radiation oncologist is familiar with these issues and is willing to discuss with you how they plan to best protect your heart and lung.[26]

As with all decisions related to breast cancer treatment, it ends up being a balance of risk versus benefit. When the risk of local recurrence is high enough after a mastectomy, radiation is worthwhile. Talk to your doctors and consider your own feelings, then make the decision that feels best for you.

What becomes more complicated is how to integrate postmastectomy radiation therapy with potential reconstruction. If you fit in this category, it is best that your surgeon, radiation therapist, and plastic surgeon work collaboratively to ensure the best result.

AXILLARY SURGERY: CHECKING THE LYMPH NODES

As discussed earlier, along with getting rid of the cancer, we usually try to discover whether there are affected lymph nodes in the armpit area (axilla). Aside from preventing recurrence in the armpit, the other purpose for doing axillary surgery is to help decide the stage of the breast cancer. If a patient has palpable (feelable) lymph nodes in their axilla, an ultrasound-directed fine-needle aspirate or core biopsy should be done to help determine whether those nodes represent cancer (see Chapter 8). If this does not show cancer, surgery should still be done as the needle biopsies may miss small areas of cancer within a lymph node.

The only people who need to have all their armpit nodes removed are those with large tumors (T3/T4), inflammatory breast cancer, or lymph node involvement determined by needle biopsy. Most people can undergo a sentinel node biopsy with less surgery and fewer complications. The concept of sentinel node biopsy is pretty straightforward.[27] It is based on the theory that there are one or more nodes to which a breast cancer is most likely to spread. During or just before surgery, the surgeon injects a small amount of blue dye and radioactive tracer into the breast and follows it as it travels to the lowest draining lymph node or nodes (see Figure 11.3). These nodes are then the ones that are removed for examination, with the idea that they would be the cancer's first stop on its way out of the breast and into the body (see Chapter 13). If these nodes are found not to have any cancer, the rest of the axilla is left alone. This is another example of more is not better. We find the nodes that are most likely to have cancer, so we don't worry that we may miss a node that's hiding in a corner somewhere. And because the pathologist knows that this is the node to check, it will be checked more thoroughly than the many nodes in a regular node dissection (see Chapter 13). Thus, there's less room for error. Because the surgery is less extensive, sentinel node biopsy is also associated with fewer complications. There is no need for an axillary drain after the surgery, less patient discomfort, decreased incidence of lymphedema (see Chapter 18), and less chance of inadvertent damage to nerves and blood vessels.

Over the past decade we have made even more progress in limiting the amount of surgery to the armpit. We initially thought that finding positive sentinel nodes indicated a need to remove all the lymph nodes to make sure there were not others involved. This was challenged by a study called Z0011[28] in which patients undergoing breast-conserving therapy (lumpectomy followed by radiation) with tumors measuring less than five centimeters and no palpable lymph nodes in their axilla underwent a sentinel node biopsy. If up to two sentinel lymph nodes were positive, they were randomized to have a traditional axillary dissection (all the nodes removed), in case there were some positive nodes left behind, versus no further axillary surgery. The researchers knew that some of the patients who did not have additional axillary surgery would have some cancer in

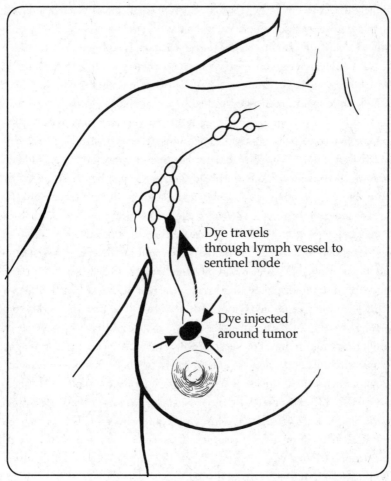

Dye travels
through lymph vessel to
sentinel node

Dye injected
around tumor

Figure 11.3

the other lymph nodes, but many of these are treated in the normal breast
radiation fields and all would be treated by the appropriate systemic therapy that patients get to treat the whole body. They sought to determine
whether the additional surgery improved survival and decreased local recurrence. Much to everyone's surprise, it made no difference after an average of six years' follow-up! This is good news indeed, as it suggests that
patients with up to two positive sentinel nodes who plan to undergo breast
conservation and systemic therapy can avoid further axillary surgery.

An international trial called AMAROS[29] included patients with
more than two positive sentinel nodes and randomized them between

traditional axillary dissection and no further surgery but with a directed field of radiation to the lymph nodes. The results were similar to the Z0011 study, again showing that more surgery was not better. Current studies are looking at the safety of sentinel node procedures in patients who had known positive sentinel lymph nodes at the time of diagnosis, had preoperative chemotherapy, and at the time of surgery have lymph nodes that feel normal.

Since the last edition of this book, an approach called targeted axillary dissection (TAD) was introduced that involves inserting radiotracers in positive lymph nodes before chemotherapy. When the therapy is finished, surgeons remove the marked nodes to see if there is still disease. Often the chemo takes care of it, meaning fewer lymph nodes would need to be removed. The reaction of the positive lymph nodes to therapy also provides useful information as to the best treatment strategies going forward.[30]

Under the traditional approach, patients who still require axillary dissection are those with positive lymph nodes on physical exam, those who have a lot of involvement of their sentinel nodes (usually an unexpected finding), or those whose medical oncologist is using the information to decide whether more systemic treatments are necessary and the additional lymph node information will help. As you will see when we discuss the collateral damage from surgical treatment in Chapter 18, this decrease in the amount of surgery in the armpit will have large benefits for at least some patients.

Sentinel node biopsy can be used effectively in all age groups with breast-conservation surgery or mastectomy at the time of primary excision or re-excision in unilateral or bilateral breast cancer. It is also effective in pregnant women with breast cancer (using radioactive seeds rather than blue dye),[31] after long-interval reduction mammoplasty, and with breast implants. The technique also works with most types of tumors, including those that have been treated with chemotherapy to shrink them before surgery (examined later in this chapter).

GUIDELINES FOR LOCAL CONTROL

In 1996 with colleagues at UCLA, I published the first practice guidelines for breast cancer treatment.[32] Since then, many more have been developed. The most all-inclusive are those of the National Comprehensive Cancer Network (NCCN), which can be found free in a patient-friendly version in English and Spanish at www.nccn.org.

The first step for local control is definitive surgery. This means either operating to remove the tumor with clear margins (wide excision or lumpectomy) or mastectomy, using sentinel node biopsy to determine if axillary dissection is called for. If the margins are clean after wide excision, the patient is a candidate for radiation therapy without further breast surgery, although they may still need an axillary dissection if they have extensive sentinel node involvement.

Any patient whose cancer was discovered through suspicious microcalcifications on a mammogram should follow up with a core biopsy. Mammograms are usually performed immediately after any type of core biopsy (including stereotactic, tomosynthesis, ultrasound, MRI, and so on). This mammogram can determine if any calcifications remain and can help plan next steps.

If the patient has a lumpectomy and the margins are involved in more than one spot, or the postbiopsy mammogram shows residual disease, the surgeon usually suggests more surgery. This step gathers further information on the cancer. If the new margins are clean, the patient is a candidate for radiation therapy; if not, they may need another re-excision or mastectomy. If the tumor is too large compared to the size of the breast to perform lumpectomy, the patient may be a candidate for neoadjuvant therapy, or chemotherapy or hormonal therapy before surgery, to shrink the tumor before the operation described next. All patients who choose mastectomy should be offered the option of reconstruction, either immediately or, if they prefer, at a later time.

CHOICES ABOUT MASTECTOMY

What are some of the factors that may influence your choice? There's a tendency to think that mastectomy is more aggressive because it's more mutilating. Actually, the combination of lumpectomy and radiation is more aggressive than mastectomy without radiation. Lumpectomy and radiation treat all the breast tissue. The field of radiation may encompass all the tissue that even extensive surgery misses. Some patients choose mastectomy because they do not want to make daily trips for radiation therapy; others may want to get it all over with as soon as possible and get back to their lives as though it never happened. That is always a very individual decision, but you need to remember that, as I said earlier, it *has* happened, and you can never go back to your life exactly the way it was.

There are important drawbacks to mastectomy. It's less cosmetically appealing except with the very best reconstruction. And even with re-construction (see Chapter 13), you are left with no sensation in the nip-ple, breast, or breast area. Lumpectomy and radiation leave you with a real breast that retains its physical sensation.

Some patients choose mastectomy without radiation (if they do not need radiation as discussed earlier) because they don't want to take more time off from a demanding profession than is necessary. This may make sense for some, but most women are relieved (and surprised) to learn after talking to their radiation oncologist that almost everyone can con-tinue to work through all or most of their radiation therapy course. In addition, if they do need radiation, they can also consider a hypofraction-ation schedule or one of the partial-breast irradiation (PBI) approaches, which will allow them to be treated in a much shorter time, sometimes as little as a few days. The recovery time for mastectomy is about ten days to two weeks and, with reconstruction, often means four to six weeks away from work, depending on the type of reconstruction and activity level of work, whereas lumpectomy is usually a few days.

The availability of one kind of treatment or another is also a factor. In some geographical areas radiation centers are far apart, and access can be an issue. In others it is available but is not especially good: a radiation on-cologist has to know the technique to get good results. For some people, however, their breasts are an integral part of their sexuality and identity and they are willing (and able) to go to great inconvenience to save them. One of my patients lived in a small town in the Central Valley of Califor-nia, too far to commute to my breast center in Los Angeles. So she and her husband drove down in their van and lived in the hospital parking lot for six weeks until her treatment was completed. I've had patients whose cancer recurred after lumpectomy and radiation, and even though they finally had a mastectomy, they were grateful for an extra few years with both breasts.

Regardless of the medical facts, however, you need to feel safe with your choice. A few of my patients who had lumpectomy and radiation would wake up every morning sure that the cancer had come back. They worried every year about their mammograms, even though they knew that they had a 94 percent chance the cancer would never come back. For women who have this level of extreme anxiety about their lumpectomy choice, perhaps they would have "felt" better with mastectomies in the first place, even though the recurrence rates are the same.

Remember above all that it's your body and no one else's. Don't decide on the basis of what anyone else thinks is best. Get information from all the kinds of doctors—medical oncologists, surgeons, and radiation oncologists—and maybe even get two opinions from each. And by all means talk to your friends, your family, and your partner, and think about what they say. But make your own decision. As I said earlier, partners come and go, but your body is with you all your life. A truly caring mate will support whatever course you think is best for you.

The next issue that may come up at decision-making time is whether to have a *prophylactic mastectomy* on the other breast at the same time. This is not usually necessary or even contemplated unless the patient is a carrier of a BRCA 1 or BRCA 2 mutation (see Chapter 5) or had thoracic irradiation for diseases such as Hodgkin lymphoma in the past, and even then it's certainly not mandatory. People with a new diagnosis of breast cancer and a family history suggestive of a BRCA 1 or BRCA 2 mutation could choose to have a lumpectomy and lymph node surgery, then undergo testing and have chemotherapy while waiting for the genetic test result (it takes about two to three weeks). If the test is positive they can, if they wish, undergo bilateral mastectomy with or without reconstruction following the completion of chemotherapy. If the test is negative or they decide to be followed closely, they can go on to radiation following the completion of chemotherapy. Remember, there is no urgency over prophylactic mastectomy, and you may want to get the cancer therapy taken care of first; then, when the timing is convenient, if you still want it, you can have your breasts removed. It is important to remember that BRCA mutation carriers are also at increased risk of ovarian cancer, and removal of the ovaries by age 40 (or sooner) is recommended to reduce the risk of ovarian cancer. In such people who have not reached menopause, prophylactic removal of the ovaries can reduce the risk of breast cancer as well as ovarian cancer.

Remember that in addition to the well-known BRCA gene mutations, there are more than a dozen other inherited or germ-line mutations you can be tested for that increase breast cancer risk, and the list continues to grow.

The risk to the other breast in nonmutation carriers averages about 0.8 percent per year and an estimated 2 to 11 percent over a person's lifetime.[33] A nonrandomized study compared 1,072 women who had undergone prophylactic mastectomy in the other breast to 317 who had not. After 5.7 years of follow-up, 2.7 percent of participants who had not had the preventive surgery developed a second cancer compared to 0.5 percent of those who had it.[34] This suggests a small benefit in decreasing new breast cancers from the surgery; however, prophylactic contralateral (on both sides) mastectomies did not make a difference for the 10.5 percent of participants who developed metastatic disease or the 8.1 percent who died. And the current use of hormone therapy in most patients with hormone-sensitive tumors has the added benefit of reducing the risk of cancer in both breasts by at least 50 percent. It is important to be realistic about the risks and benefits in your own case before jumping to extra surgery in an effort to do "everything possible."

Some plastic surgeons encourage removing both breasts at once because breast reconstruction surgery is easier when they don't have to match an existing breast. Although this is worth considering, I don't think it should be the main factor in making the decision. Remember there will be no sensation, and it will not be like having the breasts you are used to, but more like having your prosthesis glued to your chest.

Finally, neither reconstruction nor prophylactic mastectomy has to be done immediately. Sometimes all the decisions you have to make are overwhelming, and it helps to leave a few for later. A woman I once counseled had dirty margins and a positive sentinel node. She was agonizing over whether she should have a prophylactic mastectomy on the other side and immediate reconstruction at the same time. Once she realized that she did not have to make that decision right away, she was quite relieved. She decided to go ahead with the mastectomy and axillary dissection and then chemotherapy while getting genetic testing (she had a family history of breast cancer) to find out what the risk really was to the second breast. After her systemic therapy was over, she went on to consider prophylactic mastectomy on the other side and research the best type of reconstruction for her.

CHOICES ABOUT RADIATION THERAPY

Similar to systemic therapy, radiotherapy has precise indications and different techniques. The recommendation for different radiotherapy protocols depends on the stage of your disease and the type of surgery you have received. Importantly, some types of radiotherapy are more established (there is more data regarding their safety and efficacy) than others. We have been giving a six-week course of whole-breast radiation for many decades—we know exactly what to expect from radiation in terms of safety, effectiveness, and long-term side effects. Shorter courses of radiation have a shorter track record but show great promise. Remember to ask your doctor whether what they are offering is part of clinical trial or is standard care. What is established is the importance of using techniques that best avoid giving radiation to the heart and lung while treating the area at risk of recurrence. This can be done by having you lie on your stomach or through breath-holding techniques. A technique called respiratory gating may be used, which uses a device to time the radiation with your breathing. Much of your discussion with the radiation oncologist should cover these issues: How will they protect your heart and lung while being sure the breast tissue is maximally treated? Will they use special blocks called MLC leaves? Do they use breath-holding techniques? Do they use a special form of radiation planning called intensity-modulated radiation therapy (IMRT)? Will you have a better treatment plan if you are treated on your stomach (prone)? Some medium- to large-busted people (that is, those who wear a C cup or larger) need to lie prone to best avoid the heart and lung (see the previous discussion). Sometimes this involves lying on a special kind of board for "prone treatment," and the main maker of radiation machines in the United States currently offers a modification of the radiation table to accommodate prone breast radiotherapy.

SYSTEMIC THERAPY

Systemic therapy used to be the second set of decisions you needed to make, and indeed it often still is but not always. As mentioned earlier in the chapter, it sometimes makes sense to have your chemotherapy or hormonal therapy first to shrink the primary tumor and give you an idea as to whether your cancer is sensitive to the drugs you are taking.

Systemic means something that creates its effect by circulating throughout your body; *local* treatments are applied only to the area in question. Systemic treatments include chemotherapy (drugs that kill cancer cells and are known as cytotoxic drugs) and targeted therapies such as hormone therapies (treatments that are hormones or affect your body's hormones) and blockers of HER2/neu. They can also include alternative and complementary therapies (see Chapter 16). Drugs given at the time of diagnosis when there is no known metastatic disease are considered adjuvant treatment. If they are given before surgery they are called neoadjuvant. The same drugs are just called "treatment" when metastatic disease is clearly present.

The reason for adjuvant or neoadjuvant systemic therapy is the fact that breast cancer deaths rarely occur because of what is in the breast. You could have a lump as big as a basketball, and it would not kill you. What kills people with breast cancer are the breast cancer cells that are in other, more important parts of the body such as the lungs, liver, bone, or brain. This became all too clear in the 1930s when the ten-year results from a radical mastectomy study revealed a 12 percent survival rate. Needless to say, this was well before the days of mammography, and most tumors were larger than those we deal with today. However, even in modern times, up to 20 to 30 percent of women with negative lymph nodes at the time of diagnosis and up to 75 percent of those with positive ones will die of their disease within ten years if they are treated *only* with local therapy (surgery or surgery and radiation alone). Obviously many patients have undetectable microscopic cells in other parts of their bodies at the time of diagnosis; in fact, that is one of the reasons that we are comfortable taking time to perform a thoughtful workup prior to surgery and taking time for second opinions: we know that cells have circulated well before the cancer was discovered. The question isn't whether they have circulated but rather whether the cells that have circulated have done anything bad. Adjuvant systemic therapy is actually the acknowledgment that we need to treat these cells by killing them, by changing the environment in which they exist, or both. The success of this approach is the fact that we currently can cure over 80 percent of breast cancers.

One of my surgical friends suggested that when a surgeon pushes for surgery being done "right away" (rather than within a month or so), they may be worried about second opinions that will take the patient in a different direction. If the concern about getting going is so high, then a deep breath and preoperative chemotherapy (neoadjuvant therapy) should probably be considered.

Although the first randomized trial of systemic adjuvant therapy was in 1948 when ovaries were removed to change the hormonal environment, only recently has it become a mainstay of treatment. Initially adjuvant therapies were given to all patients with positive nodes. As newer drugs have been developed, they have been added to the mix and are often given to patients with negative nodes as well. As we have figured out the different types of breast cancer, we have been better able to match the treatments to the patients in terms of both their risk of recurrence and the potential benefit of the therapy. This is important because none of the systemic therapies are without side effects, some of which can be quite significant. If a drug has prolonged your life, you may well put up with secondary heart problems or surgery for uterine cancer. If, however, you really did not need or benefit from chemotherapy, then developing leukemia as a result would be tragic. Although we are better nowadays at matching treatment with patient, there is still a gray zone. How much risk of recurrence is enough to justify a treatment? Physicians frequently use the threshold of greater than 90 percent disease-free survival at ten years with local therapy alone to define patients whose prognosis is too good to justify systemic therapy. Depending on your age, general health, and outlook on life, this may be what you would choose as well. However, it is worth taking the time to think about what you are willing to undergo for a statistical improvement in your odds. It is, after all, a bit of a gamble. For example, if we consider that chemotherapy reduces the risk of recurrence by about a third,[35] that means that the higher the chance of recurrence, the more beneficial the chemotherapy is likely to be for you. If you have a 60 percent chance of recurrence, a one-third risk reduction means chemo will reduce that chance by 20 percent, but if you have a 9 percent chance of recurrence, the one-third reduction is only 3 percent, although the effects are not perfectly linear. We tend to equate recurrence with death because at this time we are not able to cure a patient whose breast cancer comes back outside the breast or axillary lymph nodes—known as a distant recurrence. But research on new drugs and treatments continues and perhaps one day that will change (see Chapter 20).

Although I think it is important to ask about statistics to get a sense of the seriousness of your situation, it is also important to repeat my refrain about statistics: Remember that whatever happens to you is 100 percent! If 99 percent of patients live and you die, you are still dead. And if 99 percent die and you live, you are still alive. This is an important concept to understand when trying to weigh risks and benefits. I think it is always better to look at the absolute benefit of chemotherapy. In other words, if your chances of dying in the next ten years were 50 percent and you had a treatment that reduced the risk of mortality by 50 percent, your absolute benefit at ten years would be 25 percent. Another way to say this, for those of you who find percentages difficult to follow, is if there were one hundred people with the same cancer as you, then fifty of them would be dead at ten years, having died within that time frame. If a treatment reduced the chance of dying by 50 percent, then 25 of them would be dead at ten years. And we have to remember that *there are other things that can kill us, from car accidents to pneumonia.*

Not all oncologists agree with this way of looking at the figures, and there is a bit of wishful thinking in their approach to chemotherapy. They want it to work and so they hope that it works better than it does, or they just don't understand statistics. And they make their income by giving chemotherapy. In a 1994 study by S. Rajagopal, oncologists were presented with certain scenarios and for each one were asked whether they'd give chemotherapy.[36] Then they were asked what percentage of improvement in survival they thought the patient would have. Overall, they estimated a three-times-greater improvement than the available evidence justified. Thus you need to pin your oncologist down so that you are realistic about the benefits of chemotherapy in your case. If your oncologist is not sure of the absolute benefits, you can suggest that they go to an online tool such as the UK's Predict Breast (https://breast.predict .nhs.uk/tool). This program allows your physician to put in your information regarding the stage and type of cancer as well as your age and health. Then it shows how different treatments may improve survival. A similar online U.S. tool, at www.adjuvant.com, was under construction as of this writing and may be working when the book is out. I have found that these tools help many patients gain perspective on their odds as well as the benefits they can expect. It does not, however, include the potential side effects of the therapy, a point too often glossed over. I discuss this at length in Chapters 15 and 18.

Systemic therapy does not guarantee that your cancer will be cured; it may simply prolong the time to recurrence. But that in itself can be a worthwhile goal. The key, however, is to actually understand what the treatments are buying and weigh whether they are worth it. A few years ago a sixty-eight-year-old woman with an ER-negative tumor called me for advice. Her oncologist thought she should be on chemotherapy because her chance of dying in the next five years was 15 percent without it. So she thought she might try it. I asked whether the doctor had told her what her chance of dying in the next five years was even if she did take chemo—he hadn't. "I assume it means I have a 100 percent chance of surviving the next five years," she said. I told her that wasn't accurate: her chance of dying from breast cancer, with chemo, was 13 percent. She paused. "Then forget that!" she said finally. "I don't want to go through that for a 2 percent better chance!" However, studies have shown that some patients will choose chemotherapy even for a 1 percent improvement in survival. What matters is that each person has accurate knowledge to work with.

Combinations of Systemic Therapy

We can classify most cancers into one of the five categories described previously and from there come up with the likely combination of drugs (see Table 11.1). Patients with ER-negative tumors will be offered chemotherapy with the addition of Herceptin (trastuzumab) if their tumor shows high levels of HER2/neu. Patients with an ER-positive tumor that is over a centimeter in size will be offered hormonal therapy and possibly chemotherapy, depending on their risk (see Chapter 10 for a discussion of Oncotype DX and MammaPrint). If the tumor is also HER2/neu-positive, then Herceptin and probably Perjeta (pertuzumab) will be added to chemotherapy. Although early studies suggested that chemotherapy worked better in premenopausal patients, it now looks like the hormone receptor status of the tumor is also important, and these combinations are recommended across all ages. Although patients over age 70 are not generally included in studies, if you are over age 70 and in good health, it is probably reasonable to undergo the same regimen as a

Table 11.1 New Subtype Treatments

Molecular Type	Hormonal Therapy (tamoxifen, ovarian, ablation, AI)	Chemotherapy	Herceptin
ER+ and/or PR+ HER-2– (low recurrence score)	Yes	No	No
ER+ and/or PR+/ HER-2– (high recurrence score)	Yes	Yes	No
ER+ and/or PR+/– HER-2+	Yes	Yes	Yes
ER– and PR– HER-2+	No	Yes	Yes
ER– and PR– HER-2–	No	Yes	No

younger person. It is not your numerical age but any other conditions and life expectancy that should affect your decision to undergo toxic therapy for small improvements in survival. Researchers recently created a useful tool to gauge the effects of different chemotherapy regimens on women over age 65. If you want to check it out, go to the website of the Cancer and Aging Research Group and click on the Chemo-Toxicity Calculator.

Types of Chemotherapy

The effectiveness of chemotherapy depends on which drug or drug combination you use. At the time of this writing, the best results come from the use of sequential combination chemotherapy containing anthracyclines, alkylating agents, and taxanes. New studies base adjuvant therapy on the genetic signature of the tumor (TAILORx for node-negative, ER-positive, and RxPONDER for node-positive), which signals a more precise approach to therapy. As we become more successful in treating breast cancer, the side effects of various therapies acquire more importance and must be weighed in a risk-versus-benefit equation. Make sure your oncologist discusses the short- and long-term side effects of the therapy being proposed, so you won't be surprised later.

Because there are choices to be made among different chemotherapy drugs, it's especially important for the patient to participate in the decision-making process. Ask why your doctor has chosen a particular treatment regimen and ask to see studies that back it up. Find out exactly what the differences are in efficacy and side effects. For example, as I explain later, some drugs are more likely to put you into menopause and render you infertile than others (see Chapters 15 and 18). If you are premenopausal and still want to have children someday, tell your oncologist and turn to page 320 *now*—fertility preservation should always come first! Some drugs, like Adriamycin (doxorubicin), can be more toxic to the heart. If a clinical trial is available, consider participating so that we will get some answers (see the discussion later in this chapter). You can get accurate survival or recurrence statistics for your own case in several ways. There are online predictive nomograms and tools available to oncologists that can make precise calculations for you. Ask your oncologist to provide you with the data. You are more than capable of taking control of this decision.

Timing of Chemotherapy

Classically, chemotherapy treatment follows surgery and is virtually always before radiotherapy. But another course is *neoadjuvant* (or *preoperative*) chemotherapy. This means that chemotherapy is given before surgery, after a diagnosis is made with a core or needle biopsy. Because chemotherapy is the most important treatment dealing with the life-threatening element of the cancer, some of us thought that giving it first might make a difference in survival. Unfortunately none of the studies have shown this to be true. However, there are advantages. For starters, we can see whether the chemo works. If the tumor starts melting away, we know the chemotherapy is working. Interestingly, this approach appears to be most effective in the most aggressive tumors, the triple-negative and ER-negative HER2-positive tumors where neoadjuvant chemotherapy plus Herceptin (trastuzumab), when indicated, showed a complete response in 28 to 32 percent of patients. This means that doctors couldn't detect any cancer but also couldn't rule out the possibility of dormant cells still existing in the body. Unsurprisingly, patients who had no residual cancer in their breasts also had a much better outcome.[37] In a meta-analysis of fifty-two studies on preoperative chemotherapy, researchers found that 88 percent of patients who had a complete response had five years without invasive breast cancer recurrence compared to 67 percent of those who did not have a complete response.[38] If the preoperative chemotherapy does not result in a complete response, another bout of chemotherapy may help. In a study of HER2-positive women who had residual invasive disease after completion of preoperative (neoadjuvant) therapy, changing from Herceptin alone to a Herceptin-chemotherapy combination drug called Kadcyla lowered the risk of recurrence by half. In this study, called the KATHERINE study, half of the 1,486 patients with residual cancer received neoadjuvant Herceptin (trastuzumab) alone and the other half Kadcyla (ado-trastuzumab emtansine). The risk of recurrence of invasive breast cancer or death was 50 percent lower with Kadcyla than with Herceptin alone.[39] As this edition was being updated, yet another option was being tested for therapy on patients who had already received the additional Kadcyla therapy. Based on the positive results of Enhertu (trastuzumab deruxtecan) in the studies Destiny Breast 03 and Destiny Breast 04, the study Destiny Breast 05 is looking at Enhertu for patients with residual disease after neoadjuvant chemotherapy compared to Kadcyla.[40]

Today, most surgeons will consider preoperative chemotherapy plus anti-HER2 therapy, if indicated, for tumors over two centimeters in patients who wish to have a lumpectomy or have positive lymph nodes. It is better to wait until after the surgery in smaller tumors, which qualify for a lumpectomy anyway, and in cases where doctors are unsure before surgery whether chemotherapy will be required.

The caveat to this recommendation is that in some tumors, particularly those that are estrogen sensitive like lobular cancers, preoperative chemotherapy may not shrink the tumor.

But a Japanese study showed that additional chemotherapy after surgery in these cases can help. Researchers in a study called CREATE-X tested a drug called Xeloda (capecitabine) in women who still had residual disease after neoadjuvant chemotherapy and surgery. A control group received no additional therapy. The three-year rate of disease-free survival was 9 percent higher in the capecitabine group. The disease-free survival of patients with triple-negative disease was 70 percent in the capecitabine group and 56 percent in the control group.[41]

There is also the option of hormone therapy, particularly with aromatase inhibitors, which has been effective in postmenopausal women. In a Dutch study, an aromatase inhibitor called Aromasin (exemestane) given neoadjuvantly for six months improved the breast conservation rates by 10 percent.[42]

TARGETED THERAPIES

Hormone Therapy

Since 1890, doctors have been interested in the hormonal manipulation of breast cancers. In fact, the first adjuvant therapies were based on changing the body's hormonal milieu. If a premenopausal patient had a "bad" cancer, their ovaries were removed in an attempt to decrease the total amount of estrogen in their system. The idea was good, and recent studies show a survival difference between patients who had ovarian ablation (either removing the ovaries, radiating them, or suppressing them with medication) and those who did not (see the following discussion). This difference is as great as, or greater than, that with chemotherapy.[43]

Now we can predict who is likely to benefit from adjuvant hormone therapy by using the estrogen and progesterone receptor test discussed in Chapter 10. In patients with hormone-sensitive tumors, we can use a hormone treatment as adjuvant therapy, though it is useless and even potentially harmful in patients whose tumors are not sensitive to either estrogen or progesterone.

We are also starting to understand how these hormone therapies work. What they probably do, at least in part, is change the environment around the cell, resulting in control or even death of the cancer cell (see Chapter 3). This can happen in a number of different ways. Currently we have two different adjuvant hormone approaches: reducing the production of estrogen or blocking the estrogen receptor on the cell.

Nolvadex (tamoxifen)

You sometimes hear that Nolvadex (tamoxifen) throws premenopausal people into menopause. Actually, it's more complicated than that. Nolvadex stimulates the ovaries to make more estrogen. While blocking estrogen receptors in the breast, it is acting *like* estrogen in other organs, such as the bone and uterus (see SERMs, Chapter 6). This trait is responsible for both its negative side effects, such as uterine cancer and blood clots, and its benefits, such as increased bone density and lower cholesterol. Nolvadex is still the hormone treatment of choice for premenopausal patients with or without functional ovaries (see the following discussion). Sometimes patients and doctors act as if it is not as good as some of the newer drugs because it is old and has been around a long time. This is certainly not true. In fact, because it is an old drug, we know a lot more about it. We know all its side effects as well as its benefits. We have a lot less experience with some of the newer aromatase inhibitors. (An added benefit with Nolvadex is financial: because it's been around so long it has become a generic drug.)

The 2004 overview of treatment for early breast cancer found, not surprisingly, that Nolvadex (tamoxifen) doesn't help with ER-negative tumors.[44] But with ER-positive tumors, it has a benefit across the board. The reduction in the odds of recurrence is 29 percent, and the reduction in the chance of death is 24 percent in women between ages 40 and 49. This means that while people are on Nolvadex, one of every three recurrences and approximately one of every four deaths are prevented. Looking at absolute reductions, we find an 11 percent decrease in recurrence and a 6.8 percent reduction in death at ten years for premenopausal patients who have taken Nolvadex (with or without chemotherapy as well) for five years. For postmenopausal patients it is a 15 percent decrease in recurrence and an 8.2 percent reduction in death at ten years. As I pointed out earlier in the chapter, the absolute benefit depends in part on the risk and may not be proportional: the benefits may not be as good for a high-risk patient as for a low-risk one. The aromatase inhibitors are a fairly recent addition for postmenopausal patients and will be discussed shortly.

When I lecture, people often come to me and say they're taking Nolvadex (tamoxifen) but having side effects, and they want to know whether they need to continue on it. I suggest they check with their oncologist about why they're taking it. Oncologists tend to put every ER-positive premenopausal patient on it because it benefits everyone.

But it benefits by different amounts, and if you're in a category in which the benefit is only 1 to 2 percent and it's making your life miserable, you may not want to stay with it. An Italian study showed that a lower dose of Nolvadex in patients with DCIS for a shorter period of time can still reduce the recurrence rate compared to not taking any at all. Normally 20 milligrams of Nolvadex is given daily for five years, but researchers confirmed that 5 milligrams a day for three years can still halve the recurrence rate.[45] A Swedish study showed that an even more modest 2.5 milligrams of Nolvadex reduced breast density in premenopausal patients unaffected by breast cancer by some 20 percent. The reduction in density improved mammographic screening and potentially reduced risk of undetected cancer. Side effects and hot flashes were also reduced by 50 percent with the lower dosage.[46]

Ovarian Ablation

Blocking the estrogen receptor is one way to deprive the breast cancer cell of estrogen; another is to remove the source of the hormones. In premenopausal people, this is the ovary. There are three ways to do this: surgery, radiation, or hormonal manipulation—all these are known as *ablating* the ovaries. Unless you are a carrier of one of the BRCA genes or another inherited mutation, and therefore at higher risk of subsequent ovarian cancer, surgery probably is not the best way of doing this. The surgery is irreversible: if it doesn't help with the cancer, we can't return your ovaries to you. So you're stuck with all the consequences of having no ovaries—a condition that studies have shown increases overall mortality.[47]

Sometimes doctors can irradiate ovaries instead of removing them, saving the patient the pain of surgery. This isn't done much anymore as it takes a while to have an effect, means multiple visits, requires technical expertise, and, like surgery, is permanent. But that's one option.

More commonly we can use gonadotropin-releasing hormone (GnRH) agonists, originally developed for endometriosis, that block the ovaries and essentially put you into a temporary menopause. This approach seems to work as well as surgery or radiation and has the advantage of being reversible.

The most thoroughly tested drug for doing this in breast cancer is Zoladex (also known as goserelin). In a 1998 study, patients were put on

Zoladex (goserelin) for three to five years to see if it had the same effect as oophorectomy, and it did.[48] In the study, premenopausal node-positive and ER-positive women were randomized to take CMF (cytoxan, methotrexate, 5-fluorouracil) chemotherapy or goserelin for two years. After more than seven years of follow-up there has been no difference between the two groups. Most interesting to me was the fact that most of the participants on Zoladex got their periods back after the therapy was completed and still did just as well as those on CMF, who stopped menstruating permanently. In other words, just as with Nolvadex (tamoxifen), a short time (my approach is two to three years) of decreased estrogen production was enough to change these patients' prognosis. However, the ER-positive patients who did not become menopausal on CMF did significantly worse than those who stopped menstruating.[49] Obviously part of the benefit of the chemotherapy was that it put these patients into menopause. Further studies have shown that adding an aromatase inhibitor (see the following discussion) but not Nolvadex to the Zoladex is even more effective.[50] The benefits of even temporary ovarian suppression are worth discussing with your doctor.

Aromatase Inhibitors

Removing the ovaries or blocking them with drugs has much less effect on people who are already postmenopausal: their main source of estrogen is no longer their ovaries. Instead, the precursors of estrogen, such as testosterone and androstenedione, are produced in the ovaries and the adrenal glands and then secreted into the bloodstream, where specific organs pick them up and convert them into estrogen through an enzyme called aromatase. This enzyme has been found in the adrenal glands, fat, breast, brain, and muscles, and is responsible for much of the local estrogen in postmenopausal people. (Other enzymes such as sulfatase may also be important in this regard.) In addition, fairly recent studies show that postmenopausal people with breast cancer have aromatase in their breast tissue, giving the breast its own supply of estrogen.[51] So to reduce estrogen levels in the tissues of postmenopausal people we need to block aromatase. A class of drugs called aromatase inhibitors can do this with minimal side effects.

Three aromatase-blocking drugs are available clinically. Arimidex (anastrozole) and Femara (letrozole) work by reversibly blocking this enzyme, while Aromasin (exemestane) binds to the enzyme and inactivates it permanently. These drugs were first tested in patients with ER-positive metastatic disease. All of them had favorable effects (see Chapter 15). Arimidex was then studied head-to-head against Nolvadex and showed a small advantage. Randomized trials have shown that initial treatment with an aromatase inhibitor or the sequence of Nolvadex (tamoxifen) followed by an aromatase inhibitor are acceptable strategies. Unlike Nolvadex, aromatase inhibitors have no estrogenic effects but also produce no blood clots or endometrial cancer. Instead they have a whole different set of side effects, including bone and joint pain and, more significantly, increases in fractures due to a decrease in bone density (see more on bone health on page 438). Interestingly, the patients who took both Nolvadex and Arimidex at the same time did no better than those who took only Nolvadex. One theory is that Nolvadex acts more like estrogen when total body levels of estrogen are low.

Two large international studies compared adjuvant Aromasin (exemestane, an aromatase inhibitor) with ovarian suppression to Nolvadex (tamoxifen) plus ovarian suppression in people who are still having their periods. In the first study, called TEXT, the ovarian suppression was achieved with a GnRH inhibitor called triptorelin (similar to goserelin) or through ovarian radiation. After five years, 92.8 percent of participants who had taken Aromasin had no signs of breast cancer recurrence compared to 88.8 percent of participants who had been on Nolvadex.[52] Overall survival was the same in both groups, and side effects were significant in about 30 percent of participants in both groups. Although this study certainly shows that the aromatase inhibitor Aromasin was better at preventing recurrence, it was not by much. Shortly after the TEXT study, we got the results of the second trial, called SOFT, which compared Nolvadex alone to Nolvadex plus ovarian suppression or Aromasin plus ovarian suppression.[53] The analysis included patients who had not received chemotherapy as well as those who had received chemotherapy but had remained premenopausal. The researchers found that adding ovarian suppression to Nolvadex did not provide a significant benefit in the overall groups. However, for the patients who had undergone chemotherapy and were still having periods, the addition of the ovarian suppression—particularly along with Aromasin—improved their survival. A combined analysis of both trials found a 1.8 percent difference in twelve-year-distant metastasis-free survival in favor of the

Aromasin-plus-ovarian-suppression group. But no significant difference in overall survival was observed between the two groups.[54]

In a meta-analysis of these and another two studies at a recent breast cancer conference, researchers found that the annual rate of breast cancer recurrence was one-fifth lower with an aromatase inhibitor compared to Nolvadex (tamoxifen). After ten years the rate of recurrence for the aromatase inhibitor and ovarian suppression group was 14 percent compared to 17.5 in the Nolvadex group.[55]

Nonhormonal Targeted Therapy

Herceptin (trastuzumab)

In addition to efforts to destroy cancer cells or change their hormonal milieu, there is a newer form of drug designed to attack a target on the cancer cell in hopes of reducing its malignant potential.

Herceptin (trastuzumab) is the first drug of this category in clinical use. It is the antibody to the HER2/neu receptor, which is overexpressed in 20 percent of women with breast cancer. It was first tested in women with metastatic disease and shown to have a beneficial effect, both alone and with chemotherapy.[56] Subsequent studies have shown its benefits as an adjuvant therapy in combination with chemotherapy, as it reduces recurrence by one-half at three years after administration.[57] All women with tumors over one centimeter or positive nodes whose tumors overexpress HER2/neu are now given one year of Herceptin, or Herceptin in combination with chemotherapy for a shorter period, unless there is a contraindication, such as cardiac disease. Some doctors may recommend Herceptin for even smaller tumors, based on new data that indicate that HER2-positive tumors pose a significant risk for spreading, even when caught early.[58] Ongoing studies are evaluating shorter and longer durations of therapy. Herceptin can be given at the same time as some drugs but not others, depending on the specific drug and possible interactions (see Chapter 15).

There are now other inhibitors of HER2/neu: Tykerb (lapatinib), Nerlynx (neratinib), and Perjeta (pertuzumab). Several studies have shown that Tykerb-based therapy is no better than Herceptin and likely not as good. However, as suggested in women with metastatic disease, a combination of the two HER2 inhibitors that have different mechanisms of action, known as dual-blockade, works better—at least in the short term. A study called exteNET proved that Nerlynx significantly improved invasive disease-free survival in HER2-positive, hormone-positive, early-stage breast cancer. It also proved to be effective as therapy in early-stage breast cancer after patients completed a full year of Herceptin.[59] Unfortunately one of its side effects is a high incidence of diarrhea, but there are measures that can be taken to reduce this. As with all drugs, the stronger the dosage, the greater the side effects. Perjeta (pertuzumab) uses yet another mechanism to block HER2 and has proved to be effective in a dual blockade with Herceptin. In a study of 4,805 women, Perjeta added to Herceptin and chemotherapy slightly improved invasive disease-free survival among patients with HER2-positive operable breast cancer. The three-year disease-free survival rate with the dual blockade was 94 percent, while in the placebo group it was 93 percent. In participants with node-positive disease, the result was 92 percent in the dual-blockade group and 90 in the placebo group.[60]

Perjeta has also been shown to augment the effectiveness of Herceptin in metastatic disease. The median overall survival in the Perjeta group was 56.5 months compared to 40.8 months in the placebo group.[61]

The combination of Herceptin and Perjeta would be relevant for patients with tumors larger than three centimeters and/or positive nodes. Patients and their doctors could consider a combination of chemotherapy with a taxane and HER2 blockade neoadjuvantly followed by surgery. Depending on their stage at presentation, what chemotherapy is added to the Herceptin will be variable. Alternatively they could go on a trial to see whether the combination of anti-HER2 drugs post-chemotherapy and primary surgery are also better. Finally, they could choose to receive adjuvant chemotherapy with a year of Herceptin. This is an area that is continually changing as new treatments are explored, so make sure you ask what has been shown to be the best option at the time of your diagnosis.

Bisphosphonates

Another way to change the environment to make it less supportive of cancer is with the use of bisphosphonates. Bisphosphonates are drugs like Fosamax (alendronate), Zometa (zoledronic acid), Prolia or Xgeva (denosumab), Bonefos (clodronate), or Boniva (ibandronate), commonly used to treat osteoporosis and prevent bone loss. Because they function well in protecting bone from absorption, they were first used to treat bone metastases and had some success. Studies were then launched to see if they could prevent breast metastases as well. A Canadian study of 6,097 patients in their fifties with stage I to stage III breast cancer tested three different bisphosphonates in adjuvant therapy. After five years, all three groups differed little in disease-free survival, with Zometa at 88.3 percent, Bonefos at 87.6 percent, and Boniva at 87.4 percent.[62] After several studies, it appears bisphosphonates are useful primarily in postmenopausal patients or those on ovarian suppression with early-stage breast cancer.[63] The rare but serious side effect in some women is osteonecrosis or degeneration of the jaw, so it is important to have attentive dental care. In addition, women taking these drugs need to make sure their diet includes adequate vitamin D and calcium. Currently bisphosphonates are not yet standard of care for all patients (and the intravenous versions are not covered by many insurance programs), but for the highest-risk patients it may be worth pursuing. Updated guidelines by the American Society of Clinical Oncologists note that they should be used only in conjunction with, and not in place of, standard anticancer treatments.

Most of the treatments for hormone-positive tumors involve decreasing estrogen and therefore increasing premature bone loss. Bisphosphonates are good at preventing this in postmenopausal patients.

IMMUNOTHERAPY

In Chapter 3, I discussed the immune system at some length because the hottest new area of research is the use of immunotherapies for the treatment of breast cancer. Since the last edition, two immunotherapies for breast cancer have been approved by the U.S. Food and Drug Administration (FDA). There had initially been three, but one called Tecentriq (atezolizumab) has been withdrawn because of negative results during confirmation testing—an example of why clinical trials need to be so methodical and thorough.

Keytruda (pembrolizumab) is used in combination with chemotherapy and is particularly effective when treating triple-negative breast cancer. But it also has some benefit with other types of breast cancer. As you may recall from Chapter 3, the immune system's T cells are the ones with a "database" of previous threats like viruses, and they respond to each with specific antibodies. These cells have a special link called PD-L1 that attaches to the tumor to cause an immune response against it, but tumors hack this receptor so they can keep growing. Keytruda blocks the hacked PD-L1, allowing the immune system to slow or shrink the growth of cancer cells. This drug may also be administered as an initial treatment for some people.

Studies have shown that patients with high-risk, early-stage triple-negative disease who receive Keytruda do remarkably better than those receiving a placebo. In the initial 602 patients of a recent trial, 65 percent of those given Keytruda and chemotherapy showed no signs of cancer in tissue samples after treatment compared to 51 percent in the placebo-chemotherapy group. In a follow-up fifteen months later, 7 percent of the patients in the Keytruda group and 12 percent of those in the placebo group had disease progression, an improvement of 5 percent.[64]

For patients with advanced metastatic triple-negative breast cancer, the addition of Keytruda to chemotherapy resulted in longer progression-free survival: twenty-three months with the drug compared to sixteen months without it.[65]

Jemperli (dostarlimab) is a very specific immune checkpoint inhibitor for a rare marker that appears in less than 1 percent of advanced breast cancers. It is used to treat a mismatch repair deficient (dMMR) cancer that has grown during or after treatment, and when no other options are available.

Personalized Immunotherapy with TILs

Another exciting breakthrough in clinical trials has been the use of an individual's own tumor-fighting immune cells to fight metastatic breast cancer. These tumor-infiltrating lymphocytes (TILs) are white blood cells that recognize abnormal cancer cells and penetrate the tumor in an effort to fight the disease. But they are often thwarted by brakes in the immune system or signals from the tumor itself telling them to stop. This new immunotherapy seeks to remove and isolate these TILS from biopsied tumor tissue, multiply them, and then reprogram them to defy cancer's orders to leave it alone. These improved TILs are reinserted in the patient via blood transfusion after chemotherapy. Since the TILs are extracted from the tumor itself, they already know the enemy's weak points. Unfortunately, TILs can't always be found in biopsied tissue, but they have been located in patients with hormone-positive cancers— previously thought incapable of an immune response and thus not responsive to immunotherapy. In a clinical trial of forty-two women with metastatic breast cancer, twenty-eight (or 67 percent) generated an immune reaction against the cancer. Six participants were treated, half of whom experienced measurable tumor shrinkage.[66] This therapy may be an option for women with metastatic breast cancer whose previous treatments have failed. As I write this update, TILs immunotherapy is available only in clinical trials.

Other Research in the Works

An entirely different approach to destroy cancer tumors has been adopted by scientists at Purdue University, who are targeting nonmalignant immune cells found in cancer tumors. Using an old analogy, if the tumor were the headquarters of a terrorist group, the new drug would be focused not on the leaders but rather on citizens they've co-opted to ensure their safety and well-being. The potential new drug would destroy any loyalty to the terrorists and incite them to attack instead. Purdue chemist Dr. Philip Low noted that depending on the type of cancer, 30 to 80 percent of the cells in a solid tumor are not cancer and are used for other functions. These nonmalignant cells are very similar from one tumor to the next, so a drug that corrects their misbehavior can be used to treat most solid tumors. Development of the drug is still in the early stages, but tests in the laboratory and in human tumors in animals have shown effectiveness in six different cancer types, according to lead scientists who predict it will be ready within the next decade. The essential part of the anticancer drug is quite toxic, but it would be linked to folate, a type of vitamin B, which only the corrupted immune cells consume.[67]

Vaccines

Vaccines for the prevention of breast cancer recurrence got a jump start in the wake of the COVID pandemic, with new research prompting more than forty different clinical trials.[68] Some immunotherapy approaches under study include vaccines focused on HER2,[69] mammaglobin,[70] and MUC1.[71] So far none of them is ready for prime time. Until now, the antitumor activity triggered by potential vaccines has not lasted long enough for significant benefits in survival. This may be caused by the formula of the vaccines themselves, a developed tolerance to them, or the tumor's effectiveness in suppressing the immune system.[72]

One vaccine trial that is sparking increased interest is aimed at women with triple-negative cancers, targeting a protein involved in milk production that is overexpressed in these breast tumors. As I write this, the α-lactalbumin vaccine is still in initial stages of testing for safety and dosage. These phase 1 trials are the first tests in humans and are usually too small to measure the vaccine's anticancer effects.

Because so many vaccine clinical trials in different stages are under way, you may want to investigate them once your primary treatment is done.

LIFESTYLE CHANGES

Growing data suggest that lifestyle changes can further add to the adjuvant effect. The ones that have been studied the most at this point are weight loss, diet, and physical activity. The influence of excess weight on breast cancer outcomes was examined in a group of 14,709 women with localized disease. Being overweight increased the chances of metastases, second cancers in the other breast, and decreased overall survival. In the Nurses' Health Study, higher weight at diagnosis was associated with decreased survival, and another study of 3,924 women with localized breast cancer showed that women with a body mass index (BMI) over 30 were more likely than lean women to die of their breast cancer.[73] Several other studies have confirmed this effect. There have been two randomized controlled studies called WINS (The Women's Intervention Nutrition Study) and WHEL (Women's Healthy Eating and Living). WINS was designed to test a low-fat intervention. After five years there was a significant reduction in dietary fat intake as well as a resulting decrease in weight in the intervention group. Initially there was a significant difference in recurrence in the control group, but it was no longer significant after three more years. Interestingly, there was a bigger effect in the participants with ER- and PR-negative cancers than in the hormonal ones.[74] The WHEL study randomized participants to a diet high in fruits and vegetables and low in fat, or nonfat. Although the fruits and vegetables didn't seem to have an impact, weight and exercise did. A recent meta-analysis of eighty-two follow-up studies showed that obesity is associated with poorer health overall and less breast cancer survival in pre- and postmenopausal people. Participants who were obese (BMI over 30) had a 41 percent increase in mortality.[75] It's amazing that we are willing to take poison to reduce our chances of recurrences or have our breasts cut off but balk at losing weight. It probably is the most important thing you can do! In addition to obesity, another danger is a diet with a high glycemic index—carb-heavy foods like cakes and cookies, bread, potatoes, chips, white rice, and sugary sodas. A study of the diets of more than eighty thousand cancer-free women with no prevalence of diabetes showed that a high-glycemic diet increased breast cancer risk. Foods heavy in carbohydrates are broken down quickly and increase blood sugar. Avoiding or cutting down on such foods is one way to reduce your breast cancer risk.[76]

Another key to reducing risk is physical activity. Here the data are similar: several studies show that women who participate in physical activity at least thirty minutes a day have a lower likelihood of recurrence than couch potatoes, and this is true regardless of weight. Lean women who exercise do better than lean women who don't exercise, and heavier women who exercise have better outcomes than women who lead sedentary lives. The more activity, the better the outcome. So get moving!

While the benefits of exercise are indisputable, those of dietary supplements are in question. It is essential to check with your doctor or care team before taking any herbal or dietary supplements, because many can hinder treatment—particularly chemotherapy. A randomized controlled study has shown that breast cancer patients who take different dietary supplements before and during chemotherapy have an increased risk of recurrence. These include antioxidant supplements such as vitamins A, C, and E as well as vitamin B12 and iron.[77]

GUIDELINES AND CHOICES

This chapter has spelled out the menu of treatments. At this point you and your doctor will need to consider them in relation to your situation and particular kind of breast cancer (see Chapters 10 and 12). We are moving into the era of personalized medicine rather than one-size-fits-all. So the global recommendations that you may have found in previous editions of this book have given way to describing particular scenarios. That being said, I will try to summarize where we are in general, so that you have a place to start.

Local treatment for small tumors (less than two centimeters) and no suspicious lymph nodes on examination is usually breast conservation with sentinel node biopsy followed by adjuvant treatment, depending on hormone status and HER2/neu. Mastectomy is also a choice, although it has no additional benefit to breast conservation and the downside of additional surgery with the attendant risks. Radiation therapy may follow depending on the location of the tumor and the risk of local recurrence. Tumors larger than two centimeters can be treated first with excision and sentinel node biopsy, unless the size of the tumor compared to the size of the breast suggests the use of neoadjuvant therapy to shrink the tumor with chemotherapy, and Herceptin if indicated, or even hormonal therapy. If mastectomy must be done, then it can be done before or after systemic therapy. Reconstruction can be immediate or delayed.

Women with positive lymph nodes are generally given chemotherapy regardless of their hormone status. However, the twenty-one-gene RT-PCR assay (Oncotype DX) test can be used in postmenopausal patients to judge the possibility of forgoing chemotherapy if the recurrence score is low (see Chapter 10). If the tumor overexpresses HER2/neu, you will also be given Herceptin for one year and Perjeta. If you are ER-positive, you will also probably receive a hormonal regimen such as Nolvadex, ovarian ablation, and/or an aromatase inhibitor.

All this means that deciding whether to have systemic treatment, and if so which kind, is complicated. You may want to look at the practice guidelines from the NCCN online at www.nccn.org. And you certainly will want to discuss with your doctor all the prognostic information you can (Oncotype DX testing if done, HER2 status, grade of tumor, and so on). This can all be helpful in understanding your individual risks and benefits.

And don't forget to exercise and lose weight if need be. Find a local group of survivors that walk, run, or even do dragon boating! Exercise, get support, and lose weight all at once. Others will be doing a lot to you, but this you can do for yourself.

SECOND OPINIONS

It's always wise to consider getting a second opinion, no matter how much you trust the advice of your surgeon or oncologist. The preference for a treatment is always somewhat subjective, and you're entitled to consult with more than one expert. Furthermore, special kinds of cancer may require approaches different from your doctor's, and different institutions may be involved in different research with new treatments you may be interested in.

Several breast centers in the United States have multidisciplinary programs in which you can meet with all the specialists involved in your care at the same place. Sometimes these are called *multimodality breast clinics* or *second opinion centers*. And the National Accreditation Program for Breast Centers (https://www.facs.org/quality-programs/cancer-programs/national-accreditation-program-for-breast-centers/) lists centers where you can be assured of a certain level of quality. In most of them you can be self-referred—you don't have to be referred by a doctor. I would recommend that anyone who has breast cancer should investigate the possibility of hooking up with one of these centers.

If looking to a multidisciplinary program for a second opinion seems complicated to you, try a single expert who knows the field and specializes in breast cancer. Either a breast surgeon or a medical oncologist specializing in breast cancer is more likely to be able to talk to you about chemotherapy and radiation therapy than a general surgeon.

And don't be afraid of hurting your original doctor's feelings. Most doctors welcome another point of view—and if yours doesn't, you should probably be looking for another doctor anyway.

This field is changing constantly. Yesterday's answer may be passé today. I suggest you supplement the information in this book with other sources and especially the Internet. On my website, www.drsusanlove searchfoundation.org, or on the NIH website, www.cancer.gov, you can find the latest studies and up-to-date information to supplement the overview given here. And don't be in a hurry—take all the time you need to get all the information you need. Breast cancer is rarely an emergency, so you should feel free to seek out multiple opinions until you come up with a plan that you're comfortable with.

STATISTICS

Several software programs add more factors to the survival data shown earlier. You can ask your physician to go to the PREDICT website (https://breast.predict.nhs.uk) to check your particular factors. This kind of evaluation of the cancer is what we're currently using to decide what seems to be the most medically sound course of treatment because it encompasses as much as we know to date about the natural history of the disease and the biology of the tumor. Remember that these statistical tools apply only to populations and so can only give you an overall picture of what is likely; what happens to you may not fit the norm.

Even considering the different types of breast cancer, it is impossible to tell what is going to happen with any one person. Two people may have the same genetic mutations, but the factors affecting the microenvironment (neighborhood) in which those cells live will vary. This explains why a doctor can say that someone with advanced metastatic disease can still "beat the odds." All our prognostications are, of necessity, based on large statistical groups of patients and the long-term survival rates of the different kinds of breast cancer. You can see that if triple-negative patients get through the first five years, they do very well, while patients with ER-positive tumors can have recurrences after five years! These prognostications have some use—as long as you realize they don't absolutely predict the course of your particular disease. I realized this myself when I was diagnosed with leukemia. It is good to know how serious the situation could be, but whatever happens to you is 100 percent! If 99 percent of people with tumors like yours die and you survive, you have beaten the odds. On the flip side, the majority of patients can be cured and if your cancer comes back, you are in the unlucky small percentage. I think it is important to look at the statistics and get a sense of how serious the situation is so that you can take care of what you need to, but then you should forget them because whatever happens to you is what is important, *not* the statistics!

TREATMENT STUDIES: CLINICAL TRIALS
AND RESEARCH PROTOCOLS

In making all the decisions that we have been talking about, you will be relying on information from research studies and the people who agreed to participate in them. It is important to understand how studies are done and the terminology used in describing these results, and even whether you want to participate in one yourself.

The most important studies involving the treatment setting are clinical trials. These types of studies (also known as interventional studies or research protocols) are prospective trials that evaluate a new treatment by having one group of participants get the treatment while another group, known as the control group, gets the standard treatment or, in some cases, a placebo (an inert pill). To be clear, a placebo is used in a trial only when no standard exists. It is in clinical trials that we actually test our hypothesis that a treatment has an effect. The people are followed closely for a given period of time, after which researchers compare the two groups. For example, let's say a new drug (or an older drug used for a new purpose, such as Nolvadex [tamoxifen]) is now being considered for prevention rather than just treatment. In the study the experimental group would be given the drug and the control group would be given a placebo, and no one would know which group was which. If 20 percent of the participants who received the drug developed breast cancer, and 40 percent of those who got the placebo did, we'd know that the drug did some good. If there is a standard therapy, the new treatment will be compared to it. In studies of the new aromatase inhibitors, for example, the inhibitors were compared to Nolvadex, the standard therapy. (See Chapter 15.) When there is no standard therapy, we use placebos.

These studies are usually randomized. This means that each participant's treatment is picked at random, usually by a computer, so there is no possibility that participants will be chosen based on certain aspects of their disease. If, for example, more people with atypical hyperplasia are chosen for a treatment regimen to prevent breast cancer and fewer people without it are put on another, the second treatment will end up looking better than it really was.

It's important that neither the researchers nor the participants know who's getting the new treatment and who's getting the placebo (or the standard treatment). That way the participants won't be tempted to alter their behavior based on the treatment they're getting or to unconsciously misreport symptoms, and the researchers won't be tempted to treat one group differently or interpret the results differently. Because neither researcher nor participant knows who's getting the treatment until after the study is completed, these studies are called double-blind. Not all studies can be double-blind. An example is the Veronesi study comparing radical mastectomy to quadrantectomy (see earlier in this chapter) for early breast cancer.[78] Surprisingly, this form of extensive lumpectomy had better medical results than mastectomy.

The controlled study that is prospective (planned from the beginning and not looking back at past results), randomized, and double-blind has the fewest potential flaws, and so it's the most reliable. It's still not perfect, however, because people who decide to participate in a study like that may not be like most of us—usually people prefer to know what treatment they're getting and don't want to risk being given a new drug that may not work as opposed to the tried-and-true treatment. But it's the closest we can get to good data.

An example of the problems that can arise when a study is not randomized is the clinical acceptance of high-dose chemotherapy with stem cell rescue after initial studies in the early 1990s. These studies compared women who had undergone this very toxic therapy to what we call historical controls—women with similar cancers that had been treated in the past. The findings suggested that the high-dose chemotherapy was better and appeared to confirm the largely accepted hypothesis that more aggressive treatment was better and that killing all the cancer cells was key.[79] When the randomized controlled studies comparing high-dose chemotherapy to standard chemotherapy were later completed, they showed no benefit from the high-dose regimen.[80] How could this happen? We don't know for certain, but probably the participants in the original study were screened extremely well to make sure that they had no obvious microscopic spread of their disease before they were enrolled in such a dangerous treatment, while the historical controls were not.[81] Also, treatments in general had improved over time, so the new therapy looked better than it actually was. It took the later, randomized study to bring out the truth. Thus the main job of randomized controlled trials is to correct or confirm the results of nonrandomized studies.

What, then, is the good of nonrandomized studies? They are a valuable first step for medical scientists. Randomized studies are difficult and expensive. So we do one only if we have good reason to believe it will contribute to our understanding of the disease. An early study may rule out the use of a randomized study. If, for example, those first studies on high-dose chemotherapy with stem cell rescue had shown no improvement, we could have ruled out the treatments without undertaking larger studies. We are lucky because hundreds of randomized controlled studies have been done on breast cancer treatments, and our current approaches exist thanks to participants who were willing to be randomized. This is a significant benefit to patients who are diagnosed today. Ongoing and future studies will continue to improve treatment for people with breast cancer.

Endpoints of Clinical Trials

We need to spend a moment looking at what the numbers mean so you can evaluate information from available studies and understand the figures your doctor may quote you. Research studies about cancer therapy can be confusing. The first thing to look at is a given study's endpoint. Endpoints represent the outcome that is being compared in the two treatments. For example, one study may be looking at whether a cancer came back in the breast, which is very important, but you yourself may be more concerned with whether it prevents the spread of cancer to the rest of the body.

The most important endpoint to most patients is overall survival (OS). The time frame is the beginning of the participant's entry into the study to their death from any cause. This may seem odd—if someone who has had breast cancer dies of heart disease, why is that relevant to the study? It may not be—but it is possible that the treatment that cured their breast cancer caused the disease that eventually killed them. An example of this is the postmastectomy radiation therapy that was used in the 1970s. Although the patients had fewer recurrences, those treated on the left side had more heart disease twenty years later (see Chapter 18). This endpoint also takes into consideration the treatment for any recurrence. But the question then arises: How long do you have to follow a patient to measure overall survival? (This is where arbitrary numbers like five years come in.)

Because we want to evaluate the studies as soon as possible, we have other endpoints as well as OS. Disease-free survival (DFS) measures the time from randomization to the first evidence of recurrence or death. This figure reflects the number of participants at a particular time who have no recurrence of breast cancer in the breast, in the chest wall (after mastectomy), or elsewhere in the body. It presumes that the more participants who are disease free, the better.

Local recurrences (see Chapter 19) aren't always as serious as disease that spreads to the rest of the body. As a result, this is sometimes further modified in a third endpoint, distant disease-free survival (distant DFS), which indicates the time until the first recurrence outside the breast. Here we are looking at how many participants are alive without metastases at a particular point in time.

All these endpoints have their limitations. DFS is a good measure of how effective the treatment is, but it doesn't consider what happens to the patient after they have a recurrence. Although it usually translates into OS eventually, a treatment could put off recurrence but cause such serious side effects that the patient would die sooner than someone whose cancer recurred sooner and lived for a long time with their recurrence. Two treatments may not show a difference in overall survival, yet one may prolong the time the patient is symptom-free. Although lengthening the time to recurrence isn't a cure, it is important. For example, let's say you were diagnosed with a breast cancer that, with the old treatment, would have killed you in one year. A new treatment increases your time to recurrence, or disease-free survival time, by three years, and so you die four years after your diagnosis. Your survival at five years would be zero either way, but you have had three extra years of quality time. Improving DFS or OS does not guarantee that the patient will not die of breast cancer eventually; it just makes it less likely to happen within the time frame of the study. For some patients, a longer life may be worth the side effects of the treatment even if it is not ultimately lifesaving.

When studies are reported in the medical literature, they are often viewed as survival curves. This is the percentage of participants alive in each arm (treatment) of the study at set time periods (see Figure 11.4). This shows you graphically (these are not real statistics) the difference between the two curves in general and the absolute difference between them at any one point in time. The overall difference may be that in one arm of the study a large number of participants die in the first few years, but then anyone who gets past that has a good chance of survival, whereas on the other arm the benefits decrease much more gradually (see the

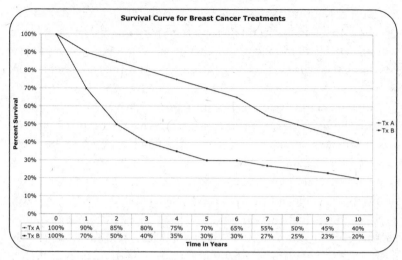

Figure 11.4

previous discussion). The absolute difference would be the difference in survival at any one point in time. In this figure, the absolute difference in survival at three years may be 40 percent, while at ten years it may be 20 percent because the patterns of the curves are different. Disease-free survival refers not to death as the endpoint but recurrence of disease—that is, metastases or recurrence in the mastectomy scar or breast. Most people who have a recurrence of breast cancer will ultimately die of it, and so the curves are often similar; however, recurrence happens sooner, so they can end the study sooner and report results sooner.

Another way data are presented is in terms of a hazard ratio. You see the risk of a recurrence at a particular moment in time for a person who is still surviving, depending on which of the two treatments they took. You then see the risk for a surviving person taking the other treatment. These two are compared in the form of a ratio. Using the preceding example, the hazard ratio at three years would be 40/80 or .5; in other words, only 50 percent of people with treatment B are alive versus those with treatment A. At ten years, this would also be 20/40, or .5, or 50 percent. Although this is useful for scientists (and drug marketers), it is less so for the person with cancer. It tells you only that one treatment is relatively better than the other, not whether either is especially good. What is better for you is to look at the absolute difference in the treatments at a point in time. That time needs to be long enough for at least half the people in the study to have reached it. On our survival curves, the absolute difference at three years is forty people, while at ten years with the same hazard ratio it is twenty people. They are saying only that treatment A is twice as good as treatment B, but by ten years neither one is that good.

Unfortunately not all studies are reported that way. Some studies refer to the *percentage reduction in mortality*. This refers to the percentage of patients who died compared to the number of deaths that were expected. For example, if a study showed that eight patients died in the control group and only six in the study group, there were two fewer deaths than would normally be expected. This is then reported as a 25 percent reduction in mortality, or two divided by eight. A similar study with more patients might show that forty patients died in the control group compared to thirty in the study group. The reduction of ten deaths over a possible forty is still 25 percent. In the second study, ten patients' lives were saved, while in the first it was only two. You should always try to get the absolute benefit rather than the relative one if you are comparing treatments. If your oncologist or surgeon does not know the absolute figures, they can get them online and print them out for you.

Even here there are limitations. In the study we are analyzing, people who died of cancer within ten years on treatment A still may have had their lives prolonged by the treatment. A way to get at this is to compare median DFS and OS. That is the time in which half the patients in the study had had recurrences or had died. In a study of one particular chemotherapy, the median time to recurrence was three years in the control group and seven years in the chemotherapy group. The difference in median survival was eight years and fifteen years, respectively. Clearly there were some people who benefited from a longer time before their cancer recurred who were not measured by looking at the data at fifteen years.

Another important study tool is the meta-analysis. Sometimes a study is too small to show an effect. For example, let's say that twenty people are studied, ten on the new treatment and ten on the old. It appears that there is no difference. But if the study had included one hundred in each category, five more people would have been seen to survive on the new treatment. By combining many studies looking at the same question, a meta-analysis can come up with more precise figures. The Early

Breast Clinical Trialists' Collaborative Group[82] combines studies looking at chemotherapy and hormone therapy for a large analysis about every five years and has come up with statistics that none of the small studies found individually.

Understanding the value of various treatments will help you understand what your doctor is suggesting, and why. It will also help you decide the treatment *you* want—and they may or may not be the same thing. If, for example, the treatment has comparatively little chance of keeping you alive for a substantial length of time, you may decide that painful chemotherapy will ruin the time you have left to live and that you'd rather risk a shorter, more comfortable life span. The writer Audre Lorde, who died in 1992, explained her reasons for making this choice in her book *A Burst of Light*: "I want as much good time as possible, and their treatments aren't going to make a hell of a lot of difference in terms of extended time. But they'll make a hell of a lot of difference in terms of my general condition and how I live my life."[83]

However, a year or two may feel like "a hell of a lot of difference" to you. You may decide that the possibility of living a little longer is worth the limited suffering that chemotherapy entails. There are no right or wrong decisions here; there is only your need and your right to have the most accurate information possible and to decide based on who you are and what choices make the most sense for you.

BECOMING PART OF A STUDY

Learning what studies mean is vital for every person who is considering using a study as part of any decision they make. But you can also take a further step and become part of a study—helping others and very possibly helping yourself.

When you participate in a clinical study, you join a protocol—a program designed to answer specific questions about the effectiveness of a particular approach. The questions can be about methods of diagnosis, types of treatment, dosage of drugs, timing of administration of drugs, or type of drugs used. Let's say you're involved in a protocol for breast cancer treatment to compare two new hormone therapies. You'll be one of a large group of patients who fit the criteria and randomized to take one drug or the other. Both groups will be followed just as rigorously.

What makes it a clinical study is the fact that it is asking a question, for example: Will the people receiving drug A do better than the people on drug B? By participating in such studies you and the other participants will get reasonable treatment and at the same time help us figure out the answer.

If you're considering taking part in a study, you have a right to know everything about it. Ask the researchers what exactly they're giving you, find out the possible side effects, find out what they know and don't know. The researchers are required to prepare an informed-consent form, giving participants complete information about the study. It is often very long. (The form for the study of high-dosage chemotherapy was twenty-seven pages.) Before signing it, read it thoroughly—it's worth the effort. Write out your questions. Sit down with the investigator and/or your doctor and go over questions about anything that's unclear. Also, if the study has been ongoing, ask to speak to another person with breast cancer who has gone through the same program ahead of you.

There are safeguards in most trials. In addition, there is a human participants protection committee (often called an institutional review board or IRB) in every hospital that does research. These committees review each protocol to make sure it is safe and well designed. They oversee all clinical trials and make sure that the informed consent is readable and the potential benefits of the study outweigh its risks for the people being studied. Of course, you'll always be given the choice. It's both unethical and illegal for a doctor to put you on a protocol treatment or clinical trial without your full and informed consent, and you have every right to refuse. If you're in an experiment and become convinced that it's harming you, you can leave it. You and your doctor both have the right to take you off the study at any time.

There are very good reasons for participating in a protocol. Aside from its usefulness to people in the future, studies done at top-notch cancer centers and hospitals may assure a patient of up-to-date care. For these reasons many people are eager to be part of studies.

One woman who was diagnosed in 1990 with a stage III cancer became involved in a phase 2 study using far higher doses of chemotherapy than the standard—the dose was adjusted upward as far as the patient's tolerance allowed. Along with the treatments in the hospital, which occurred every three weeks, she gave herself nightly injections of a material that stimulated the growth of bone marrow destroyed by the chemotherapy.

She had a difficult time with the treatment, throwing up so often that she slept on the bathroom floor for weeks. "They called me the nausea queen," she recalls ruefully. But her experiment paid off. Although in this study the patients went straight into chemotherapy without having surgery or radiation beforehand, they had been warned that they would probably require both when the chemotherapy course was over. But her tumor shrank so dramatically that she did not need either. "I feel that the only reason I'm alive is because I did that trial," she says. One of the other women in the trial, with whom she became close friends, survived in spite of the fact that she had aggressive inflammatory cancer. Still other studies have not demonstrated benefits or even shown harm. A study, after all, is still the luck of the draw.

Some studies are actually begun by patients themselves. You can get a group in the community together and initiate a study on your own terms. For example, if you want to research lesbians and breast cancer, you can go to the local medical school or a researcher and say, "This is a study we want to see done. We'll supply the participants—do you have anyone who can work with us?" A number of recent studies have begun that way. For example, a group of women in Long Island were disturbed at the high level of breast cancer in their community. They lobbied the National Cancer Institute and got a study that investigated a possible relationship between environmental pollutants in Long Island and breast cancer. Women on Cape Cod set up a similar study for Massachusetts.

So far, we haven't done enough to encourage people to participate in studies. Only about 3 percent of breast cancer patients in the United States participate in protocols—much lower than in Europe. And this is true of patients with many diseases. But we can't wholly blame the patients for this; many hospitals or doctors don't offer protocols. If you're being treated at a research hospital or major cancer center, you'll usually be offered protocols if you qualify, and large numbers of patients there do participate. People who choose such hospitals for treatment tend to be those who seek out the most advanced, sophisticated treatments. They feel safer in an environment where the major purpose is to study and fight cancer. But the ability to offer protocols isn't limited to these hospitals. There is now a mechanism allowing community hospitals to offer participation in protocols through a program called CCOP (Cancer

Center Outreach Program) that links community hospitals with large medical centers and allows you to participate in the same studies in your local area. Participation ensures that your doctor is keeping up-to-date and helping develop the best that medicine has to offer.

If you're a patient, please seriously think about joining a study. If you ask about trials and your doctor doesn't know of any and doesn't want to bother finding out, you can check out www.breastcancertrials.org or check the National Cancer Institute's website at www.cancer.gov. You can obtain a list of every clinical trial you're eligible for. You'll also find out the trial locations so you'll know whether a given study is being conducted near you. Then you can go with that information to your doctor and work with it from there.

The financial aspects of studies vary greatly depending on the nature of the study. For a study that offers no benefit and some inconvenience to the participant, payment may be offered as an incentive—those are the studies college kids often get into to earn a few hundred dollars. (I participated in a study of diethylstilbestrol (DES) as a contraceptive to help pay my tuition when I was in medical school.) Studies that may benefit the participant or cause the participant no inconvenience involve no financial exchange at all. Occasionally a study of a treatment that can benefit the patient will offer a reduced fee for the treatment, like an asthma and visualization study my coauthor participated in. Finally, as is the case with the chemotherapy studies comparing drugs already approved by the FDA, the patient (or the insurance company) pays the full price for the procedure. When new drugs are being tested, the drug company generally pays for the treatment. Many hospitals will not allow studies involving an experimental drug or device in which the patient must pay. Political action has led some states to mandate that insurance coverage and Medicare cover the standard cancer care that is part of the clinical trial.

Unfortunately, even when they're offered protocols, only a small percentage of patients accept the offer. Here too there are a number of reasons. Some people are afraid of being randomized. They want to get the best treatment and they find it hard to believe that the medical profession doesn't know what that is. Or they have strong feelings about getting a particular treatment and they don't want to experiment with anything else.

"I'd be in a study comparing chemotherapy and an aromatase inhibitor," a woman will tell me, "if I could choose which one I'll get." That can't be done in a study as the treatments need to be chosen randomly for the study to be valid.

Some people don't participate in clinical trials because they think we already have the answers. For example, they assume that the standard treatments will save their lives, and they don't want to rock the boat with something new. But it's precisely because the standard treatments *don't* always work that we do experiments. The courageous people who participated in the phase 1 and phase 2 trials of Adriamycin and Taxol benefited not only themselves but the many people who followed them. Often once a study is over, the drug is made available to the people who had not received it as compassionate use.

Some people fail to understand the whole idea of a study. They want to choose their own treatment and after the treatment is finished, they want that treatment and its effects on them to be studied. But of course, that isn't the way it works. For a study of a treatment to give us clear information, it must be done under controlled circumstances, defined by the researchers, and strictly followed. After-the-fact statistics have their use, but we can never get the same level of information with this kind of observational study that we can with randomized control studies.

Ironically, some people swing to the other extreme. Once in a while a highly publicized experimental procedure comes along that people think is the miracle we've been searching for. Then the attitude toward being in a study turns around. Instead of fearing being part of an experiment, people demand what they think will be their share of the miracle.

After learning what protocols are available, you may decide that none of them offers the treatment you want. But before you decide, you owe it to yourself and other women to find out what protocols you are eligible for and what they involve. My patient who took part in the high-dose chemotherapy experiment says that if she had a friend newly diagnosed with breast cancer, she would strongly urge her to look into protocols. "I'd tell her not to jump into anything," she says, "but to explore everything. Find out what's there; weigh it in your mind. 'Latest' isn't always best, and it may be that what you find isn't right for you. But there's a very good chance that you'll find that what's best for you is in a clinical trial."

Whether or not you decide to become part of a clinical trial in terms of your treatment, there's another way you can contribute to breast cancer research and do yourself a favor as well. If you have any surgical procedure—whether a biopsy, a wide excision, a mastectomy, or even breast reduction—ask whether the tissue removed from your breast can be deposited in a tissue bank (see Chapter 5). This is becoming increasingly possible because one of the things we're pushing for politically is regional and national tissue banks. You can have this done in any hospital. Both benign and cancerous tissue are useful in medical studies.

We have no guaranteed cures. If we did, there'd be no need for trials. But trials ensure that we are doing all we can to help people in the future. Already we see some of the trial results. Not too long ago a person with breast cancer had no choice but to lose their breast. But a number of people participated in the first breast conservation studies and were randomized to get either mastectomy or lumpectomy and radiation. They were very courageous people, going against the standard thinking to see if there was an alternative. Thanks to them, thousands of people today have saved their breasts. As you make the complex, difficult decisions about your own treatment, keep those people in mind—the brave experimenters and all of us who have benefited from their courage.

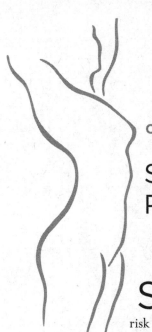

CHAPTER 12

Special Situations and Populations

So far, I've talked about breast cancer in general, the overall benefit of various treatments, and the risk of getting the disease. But it is important to remember that all breast cancers are not the same. They can vary in their molecular biology, the way they are diagnosed, or even in those affected. I wish I could tell you exactly how we'd treat your ER-positive, HER2/neu-positive cancer when you're a 40-year-old vegetarian who has had her ovaries removed and had her first child at age 20. In other words, I'd like to be able to give each of you a prescription for your best treatment. But since that's not possible, I'll do the next best thing and at least home in on characteristics and treatments for various specific forms of breast cancer.

NONINVASIVE PRECANCERS: DCIS AND LCIS

In ductal carcinoma in situ (DCIS) and lobular carcinoma in situ (LCIS), you have cells that appear to be cancer with their characteristic molecular changes but are completely contained within the lobule or duct (Figure 12.1). These tumors are called noninvasive breast cancer because they haven't spread outside their normal territory into the stroma. And until they do that, they cannot enter a blood vessel and spread to the rest of the body. Current thinking is that it is not the cells that develop the ability to break out of the duct but rather the neighborhood that allows or even invites them out (Figure 12.2). Think of a prison surrounded by ferocious guards keeping the inmates within the

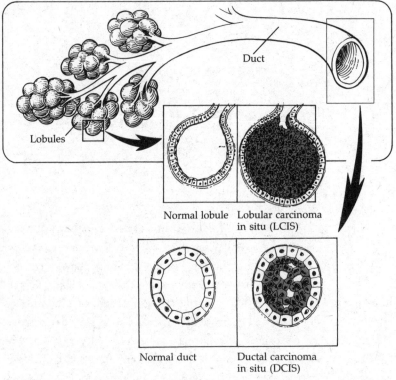

Figure 12.1

walls. Then someone comes around with a jug of whiskey and gets the guards drunk, and before you know it they are inviting the prisoners out. How this happens is not totally clear, but what *is* clear is that not everyone who has DCIS or LCIS will go on to develop invasive cancer. As I will explain at length later, the treatments include strengthening the neighborhood cells with Nolvadex (tamoxifen) and/or removing mutated cells so they can't cause trouble.

Although we have worked out differences among breast cancers with respect to invasive tumors, we are only just beginning to apply this understanding to the noninvasive lesions. The earlier jailbreak story offers a nice analogy for atypical ductal and lobular cells that have overgrown (hyperplasia), and how they lie in a continuum leading to carcinoma in situ and, ultimately, invasive cancer. But studies of DCIS have found many of the same types of cancer cells that are also seen in invasive disease, although distributed differently. Recent studies of molecular markers have led scientists to look at this in another light. DCIS has different

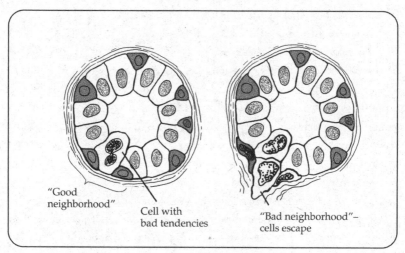

"Good neighborhood"

Cell with bad tendencies

"Bad neighborhood"– cells escape

Figure 12.2

subgroups just as invasive cancer does. Remember the different molecular categories described in the previous chapter based on ER, PR, and HER2/neu? We can also divide these precancerous or noninvasive lesions into categories, based on how the cells look and their molecular and immunologic markers.[1] The low-grade (not so worrisome) group includes atypical hyperplasia, low-grade DCIS, LCIS, and their invasive counterparts. These are hormone-sensitive lesions (ER-positive) that are HER2-negative, with no basal markers. The high-grade DCIS lesions encompass a more varied group that lacks estrogen receptors, may or may not be HER2/neu-positive, and could be triple-negative with basal markers. Those of you who have waded through Chapter 10 will recognize the luminal B, HER2-positive, and triple-negative tumors.

Interestingly, these precancerous lesions do not have the same distribution of markers as invasive disease. For example, DCIS shows a higher percentage of luminal B and HER2/neu-positive tumors and a bit less luminal A and basal than invasive ductal cancer. Consequently, there may not be a direct route from one to the other. You could not say, for example, that all luminal A DCIS that grew into cancer became luminal A invasive ductal cancer.[2] An intriguing study by Dr. Craig Allred from Washington University in St. Louis suggests that at least a third of DCIS showed a combination of types.[3] He proposes that only the most aggressive, or "fittest," cells or types go on to become invasive. What makes these types so interesting is that they could direct therapy in the future for these lesions, just as they do for invasive cancer. And they may also give us some clues about the causes of the disease.

How many of these in situ lesions progress to cancer? A 2014 Canadian study[4] looked at this question. Although women with carcinoma in situ treated with breast cancer conservation alone or with radiation had a higher risk of developing invasive breast cancer over the next twenty years than women without these lesions, more than 80 percent remained free of invasive cancer. This matches other studies and suggests that DCIS and LCIS should be considered risk factors for later breast cancer but certainly not cancerous lesions.[5]

I debated whether to discuss these "noninvasive cancers" in the chapter about prevention or in a chapter about cancer. I've settled on describing them as a special type here because most patients diagnosed with LCIS or DCIS think of themselves as having cancer, and, indeed, in medicine we've tended to move from the language of "precancer" into that of "noninvasive cancer." Still, I prefer the term "precancer" which is much less formal, so I will use both terms.

Lobular Cancer In Situ (LCIS)

Under the microscope, LCIS appears as a bunch of small, round cells stuffing the lobules, which normally don't contain any cells (Figure 12.3). Such clusters of cells have been termed "multicentric" because they can be scattered throughout both breasts. However, no one has tied them to a particular ductal system as we have with DCIS. We may not be accurate in this: because the lobules are at the periphery of each ductal branch, the LCIS could appear scattered while actually being part of the same branch of ducts. Picture the leaves that are attached to one branch of a tree. If you only looked at the leaves, they would seem to be spread all over, but if you examined the branch, you would see they are all attached. This is another reason to map the anatomy of the breast ducts.

We thought we knew the natural history of LCIS based on studies by Cushman Haagensen in 1978, but recent work has challenged our previous ideas. The old theory was that LCIS doesn't grow into cancer but rather signals a possible danger—the way, for example, an overcast day warns you it may rain. Because of this, many experts believed that LCIS wasn't a true precancer but more of a risk factor. As I noted earlier, this

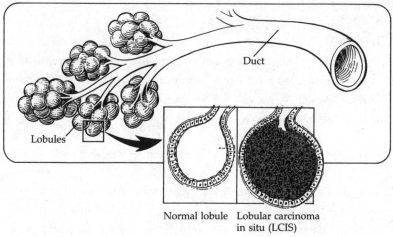

Normal lobule   Lobular carcinoma
in situ (LCIS)

Figure 12.3

may not be the case. The first evidence that LCIS can progress to invasive lobular cancer came from a 2004 analysis of 180 women who had participated in a study of the National Surgical Adjuvant Breast and Bowel Project (NSABP).[6] Overall, they found, after twelve years of follow-up, that nine (5 percent) invasive breast cancers had developed in the same breast as the original lesions, and eight of these (89 percent) were invasive lobular cancers, located in the site of the original LCIS. A second piece of evidence was a study of women who had both LCIS and invasive lobular cancer in the same breast. The pattern of mutations in the involved cells was very similar, suggesting that one had indeed evolved from the other.[7] Molecular studies have shown that both LCIS and infiltrating lobular cancers are ER-positive and HER2/neu-negative and lack expression of a certain protein, E-cadherin,[8] which helps cells stick together. Its absence may help explain why lobular cancers don't cling together in a nice lump but instead march cell by cell through the stroma in single-file lines, forming a diffuse pattern that is difficult to detect.

A twenty-nine-year longitudinal study on women with LCIS sponsored by the National Institutes of Health found a continuous 2-percent-per-year risk of developing invasive breast cancer.[9] This risk can be compounded by other risk factors for breast cancer. Interestingly, women with LCIS develop ductal as well as lobular cancers, although all of them are of the ER-positive variety. This means they are slow growing, less aggressive, and easier to pick up on screening mammograms.

Options

What can you do if you have LCIS? Basically you want to prevent yourself from getting invasive breast cancer. There are a number of options; the most drastic is bilateral prophylactic mastectomy. Why bilateral (both breasts)? Because the risk occurs in both breasts. In the NSABP study mentioned earlier, there was a 5 percent chance of getting an invasive cancer in the same breast and a similar 5 percent chance of getting an invasive cancer in the opposite one.

Some patients choose bilateral mastectomies because they want to know they've done everything possible. That way if they do get breast cancer, they feel that at least it isn't their fault. If they hadn't had this surgery and then developed the disease, they'd always wonder whether they could have prevented it. In the mid-1980s a patient told me, "I knew instantly what my decision should be. I was astounded to see how greedy for life I was." This woman was in a high-risk group because of her family history; she had relatives with breast cancer and was determined to do all she could to avoid getting it herself. She was uncomfortable with the studies about monitoring, which she considered too recent, while mastectomy had been around a long time. She was helped by the knowledge that she could then have breast reconstruction, which we'll talk about in Chapter 13.

A *pleomorphic* subtype of LCIS, with cells in multiple shapes and sizes, is treated with surgery as there is a risk of breast cancer already existing at the biopsy site. This is different from the classic type of LCIS, which does not require surgery, but it still represents a risk factor for future cancer in either breast.

The alternative to surgery is close monitoring: follow-up exams every six months, with a yearly mammogram. MRIs have not been shown to add any benefit to monitoring in patients with LCIS[10] if their overall risk is relatively low. However, high-risk screening with MRI is recommended for patients with a greater than 20 percent lifetime risk of breast cancer. Because the type of cancers that develop from LCIS appear to be the less aggressive, slower-growing, hormone-positive tumors, this seems a reasonable course. That way if a cancer does develop, you're likely to catch it and can then decide if you want a mastectomy, or a lumpectomy and radiation (see Chapter 11). If a cancer doesn't develop, you've been spared the ordeal of major and disfiguring surgery. This approach is what most surgeons recommend and is supported by the NCCN guidelines.[11]

Another alternative to mastectomy is taking Nolvadex (tamoxifen) or Evista (raloxifene) (in postmenopausal patients) for five years to prevent the future development of breast cancer. These estrogen-blocking drugs have been shown to reduce by 56 percent the chance of getting breast cancer in women with LCIS. Remember this means that the risk then becomes half of the original risk—about 0.5 percent a year as opposed to 1 percent per year. All these drugs have side effects that must be taken into consideration (see Chapters 15 and 18). They aren't safe to take if you are trying to get pregnant; Nolvadex (tamoxifen) taken during pregnancy can cause birth defects. Not all the side effects are bad, however. In postmenopausal people, both Nolvadex and Evista (raloxifene) can help prevent fractures. Like other decisions regarding treatment, taking these drugs depends on how you personally weigh the pros and cons.

If you're diagnosed with LCIS, give yourself time to think about what you want to do. LCIS doesn't call for an immediate decision. A woman once called me in a panic because she had been diagnosed with LCIS and was told by her oncologist that she should start on Nolvadex (tamoxifen) immediately. She was appropriately uncomfortable with this. He was treating it as if it were cancer and not a precancerous or noninvasive lesion. The risk of developing invasive cancer is 2 percent per year, so there is no rush to begin a treatment. I suggested to this woman that she take the follow-up route initially, and see how she felt about it in six months or a year. If she was comfortable living with it, then she could continue this course for the rest of her life, or until a cancer occurred. You can always decide to take Nolvadex or undergo a mastectomy later, but you can't undo a mastectomy, and you may not be able to undo some of Nolvadex's side effects. However, if a patient finds themself living in a constant state of anxiety, waking up every morning thinking, "This is it—this is the day I'll find the lump," then maybe a bilateral mastectomy is best for them. Invasive lobular cancers are much more common in women who take hormone therapy, so HT is not a good idea for women with LCIS.

Sometimes when a patient has a lump that turns out to be cancer, the pathologist will find LCIS in the adjacent tissue. What does this mean? In essence it suggests that the patient was at a higher risk of getting breast cancer and, sure enough, they got it. A number of studies show that women with LCIS associated with their invasive cancer who get a lumpectomy have the same risk of local recurrence and contralateral breast cancer as those without LCIS—that is, 1 percent a year.[12]

Ductal Carcinoma In Situ (DCIS)

Ductal carcinoma in situ (DCIS) is more common than LCIS and is more likely to grow into an invasive cancer. DCIS rarely forms lumps, but it does sometimes form a soft thickening (caused by the pliable ducts becoming less pliable because they're filled with cells; see Figure 12.4). DCIS is now found far more frequently because of mammograms, where it appears as little specks of calcium known as microcalcifications. A full 20 percent of malignancies detected by screening mammography are DCIS. In fact, it's probably even more common since not all DCIS demonstrated microcalcifications. Autopsies done on women who died from different causes show that between 6 and 16 percent had DCIS.[13] This suggests that many of us have it unknowingly and it is probably not as rare a condition as we used to believe.

In the past, standard treatment was a mastectomy of the breast with the lesion. That worked most of the time, but it probably wasn't necessary. Unfortunately, since the breasts had been removed, we had no way of studying what happened when a breast that had DCIS wasn't removed.

A few small studies, however, have given us a clue. Two followed people who were biopsied and thought to have something benign. Reviewing the pathology years later, these lesions were reclassified as being DCIS.

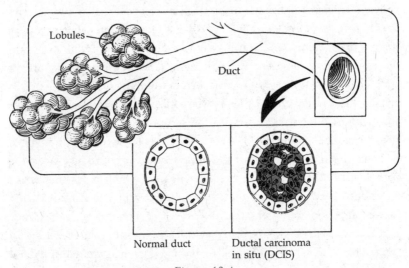

Normal duct   Ductal carcinoma
                       in situ (DCIS)

Figure 12.4

Follow-up of the patients has led us to believe that about 20 to 25 percent of women with untreated, low-grade DCIS will go on to get invasive cancer up to twenty-five years after the initial biopsy, and in the same area of the breast in which the biopsy was done.[14] Furthermore, their lesions were on the border between atypical hyperplasia (see Chapter 5) and DCIS, or they would have been diagnosed initially. What is clear from these studies, however, is that untreated DCIS can progress to invasive breast cancer, but in the majority of women it does not seem to do so. This matches the numbers quoted at the beginning of this chapter that about 20 percent of women treated for DCIS with excision and/or excision and radiation therapy developed invasive cancer over the next twenty years.

Unfortunately, we don't know how to tell which cases will become invasive and which won't. The other critical question is anatomical, whether DCIS is confined to one "sick duct"[15] or represents changes that are going on throughout the whole breast (multicentric). This is important not only in terms of our scientific understanding of DCIS but also in an immediate way for patients diagnosed with the disease. If it were multicentric, it would lend itself to the argument that you may as well have a mastectomy because it is only a matter of time until it pops up somewhere else. But if DCIS is actually unicentric, the wiser treatment would be to remove the one affected section of the affected breast.

Most high-grade lesions tend to be continuous and well marked by calcifications that are visible on a mammogram. However, low- to intermediate-grade lesions can be sneakier, with discontinuous

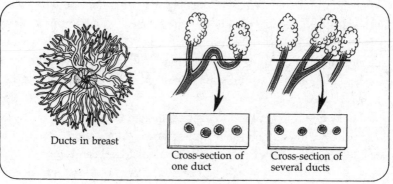

Ducts in breast

Cross-section of
one duct

Cross-section of
several ducts

Figure 12.5

intraductal spread, often with gaps of up to one centimeter between areas of involvement.

Our current approach is a wide excision based on our best guess of the extent of disease. We arrive at this guess by looking at the preoperative mammogram and magnification views, and then studying the tissue we remove from the breast. Although over 80 percent of DCIS is diagnosed by the presence of microcalcifications on a mammogram, there are some parts of the DCIS that may not have microcalcifications and so are essentially invisible to the surgeon. That can make it tricky to know exactly how much breast tissue to remove (Figure 12.5).

In making a decision, we look at the margins (see Figure 10.6, page 214) and look for a normal rim of tissue (one millimeter) around the disease. This is not perfect, however, so when there's a "recurrence" of DCIS, it's often not a recurrence at all; it's DCIS that we left behind in the first place, in spite of what we thought were clean margins. This doesn't happen frequently, but often enough (about 10 to 20 percent of the time) to make it significant. That's why surgery is often followed with radiation therapy. And also why mastectomy, though imperfect, tends to give a lower recurrence rate—it's the widest excision possible.

Surgeons often have the bad habit of saying they "got it all," which is misleading. People tend to think of cancer as a pea that expands to a marble and ultimately a golf ball. Dr. Stephanie Graff, a medical advisor for our research foundation and professor at Brown University, tells patients cancer is much more like a pile of salt. "And if you hold your salt shaker upside down on your kitchen counter, you get a pile of salt—the bigger it is, the more it spreads," Graff explains. "So when your surgeon says 'I got it all,' what they mean is 'I cleared up your pile of salt,' and your radiation oncologist is then the one who clears up the salt sprinkles that are all over the kitchen, which in this analogy includes your skin, the remaining breast, the muscle of the chest wall, and the fat and structures of the armpit." All these areas could be at risk depending on the size of your initial "pile of salt," as well as other features of your cancer.

It can be useful to get a follow-up mammogram after surgery. Because DCIS usually shows up on the mammogram as calcifications, it's important to ensure that all suspicious calcifications have been removed with the surgery. As already noted, however, DCIS can be present without calcifications.

Options

The current goal of treating DCIS is prevention. When the lesion is completely removed, it can neither come back nor become invasive. The question is how much surgery is necessary. Reasons for mastectomy are the same for DCIS as they are for invasive cancer: if the extent of the lesion is too large to allow a cosmetic excision, then a mastectomy (with or without immediate reconstruction; see Chapter 13) is indicated. This can sometimes be predicted before the operation when there are extensive malignant-appearing calcifications throughout the breast. In other cases, several attempts are made to excise all the disease, but the margins remain positive. Because DCIS can fill a whole ductal system, some of which take up a third of the breast, these lesions can be fairly extensive in their reach. Dr. Monica Morrow from Memorial Sloan Kettering found that about 33 percent of women with DCIS ended up needing mastectomies while women with stage I invasive cancers forming very discrete lumps required mastectomy only 10 percent of the time.[16] While you may think that an MRI would be as good as or better than a mammogram at predicting the extent of disease, this has not proved to be the case for DCIS.[17]

At the Dr. Susan Love Research Foundation we are trying to use ultrasound to map DCIS in the breast prior to surgery. Although we are well underway, technical difficulties in imaging the duct have slowed us down. Once we have a map of the disease, we can increase the effectiveness of surgery and maybe even consider watchful waiting.

Although mastectomy is sometimes required, wide excision is a reasonable choice to treat DCIS when the margins of resection are clear (see Chapter 13). Wide excision is usually followed with radiation therapy. Four randomized controlled studies have compared wide excision alone to wide excision and radiation for DCIS.[18] All these studies found that the addition of radiation therapy reduced the risk of recurrence by 50 to 60 percent. In the NSABP B 24 trial, the twelve-year rate of an invasive recurrence was 18 percent with lumpectomy alone, which was reduced to 8 to 9 percent when combined with radiation therapy.

The second question regards the use of Nolvadex (tamoxifen). In the same study, Nolvadex was shown to be beneficial for women with ER-positive DCIS, further reducing the risk of recurrence when combined with radiation by 2 to 3 percent. As with all other treatments, the higher your risk, the more you stand to gain.

Can we predict which women with DCIS can do without radiation? After all, 75 to 80 percent of the DCIS never recurred in those biopsy-alone studies mentioned earlier. The predictors of recurrence after breast-conserving surgery have been studied extensively. In addition to the markers I mentioned at the beginning of the chapter, the predictors of recurrence are whether the cells are high-grade and necrotic (dead-looking). In addition, young women have a greater rate of local recurrence than older ones. A new test developed by Genomic Health, the DCIS Score, looks at molecular markers in a DCIS biopsy and can categorize the risk of recurrence. A study from Ontario, Canada, applied this test to 718 women who had had wide excision alone. The women who were designated low risk by the Oncotype DX test were significantly less likely to develop a recurrence of DCIS or invasive cancer over ten years (12.7 percent) than those with an intermediate risk or high risk (27.8 to 33 percent).[19] Whether you consider 12.7 percent a low or high risk depends on your frame of reference. Nonetheless, this test has the potential to add key information in deciding the best treatment approach.

There is no reason to remove lymph nodes for small areas of DCIS because noninvasive cancer can't spread at this stage. But if the lesions are big (greater than five centimeters), some experts think they may hide microinvasion and recommend removing the lymph nodes as well. (Sentinel node biopsy, discussed in Chapter 13, is a good option here; most experts agree that removal of all the lymph nodes is not necessary unless the sentinel node contains cancer.) However, many surgeons will forgo lymph node surgery in this group as well, as even with microinvasion, the chance of having positive nodes is so low.[20] The NCCN guidelines recommend not doing a sentinel node biopsy with breast conservation for DCIS. If the wide excision demonstrates invasive carcinoma, the surgeon can go back to the few patients with invasion rather than increase the risk of lymphedema (see Chapter 18) if there is none.

It appears we are getting better at both finding and treating DCIS. The Cancer Research Network consortium reviewed 2,995 women with DCIS treated between 1990 and 2001. The women received a variety of treatments, from lumpectomy alone to lumpectomy, radiation, and Nolvadex (tamoxifen). The consortium found that the five-year risk of recurrence decreased from 18.5 percent for women diagnosed in 1990–1991 to 11 percent in women diagnosed in 2000–2001.[21]

What does all this mean for you? How should you proceed? First, if your routine mammogram has shown a cluster of microcalcifications, you'll need to have a core biopsy. This will determine whether you have DCIS. If the core biopsy does show DCIS, make sure your pathology report includes information regarding the grade, presence of necrosis, and ER status. Then you've got the four choices described earlier: wide excision alone, wide excision and radiation, a combination of both with Nolvadex (tamoxifen), or mastectomy.

Most surgeons recommend a wide excision. This means taking out the area with a centimeter-wide rim of normal tissue around it (margin). Sometimes this has been done on the first operation, and other times it has been necessary to go back and remove more tissue (a re-excision). This is usually followed by radiation therapy. You can add five years of Nolvadex (tamoxifen) to any of these choices if the DCIS is ER-positive (a bonus of doing this may be not only in treating the DCIS but in preventing an invasive cancer or one in the other breast).

Mastectomy, as noted earlier, is the ultimate wide excision. Most of the time this will be more than adequate, but there have been reports of DCIS recurring in the remaining breast tissue.[22] It happens in about 3 percent of cases followed for ten years. Generally we do a mastectomy only if the DCIS is so extensive that it's the only choice or if the patient strongly wants it.

One final alternative to these standard treatment options for DCIS is a plan of "watchful waiting" for low-risk DCIS, as is commonly used for early-stage prostate cancer. A study of low-risk DCIS in postmenopausal people found that close monitoring with the option of hormone therapy is a rational alternative to surgery. Of sixty-seven postmenopausal people who were given six months of Femara (letrozole), 15 percent had no signs of detectable cancer and 75 percent of those with low-grade disease had a pathological complete response—the absence of all signs of cancer in tissue samples.[23]

Researchers suggest a more individualized approach to DCIS, taking into account the projected risk of invasive progression of the disease rather than the diagnosis alone.[24]

If we develop the map of the disease mentioned earlier, it will allow us to test a variety of other approaches by offering us a clearer way to monitor the disease.

LOCALLY ADVANCED BREAST CANCER

Once in a while, a breast cancer isn't discovered until it's fairly big—a stage III cancer. It is larger than five centimeters (two inches), with positive lymph nodes, or it has one of the other features that we think give it a bad prognosis, like swelling (edema) of the skin or a big, matted cluster of lymph nodes under the arm. It may be stuck to the chest muscle or breaking through the skin. As with other situations, the first step is one or more core biopsies for diagnosis. These can also be used to determine the type of cancer with biomarkers such as hormone receptors, HER2/neu, and nuclear grade (see Chapter 10). Tests such as mammogram, ultrasound, PET/CT, and often MRI are done to rule out obvious spread.

The clinical indications, however, suggest that the locally advanced cancer is likely to have spread elsewhere in your body, at least microscopically. After imaging has shown the size of the cancer, we often go straight to systemic therapy to destroy the cells and try to shrink the tumor. Surgery and radiation therapy then follow the chemotherapy or hormone therapy. As mentioned in Chapter 11, this is termed "neoadjuvant therapy." Some patients are nervous about leaving the tumor in the breast and want a mastectomy right away. This is a bad idea for two reasons. First, the tumor often shrinks with chemotherapy or hormone therapy, making it more possible for doctors to do breast conservation surgery rather than a mastectomy. Even if lumpectomy is not possible after chemotherapy, it is more likely that all the cancer will be removed with negative margins. Second, the tumor's response to the chemotherapy can be a test of whether it responds to a particular combination of drugs and allows them to be changed if it does not (see Chapter 15). This approach results in major shrinkage of the tumor for 75 to 95 percent of patients. Sometimes even moderate-size tumors (three to five centimeters in a small breast) may behave like locally advanced tumors and respond best to a combined approach.

The group at MD Anderson has the most experience with this approach and has found that giving two different regimens of chemotherapy before surgery maximizes the response.[25] They usually start with four cycles of FAC (5-fluorouracil, Adriamycin, and cyclophosphamide) and follow with a second regimen containing taxane. If the tumor does not seem to be responding to the FAC after a cycle or two, an alternate

chemotherapy such as Taxol can be tried sooner. Whether all the chemotherapy is given at once or one regimen before and another after does not
seem to alter the outcome. If the tumor overexpresses HER2/neu, Herceptin (trastuzumab) is added preoperatively.[26] A potential problem with
surgery can be finding the tumor. In 30 percent of women treated with
chemotherapy and up to 60 percent who receive Herceptin, the tumor
can't be seen on exams and imaging. This is one reason the radiologist
usually places a clip in the tumor under imaging during the initial needle
biopsy—to facilitate systemic therapy later.

Although chemotherapy is most often used for neoadjuvant therapy,
occasionally hormone therapy (Nolvadex or an aromatase inhibitor)
may be used, especially in older women with hormone-positive tumors
who may not tolerate the chemotherapy as well. It is also capable of
shrinking the tumor and allowing less surgery. Recent data suggest
that women with tumors over three centimeters who have a low recurrence score on Oncotype DX or MammaPrint (see Chapter 10) and/
or are ER-positive with low-grade, low-proliferative tumors have a low
chance of responding with neoadjuvant chemotherapy (7 percent) but
do well with hormone therapy. However, patients with tumors that
were ER-negative, high-grade, and with high-proliferative markers did
very well with chemotherapy up front, with 45 percent of patients having no apparent tumor when the area that had been involved was removed. So yet again it is important to know the biology of the tumor
rather than just the size.[27]

After neoadjuvant therapy, recommended options are surgery alone,
radiotherapy alone, or a combination of both. Surgical therapy may involve a total mastectomy or only a wide excision for the breast, with
sentinel node biopsy or axillary dissection for the lymph nodes. The main
criterion for breast-conservation therapy is that the remaining tumor, if
any, be removed with negative margins without disfiguring the breast. In
this setting, the local recurrence rate and ten-year overall survival rate
after breast-conservation therapy are equivalent to those of early-stage
disease.[28]

If the tumor has shrunk, we often have the option of doing a lumpectomy; if there is no change, we would still do a mastectomy. Even when
the tumor seems to have disappeared—we can't feel it or see it on a
mammogram—there may still be some cancer cells present. So we always want to do a lumpectomy at least on the spot where the tumor had

been to see what's actually left. (This procedure is rather imaginatively called a ghostectomy.) If the ghostectomy is clear or shows clean margins, the patient is a candidate for radiation. Similarly, if we can do a lumpectomy and get clean margins because the lump is small, it is sensible to follow that with radiation. If there is still a large lump or a lot of cancer at the margins, it may be best to do a mastectomy with or without immediate reconstruction. In the case of an ulceration that doesn't leave enough skin to sew together, breast reconstruction provides medical as well as cosmetic benefit, since reconstruction usually takes skin from another part of the body, allowing the wound to be closed (see Chapter 13). At this time the lymph nodes are also checked. Although the significance of negative nodes is not the same after someone has received chemotherapy, it is still a prognostic marker of the likelihood of recurrence. Finally, after either form of surgery, the patient will have radiation therapy to reduce the chances of cancer coming back in the breast or chest wall. And if the tumor tested sensitive to hormones, either Nolvadex (tamoxifen) or an aromatase inhibitor will be given for five to ten years, usually starting after radiation.

Locally advanced cancers usually fall into one of two categories, though both are generally treated the same way. Sometimes a very aggressive cancer seems to come up overnight as a large and evidently fast-growing tumor (although it's been there undetectable for a while). At other times, the tumor has been present for years and the person lacked insurance, was a victim of racial health disparities or possibly misdiagnosed, or had no follow-up until the tumor was huge or ulcerating through the skin. We call this last one a neglected primary—it's not an especially aggressive cancer, just especially big because treatment was not received earlier. Patients with a neglected primary cancer often do better than you may expect: if you've had an untreated cancer for five years and it hasn't killed you or obviously spread anywhere, it's clearly a slow-growing cancer.

If you've been putting off seeing your doctor about a lump that's been growing, or if you're suddenly faced with a new large or ulcerating tumor, don't ignore it and assume you're dying—get it diagnosed and start your treatment right away. Your prognosis may not be as good as it would be with a smaller tumor, but the cancer may very well be curable, and the sooner you begin to take care of it, the better your chances are.

INFLAMMATORY BREAST CANCER

One rare kind of breast cancer is termed "inflammatory," as the first symptoms are usually the rapid development (within three months) of redness and warmth in the skin of over one-third or more of the breast. There is also edema or swelling of the skin of the breast, often without a distinct lump. Frequently the patient and even the doctor mistake it for a simple infection, and the patient is put on antibiotics. But it doesn't get better and may well get worse, and that's the tip-off: an infection usually gets better within a week or two of antibiotics. If there's no change, the doctor should order imaging including mammogram, ultrasound, and MRI. The imaging can help find a suspicious area of the breast tissue that can be biopsied to see whether it's cancer. Two of my patients who have had this cancer had similar stories. One had been breastfeeding and developed what her doctor thought was lactational mastitis (see Chapter 2). It never cleared up and didn't hurt much; there was no fever or other sign of infection. The other patient, not breastfeeding, noticed that one breast had suddenly become larger than the other, and there was redness and swelling. Here too, the doctors at first thought it was an infection. So if you have such symptoms and they continue after one course of antibiotic treatment, you should ask to have imaging and a biopsy of the breast tissue and the skin. With inflammatory breast cancer, you have cancer cells in the lymph vessels of your skin. The skin is red because the cancer is blocking the drainage of fluid.

The incidence of inflammatory breast cancer is more common in Black women than Caucasian ones and is more common in the Middle East and Northern Africa, as well as in geographic areas of lower socioeconomic level in the United States. Other risk factors are higher body mass index (BMI), earlier age at first period, and earlier first pregnancy. Genetic alterations that may be predictive for inflammatory breast cancer have been identified in a Danish study. Further studies are needed but one particular protein, MDM4, is considered an interesting therapeutic target for treatment.[29]

This type of breast cancer is one of the most aggressive. Almost one-third of women with inflammatory breast cancer already have identifiable metastasis at the time of diagnosis. For this reason it is important to have imaging tests looking for spread including PET or PET/CT scan of the chest, abdomen, and pelvis as well as a bone scan before starting treatment.

Inflammatory breast cancer is uncommon enough and complicated enough that it is important to be seen at a cancer center that has a multidisciplinary team with a surgeon, radiation therapist, and oncologist experienced in treating it. If you are unsure, ask your doctors how many cases of inflammatory breast cancer they see in a year. Since it comprises only 1 to 5 percent of breast cancers in the United States, most local hospitals will not have the expertise you need. In the past this cancer has been diagnosed as everything from shingles to poison ivy to spider bites. This is one time when it may be worth traveling to find what you require. An experienced team will be able to integrate the different treatments in the most effective way and monitor your progress.

You would think that this aggressive cancer would have a specific molecular signature (see Chapter 10); however, sadly this is not the case yet. It can be sensitive to hormones or triple-negative but often is HER2/neu-positive. Inflammatory breast cancers are currently treated with a neoadjuvant therapy protocol. This means that we start with three or four cycles of AC, which stands for doxorubicin hydrochloride (Adriamycin) and cyclophosphamide (Cytoxan), followed by paclitaxel (Taxol) or docetaxel (Taxotere). Then we'll do a local treatment, usually mastectomy followed by radiation. Tumors that overexpress HER2/neu can also be treated with adjuvant Herceptin or other HER2/neu-targeting therapies such as Perjeta (pertuzumab). If the tumor is sensitive to hormones, then either Nolvadex (tamoxifen) or an aromatase inhibitor will be added to the mix. A number of other treatment combinations are being tried for inflammatory breast cancer as well.

One report followed 61 women with inflammatory breast cancer who had received multimodality (several types of treatment) and found that the five-year survival rate was 47 percent. Over 40 percent of the women who received trimodality (chemotherapy, radiation, and surgery) were free of disease at five years.[30]

Although this is encouraging, it is not good enough, and the number of research and clinical trials focused on this disease is high. There are new targeted drugs as well as other novel approaches, and I would strongly suggest that anyone with this diagnosis check out the website of the Inflammatory Breast Cancer Research Foundation at www.ibcresearch.org for up-to-date information and support. This disease is serious, but great progress is being made and the prognosis is much more positive than it was when the first edition of this book was published.

THE UNKNOWN PRIMARY

"The unknown primary" may sound like the title of a murder mystery, but it's the name we give another kind of mystery—a cancer that has spread to a lymph node in the armpit without an obvious primary tumor. In women this type of tumor (also called occult primary) almost always originates in the breast.

This is a rare form of breast cancer, accounting for less than 1 percent of cases. Someone shows up with an enlarged lymph node, usually in the armpit. A biopsy finds breast cancer cells, but there are no breast lumps. Sometimes we call this *axillary presentation of breast cancer* and it is staged as T0 and either N1 or N2 (see Chapter 10). Modern imaging techniques have helped in finding the original tumor. A patient in this situation is first sent for a mammogram and ultrasound. Looking for a cancer that we suspect is there is always different than screening, and many tumors are found on repeat study. If that doesn't show a tumor, then an MRI is done.

Although an MRI is not yet optimal as a general screening test for those with average risk, it is recommended for people with high breast cancer risk and does help in this situation. Recent studies of MRI have shown that it can detect the tumor in the breast in 70 to 95 percent of women.[31] If the doctors can find the primary cancer, then the patient has the option of getting a lumpectomy and radiation; otherwise, they can have either a mastectomy or whole-breast radiation.

Systemic therapy is given according to the type of tumor. Contrary to what you may expect, the survival rate in cancers that show up in the nodes but not in the breast is actually a bit better than it is for cancers that show up as both a breast lump and an enlarged node.[32]

PAGET'S DISEASE OF THE BREAST

Dr. James Paget (1814–1889) has gotten his name on any number of diseases: there's a Paget's disease of the bone and a Paget's disease of the eyelids, as well as a Paget's disease of the breast. The diseases have no relation to one another, except for their discoverer. In the breast, Paget's disease refers to a form of breast cancer that shows up in the nipple as an itchiness and scaling that doesn't get better.

As I was researching this section, I was amazed to find that the first description of this rare type of breast cancer was by John of Arderne in 1307. John described a nipple ulceration in a male priest, which over several years without treatment (there weren't many treatments available in 1307) went on to become full-fledged breast cancer.[33] Luckily we can now do more than just observe someone with Paget's.

There are two theories about this type of breast cancer. One is that the cancer cells start in the lactiferous sinus (see Chapter 1) and travel up to the nipple openings. This explains why the nipple itself rather than the areola is the first spot of irritation noted in Paget's, as well as the fact that people with Paget's disease often harbor cancers with similar cell types elsewhere in the breast.[34] The other theory is that the cancer cells actually start in the nipple openings. This correlates with the fact that some people with Paget's disease have no sign of cancer elsewhere.[35] Further study will tell us whether either or both theories are correct.

Usually Paget's disease presents as redness, mild scaliness, and flaking of the nipple skin and gradually goes on to crusting, ulceration, and weeping. It can be itchy, hypersensitive, and painful. It's often mistaken for eczema of the nipple, a far more common occurrence. Paget's disease is almost never found in both breasts, so if you have itching and scaling on both nipples, you probably have a fairly harmless skin condition. In addition, the fact that Paget's usually starts in the nipple and not the areola can be a telling sign. However, if it doesn't get better, you should get it checked out, whether it's on one or both nipples, or even on the areola.

First the skin on the nipple will be biopsied. This can be done in the doctor's office with local anesthetic; either a nipple scrape or a punch biopsy can make the diagnosis. If it's Paget's, the pathologist sees little cancer cells growing up into the skin of the nipple—that's what makes the skin flake and get itchy. Then you will need a mammogram to look for cancer in the breast itself. As with the unknown primary tumors previously described, you may want to have an MRI if the mammogram is negative. An MRI can be especially useful in making sure that there is no area of disease other than the nipple. If these imaging tests detect something, then a biopsy of the lesion is necessary. Paget's can indicate the possibility of a further breast cancer. Dr. Carolyn Kaelin, a Boston breast surgeon, combined several studies of Paget's disease and found that out of 965 patients, 47 percent had a breast mass as well as the nipple symptoms, and 53 percent had no mass. Of the patients with a mass, 93 percent had invasive carcinoma of the breast and 7 percent had noninvasive cancer. Among those with no mass, 34 percent had invasive cancer, 65 percent had DCIS, and 1 percent had only Paget's disease with no cancer in the breast.[36]

The treatment of Paget's disease depends on whether it is associated with DCIS, invasive cancer, or neither. By itself, Paget's disease is low-grade and not aggressive. If there is an invasive or a noninvasive cancer near the nipple, a lumpectomy that includes the nipple and areola can be performed, followed by radiation. Sentinel node biopsy can be added if it is invasive. If the invasive cancer lump is far from the nipple, a mastectomy may be necessary to get both areas out; otherwise, wide excision and radiation is a reasonable alternative. If just the nipple is involved, then removing the nipple-areolar complex and adding radiation has shown excellent results.[37]

As you might guess, Paget's disease that involves only the nipple has a better prognosis than other types of breast cancer. Usually the lymph nodes turn out to be negative. Because of its rarity, most doctors do not see many cases of it, and many assume that it requires a mastectomy— they seem to think that if you can't keep your nipple, your breast doesn't matter.[38] Most patients, of course, know better.

This has long been a campaign of mine, and a few years ago some of us managed to convince the rest of the medical establishment that removing the nipple and areola is sufficient treatment, and that many women prefer to keep the rest of the breast if they can.[39] True, your breast looks a bit funny after the nipple has been removed, but it has sensation and is still there. A plastic surgeon can make an artificial nipple (see Chapter 13), or you can get one tattooed.

PHYLLODES TUMORS

A phyllodes tumor is another rare type of breast tumor, occurring less than 1 percent of the time. It's usually fairly mild and takes the form of a malignant fibroadenoma (see Chapter 2). It shows up as a large lump in the breast—it's usually lemon-size by the time it's detected. It feels like a regular fibroadenoma—smooth and round—but under the microscope some of the fibrous cells that make up the fibroadenoma are bizarre-looking and cancerous. It's not very aggressive and rarely metastasizes; if it recurs at all, it tends to do so only in the breast. In the past it was usually treated with wide excision, removing the lump and a rim of normal tissue around it.[40] If the phyllodes tumor is large in comparison to the breast, oncoplastic surgery is a good consideration (see Chapter 13). This includes removing the tumor cosmetically and then reducing the other breast to match. Not all surgeons have been trained in this approach, and it may be worth investigating where it can be done. This type of lesion is not fast growing, so you have time to get a second opinion.

Phyllodes tumors don't require radiation at initial diagnosis and treatment, and we usually won't check the lymph nodes, since when the tumor does metastasize it is usually to the lungs. A patient once came to see me because her phyllodes tumors had recurred three times, and her surgeon told her she'd have to have a mastectomy because it kept coming back. I told her I thought we should wait and see if it did come back, and in the six years I followed her, it didn't recur. Chemotherapy is almost never recommended for these tumors. In the extremely rare case of metastatic phyllodes tumors (*malignant phyllodes*), the type of chemotherapy used for sarcomas (a kind of skin cancer) rather than breast cancer is used.

The medical literature sometimes talks about *benign*, *borderline*, or *malignant* phyllodes tumors, based on a subjective interpretation of how cancerous the cells appear. The implication is that malignant cystosarcomas behave more aggressively. About 95 percent are benign. And the 5 percent that metastasize and ultimately kill the patient are hard to predict accurately in advance. Metastases are unusual, even with the malignant variants. Although many surgeons suggest the more aggressive approach of mastectomy if the pathologist feels that it is malignant, this approach is not justified by data. A wide resection with lumpectomy is likely as effective as mastectomy as long as reasonable negative margins are demonstrated. These cancers are sufficiently rare that you should definitely get a second opinion on the pathology from a specialist at a major medical center before embarking on a more aggressive therapeutic approach. Some potential biomarkers have been identified for this cancer, but further study is still needed.

CANCER OF BOTH BREASTS

Once in a while (3 to 5 percent of the time) a person is diagnosed as having a cancer in both breasts at the same time. Typically they find a lump in one breast, get a mammogram, and learn there's also a lump in the other breast. Biopsy shows both to be cancer. Although the patient can despair, thinking their situation is twice as bad, that actually isn't the case. The prognosis is based on the stage of the more aggressive of the two tumors. A review from Milan reported that these tumors are more likely to be small, invasive lobular, low-grade, and sensitive to estrogen.[41] Such tumors are thought to reflect a situation in which a person's particular hormonal environment is conducive to developing cancers. Or there may be some external environmental risk/cause.

Does one cancer spread from the other? Most studies have found noninvasive cancer associated with each of the two tumors, suggesting that it does not. They're both treated the same way: we do a lumpectomy or mastectomy and lymph node dissection on one and then the other side. Usually the surgeon first looks at the lymph nodes on the side that appears worse. If the nodes are positive and require chemotherapy, the other nodes won't necessarily have to be dissected if the second cancer has a low likelihood of spreading to the nodes. Unfortunately the surgeon's guess isn't always right. Many years ago I had a patient with three cancers: she had a lump in the top of her right breast, and the mammogram showed two densities in the bottom of the left breast. They'd all been biopsied with needles. She wanted to keep her breasts, so I did a wide excision of the right breast and sampled the lymph nodes, which were fine. Then I did a wide excision of the two cancers in the left breast, and on the left side she had positive lymph nodes and went on to receive chemotherapy. For this reason many surgeons will do bilateral sentinel node biopsies.

You can have radiation treatment on both breasts at the same time, but the radiation therapist has to be very careful that the treatment doesn't overlap and cause a burn in the middle area.

It isn't necessary to have the same treatment on both breasts. You may decide on a mastectomy on one side and wide excision plus radiation on the other.

CANCER IN THE OTHER BREAST

Sometimes a person who has had cancer in one breast turns up later with cancer in the other breast. Usually this isn't a recurrence or a metastasis; it's a brand-new cancer, and the likelihood of finding yourself in this situation is estimated to be about 0.5 percent per year. It's possible for breast cancer to metastasize from one breast to the other, but it's rare. A new primary cancer has a different significance than a metastasis. It suggests that your breast tissue, for whatever reason, is prone to develop cancer, so you developed one on one side and then several years later the other side followed along. As with any new cancer, it's biopsied and removed, your lymph nodes are checked, and you're treated. Your prognosis isn't any worse because you developed the second breast cancer; rather, as with cancer of both breasts, it's only as bad as the worst of your two. You can still have breast conservation; you don't have to have a mastectomy if you don't want it. People who have second cancers are more likely to have a hereditary predisposition to breast cancer, so people in this situation should ask their doctor whether they should go to a genetic counselor (see Chapter 4). Some people with cancer in one breast are so scared of getting cancer in the other that they consider having a prophylactic mastectomy to prevent it, and more and more people are choosing this option (see Chapter 11). Yet in people without a genetic mutation that causes breast cancer, prophylactic mastectomy has not been shown to improve the chances of not dying from breast cancer.

BREAST CANCER IN VERY YOUNG WOMEN

As noted earlier, breast cancer is most common in women over age 50 in countries that perform population-based screening mammographically, and there are many cases in women in their forties. It's rare in women under age 40, but it does occur. Only 5 to 7 percent of women in the developed world are diagnosed with breast cancer before age 40. For this reason we tend to be particularly shocked when breast cancer occurs in a young person.

Usually in these situations it's detected as a lump, as we generally don't do screening mammography at those ages for the reasons discussed in Chapter 7. Often a young person gets misdiagnosed. They detect a lump or a thickening, and they're told it's just lumpy breasts, or "fibrocystic disease," and it's followed for a while until doctors realize it's serious. The vast majority of lumps in women under age 35 are benign, and the risk of cancer is very low. Still, it's important for doctors to be vigilant and bear in mind that young women can develop breast cancer.

Luckily we can easily determine which lumps are significant and which are not with a diagnostic mammogram and ultrasound. And it is easy to do a needle biopsy (see Chapter 12) to obtain a diagnosis without surgery. This is indeed an improvement over the approach we would have taken twenty-five years ago when you would have to have surgery to know whether a lump was cancer, and watchful waiting was more acceptable.

The youngest patient I ever diagnosed was twenty-three. She was on her honeymoon when she discovered a lump. We diagnosed the cancer; she had a positive node, and she underwent lumpectomy, radiation, and chemotherapy. Ten years later she developed a local recurrence that required a mastectomy. She is now the mother of three grown daughters and a friend of mine on Facebook.

Breast cancer in younger women is more likely to be hereditary.[42] If you've inherited a mutation (and you need only one or two more mutations to get cancer), you're one step closer and likely to get there sooner, whereas if you have not inherited any mutations, you still need to get all of the mutations for cancer to develop. That does not work all the time. Like older women, the majority of younger women with breast cancer have no family history of it. But if you have a BRCA mutation in your family, you're more likely to get breast cancer at a younger age than if you don't. It is advisable for very young women to have genetic counseling and consider being tested for the BRCA mutations, particularly if they feel the result would affect their treatment decisions.

Compared to that of older women, breast tissue in young women is subject to more changes, including monthly cycles, pregnancy, and breastfeeding. This undoubtedly affects not only the development of cancers but also their behavior. Several large studies examined the different subtypes of breast cancer in relation to age. Young women have more basal-like tumors (34.3 percent) that are not sensitive to estrogen or progesterone and are HER2/neu-negative. These are sometimes termed "triple-negative tumors" (see Chapter 10). This is also the most common type encountered in women who have mutations in BRCA 1 and develop breast cancer at an early age.[43] This type becomes more common with age. There are also more HER2-positive tumors in young women but fewer luminal A tumors (ER-positive, PR-positive, and HER2-negative).[44]

Pregnancy and breastfeeding affect the different types of breast cancer differently.[45] Pregnancy decreases the chance of developing hormone-positive tumors but increases triple-negative ones, especially if you don't breastfeed. This is true even if you are BRCA positive. But breastfeeding for at least a year reduced the risk of triple-negative cancer by 31 percent overall, according to a study on reproductive factors and risk. But the benefit was far greater for Black women aged 20 to 44, where an 82 percent reduction in risk was seen in people who breastfed for six months or longer compared to their nonbreastfeeding peers.[46]

Both lumpectomy with radiation and mastectomy have special implications for younger women. There appears to be a higher local recurrence rate in young women who get lumpectomy and radiation than in women in their forties and fifties. Recent data have suggested that younger women benefit significantly from a radiation boost, which reduces this risk considerably.[47] No evidence exists to suggest that mastectomy in young women is better for survival than breast conservation, probably because the risk of metastatic disease is higher than the risk of local recurrence. Nor are double mastectomies necessarily indicated in people who do not carry mutations. Yet many young women have been choosing them. The incidence of breast cancer in the other breast is about 0.8 percent per year, which usually maximizes out to about 10 to 15 percent. However, women with BRCA 1 or BRCA 2 mutations (about 6 percent of women under age 36) can have a much higher chance of developing a second breast cancer in the same or other breast. Because younger women have many more years to get cancer in the opposite breast, their risk is slightly higher than that of older women. Both chemotherapy and hormone therapy reduce this risk.

Generally the systemic therapies for younger women are the same as for older women, depending on the type of breast cancer. Women with tumors that are not sensitive to hormones do well with chemotherapy and Herceptin (trastuzumab), when indicated. Controversies arise with the hormone-positive tumors. An interesting study done by the International Breast Cancer Study Group evaluated the treatment outcome for very young women compared with that for older but still premenopausal women who received chemotherapy but no hormone treatment.[48] The participants under age 35 who had ER-positive tumors did worse than older premenopausal women with ER-positive tumors and older and younger women with ER-negative tumors. This surprising finding led to three reviews, all of which found the same result.[49]

Another two important studies came out looking at the use of "ovarian ablation," a medical term for inducing menopause either temporarily or permanently. This is done by surgically removing ovaries, radiating ovaries, or poisoning ovaries (chemotherapy), or through a temporary blocker of menstruation (GnRH agonist). The Suppression of Ovarian Function Trial (SOFT) showed that adding ovarian suppression to Nolvadex (tamoxifen) did not provide a significant benefit overall. This was particularly true for participants with negative lymph nodes and smaller tumors. However, in those who had received adjuvant chemotherapy and were still menstruating, ovarian suppression combined with Nolvadex (tamoxifen) was better than Nolvadex alone, and an aromatase inhibitor with ovarian suppression was even better.[50] Although this is important information, we need to put it in perspective. Most recurrences occurred in women who received chemotherapy, probably because they were considered to have a higher risk of recurrence to begin with. The number of women without a recurrence of breast cancer at five years was 82.5 percent in the Nolvadex-ovarian-suppression group, 78 percent in the Nolvadex-only group, and 85.7 percent in the Aromasin (exemestane)-ovarian-suppression group. These kinds of numbers are enough to impress oncologists, but in weighing these approaches, you should take into account their side effects and how they may affect the quality of your life.

A twenty-one-gene expression test to assess recurrence risk was used by two large studies to evaluate the benefits of chemotherapy in addition to hormone therapy. They used a 0–100 scoring system, with a low score at 10 or under, a mid score at 11–25, and a high score over 25. The TAILORx study combined recurrence score with clinical risk, which is high or low depending on tumor size, appearance, and growth. In early-stage ER-positive, HER2-negative, and node-negative breast cancer, the study found that treatment after surgery with chemotherapy and hormone therapy is not more beneficial than treatment with hormone therapy alone.[51] The RxPONDER trial found that premenopausal patients with one to three positive lymph nodes and a recurrence score of 25 or lower actually did better with chemotherapy plus hormone therapy after breast cancer surgery.[52] A third study examined chemotherapy for those who find themselves in a midrange of risk, with scores at 11–25. In this group both hormone therapy alone and HT combined with chemo had similar efficacy, but women age 50 or younger had some benefit with chemo.[53]

Fertility is a problem with both chemotherapy, which can induce menopause, and ovarian suppression. This plays out in two ways. First, breast cancer treatment with all the components can take several years. Herceptin (trastuzumab) is usually given for a year following the six months of chemotherapy, and Nolvadex (tamoxifen) can be given for ten years. During this time, when pregnancy is dangerous because of the drugs, a person's fertility will already be declining because of age. Often chemotherapy will prompt premature menopause, even when it does not bring it on directly. The risks of menopause range from 10 to 90 percent depending on the drugs, the person's age, and the definition used for menopause. Although this sounds odd, some studies say that you are in menopause if you do not have a period for six months to a year. But many people get their period more than a year later. Even blood tests are not that accurate at predicting whether your menopause is temporary or permanent.

If you wish to have a biological child in the future, advise your doctor very early in your consultations. Be sure to ask about the statistics for the treatments being recommended so that you have a realistic assessment of the risk. In the end you will decide what matters to you, and you may want to try a different regimen if it will be more likely to preserve your fertility. Go back to the discussions in Chapter 11 and earlier in this chapter regarding the absolute benefit you'll receive from adjuvant therapy so that you have a realistic idea of the risks versus benefits.

One encouraging review in 2018 studied five trials measuring the effect of adding Zoladex (goserelin) to chemotherapy to preserve ovarian function and potentially improve future fertility. Half the patients were randomized to the Zoladex and chemotherapy group and the rest were in the chemo-alone control group, regardless of cancer subtype or age—although the average patient was age 38. Of the patients they followed for two years, 18 percent of the goserelin group had yet to get their period, while 30 percent of the control group had not. More heartening still, in the Zoladex group 10 percent had at least one post-treatment pregnancy, while in the control group the rate was 5 percent.[54] Of course, in these five studies the final objective wasn't to get pregnant, but it is worth mentioning Zoladex to your doctor if you want to maintain your fertility.

The likelihood of chemotherapy-induced menopause has led some patients to consider freezing eggs or ovarian tissue before the treatment so they can still have children later. Doctors are often reluctant to give the high doses of hormones needed to stimulate production of eggs to patients who have cancer, especially those with hormone-positive tumors. However, in early studies Nolvadex (tamoxifen) and/or Femara (letrozole) have been used with no increased incidence of recurrence.[55] Cryopreservation of embryos is a more standard path but requires a male partner or sperm donor and also hormones for egg stimulation. These approaches take two to three weeks and can be done either before or after surgery but prior to starting systemic therapy. It is important to have a conversation with your team, however, so that they take your wish to do this into consideration during treatment planning.

The question then arises whether a pregnancy after breast cancer treatment increases the risk of recurrence. The studies that have looked at people who did have pregnancies after breast cancer have not shown an increase in recurrence; in fact they showed a decrease.[56] It is important to bear in mind that people who go on to get pregnant are often less likely to be at risk for recurrence; otherwise, they probably would not have gone ahead with it. Yet it is reassuring that the risk does not seem to increase markedly. In people who do give birth after treatment, the ability to breastfeed may well be compromised by the radiation and surgery they received for their initial cancers. This varies according to the extent of the surgery and whether the nipple and ducts have been disturbed. Remember that breast MRIs should be avoided during pregnancy due to the contrast "dye" that is used for this kind of imaging.

This is obviously a moving target. Again, if this is an issue for you, make sure you check out your options before undergoing chemotherapy. (The website www.youngsurvival.org is a good source for up-to-date information on this topic.) And remember that there are other ways to have children. Losing your fertility does not mean losing all chances to be a parent.

CANCER DURING PREGNANCY

Once in a very great while a patient develops breast cancer while they are pregnant or breastfeeding. The studies are contradictory. The problem for diagnosis is that when you're pregnant, your breasts are going through a lot of normal changes, which can mask a more dangerous change. For one thing, breasts are much lumpier and thicker than usual. Similarly, when you're breastfeeding, as I discussed at length in

Chapter 1, you tend to have all kinds of benign lumps and blocked ducts, and you may not notice a change that otherwise would alarm you. Infections are common when you're breastfeeding and can mask inflammatory breast cancer, so the physician may also find diagnosis of inflammatory breast cancer difficult.

Recent research suggests another hypothesis. With pregnancy the breast undergoes a lot of changes in order to accommodate its new function, making milk. This involves an increase in the numbers of cells, remodeling, and lots of hormonal stimulation. If there are any mutated cells around, they could be stimulated to grow as well. At the end of lactation there is also a massive cleanup so the breast can get ready for the next baby. During the cleanup there is stimulation of cells, growth of new blood vessels, and inflammation—all of which can stimulate cancer cells as well as normal ones.

A meta-analysis of thirty studies found that people who were diagnosed with breast cancer while pregnant, or within four years thereafter, did indeed have a higher risk of death.[57] As more people are having later pregnancies at an age when breast cancer becomes more common, this may become a bigger issue. Contrary to what you would think, people who abort their fetuses do not have a better prognosis. The treatment can start during pregnancy, and terminating the pregnancy does not seem to affect the outcome.

If there is a question of a breast lump, you should have a mammogram and ultrasound. It has been shown that the radiation to the fetus is negligible with a mammogram. Breast MRIs should be avoided during pregnancy because of the contrast dye that is used for this kind of imaging.

The diagnosis can be made with a needle or core biopsy. The treatment will depend on what kind of cancer you have and how far along you are in your pregnancy. First, assemble a team that includes an obstetrician as well as medical, surgical, and radiation oncologists. Surgery can be a mastectomy or lumpectomy, depending on the size of the tumor. Chemotherapy (doxorubicin) can be given after the first trimester and prior to the thirty-fifth week of pregnancy. Radiation therapy, additional chemotherapy, and Herceptin or hormone therapy can be given postpartum as indicated.

If you're in your third trimester, we can do a lumpectomy, or, if need be, a mastectomy and possibly chemotherapy, then wait for further treatment like radiation and/or Nolvadex (tamoxifen) until after the child is born. We can begin chemotherapy if it's important to get going right away. If you are close to your due date, your obstetrician can induce labor as soon as the baby can be expected to survive well outside the womb (as early as thirty-three to thirty-four weeks if needed), or do a cesarean section and then start you on chemotherapy and radiation after delivery. Sometimes the due date can be moved up with medication to increase the lung maturity and allow earlier delivery.

In the mid-1990s I saw a woman who had been diagnosed twenty years earlier, when she was seven months pregnant. She had undergone a radical mastectomy and then had radiation with cobalt (a chemical used in the mid-twentieth century) while she was pregnant. She said she had to have a dose monitor in her vagina to keep track of the amount of radiation her fetus was receiving. Nonetheless she carried the baby to term and both were fine twenty years later.

BREAST CANCER DURING LACTATION

Breast cancer during lactation isn't quite as complicated, since you can always stop breastfeeding and start your child on formula or donor milk. Radiation will probably make breastfeeding impossible, and you won't want to breastfeed if you're on chemotherapy, since the baby will swallow the chemicals.

There are some misconceptions about cancer and breastfeeding that need to be addressed. The first is that a child who drinks from a cancerous breast will get the cancer. This theory is based on a study of one species of mouse, which does transmit a cancerous virus to its female offspring through breastfeeding. At this time, it hasn't been found in any other species of mouse, or in any other animal.

Another notion is that a baby won't drink milk from a cancerous breast. Normally this isn't so. If a breast has a lot of cancer, it probably won't produce as much milk, so the baby will, quite sensibly, favor the milkier breast. There's nothing wrong with this. Many babies prefer one breast to another even with a healthy breastfeeding parent.

We're not sure yet whether lactation affects the cancer. I've had two patients whose breast cancer showed up while they were lactating. Both were treated, both stopped breastfeeding, and both did well without a recurrence for several years. After much debate both women decided to get pregnant again. One had a recurrence during the second pregnancy; the other had a second primary develop in the other breast while she was lactating. This leads me to wonder whether, if a cancer shows up while a person is pregnant or lactating, there is a higher risk of a recurrence in another pregnancy. However, I have no data for this. Obviously we can't do a randomized study, and it's too unusual an occurrence to draw any conclusions. Our evidence is purely anecdotal. For now, all I can suggest to someone who has developed breast cancer while pregnant or lactating is to seriously consider not having another pregnancy in case it affects the chance of a recurrence.

However, pregnancy after breast cancer treatment appears to have no effect on long-term survival according to a large international review and analysis. The 2021 review of thirty-nine clinical studies concluded that people who have had breast cancer are less likely to get pregnant and their babies are smaller but birth does not have a negative effect.[58] It may be that getting cancer while you're pregnant has a different effect than getting it afterward;[59] we don't have the full answer yet.

BREAST CANCER IN ELDERLY WOMEN

Just as very young women can get breast cancer, so can women over age 70, and they share some issues. Neither end of the extreme always fits our general models. As opposed to young women, those over seventy are less likely to develop the more aggressive cancers and more likely to have hormone-positive cancers (luminal A or B) that are slower growing. That being said, more aggressive cancers such as the triple-negative and HER2-positive tumors do occur even in the oldest women.

There are studies showing that older women aren't treated as aggressively. There's a tendency to restrict the options for treatment: "Well, they're old—they don't really want chemotherapy."[60] I think a special effort has to be made to ascertain what the patient wants, what is appropriate for their cancer, and what their state of health can handle, and not permit physicians to act solely on their own assumptions.

In addition, there's a tendency to do mastectomies on older patients without offering them breast conservation or reconstruction treatments, assuming that elderly patients don't care as much about their looks. In fact, breast conservation with sentinel node biopsy is less disruptive and can often be done as an outpatient. Older people tolerate breast irradiation as well as younger people, but studies have shown that it may not be necessary. Postoperative radiotherapy may often be omitted altogether in low-risk patients.[61] Older patients are good candidates for local partial-breast radiation, intraoperative radiation, or even once-weekly radiation (see Chapter 14).

Not only do many doctors neglect to mention lumpectomy and radiation to older patients; they also neglect to offer reconstruction for those urged to undergo mastectomies, again assuming that they won't care enough about their looks to want it. Again, that assumption is totally off base. I remember one patient in her mideighties with large, droopy breasts, who had always wanted to have a reduction but thought it was too dangerous. She got a cancer at the upper end of one of her breasts. She wanted breast conservation; she didn't want a mastectomy. It seemed foolhardy to us to radiate this entire breast when most of it showed no cancer. So after discussing it with her, we did a lumpectomy and bilateral reductions, and then radiation. She was delighted; when the radiation was done she went off on a cruise and found a new boyfriend. So you can't make any assumptions.

The recommendations for older patients, of course, have to consider their overall health. The late Dr. Arti Hurria of the cancer center City of Hope developed a particularly useful Chemo-Toxicity Calculator for elderly women with breast cancer. The tool was able to predict toxicity through eleven questions, including five on geriatric assessment and six that were clinically related. Patients with high predictive scores may have their treatments adjusted to reduce toxicity.[62] As with younger patients, larger tumors can be treated with systemic therapy in an attempt to shrink them enough to allow breast conservation. This can be done with an aromatase inhibitor or, if the patient is fit enough and the tumor is not sensitive to estrogen, chemotherapy. If the tumor is small, then either breast conservation with sentinel node biopsy or mastectomy are both options. The use of systemic therapies after local treatment again depends on the patient's health. If they have a hormone-negative tumor and can tolerate chemotherapy, it certainly should be an option. But if they have other serious health problems, it may not be wise. Hormone therapy is easier to take and should probably be used in most patients with hormone-positive tumors.

In one of the few studies directed specifically to women over age 70, patients who had undergone lumpectomy were randomized to have either Nolvadex (tamoxifen) alone or Nolvadex plus radiation therapy. There were small differences between the two groups, suggesting that radiation therapy may not be necessary in this situation in people with multiple health problems.[63] One would suspect that similar results would be obtained with an aromatase inhibitor.

Part of the problem in studying women over age 70 is that we really can't evaluate long-term survival as elderly people die from many illnesses. But not all elderly people are frail. I had a ninety-five-year-old breast cancer patient in Boston who was very active. I did a lumpectomy and put her on Nolvadex. Unfortunately she couldn't tolerate the Nolvadex and dropped it. She was fine for about a year and a half; then her cancer recurred locally. I did another lumpectomy, and this time I really tried to get her to stick with the Nolvadex, and she did for a while. The last I heard she was still going strong. So when we look at how to treat elderly people, we need to look at how frail they really are: people vary greatly. Those who live into their nineties tend to be healthy, or they wouldn't live to that age. We can't just assume, as many doctors do, that they'll be dead in a year or so and forget it—more and more of them are now living to over one hundred. Some ninety-year-olds are healthier than some people at sixty.

PEOPLE WITH IMPLANTS

There's no evidence that people with implants have a higher vulnerability to breast cancer than other people, and some evidence that it may actually be lower.[64] Sometimes cancer is detected on mammograms, and sometimes the lump is palpable. It's diagnosed in the same way as any breast cancer—with a biopsy. We may be able to do a needle biopsy, depending on where the lump is. We don't want to stick a needle into the sac and release the silicone or saline into the breast. Breast MRI is helpful for screening in patients who have silicone injections, in other words silicone droplets injected directly into the breast tissue. These droplets dramatically reduce the efficacy of mammograms and even ultrasounds. Silicone injections are not allowed in medical facilities, yet some patients seek this dangerous treatment in nonmedical settings.

The treatment options are the same. You can have lumpectomy and radiation.[65] You can radiate with the implant in place. There is a higher incidence of encapsulation (see Chapter 14), but other than that there's no problem. You may think that cutting into the breast would break the silicone cover, but there are a couple of ways around that. For example, we can use the electrocautery instead of the scalpel, and that can't cut into the implant.

If you had silicone injections back in the 1960s when they were legal, the same applies. They make detecting cancer on a mammogram more difficult, since it's hard to tell what is silicone and what's something else. So you need to go to a high-quality center where you can be carefully monitored. It's very important to have the mammograms serially, comparing one year's to the next, because that's what can tip you off: one of these lumps that you were calling silicone is growing. You can then have a lumpectomy and radiation.

BREAST CANCER IN MEN

This book addresses breast cancer in women because it is the most common malignancy in women. Among men it accounts for less than 1 percent of all cancers. Overall there are fifteen hundred cases a year in men and over two hundred thousand in women. In men, breast cancer usually occurs at a later age than in women, with the average being age 72. There is a different distribution among different racial and ethnic groups, with Black men having the highest rate, followed by non-Hispanic whites, then Hispanics, and, finally, Pacific Islanders. The subtypes (see Chapter 10) are also different, with the vast majority being hormone-positive at around 80 percent; HER2-positive subtypes account for 15 percent and triple-negative about 4 percent.[66] Non-Hispanic whites have the highest rate of hormone-positive cancers, whereas Black men are most likely to be triple-negative.

The risk factors for male breast cancer are the same as their female counterparts: obesity, lack of physical activity, and alcohol use. However, more of male breast cancer appears to be hereditary, with 15 to 20 percent of men with the disease belonging to families with a history of female breast cancer.[67] Not surprisingly, many men who develop breast cancer are also carriers of mutations in the BRCA genes, most commonly

BRCA 2 (see Chapter 4). The NCCN guidelines suggest that all men diagnosed with breast cancer should undergo genetic testing.

There's also a theory that it's connected to gynecomastia—enlarged
breasts (see Chapter 1), either now or during puberty, but so far we have
no proof of this. We do have proof that men with Klinefelter's syndrome,
a chromosomal problem in which not enough testosterone is produced,
are susceptible to breast cancer.[68] Interestingly, risk factors for women
such as early exposure to radiation[69] and higher estrogen exposure in
utero and estrogen-mimicking chemicals also seem to be relevant to men.

For a time there was concern that men who got estrogen treatments
for prostate cancer were more vulnerable to breast cancer, but this
doesn't seem to be the case; rather, prostate cancer can metastasize to the
breast.[70] (Remember that it remains prostate cancer, not breast cancer.)

Breast cancer in men shows itself in all the ways it does in women—
usually as a lump—but it tends to be diagnosed later because men
ignore symptoms, put off going to the doctor, and are not routinely
screened with mammograms. The treatments are the same as well.
Men can undergo sentinel node biopsy[71] (see Chapter 11), and either
lumpectomy and radiation or mastectomy. There is a tendency to overtreat men with postmastectomy radiation because surgeons see these
cancers so rarely. Breast cancers in men more frequently involve the
skin or chest wall, probably because of the relatively small amount of
breast tissue, and this can be an indication for radiation. Recent data
demonstrate that local recurrences in men are rare even in stage III
disease and that the same indications should be used that are employed
in women (see Chapter 14).[72]

One issue that is often not addressed, however, is the fact that the
cosmetic implications are somewhat different for men. On the one hand,
they don't tend to regard breasts as crucial to their sexuality the way
women do. On the other hand, their naked chests are more likely to be
visible. It can be more awkward for a man to have a scar, to lack a nipple, or to have a deformed chest than it is for a woman. So a man may
prefer lumpectomy and radiation to mastectomy. The one extra consideration is hair. After radiation therapy a man loses most of his chest hair
on that side. If he is very hairy, a mastectomy with the scar hidden in hair
may prove more cosmetic. Depending on where the tumor is, the nipple
can often be conserved. If he loses the nipple, a plastic surgeon can give
him an artificial one. When I worked at UCLA, a golfer with a small

breast cancer came to me. He was distressed that the only option he had been given was a mastectomy. After a lumpectomy and radiation, he was very happy and felt normal on the course and sometimes swam without a shirt.

In addition to local treatments, men are also given systemic therapies similar to those given to postmenopausal women with the same stage and type of cancer. This is in part because the situation is similar but also because there are few randomized clinical trials of treatments in men with breast cancer, and so we have to extrapolate. As we mentioned earlier, most breast cancers in men are ER-positive, either of the luminal A or luminal B type. Interestingly, Nolvadex (tamoxifen) works in men with ER-positive tumors. Aromatase inhibitors may need to be combined with a treatment to block testosterone as for premenopausal women. Aromatase inhibitors alone won't stop hormone-related cancer growth in men according to guidelines by the NCCN.

There is a lot of data on men taking Nolvadex. Men do get hot flashes, weight gain, sexual dysfunction, and increased blood clotting, but they can't get vaginal dryness or endometrial cancer, or any male version of those.

Usually, however, when a man or boy has a breast lump, it isn't cancer but unilateral gynecomastia, which literally means "breast tissue like a woman's." It can happen anytime in a man's life, especially if he's been on some of the drugs used to treat heart conditions or hypertension, smokes marijuana, or does anything else that increases estrogen levels. It's never a cyst or fibroadenoma—men don't get those.

BREAST CANCER IN TRANSGENDER/ NONBINARY INDIVIDUALS

As gender-affirming hormone treatments and surgeries increase together with public acceptance, transgender individuals' breast cancer risk has become a topic of concern. Transgender people experience an incongruence between the sex assigned to them at birth and their expressed gender identity, and some get hormone treatment to induce some desired changes in their bodies. Concerns that this may increase cancer risk were allayed in a large Dutch study. Transgender women with an average of thirteen years of hormone treatment had an increased risk of breast cancer when compared to the general (cisgender) male population, but a lower risk than the general (cisgender) female population. Of the 2,260 transgender women followed, fifteen had cases of invasive cancer, most of them hormone-positive. Of the 1,229 transgender men, with an average of eight years of hormone treatment, four cases of invasive breast cancer were found—a lower rate of breast cancer than (cisgender) women in general.[73]

Once cancer is found, it is treated on the basis of the type of cancer, regardless of gender identity.

People who were assigned female gender at birth who are receiving male gender affirmation treatment who do not undergo mastectomy remain at their previous risk for breast cancer and should follow screening guidelines for the general (cisgender) female population. If they opt for top surgery to remove their breasts, no reliable evidence exists yet for screening, but some residual breast tissue may remain, and with it any inherited risks. It is wise to consult with your doctor, particularly if you have a BRCA 1 or BRCA 2 gene.

Transgender women with more than five years of hormone therapy should get annual or biannual screening starting at age 50, depending on other risk factors.[74]

In the 2019 documentary *Trans Dudes with Lady Cancer* (www.transdudes withladycancer.org), trans rights activist Yee Wong Chong describes getting breast cancer four years after having top surgery so his body would match his gender identity. He initially got a lumpectomy and later a double mastectomy to remove any remaining breast tissue. "If we have the part, we have to get it checked, no matter how uncomfortable it is," said Chong.

In the film, Dr. Norma Pham Steiner of Kaiser Permanente empathized with the psychological toll of getting cancer in body parts you no longer identify with. "People may have a lot of hang-ups about coming until there is no choice, there is so much history people carry that make it emotionally difficult," she acknowledged.

Our radiology advisor Dr. Lauren Green recalls a transgender female patient who had been taking estrogen therapy for breast enlargement for several years. She came to the breast imaging department of University of Illinois Hospital after feeling a lump in her breast. A mammogram and ultrasound showed a suspicious mass, which a biopsy later confirmed to be breast cancer.

It is hard to determine the true number of transgender patients with breast cancer because of a reluctance to seek medical care, usually based on poor experiences in the past. Many health care professionals now undergo training to help provide more inclusive care to all patients.

Activists in the transgender community suggest researching providers and tapping into networks to find professionals used to treating LGBTQ and nonbinary patients. Planned Parenthood can be helpful. Come up with a plan with someone who can support you, and do a little role-playing around pronouns and other areas you believe may be problematic with your care provider.

The Centers for Medicare and Medicaid Services advises providers to use two billing modifiers for transgender patients, condition code 45 (Ambiguous Gender Category) and the KX modifier (to note that conditions specified in the medical policy have been met and documentation exists to support the medical necessity of a listed procedure). When attached to medical procedure codes, these modifiers provide additional information about the billed treatment and can prevent rejection of claims over an alleged gender/procedure conflict.

OTHER CANCERS

When I arrived at UCLA in 1992, within the first week or two I got a call to see a patient who had a breast lump. It was soft and smooth, and on the side of her breast. It felt like a cyst, but I was unable to aspirate it. Then she had a mammogram and an ultrasound, which confirmed that the lump was solid. We took the lump out under local anesthesia, and indeed it was malignant. When I talked to her afterward, I broke one of my cardinal rules—never make absolute promises. I told her that, though it was unfortunate that her tumor was malignant, it was a small tumor and I could guarantee that she wouldn't have to get chemotherapy. Since she was elderly, the most she'd need would be Nolvadex (tamoxifen).

Then we looked at it more closely under the microscope and found that it wasn't a breast cancer at all but lymphoma, a lymph node cancer showing up in the breast. Lymphoma is treated with chemotherapy. The tale has two morals. One, never break your own wise rules, and two, things aren't always what they seem. It's ironic that my first breast cancer patient at UCLA didn't have breast cancer. (I'm glad to report that she responded well to the treatment and when last I saw her she was in her nineties and doing fine.)

Occasionally other kinds of cancer occur in the breast. Since the breast contains several kinds of tissue besides breast tissue, any of the cancers associated with those kinds of tissue can appear in the breast. In addition to lymphoma (because there are lymph nodes), these include a cancerous fat tumor (liposarcoma) and a blood vessel tumor (angiosarcoma, occasionally found in patients who have had radiation). You can also have a melanoma—a skin cancer. Connective tissue in the breast, as elsewhere, can become cancerous. Usually these cancers are treated the same way they'd be treated in any other part of the body—the tissue is excised, followed by radiation and chemotherapy (the chemicals are different from those used to treat breast cancer).

When another form of cancer shows up in the breast, we know it isn't breast cancer from the pathologist's report. As I noted earlier, each kind of cancer has its own distinct characteristics, and we rarely mistake one kind for another. We choose treatment for the particular cancer rather than breast cancer treatment. We didn't, for example, do an axillary section on my lymphoma patient.

Having breast cancer doesn't immunize you from other forms of cancer. You have the same chances as anyone else of getting other cancers, though perhaps a bit higher if you have a BRCA mutation. I've had a couple of patients with breast cancer who were also heavy smokers. They were treated for their breast cancer, continued smoking, and ended up with lung cancer. A bout with any kind of cancer can provide a useful time to consider altering your lifestyle in ways that promote overall health.

PART FIVE

Treatment in the Age of Personalized Medicine

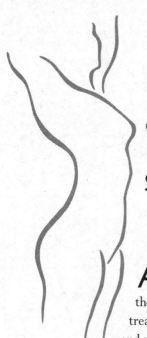

CHAPTER 13

Local Treatment: Surgery

Almost every form of breast cancer involves surgery as part of treatment. Although it is rare in the initial biopsy (when a core is not feasible), standard treatment usually includes a lumpectomy or mastectomy and possible surgery on the lymph nodes. The first concern for most people with breast cancer is maximizing their chances to live, a second and certainly important concern is how they will look after breast cancer surgery. As we have discussed in Chapter 1, our breasts carry a lot of meaning and feelings and their appearance is important to many of us. The options for creating a cancer-free as well as cosmetically appealing breast, or breast equivalent, have increased significantly over the years. A lumpectomy (also called wide excision or partial mastectomy) can be done with plastic surgery techniques known as oncoplastic surgery. You can have postmastectomy reconstruction immediately or later. Or you can use a prosthesis in your bra after mastectomy or lumpectomy (Figure 13.1). Finally, there is always the option of simply not appearing to have two symmetrical breasts. All the decisions you make about breast surgery also have implications regarding reconstruction, sensation, and body image. I will cover them all in this chapter so you can see the "menu" of options available as opposed to your surgeon's favorite approach. I think that's the best way to avoid disappointment later.

I've already discussed some general aspects of surgery in Chapter 11. In this chapter we will go over what you can expect from your surgeon and your operation for breast cancer. I'll also go into the likely side effects and the recovery process. Be warned: I will be fairly explicit because I think the more information you have, the less scared you will be. If you find surgical details unpleasant, you may skip those parts.

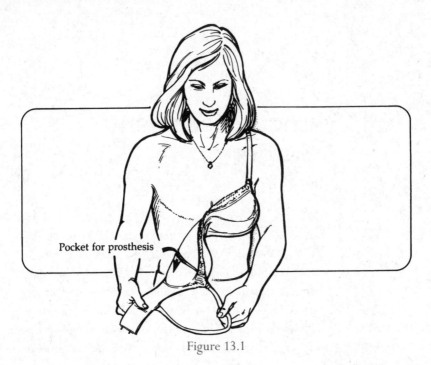

Pocket for prosthesis

Figure 13.1

When I was in practice, I would talk with the patient a few days ahead of time and explain exactly what I'd do in the operation and what risks and possible complications were involved. I'd draw pictures and show photographs, so the patient would know what to expect. At Boston's Dana-Farber Cancer Institute, my former colleague Susan Troyan, MD, and Judi Hirschfield-Bartek, RN, often encourage patients to read Peggy Huddleston's book *Prepare for Surgery, Heal Faster,* which helps them learn techniques to feel in control. Many hospitals have guided programs and workshops based on methods in this book and others to help prepare you for surgery. You can check if your doctor's facility offers them.

As with any operation, patients are asked before the surgery to sign a consent form. This can be a little scary, especially if you read all the fine print, because it asks you to state that you know you can die from the surgery or suffer permanent brain damage from the anesthetic. This doesn't mean that either is likely to happen, or that by signing the form you're letting the doctors off the hook if something does happen; rather, it's an acknowledgment that you've been told about the procedure and its risks and that you still want to have the operation. (Obviously you have to balance for yourself the risk involved in the operation against the risks of not having it.) You've probably seen many similar forms, as virtually any medical procedure—including flu shots—uses them.

It's very important to know the risks. Never permit yourself to be rushed through signing the consent form. You should be given the form well before you go in for surgery—it's hard to read small print when you're about to be wheeled into the operating room. And if no one offers to let you see the consent ahead of time, ask for it. You need to have plenty of time to ask the surgeon questions about risks and complications. If anything confuses you, be sure to ask for clarification.

Your surgeon may tell you to stop taking ibuprofen, blood thinners, vitamin E, fish oil, and some herbs/supplements at least three to seven days before surgery. All these interfere with clotting and cause more bleeding in surgery. It is important to tell both your surgeon and anesthesiologist about all drugs, vitamins, and herbs you are taking so they can check for interactions or consult with your primary MD or cardiologist if you are taking blood thinners.

ANESTHESIA

Anesthesia for breast surgery has come under increased scrutiny, leading to several changes in practice. Key to the discussion was a 2006 study[1] that showed that women who received regional anesthesia (a local block of the nerve leading to the area of the surgery) along with their general anesthesia had a 40 percent lower risk of recurrence. Although this was not a randomized study, it set anesthesiologists thinking. Obviously surgery and the pain it induces cause a stress response as well as inflammation. And some of the inhalational anesthetics (gases) have been shown to hamper the immune system in its battle with the cancer. Using the local block decreases the pain and therefore reduces the amount of general anesthesia needed.

These are valid points, but a recent international trial of more than two thousand women showed no difference in breast cancer recurrence under regional anesthesia with a nerve block or general anesthesia with opioids. They were also the same in terms of the frequency or severity of incisional breast pain.[2]

Also, several studies have shown that the more narcotics or opioids the patient takes postoperatively, the higher the recurrence rate, but it is not clear whether it is the opioids that blunt the immune system. Although this is far from resolved, many anesthesiologists are already using paravertebral blocks to reduce side effects and shorten hospitalizations. If these also decrease the chance of the cancer spreading, all the better. Meanwhile, it is important to ask about the team's pain management protocol and ask their opinion for the best strategies for pain control. This may include narcotics, muscle relaxants, and nonsteroidal anti-inflammatory drugs (NSAIDs). It can't hurt, it may well help, and it certainly can shorten your recovery.

Because anesthesia and its administration are so complicated, most hospitals will have you talk with an anesthesiologist before the operation. This is usually done during a preoperative screening appointment or, if you are healthy, through a phone call with an anesthesia team member on the day before surgery. For some less complicated operations you will first meet the anesthesiologist the morning of surgery rather than earlier. Anesthesiologists are highly trained doctors who have gone through at least three years of specialized training after internship. They often work with nurse anesthetists who are also very experienced. The anesthesiologist will take your medical history, looking for information that may suggest using, or not using, various anesthetic agents—for example, chronic diseases you may have, past experiences with anesthetic, and so on. After thoroughly exploring all this with you, the anesthesiologist will decide what to use in your operation. If you have previously undergone surgery and had trouble with the anesthesia, try to bring a copy of your anesthesia record from the hospital where the surgery was performed. Narcotics given during surgery seem to have a high rate of causing nausea after the operation among breast surgery patients. At a minimum, if you had trouble during a prior operation, remember to describe the problem(s) to the anesthesia team on the day of surgery so they can be attuned to your needs. But remember that drugs and procedures may have changed a lot since then. This interview with an anesthesiologist is very important as the risk of an operation lies as much in the anesthesia and its administration as in the surgery. When you talk to the anesthesiologist, ask questions and give any information you think may be important. Although you may have a different anesthesiologist for your operation, you can be assured that all the pertinent information will be available.

PROCEDURE

On the day of surgery you will be checked in, asked to change into a gown, and taken to the holding area. Here your doctor or an assistant will ask you which side is being operated on and mark it with an X or with their initials. This is not because they have forgotten, but to confirm that the surgeon has personally checked you and the record is correct so that no errors are made. The nurses in the holding area will again ask you your name and check your armband and what operation you're having, just to make sure that you are the patient they think you are. An IV will be put into a vein in your arm.

In some hospitals you will walk into the operating room, while in others you will be wheeled in. Different hospitals use different preoperative formulas, which can sometimes include some guided imagery, aromatherapy, and a drug cocktail. Once in the surgery suite, you will be hooked up to a variety of monitoring devices. There's an automatic blood pressure cuff that feels very tight when it's first inflated, but don't worry—as soon as it registers how big your arm is, the amount of pressure used on subsequent inflations is less. There's an EKG monitoring your heart rate, and a little clip or piece of tape is put on your finger, toe, or earlobe to measure the amount of oxygen in your blood. If the operation is a lengthy one, as when it includes reconstruction, a catheter is put in your bladder to measure the amount of urine output and make sure you're not dehydrated. Thus your bodily functions are all carefully monitored. Large pads are placed over your lower body to maintain your body temperature during the process. You'll probably wear pneumatic boots—plastic boots that pump up and down massaging your calves during the operation to prevent clots from forming during long operations (Figure 13.2). A grounding plate is put on your skin to ground the electrocautery and protect you from shock. During this time, your surgeon may or may not be with you. Some surgeons prefer making personal contact before surgery; others maintain a professional distance. Then the surgeon goes out to scrub (wash their hands).

If you are going to receive an epidural, the anesthesiologist will have you lie on your side or sit up so that they can see your back between your shoulder blades clearly. They will give you a small amount of local anesthesia to numb the skin and then place a catheter in the epidural space where the nerves exit the spinal cord. Local anesthetic is injected through the catheter, causing the area of the breast to be numb. More local can be added as needed. The numbness gradually wears off once the catheter is removed; however, it can be left in place postoperatively for pain relief if needed, as after mastectomy and immediate reconstruction. The other regional option is a paravertebral block. This does not involve a catheter but rather a series of injections of local anesthetic at several

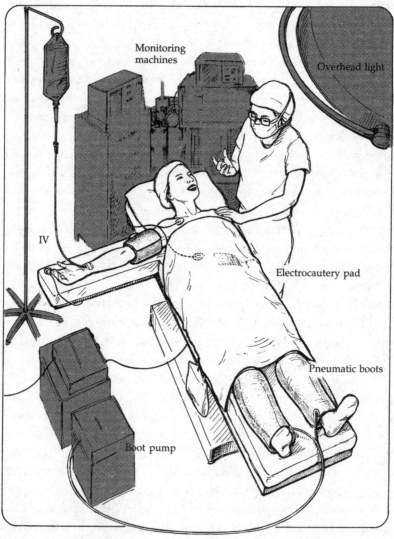

Figure 13.2

places along the back of the rib cage. The injections "block" only the nerves on the side of the chest that will be operated on and are usually given with sedation. The advantage of this approach is that the numbness lasts eighteen to twenty-four hours or more and there is much less nausea than under general anesthesia. This works well for patients who are undergoing wide excision or simple mastectomies and plan to go home the same day.

If you are having surgery under general anesthesia, you will be given propofol and go right to sleep. Even with a regional anesthetic you may well receive propofol or a sedative. Many people who haven't had surgery for thirty or forty years remember the old days of ether and are nervous about the unpleasant sensations they recall while going under. But sodium pentothal (which is almost never used anymore) and propofol work differently, and most patients report it as a very pleasant experience. You may experience a garlic taste at the back of your mouth just before you go under, and you may yawn. Propofol may burn as it goes into your arm. Pretreatment of the vein with local anesthetics before the propofol is injected helps this considerably, but if you feel it, it is only for a second or two before you go to sleep, and you probably won't remember it. Then you're asleep. People are often reassured to know that they don't talk under anesthesia, or even sedation: your deep dark secrets remain safe. With monitored anesthesia care (MAC), you may tersely answer a direct question, but you won't chat, and the questions won't be any more personal than "Do you feel this?"

After scrubbing, the surgeon returns to the operating room. The area of your body that's going to be worked on is painted with a disinfectant, and drapes are put around you to prevent infection. Prior to any incision being made, either while you are awake, after the regional anesthesia, or immediately after anesthesia is administered, a time-out is performed. This procedure has been borrowed from the checklist approach for airplanes, where everything is reviewed prior to takeoff. Everyone stops— surgical team, anesthesia team, and nursing team. They turn off the music and the anesthesiologist reads the name of the patient and identifies surgical issues, reporting the antibiotic that has been given and reminding the surgeon about any drug allergies and also if the patient is on a particular medication such as a beta blocker. (This is significant, because if you forget to put a patient back on their beta blocker post-op, they can have cardiac complications.) Then the surgeon announces what operation is going to be performed, which side, estimated operating time, and estimated blood loss. The circulating nurse is meanwhile reading directly off the consent form to verify that everything is correct.

After this thorough review, the operation is underway. Most surgical operations have traditionally been done with a scalpel or scissors. More recently, electrocautery (performed with a type of electric knife) has been used with less blood loss. Once the surgery is over and your wounds have been dressed, you are allowed to wake up.

How you wake up from the operation will depend, again, on the drugs that were used. For some drugs an antidote can be given to end the effects. For example, if you've been given a muscle paralyzer, a drug can restore your muscle mobility. As soon as the surgical team thinks you're awake enough to breathe on your own, the breathing tube that was placed in your throat while you were asleep is removed. Occasionally you'll be vaguely aware that this is happening, but usually you're still too out of it to notice. You stay a little fuzzy for a while. When the surgery is over, you're taken to the recovery room, where a nurse remains with you, monitoring your blood pressure and pulse every ten or fifteen minutes until you're fully awake and stable.

Patients used to feel cold when they first woke up, but now every patient is covered with a heating blanket and temperature is monitored. Although some of the drugs can create nausea, patients for whom anesthesia tends to create nausea can be given antinausea drugs.

You may wake up crying or shivering, but only rarely do patients wake up in great pain. You'll probably fade in and out for a while, and then you'll be fully awake. But expect to be groggy and out of it for a while. Most of the drugs take several hours to exit your system, and it's a day or more until they're all gone. If it's day surgery, you'll probably want to go home and go to bed; if you're still in the hospital, you'll sleep it off there. If you have regional anesthesia, the numbness will last for eighteen to twenty-four hours.

Even apart from the surgery, general anesthesia as mentioned is a great strain on your body, and it will cause some degree of exhaustion for at least four or five days and sometimes up to a month. People often don't realize this, especially if the surgery is very painful: they attribute all their exhaustion to the pain of the operation. But anything that puts great stress on your body—surgery, a heart attack, an acute asthma attack, or anesthetics that interfere with your body's functions—has a lingering effect. Your body seems to need all its energy to mobilize for the big stress and doesn't have any left over for everyday life for a while. You need to respect that and give yourself time to recuperate from the stress of both the surgery and the anesthetic. I also think it has some effect on brain chemistry that we don't yet understand. Previous experience is not a good guide to how it will affect you the next time, even if the same drugs are used. So don't assume that because you felt fine after your last surgery, you'll feel fine after this one. You may or may not.

There are, of course, risks involved with general anesthetic, but it's important to keep them in perspective. With the refinements in anesthesia in recent years, the risks are extremely low. As mentioned, the use of general anesthesia in breast surgery, though still very common, is being questioned. Regional anesthesia is being used more often, so check with your doctor or the anesthesiologist well before your operation to decide what is best for you.

Depending on how complicated the operation is, you will usually have surgery the same day you're admitted to the hospital, and you may have day surgery or twenty-three to twenty-four-hour-stay surgery. Hospitals often have special wings with nurses trained in post-op care to serve these patients. Many surgeons tend to do lumpectomy with axillary dissection only on an outpatient basis, so the patient has two hours of surgery, spends another few hours in the recovery room, and then goes home. Because the rate of infection is twice as high among patients who stay in the hospital, I think leaving as soon as possible is a good idea. (I understand many patients' concerns that managed care companies try to save money by sending people home too soon, but in some cases, leaving the hospital as soon as possible really can be best for the patient.) Remember that you will need to have someone drive you home from the hospital as you will not be allowed to drive yourself even if you feel fine.

A patient who has a mastectomy and expander will go home the next day, while one undergoing immediate reconstruction with autologous tissue will be in the hospital for two to five days.

One thing that keeps people in the hospital after mastectomy is learning how to manage a drain. If possible, ask your doctor to show you and your family the drain and how to empty it at the pre-op visit. The other reason to stay in the hospital is advanced age or pain control. As soon as you can take oral pain pills, you can go home and not be awakened at two a.m. for your blood pressure check!

All the procedures I've just described are done regardless of the kind of operation you're having. Now I'll describe what happens in each different breast cancer operation, starting with the simplest and moving on to those that are more complex. (Biopsies are described in Chapter 8.) I will first discuss lymph node surgery, which is done in all patients with invasive breast cancer. Then I will go into the breast procedures: partial mastectomy or lumpectomy, and mastectomy with the options of immediate or delayed reconstruction.

SENTINEL NODE BIOPSY AND AXILLARY DISSECTION

Sentinel Node Biopsy

As mentioned in Chapter 11, sentinel node biopsy has become the standard of care regardless of the type of breast surgery you choose to undergo. However, when worrisome lymph nodes are noted on a physical examination, the patient should have an ultrasound to investigate them further. If an abnormality is observed, then it can be sampled by either fine-needle aspiration or core biopsy. If the node is positive, then the patient may also have an axillary lymph node dissection and, if not, a sentinel node biopsy, depending on whether they are going to undergo mastectomy or breast conservation with radiation.

The usual practice is to do the sentinel node biopsy before attending to the breast. That way the dye is injected into an intact breast. In order to identify the nodes most likely to be involved, two different types of tracers are usually injected. Most commonly these include a radioactive protein and isosulfan blue dye. The radioactive protein is usually injected two hours before surgery or as early as the afternoon before for early-morning surgery because it lasts longer in the tissue. The injection of the radioactive tracer can be done by a surgeon, a radiologist, or a trainee. Because the injection of the tracer can be painful, some find that applying EMLA (an anesthetic cream) to your breast an hour before the injection helps. In addition, you can request Ativan (a drug used for anxiety) ahead of time if you think you will be queasy or are very sensitive to pain. The radiation is very low dose, so you don't have to worry about being radioactive thereafter or exposing others to harmful effects from your injection. Some surgeons use blue dye alone; others use it together with the radioactive tracer.

As opposed to the radioactive tracer, the isosulfan blue dye doesn't last as long in the nodes, so it is usually injected in the operating room once you are asleep, followed by a five-minute breast massage prior to operating.

A minor but potentially alarming fact is that the dye can turn your breast blue, which can take several weeks to months to fade completely. There is also a transient change in the color of your urine (blue) and stool (greenish). (See Barbara's story later in this section.)

As mentioned in Chapter 11, some surgeons are investigating an approach that they hope will reduce lymphedema, which is when your arm becomes inflamed or swells after lymph node surgery. Called reverse axillary lymphatic mapping, it involves injecting a blue dye called lymphazurin under the skin of the upper inner arm and massaging it a little. A large bright blue splotch appears on the arm, but it is gone in a day or two, unlike the residual color often seen when the dye is injected into the breast. This may allow the surgeon to differentiate the lymphatics related to the breast from those that serve the arm, which turn blue with the injection, allowing them to be avoided and, thus, protected.[3] Clinical trials have shown that this reduces lymphedema rates considerably, and when some blue arm lymphatics do get removed because they overlap with breast sentinel nodes, there is an increased risk of lymphedema.[4]

In addition to the blue dye, a small dose of radioactive materials can be injected in the tissue around the tumor, in the skin overlying the tumor, or in the periareolar area. The location of the radioactive protein can be detected by waving a handheld gamma detection probe during surgery. It identifies where the sentinel nodes are most likely to be and can also indicate when the drainage is in an unusual and unexpected direction, such as under the middle of the rib cage, suggesting a different approach. Usually, however, the drainage is to the armpit and a short incision is made (just below the hairline of the armpit) over the area with the strongest signal. The tissue is carefully dissected and the surgeon looks for the blue dye in the lymphatic vessel or the radioactive signal, which will lead to the blue sentinel node or nodes. Although we call this a sentinel node biopsy, it is really more than a biopsy and often involves more than one node, as all the nodes that are radioactive and/or blue (usually two to four but can be as few as one or as high as five) are then removed and sent to pathology for examination. The nodes can be evaluated during surgery or later with either a "frozen section" or a molecular study. These tests generally take about thirty minutes to perform and are about 90 percent accurate. If the nodes are negative, the incision is sewn closed without a drain. In some centers, the nodes are not evaluated with a frozen section test at the time of surgery. If this is the case and a positive sentinel node is found, you may be advised to have additional nodes removed in a separate operation (see the following section, titled "Full Axillary Lymph Node Dissection"). Very rarely, even if the frozen section shows a negative node, the final pathology report may show some cancer cells. Often, this situation will require a discussion with your surgeon or oncologist to determine whether additional lymph nodes need to be removed (see Chapter 11).

Several years ago Barbara, a flight attendant I met when she volunteered for my nipple fluid studies, described her experience with the sentinel node biopsy, even though she later needed a full axillary dissection. She knew that with sentinel node biopsy as part of the process, doctors would remove fewer lymph nodes. Barbara was particularly concerned, as she was afraid that with many nodes removed, she was likely to have lymphedema, which would probably be exacerbated by the constant changes of air pressure involved in her job. Fortunately she had no swelling after the procedure.

The surgery lasted several hours, and she stayed overnight in the hospital. "At nine p.m., I had to go to the john," she recalled, "and the nurse helped me. My pee was a bright cobalt blue. I had known about it, but the poor nurse hadn't, and she was really shocked." There was also some blue in her breasts, which took about a month to clear out. Rarely the dye can tattoo the breast for a year; this is still normal, and it happens when the dye is taken up by the lymphatics in the skin.

The operation on her nodes left her with several weeks of discomfort. "I felt like I had a wad of Scotch tape under each armpit," she recalls. "For about two weeks, I couldn't stand my arm and chest skin meeting." By the end of a month the discomfort subsided, and it was never bad enough to make her take the painkillers the doctors had given her.

Full Axillary Lymph Node Dissection

A full axillary dissection is done only when there are palpable nodes or a large number of nodes that have been shown to contain cancer. If the procedure is a mastectomy, then the axilla is usually approached through the mastectomy incision.

The lymph nodes, as I said earlier, are glands. Sometimes they're swollen and big, but usually they're small and embedded in fat. This lump of fat is defined by certain anatomical boundaries and usually contains at least ten to fifteen lymph nodes. We hope—but can't be sure—that we've included in this fat the significant lymph nodes. The tissue is sent to the pathologist, who examines the fat and tries to find as many of the lymph nodes as possible. The pathologist then cuts each node in half, makes slides, and examines each of them for cancer.

Some people have more nodes than others. Occasionally a patient would ask me, "How come you got seventeen lymph nodes in me and only seven in my friend?" We are all built differently. This difference was brought to my attention one time after I did a routine axillary dissection. A new pathologist was dissecting out the nodes and amazed me by finding forty in a specimen that usually would contain fifteen. She just looked harder than usual.

However, the total number of nodes is less important than the number that contain cancer (also called a *positive node*). Studies have shown that the chance of missing a positive lymph node if an axillary dissection is performed is less than 2 percent.

Some surgeons put a drain in the axillary incision afterward, and some do not. The operation takes from one to three hours. You'll go home with a small dressing on your incision. You can ask your surgeon to place a waterproof dressing over the incision and drain insertion sites, so you can shower and not have to wait until the drains are removed. Depending on the surgeon, there may or may not be sutures to remove, but in any case most surgeons like to see their patients one week to two weeks after the surgery to monitor their progress. An earlier visit can be scheduled to discuss pathology results.

Side Effects

The good news is that most studies have shown that the sentinel node biopsy has significantly fewer immediate and delayed complications than a full axillary dissection.[5] Nonetheless, because the surgery is in the same area of the body, the potential complications are the same: axillary pain, numbness, paresthesias (abnormal sensations including hypersensitivity), and arm swelling (lymphedema). The type of breast surgery does not affect the incidence of these potential complications.

One problem that can be commonly encountered in the week following surgery is fluid under the armpit (seroma). Most patients have some swelling, but sometimes a patient will get so much that it looks like they have an orange in their armpit. Usually the doctor aspirates the fluid in the office. A seroma should not be mistaken for lymphedema, which is a more generalized, long-term swelling of the arm that can occur many months or years after lymph node surgery (see Chapter 18).

Very rarely a patient gets a hematoma (collection of blood) from surgery of the breast or nodes. If it is recognized soon after surgery, the surgeon may decide to return to the operating room to find and stop the source of bleeding. A hematoma that develops days after surgery will generally improve on its own, without the need for additional surgery. You may, however, be black and blue for a few weeks. The surgical dressing tape may cause a rash known as tape burn.

Damage to a sensory nerve or nerves that pass through the middle of the fat that is removed may be longer lasting. This nerve gives you sensation in the back part of your arm, though it doesn't affect the strength and motion of your arm. If that nerve is cut, you'll have a patch of numbness in the back part of your arm (Figure 13.3). Most breast surgeons and many general surgeons try to save the nerve. Even so, it may get stretched and cause decreased sensation either temporarily or permanently. If the sensation is gone for more than a few months, the loss is

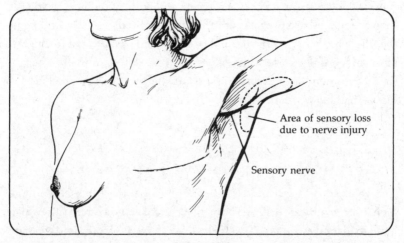

Figure 13.3

probably permanent. This problem is less common after sentinel node biopsy but is certainly not eliminated. (If this happens to you, you may want to give up shaving your armpits, or use an electric shaver rather than a razor, which is more likely to cut the skin and cause bleeding.)

Another early problem can be phlebitis in an arm vein. This usually shows up three or four days after surgery. The patient says, "I felt wonderful after the operation and now I have this tight feeling under my arm that goes down to the elbow and sometimes even to the wrist. And I can see a cord. The pain is worse and I can't move my arm nearly as well as I could before." This has come to be called axillary web syndrome and is very common but is also temporary, typically resolving within six to eight weeks.[6] I have always felt that it is an inflammation of the basilic vein, but others think it is just a general inflammation from the dissection or even a clogged lymphatic vessel. It's not serious but it is bothersome. The best treatment is ice and aspirin or an NSAID such as ibuprofen, Voltaren cream, exercise, or physical therapy. It will go away within several days to a week. Again, it's important to move your arm and keep it from stiffening. Dr. Ellen Mahoney, a breast surgeon I admire in Northern California, tells her patients to keep their hand behind their head while reading or watching TV postoperatively, to stretch the scar. Walking your fingers up the wall higher and higher can also help. If the symptoms don't improve quickly, early referral for physical therapy will usually help reduce the problem.

Both lymph node operations result in a variety of new and often unpleasant sensations in the area of the surgery. These have been reported in an article termed appropriately "Eighteen Sensations After Breast Cancer Surgery: A 5-Year Comparison of Sentinel Lymph Node Biopsy and Axillary Lymph Node Dissection." The eighteen sensations are tender, sore, pull, ache, painful, twinge, tight, stiff, prick, throb, shoot, tingle, numb, burn, hard, sharp, nag, and penetrate.[7] Although certain sensations are far more prevalent in full dissection than in sentinel node biopsy in the initial period after surgery and five years later, some sensations remain notably prevalent five years after sentinel node biopsy. Tenderness remained in 33 percent of patients after five years with sentinel node biopsy and 40 percent after full dissection.

The major complication—but fortunately one that is uncommon—is swelling of the arm, a condition called lymphedema, and nerve damage, which we'll consider in Chapter 18. Suffice it to say that a large-cohort study found the risk of lymphedema to be 5 percent after sentinel node biopsy, compared to 16 percent after full axillary dissection. But the risk of lymphedema with surgery alone doubled when adding radiation therapy and chemotherapy, especially with taxanes.[8]

BREAST ABLATION THERAPY

Breast ablation therapy is a relatively new but interesting alternative to lumpectomy for patients with small, low-risk cancers who prefer to avoid the scalpel. Once your cancer is located by ultrasound, it is either beamed with a radiofrequency, microwaved, or frozen. Several small studies have shown the effectiveness of these minimally invasive approaches, but at the time of this writing few large multicenter studies have examined them to confirm their efficacy when compared to the standard lumpectomy.

Radiofrequency ablation (RFA) uses a radiofrequency electrode guided by imaging to focus thermal energy at the tumor and destroy malignant tissue. A smaller trial of forty women comparing RFA to lumpectomy found that the surgical margins were positive for cancer in 55 percent of the lumpectomy group and 20 percent in the radiofrequency group. However, local breast inflammation and three infections occurred in the RFA group.[9]

Microwave ablation sends electromagnetic waves to the tumor by using breast imaging to place a needle that creates heat and destroys cancer cells. The dead tumor cells are gradually replaced by scar tissue. A small Chinese study of microwave ablation found that 91 percent of their 35 patients showed complete tumor cell death after treatment. Curiously, in addition to destroying the tumor, the beam also was shown to activate some of the immune system's T cells, which recognized the cancer cells as a threat.[10]

Cryoablation destroys tumor cells by exposing them to subfreezing temperatures with liquid nitrogen. In a trial of 194 patients over age 60 with early-stage low-risk breast cancer, only 2 percent experienced a recurrence thirty-five months after the procedure. Furthermore, 95 percent of the patients reported satisfaction with the cosmetic results.[11]

PARTIAL MASTECTOMY

Partial mastectomy, lumpectomy, wide excision, segmental mastectomy, and quadrantectomy are all names for procedures short of mastectomy and are used virtually synonymously (Figure 13.4). What each term means precisely depends on the surgeon who's using it. Except for quadrantectomy, none of the terms suggests how much tissue will be removed, and often surgeons use the term "quadrantectomy" when they don't necessarily mean they'll remove a fourth of the breast. With a partial mastectomy, the part removed can be 1 percent or 50 percent of the breast tissue. Lumpectomy depends on the size of the lump. Wide excision just says that tissue will be cut away around the lump—not how much will be cut. "Segmental" sounds like the breast comes in little segments, like an orange. But it doesn't, and the segment removed can be any size. Your surgeon will use whatever term appeals most to them.

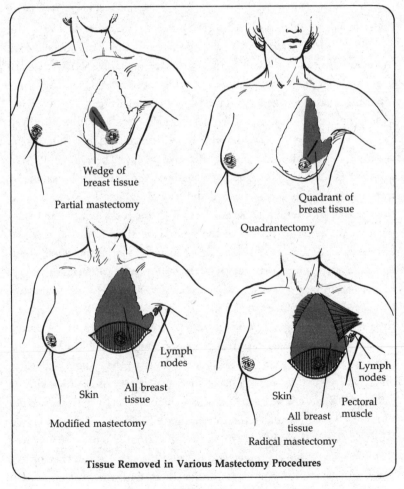

Wedge of
breast tissue

Partial mastectomy

Quadrant of
breast tissue

Quadrantectomy

Lymph
nodes

All breast
tissue

Skin

Modified mastectomy

Lymph
nodes

Skin

Pectoral
muscle

All breast
tissue

Radical mastectomy

Tissue Removed in Various Mastectomy Procedures

Figure 13.4

The goal of breast conservation is to excise the primary tumor with negative margins (no sign of the tumor on the outside rim of the tissue sample) while maintaining a cosmetically acceptable breast. If you're opting for such surgery, you need to make sure your surgeon explains precisely how much tissue will be removed and what you're going to look like afterward.

Localization of the Tumor

If your cancer cannot be felt, its position must be marked for the surgeon preoperatively. When these lesions have been diagnosed by a core biopsy under imaging guidance (see Chapter 8), a clip is placed at the biopsy site to facilitate localization later. Although this can sound scary, the clips are incredibly tiny and reactions to them are extremely rare. Often made of titanium, they are placed in all image-guided core needle biopsies; otherwise, the correct localization of the cancer can be difficult.

If a wide excision needs to be performed, the clip will be localized for the surgeon with a guide wire (needle localization) while in the mammography suite immediately before surgery. The radiologist will give you a local anesthetic and put a small needle into your breast under image guidance, pointing toward the lesion (Figure 13.5). They will then pass a wire with a hook on the end through the needle, and then position the hook so the tip of the wire is on the site of the targeted lesion. If the lesion encompasses an area larger than a centimeter or if it is elongated, more than one wire may be placed to outline the area that needs to be excised for the surgeon. Dr. Shelly Hwang, a surgical colleague at Duke, likes to think of the wires as "brackets" or "parentheses" around the area to be removed. The wire or wires are left in the breast, and you're then taken to the operating room. After the tissue and wire(s) are removed, the specimen is sent to the radiology department. There they X-ray it to make sure it includes the calcifications or lesion and then send it to the pathology department, where they make slides and look at it under the microscope. The X-ray of the specimen will tell you if the surgeon got the calcifications, biopsy clip, or area that was seen on the mammogram. Because the surgeon can't see or feel calcifications, it is also possible to miss them with the surgery. In this case the X-ray of the specimen will not show the targeted area and the surgeon may excise additional tissue.

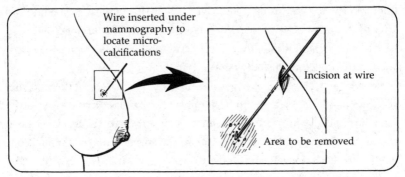

Wire inserted under mammography to locate micro-calcifications

Incision at wire

Area to be removed

Figure 13.5

Another approach for localizing small cancers for excision that is sometimes used takes advantage of a side effect of the diagnostic core biopsy used for diagnosis. After any core, there will be a small hematoma (collection of blood) in the breast where the tissue was removed. This can often be located with ultrasound, allowing a surgeon to identify the tissue to be removed without the insertion of a wire.[12]

Many medical institutions are performing seed localizations now instead of using wires. There are a few different types of seeds, and they can be placed far in advance. One popular option is a small radioactive seed that is placed in the breast for localization. A radioactive seed is a capsule that contains a small amount of radioactive material.[13] The seed is inserted into the area of the breast where the tumor is located with a small needle, under the guidance of a mammogram or an ultrasound. At the time of surgery, the same probe used to find the radioactive tracer in a sentinel node biopsy is used to detect the location of the seed. This allows the surgeon to detect the exact location of the tumor. The two advantages are that the seed can be placed anytime from a week before to the day of surgery (which allows for more efficient surgery scheduling for your surgery team) and the incision can be placed more accurately in the exact region of the tumor. In addition to radioactive seeds, there are now magnetic and microwave reflector seeds, among others. The procedures used to place and detect all types of seeds are similar.

The Procedure

The operation itself is pretty standard. It begins with carefully monitored anesthesia, either local with sedation or general anesthetic. If a sentinel node biopsy is going to be done, the surgeon starts with an injection of blue dye or radioactive tracer, if it is to be used. The lumpectomy will be done after the nodes. However, if a full axillary dissection is planned, then the lumpectomy usually comes first.

As we gain more experience with breast conservation, improved surgical techniques are leading to better cosmetic results. Incisions are often made around the nipple or adjacent to it in order to reduce scarring if the target site is not too far away. Once the surgeon makes the incision, going through skin, fat, and tissue to get to the lump isn't actually cutting; it's just spreading tissue apart until the lump is reached. The lump is then cut away from the surrounding tissue and removed (Figure 13.6). Every effort is made to take the lump out in one piece so that the pathologist can determine whether there is tumor at the edges or margins (see Chapter 10). There's little bleeding from this excision because there aren't many blood vessels here, and the cautery takes care of the few there are. Prior to closing the incision, four metal clips (like large staples) are often put in the four corners of the biopsy cavity to help the radiation therapist in directing the radiation postoperatively. The incision is then sewn up, usually in layers—tissue, then skin. The goal is to prevent a dent from forming in the breast when it heals. Most surgeons use dissolvable stitches that tend to leave less scarring. The "hidden scar" technique, as you've probably guessed, seeks to conceal the minimal scar in naturally occurring folds or skin changes. Using endoscopic instruments and robotic surgery systems, this approach takes advantage of the body's natural contours such as the crease under the breast, the armpit, and the edge of the areola. Once the incision heals, the scar is all but invisible.

ONCOPLASTIC LUMPECTOMY/ PARTIAL MASTECTOMY

Recent years have seen an increase in the use of oncoplastic surgery, a combination of cancer surgery and plastic surgery.[14] As we mentioned in Chapter 11, the oncoplastic approach applies plastic surgery techniques to the whole cancer operation including, if needed, a reduction of the other breast to match the first. Oncoplastic surgery is best done at the time of the lumpectomy, but it can still be performed a week or so later after the pathology has been reviewed. It may be used if the edges of the

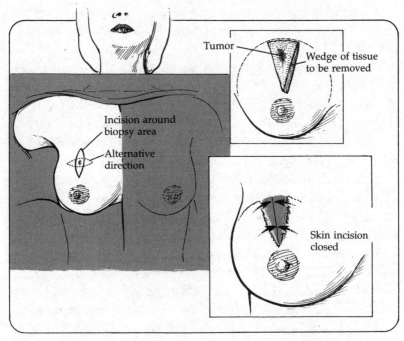

Figure 13.6

extracted tissue are not cancer-free, requiring further surgery, or at a later time to improve the appearance of your treated breast; however, doing it around the time of surgery is usually better. In this case breast size doesn't matter. Any defect resulting from tumor removal can be repaired by rearranging the breast tissue or applying techniques developed for reduction mammoplasty. Removing tissue without repairing any subsequent defect until after radiation therapy often leaves a large deformity that would then require the transfer of a flap similar to those used for total reconstruction.

If you cannot find a breast surgeon trained in oncoplastic techniques, the best alternative is involving a plastic surgeon in assisting the cancer surgeon to then balance the other breast to match. Most breast surgeons will agree to your request.

If your breasts are large and you have considered having a reduction, you should communicate this to your surgeons. My colleague in Seattle, Dr. Ben Anderson, says he is increasingly doing partial mastectomy and having a plastic surgeon do a reduction to match. This allows the surgeon to take more tissue around the cancer and get wider margins.

After the operation, the surgeon bandages the incision and will probably tell you when you can take the bandages off and shower. If not, ask.

Once the tissue is removed, it is marked for the pathologist to indicate which side is toward the head and which is toward the middle of the body. This allows the surgeon to know not only if there is tumor at a margin but also which margin. As explained in Chapter 8, the surgeon or pathologist paints the tissue with different-color ink, and then it is cut into small pieces (as seen in Figure 10.6 on page 214). It goes through several stages. First, it's dehydrated in different strengths of alcohol, then embedded in a block of paraffin wax. This is put on a microtome, a knife that cuts it into very thin slices. Each slice is then put on a slide, the wax melted away, and the tissue stained with different colors. This whole process takes between twenty-four and thirty-six hours.

When the slides are ready, the pathologist looks at them and makes a diagnosis; this takes a few hours. The pathologist then dictates a report that is sent to the doctor, who will probably have it in a week. Some doctors wait till the report comes in, but others prefer to call the pathologist the day after the operation. This is what I used to do because I liked to let my patients know what was happening as soon as possible and because for all patients, the waiting and uncertainty can be terrifying. Whatever your doctor's practice, you'll know in a week or so what the biopsy has shown, what the margins were like, and whether there was any cancer in the lymph nodes. On the basis of the pathology report, you'll discuss the next steps and whether there is a need for adjuvant therapy, radiation therapy, or both.

Since 2016, health care providers are required by law to share such test results, usually through electronic patient portals. This is thanks to the 21st Century Cures Act, which guarantees you access to your own electronic medical records without delay, free of charge, while still safeguarding your privacy. Now you yourself can forward your pertinent records to other doctors or health care facilities for second opinions or to coordinate care. But not all patients are that hands-on. Some find getting results through an online portal written in medicalese an overwhelming or scary experience and prefer not to look at alerts when they are expecting sensitive test results. And that is fine, so long as you know you can access them if you wish to.

At Home After Partial Mastectomy and Lymph Node Surgery

Once you're home, you'll be exhausted for a while. Respect that tiredness: you've just been through major surgery, general or regional anesthesia, and an emotionally difficult experience. The exhaustion often comes and goes suddenly: you'll feel fine and go do an errand; when you get home you'll suddenly feel completely wiped out and need to sleep. It may take a couple of weeks for you to feel fully recovered.

You'll have some pain but probably not a lot. Most doctors give their patients pain medication when they go home, but the majority of patients don't finish off the prescription. Occasionally people have a lot of pain, and if that's the case, it's a good idea to let the doctor know—it's often a sign of something wrong, like postoperative bleeding or a hematoma. Also be aware that if you were already taking pain medications before surgery for another condition, you may need more medications than most patients.

After a lumpectomy, you should wear a strong support bra day and night for about a week—it hurts when your breast jiggles. Another trick my patients taught me, particularly my patients with larger breasts, is that if you want to lie on your side, you can lie on the side that wasn't operated on and hold a pillow between your breasts: the pillow cushions the breast that's been operated on (Figure 13.7). If you go home with

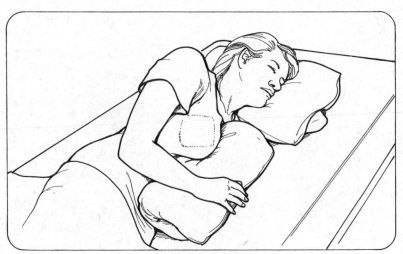

Figure 13.7

drains, there are special garments that you can get to help, with features like belts or pockets that stick to the skin. (A quick Internet search can reveal a whole new world!)

Side Effects

As with any surgical procedure, there are sometimes complications after a partial mastectomy. The two most common are hematoma and infection. If a hematoma occurs, as we mentioned after axillary surgery, it will usually be within a day or two of the procedure. Bleeding inside the area where the surgery was done causes a blood blister to form (Figure 13.8). It turns blue and forms a lump right under the skin. The body usually simply absorbs and recycles it, as it does with any bruise. But sometimes, before the body can do that, you'll bump into something or someone will bump into you, and it will burst open, causing dark blood to come out. It looks gross and disgusting and you'll think you're dying, but don't worry—you're not. It's old blood; you're not bleeding now. What you need to do is go home, clean up the mess, and take a shower. You should also call your doctor and let them know what is going on; they will probably want to see you in the office to get it checked out. Unless there is ongoing, bright red bleeding, this is not an emergency and it will eventually get better on its own, but it can take a long time to reabsorb into the body.

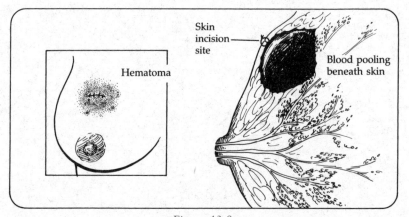

Figure 13.8

If an infection occurs, it will show up a week or two after surgery—there'll be redness and swelling and fever, and the doctor will treat it with antibiotics. Again, it's more of a nuisance than anything else. If the infection is slow to improve, you may need to be rehospitalized for a few days of IV antibiotics.

Sometimes you'll get a combination of infection and hematoma—the blood mixes with pus, like an abscess or a boil, and the doctor needs to drain it. Sometimes when stitches are removed after breast surgery—either biopsies or cosmetic procedures—a small nondissolvable stitch is overlooked and remains in the breast, which will then get infected, as was the case with one of my patients (no, I wasn't the surgeon who removed the stitches). It's easy to treat with antibiotics and removal of the stitch.

There may be some loss of sensation in your breast after a partial mastectomy, depending on the size of the lump removed. If it's a large lump, there may be a permanent numb spot, but there won't be the total loss of sensation that results from a mastectomy.

Your breast may be different in size and shape from how it was before and will probably differ from your other breast. How great the difference is depends on how much tissue was removed and how skillfully the surgery was done. If your breasts have become asymmetrical to an extent that disturbs you, you can get partial-mastectomy breast pads called shells to wear in your bra. Or you can have reconstructive surgery: a small flap of your own tissue is put in to fill things out. Or, depending on how large your breasts were to begin with, you can get the other breast reduced to create a more symmetrical appearance. Usually, however, that isn't necessary. If you have a small lump and medium or large breasts, it's often hard to tell which breast was operated on, except for the scar.

RECONSTRUCTION AFTER LUMPECTOMY
OR PARTIAL MASTECTOMY

Although the majority of people do not require additional surgery after lumpectomy to match the other side, there are certain circumstances when a patient may choose it. After radiation therapy there are sometimes changes in your breast as the tissue shrinks or contracts as it heals.

This can be avoided, as I mentioned, by a breast surgeon who knows on-coplastic techniques. The defect can be filled in with fat transfers. In this situation, fat is sucked out from other more generous areas of the body and injected into the defect. Initially this approach sparked concern that these cells might induce more local recurrences,[15] but long-term study results show that fat-grafting does not increase risk compared to other reconstruction techniques.[16] The downside, however, is that occasionally the transferred fat dies for lack of an adequate blood supply—a condition called fat necrosis. The dead cells can form hard lumps or nodules that mimic cancer recurrence, and imaging the affected breast is then necessary to rule out cancer. It is not a worrisome condition and happens around 2 to 18 percent of the time,[17] but it can cause undue stress. Medical advisors for our research foundation encountered many patients who said they would not have had the fat-grafting procedure had they known beforehand of the possibility of anxiety-causing palpable lumps as a result.

Most women can use their own breast tissue to repair unevenness, whereas those with smaller breasts may sometimes need a tissue flap from the back to fill in the defect. Results may not be satisfactory for a woman who has already undergone surgery and whole-breast radiation therapy. Although tissue rearrangement can be attempted, it has a much higher complication rate because of the previous radiation. The alternative is to use a tissue flap from another part of the body, bringing nonradiated tissue into the area. Although this can work, the flap is rarely the same color as the remaining breast tissue. Many women in this setting elect to do nothing or to have a completion mastectomy (have the rest of the breast removed) and reconstruction. Other issues come into play, of course. The most important is the size of the breast. The location of the tumor will also have an impact on how well this can be done. Bear in mind that reconstructing one breast often means surgery to the other breast to make it match. This is not usually done at the same time if there is still radiation to come, because that radiation may shrink the breast a bit. After the radiation is done, a reduction of the other breast can be performed so that it matches. If the plastic surgery is being done after radiation, then the reduction on the other side can be done at the same time.

If all this sounds like a lot of surgery, it can be, but it usually isn't. As you will see later in this chapter, mastectomy with reconstruction is also usually a multi-operation procedure. It is always easier to do the reconstruction at the same time as the lumpectomy. And it is critical that you take the time to talk to women who have been through it and get their description of what it entailed. I don't want to discourage you, but I do want to give you a realistic picture of what is involved so you can make an informed decision. Breast local reconstructive options are better than ever with a team approach and oncoplastic options. Only you can decide what is most important to you.

TOTAL MASTECTOMY

In spite of the availability of partial mastectomy and radiation, which conserve the breast, many patients in the United States choose to have total mastectomies as their initial therapy for breast cancer.

Total mastectomy should not be confused with radical mastectomy. The latter, once the norm, is now of interest for historical reasons only. It was radical because in addition to trying to remove all the breast tissue, the surgeon removed the pectoralis major and pectoralis minor muscles (see Figure 13.9) as well as all the lymph nodes in the axillary area (up to the collarbone). It was far more deforming than the mastectomy we do now. Today we almost always use neoadjuvant chemotherapy to shrink very large tumors before surgery (see Chapter 11). If the tumor is stuck

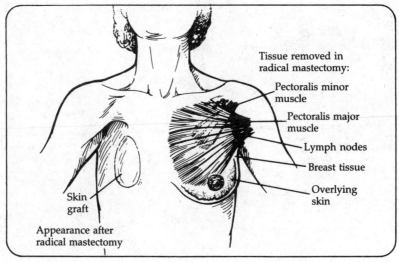

Tissue removed in radical mastectomy:

Pectoralis minor muscle

Pectoralis major muscle

Lymph nodes

Breast tissue

Overlying skin

Skin graft

Appearance after radical mastectomy

Figure 13.9

to the muscle, the surgeon must remove the muscle in order to get to the tumor. (In very rare cases the cancer spreads into the muscle.) We used to do radical mastectomies in all these cases, but now we just take a wedge of muscle under the tumor and leave the rest.

"Total mastectomy," the name usually given to the form of mastectomy used today, is a bit of a misnomer, since we can never be certain the operation is total. Our goal is to remove all the breast tissue, but we can't even be sure we've achieved that. We remove as much of the breast tissue as we can and some of the lymph nodes. It usually takes between two and five hours.

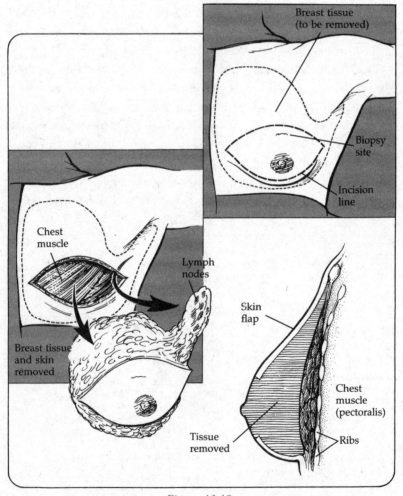

Figure 13.10

The breast tissue extends from the collarbone down to just below the fold under the breast (see Chapter 2) and from the breastbone to the muscle in the back of the armpit. The surgeon wants to remove as much of it as possible and starts with an elliptical incision that includes the nipple and biopsy scar (Figure 13.10).

With the increasing popularity of immediate reconstruction, surgeons have taken to removing as little skin as possible. We used to take out a large amount of skin when we did mastectomies in part because we liked the fact that this helped the scar close neatly. If the surgeon leaves a lot of skin and scoops out all the breast tissue, the skin looks wrinkled and baggy. Trimming the skin creates a nice neat line across the chest. But now, as immediate reconstructions are being done, the need to take off so much skin has been reconsidered. We've moved into the era of skin-sparing mastectomy and nipple-sparing mastectomy. Instead of removing a lot of skin around the breast, surgeons remove only the amount that's needed to remove the breast tissue, unless the patient is absolutely sure she never wants reconstruction, in which case it is still nice to be tidy and remove all excess skin. We've begun to view mastectomy as a very wide excision. Removing every bit of breast tissue isn't possible or necessary: it's getting the tumor out that really matters (Figure 13.11). In most cases, when the tumor is not near the nipple, the nipple can be spared as well. However, the remaining nipple will not function like a normal nipple. There will be loss of nipple sensation and erection.

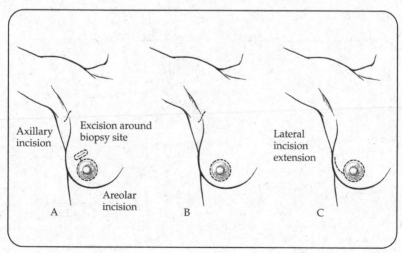

Figure 13.11

Nipple-sparing mastectomy has become more popular as it leaves you with your own nipple rather than a reconstructed nipple or nipple tattoo. Because of the need to leave a small amount of breast tissue under the nipple so that it has a viable blood supply, this approach is not used in patients who have cancers directly under the nipple or large cancers. It is worth a conversation with your surgeon about whether this is a choice for your situation.

After the skin incision has been made, we tunnel underneath the re-maining skin all the way up to the collarbone, then down to just below the inframammary fold from the middle of the sternum, and out to the muscle behind your armpit. Once the dissection is done, we dissect the breast off the chest wall muscle, leaving the muscle and skin flap behind.[18]

We send the breast tissue as well as any nodes that were removed to the pathologist, who examines it and begins the process of preparing it to make slides. Meanwhile we sew together the flaps of skin around the incision. You end up completely flat (or, if you're very thin, slightly concave), with a scar going across the middle of that side of your chest. The skin doesn't completely stick down right away; the body doesn't like empty spaces, so the area fills up with fluid. To prevent this, we insert some drains in soft plastic tubes with little holes in them, com-ing out of the skin below the scar (Figure 13.12). They help create suc-tion that holds the skin down against the muscle till it heals. Fluid will

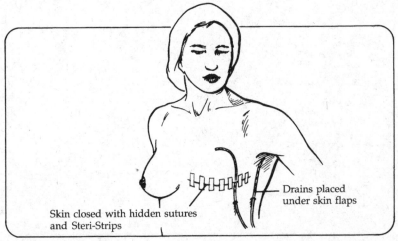

Skin closed with hidden sutures and Steri-Strips

Drains placed under skin flaps

Figure 13.12

come out of these drains—it's just tissue fluid, the kind you get in a blister. Initially there'll be a little blood in the fluid, but over time it will become clearer.

If you've decided to have immediate breast reconstruction, the plastic surgeon comes in after the mastectomy is finished but before the skin is sewn up and does the reconstruction. Alternatively, the plastic surgeon may be part of the team from the beginning, raising the tissue flap from the abdomen while the breast surgeon is doing the mastectomy. If the patient is going to need postmastectomy radiation, one option is to place a tissue expander there temporarily and then have a later flap reconstruction.

As with partial mastectomy, the pathology results will be available in four to five days.

You'll probably stay in the hospital at least overnight. When there's no longer much fluid coming out of the drains—in about seven to ten days—they will be removed in the clinic or office and the dressing will be changed. One of my colleagues, Dr. Lisa Bailey, deals with the postoperative pain with a pump that delivers continuous local anesthesia into the space between skin and muscle. This has made a big difference, as patients have little or no pain, and therefore can get out of bed and walk sooner, don't need narcotics, and so have less nausea.

Some patients want to see the wound right away; some prefer to put off looking at it for a week or two. Either way is fine; you need to decide what makes you feel best. But it's important that you look at it at some point. It's amazing how, if you're determined to avoid looking at your body, you can do so when you shower, get dressed, even when you make love. That's okay for a while, but this is the body you're going to be living with, and you need to see it and accept it. In my experience, most people are relieved when it doesn't look as bad as they feared it would.

Permanent numbness in the area around the mastectomy scar is an unfortunate result of the operation, as the breast's nerve supply has been cut. Some sensitivity remains around the outer borders of the area on which your breast was located. Sometimes the breast area is not entirely numb, however; you can tell if someone is touching you. Unfortunately this usually isn't a pleasant sensation. It can be very uncomfortable, like the sensation you feel when your foot is asleep and starts coming back again, with a tingly feeling. This is known as dysesthesia, and it will lessen but will remain with you. Often people who have had mastectomies don't like their scars being touched because it brings about this sensation. Some people will recover sensation over a long time.

Some people also experience phantom breast symptoms—like the amputee who feels itchiness in toes that are no longer there. The mastectomy patient may feel the missing nipple itch or the missing breast ache. This means that the brain hasn't yet realized what's happened to the body. The nerve supply from the breast grows along a certain path in the spinal cord and goes to a certain area of the brain. The brain has been trained over the years that a signal from this path means, for example, that the nipple is itching. When the nipple has been removed, the signal may get generated in a different place farther along the path, but the brain cells think it should be coming from the nipple, and that's the information they give you. This will gradually improve as your brain becomes reprogrammed.

Audre Lorde described these feelings wonderfully well in her book *The Cancer Journals*: "fixed pains and moveable pains, deep pains and surface pains, strong pains and weak pains. There were stabs and throbs and burns, gripes and tickles and itches."[19] In addition, some patients feel tightness around the chest as the healing starts. This will ease up over time, and all the weird sensations will start to settle down.

Side Effects of Total Mastectomy

Like any operation, mastectomy has risks. In the process of removing the breast tissue, we sever a number of blood vessels. The only ones left are those that go the whole length of the flap of skin remaining when the tissue underneath is removed. These vessels can barely get to the ends of the flap. Sometimes this doesn't supply enough blood, and the wound doesn't heal right; a little area of skin dies and forms a scab (Figure 13.13). Once healing is complete, the scab falls off. It's usually not a serious complication. If a big enough area of skin is involved or an infection develops, the surgeon may have to trim the dead tissue so the body can heal the wound. Uncommonly, a skin graft may be required to cover this area and can speed up the healing process.

A second possible complication occurs when fluid continues to collect under the scar after the drains are removed. You'll know this is happening because there's a swelling under the skin below the incision;

Two possible complications . . .

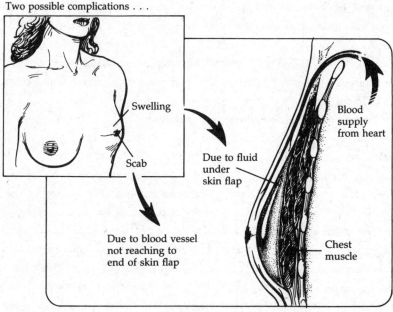

Figure 13.13

sometimes you'll hear a slosh when you're walking or you'll feel the fluid on your chest. If it's a small amount of fluid, you can just leave it alone and it will eventually go away by itself. If there's a lot of fluid, it can be aspirated with a needle: it won't hurt because the area is numb, and it usually doesn't require local anesthesia. (We try to avoid too many aspirations, as there's always the slight risk of transmitting infection through the needle.) Again, this isn't a serious complication, but it can be annoying.

Exercise After Mastectomy

Exercise is important after your treatment, and not only in terms of lymphedema. Again, some doctors can be too restrictive. After you've had a mastectomy or a lymph node sampling, your surgeon may tell you not to move your arm at all. There's a lot of controversy about how protective of the area you should be.

If you keep your arm very still at first, you'll probably have a stiff shoulder when you start moving around. Dr. Ben Anderson, a breast surgeon in Seattle, tells me that all mastectomy and axillary lymph node dissection patients treated by his group get an automatic referral to physical therapy where, at a minimum, they are taught basic exercises and also receive additional lymphedema education. As he rightly points out, physical therapy to prevent a frozen shoulder is better than having to cure one.

Certain exercises actually help your shoulder (Figure 13.14). Immediately after surgery, shoulder rolls are a good way to prevent your shoulder from getting stiff. Another exercise is called "climbing the walls." It involves walking your fingers up the wall, stretching a little bit farther each time. You can do it while you're watching TV or talking on the phone. Another good exercise starting a couple of weeks after surgery involves leaning over as if you were going to touch your toes and making bigger and bigger circles with your arm. Long-term swimming is also excellent exercise and will help maintain strength and range of motion.

If your arm remains very stiff after two or three weeks, ask your doctor to refer you to a physical therapist. It's very important to get your shoulder flexible again, sooner rather than later; otherwise, you can end up with frozen shoulder, a condition that is difficult to treat successfully.

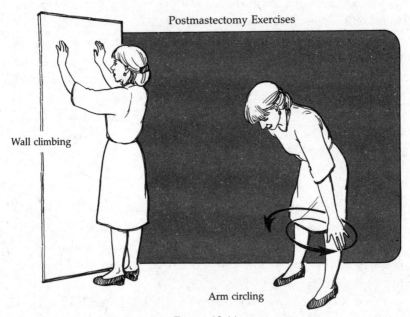

Figure 13.14

If you already have shoulder problems, see a physical therapist preoperatively for advice.

Any sport or exercise you did before your cancer, you can do now—and you should, if you want to. Studies have shown that exercising does not increase your risk of lymphedema and may actually reduce it.

Whatever your choice of surgery, it can be an emotional and difficult experience for most. Fortunately, there are more options now for people with breast cancer, and the options are more effective than ever before at maximizing cancer cure and reducing the side effects of cancer treatment. Use all the resources available to you to make a decision you will be able to live with comfortably. Your surgeon is a great resource, but it is important to try to connect with other people who have been through the experience as well. And make sure that you free up enough time and energy so you can focus on making good decisions for yourself and your family.

RECONSTRUCTION AND MASTECTOMY

Reconstruction after mastectomy is the creation of a new and natural-appearing breast by a plastic surgeon. Breast reconstruction has made a big difference both physically and emotionally for many people who have had mastectomies. But it's important to understand the limits of reconstructive surgery before you decide to have it done.

Making the Decision

What's constructed is not a real breast. It may look real, but it will never have full sensation as a breast does. Any surgeon who says "We're going to take off your breast and give you a new one, and it'll be as good as ever" is either naive or dishonest. The surgeon may tell you that the new breast "feels normal"; at best, this is a half truth. It may feel normal to the hand that's touching it, but it will have little sensation itself. However, feeling is part skin sensation and part mental experience. You may have some slight "feeling" return, but it will never feel completely real to you. As a patient told me, you need time to bond with your new breast. And as my many Facebook friends have adamantly informed me, it is *not* a free "boob job"!

Reconstruction can make your life a little easier—you can wear a T-shirt or lounge wear and not worry about putting on a bra. If the doorbell rings while you're still in your bathrobe, you don't have to deal with whether you want the mail carrier to see your asymmetry. Wearing bathing suits and other "revealing" clothes is easier. In *Why Me?* Rose Kushner explains her decision to have reconstruction. She was alone in a hotel room one night when she was awakened by a fire alarm and the smell of smoke. She jumped out of bed, threw on her clothing, grabbed her glasses, and ran. Downstairs in the lobby with the other guests, she realized that only she had gotten dressed; the others were in their robes. Then she realized why: "This 'well-adjusted' mastectomee wasn't going anywhere publicly with one breast."[20]

A reconstruction can help some people put their cancer experiences behind them. As one of my patients said, "When I was wearing my prosthesis every day, when I looked at my body and it was concave where there had been a breast, I felt that I was a cancer patient, that I was living with that every single day. With the reconstruction I feel that I'm healthy again, that I can go on with my life." Another patient says that after her mastectomy, "I always felt the hollows under my arm. After my reconstruction, I put my arms down, and something was there. That's when the tears came; it was splendid to have that back."

However, reconstruction isn't right for everybody. One of my patients regretted having it. Displeased with the appearance of her reconstructed breast, she also felt that the plastic surgery functioned as a form of denial. "It caused me to postpone the mourning I had to do over losing a breast," she says. "Instead of mourning the loss of a breast, I was thinking in terms of getting a breast. So it wasn't until the process was over, and I saw my new breast, which wasn't like my other breast, that it hit me that I'd lost a breast. If I had the decision to make now, I don't think I'd have reconstruction."

Another woman felt like she was not really given a choice. "I appreciated the option to reconstruct; however, it almost didn't feel like an option. There was definitely an assumption that I would reconstruct because of my age. I was forty. 'Here are the names of two great plastic surgeons.' I was coping with the shock and aftermath of a devastating breast cancer diagnosis. I was on autopilot." She followed the suggestion and felt all right about it. "After I completed chemo and radiation, the reconstruction [with a flap from her stomach] didn't match the remaining breast but I really could not have cared less." In spite of her plastic surgeon urging her to "do some fine-tuning," she decided she had been through enough surgery. It really bothered the plastic surgeon. The patient had problems with discomfort from the surgery for years after. "I was an active woman who mountain climbed and kayaked. If I knew then what I know now, I would not have reconstructed. To quote Popeye: 'I yam what I yam.' I would have skipped the rest entirely."

Some dissatisfaction may result from the limits of the procedure. The best reconstructions look like real breasts, but others look real only through bras or clothing. Factors that can impact the outcome of reconstruction include your body shape, the treatments you have had, and the type of reconstruction as well as the skill of the reconstructive surgeon. It's important to be realistic about your expectations. What do you hope to get from having a reconstructed breast? Some people are very concerned about symmetry; many others aren't. Do you want to look good in your clothes, or is it important that a new lover won't be put off by scars? Do you want to have your remaining breast altered to achieve a closer match? These concerns are not foolish, and you should never hesitate to look for what you want out of guilt over "vanity." You've been through an unpleasant and life-changing experience; you're entitled to do what you can to make its aftermath as comfortable as possible. Talk with your plastic surgeon about all the possibilities and decide what's best for you. Although most plastic surgeons strive to create symmetry in the nude, the most realistic goal and expectation is to obtain symmetry in a bra or clothing. Dr. William Shaw, a former colleague of mine, warned against looking for one universal operation that's best for every patient. "One of the mistakes surgeons and patients both make is to act as if breast reconstruction is some kind of product you can compare objectively—what's the best airplane? One thing I've learned over the years is that there's no one operation that's best for everyone."

And not having reconstruction at all is also an option.

When Should You Have Reconstruction?

You may not be sure at first whether you want reconstruction. Some premastectomy patients are too upset by the cancer and the prospect of a mastectomy to make yet another major decision at the time. When I come across this kind of ambivalence, I suggest the patient have her mastectomy, take whatever time she needs to deal with it, and then, when she feels ready, come back if she still wants reconstruction. (This, by the way, is equally true of surgery for lumpectomy.) You may also consider a consultation with a plastic surgeon just to obtain information, and not make any decisions.

Although plastic surgeons were once reluctant to do immediate reconstruction, it is becoming much more popular. Some surgeons recommend bilateral mastectomies with immediate reconstruction as being the easiest way to achieve symmetry. It probably *is* the easiest for the surgeon, who doesn't have to worry about the cosmetic results of breast conservation. It is also easier for the plastic surgeon, who doesn't have to worry about matching the uninvolved breast. But it may not be easier for *you*.

Make sure you think it through. There is real value in scheduling a pre-op consultation with your radiology oncologist and plastic surgeon. Planning a mastectomy with immediate reconstruction will have to allow for any needed chemotherapy and radiation. In addition you may be limited to the local surgical team that is available at the time when you need surgery. The local plastic surgeon, however, may not be the one you want to do your reconstruction, especially if you want a free flap or a muscle-sparing approach (described shortly). If you delay reconstruction, you may have a greater choice of surgeons. However, if you are going to have a nipple-sparing mastectomy it is best to do the reconstruction immediately. My surgical colleague Dr. Laura Klein suggests that putting tissue expanders in at the time of a nipple-sparing mastectomy can allow a patient to undergo postmastectomy radiation and then complete the reconstruction with a flap later, with the team of their choice. If you are going to need postmastectomy radiation therapy, it may also be better to delay because the acute effects of radiation lead to an increase in the incidence of local complications, regardless of the method of reconstruction.[21] However, if you are interested in implant reconstruction and will need radiation, delaying the reconstruction may rule out the implant option. Prior to radiation, the breast skin can be expanded quickly, leaving you with an acceptable result (although the radiation usually tightens the tissues around the implant somewhat). After radiation, however, the skin is usually not amenable to expansion and a tissue flap is typically required.

There is a pervasive bias that immediate breast reconstruction improves patient quality of life, but the few studies available do not demonstrate such a benefit and instead suggest that breast reconstruction, whether immediate or not, may actually impair quality of life.[22] It is well-documented that surgical complications have a big effect on quality of life. One study that looked back on patients who had undergone mastectomy and reconstruction found that dissatisfaction with the operation was associated with unhappiness with appearance, complications from reconstruction, having prophylactic surgery, and an increased level of stress.[23] Data from the Mayo Clinic demonstrate substantial postoperative complications after mastectomy with immediate reconstruction. This is in contrast to the much less common and less severe complications after wide excision and radiation or mastectomy alone, which rarely require further surgery.[24] Delayed breast reconstruction in general is associated with fewer postoperative complications as well.

There is no time limit for reconstruction. In fact, current techniques have made it a better option than it used to be. If you had a mastectomy in the past and are now thinking about reconstruction, you should feel encouraged. Even with a radical mastectomy, reconstruction is still possible. Or if you originally decided against reconstruction and now want to reconsider, that's also fine. (Some of my patients had their mastectomies in the winter and didn't want reconstruction but changed their minds in the summer, when they wanted to wear bathing suits and sundresses.) However, you can't think of it as a "boob job"! You had breast cancer and things will never be the same.

Types of Postmastectomy Reconstruction

Reconstructive surgery is done in a number of ways. It has at least two components: reconstruction of the breast mound and reconstruction of the nipple-areolar complex. The reconstruction of the breast mound can be done with either artificial substances, your own body tissues, or both.

Implants and Expanders

Of the more than 100,000 breast reconstructions done a year, 75 percent are done with saline or silicone implants.[25] Current options for implant-based reconstruction include immediate or delayed reconstruction with a standard or adjustable implant, two-stage reconstruction with a tissue expander followed by an implant, or reconstruction with the combination of an implant and your own tissue. One-stage implant reconstruction is gaining popularity, although results are best in highly selected patients, typically a C/D cup patient with minimal droop who wants to be a cup size smaller and higher. In the right situation the results can be excellent, although sometimes you may still need a second surgery for revision if your nipple isn't in the right place.

More commonly, a tissue expander is placed under the muscle at the time of the mastectomy. After initial healing, the expander is inflated over time with saline during weekly office visits. This process can be quite uncomfortable as the tissues are stretched out over six to eight weeks. The expander can be used while you are receiving chemotherapy. Once the expansion is complete, the tissues are allowed to relax and adjust to the new position for another one to two months or until chemotherapy is finished. At that point the tissue expander is exchanged for the final implant in an outpatient surgical operation (Figure 13.15).

This two-stage technique of expander-implant reconstruction has become the most common approach to implant-based reconstruction. The final implant is either saline or silicone and is placed behind the pectoralis muscle (Figure 13.16), but if there are problems, it can also be placed over the muscle. The outer shell is always silicone and can be either textured or smooth. Most plastic surgeons think that silicone implants tend to provide a softer, more natural feel and maintain their shape better than

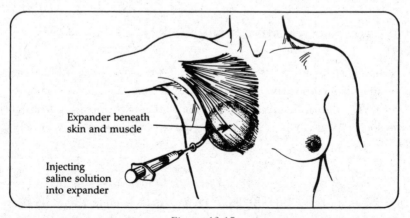

Expander beneath
skin and muscle

Injecting
saline solution
into expander

Figure 13.15

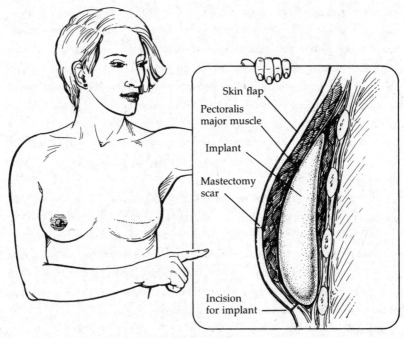

Figure 13.16

saline implants. Saline implants tend to be firmer and to provide less natural fullness in the upper portion of the breast, and they are much more likely to produce visible rippling. Nevertheless, silicone implants are not without some drawbacks. If a saline implant ruptures, the fluid leaks out, your body absorbs it, and it is immediately obvious. If a silicone implant ruptures, you may or may not detect it. However, the newer implants have thicker silicone, making this less likely.

Generally the expander-implant reconstruction will be completed in two steps if you have had a nipple-sparing mastectomy, or four steps if not. Stage one is the immediate reconstruction with an expander; stage two is converting it to the final implant; stage three is nipple reconstruction (when needed); and stage four is the tattoo of the areola (when needed). The advantages of this approach, particularly with a nipple-sparing mastectomy, is that it is simple and that most plastic surgeons are comfortable with it, so they can do it without a special team. There are no scars elsewhere as there would be if your own tissue were used. The disadvantages include the long time it takes to get a breast mound and multiple visits to the plastic surgeon every week or two for inflation. Early complications include bleeding (hematoma) and infection, the latter sometimes requiring implant removal. Although many patients are under the misconception that they are "rejecting" the implant, this really is not true. In fact, in most cases the problem is an infection around the implant or a capsule contracture (a firm scar forms around the implant). Surgery always carries the danger of postoperative infection. An expander or implant can make infection more difficult to treat. Since they are foreign to your body, an infection will not heal by itself. One of my patients developed a very bad infection and had to have the expander removed.

An option that reduces the use of expanders, or omits them completely, is the prepectoral implant reconstruction. This involves placing the implant on top of the chest muscle instead of underneath. The surgeon will not have to cut or divide muscle to insert the implant, and recovery is faster. The implant is usually reinforced and protected by a biological or synthetic mesh, which keeps it attached to the bottom half of the breast. Rippling is a recognized side effect, depending on the type of implant.

About 30 percent of all implant operations are repeat surgeries for complications, according to statistics by the National Breast Implant Registry. Of these, 89 percent were for capsular contracture, followed by hematoma, infection, seroma, skin necrosis, and wound problems.[26]

Implants or expanders are more likely than other procedures to necessitate your having something done to the other breast to make it match. They're going to give you a nice, perfect, seventeen-year-old's breast, but you're probably not a nice, perfect seventeen-year-old. Because the reconstructed breast doesn't sag much, it may be higher than you want it to be. One of my patients found this particularly displeasing. "The reconstructed breast didn't look like my real breast, and it was much higher," she says. "I had to start wearing a bra, which I don't like at all." Thus unless the reconstructed breast matches the remaining one, you may need to have the remaining one operated on to match. Dr. Ben Anderson says that it is important to remember that an implant reconstruction is not the same as cosmetic implants where the breast tissue is still in place. The implant without normal breast tissue between the skin and implant feels more like a balloon.

So when plastic surgeons tell you implants are the easiest form of reconstruction, requiring the least amount of surgery, it's true as far as it goes. This approach is the simplest at the time of surgery but may well need additional operations to refine the result, as well as surgery to the other breast so that it will match.

It's important to let the plastic surgeon know what size you want to be. I had a relatively flat-chested patient who wanted an implant. She wanted to stay flat-chested; that was what she was used to. But the plastic surgeon was conditioned to think that all women want large breasts. He kept trying to persuade her to let him give her a bigger implant and then enlarge her other breast to match it. Another patient had silicone implants, and the implant on one side encapsulated. But she liked the hard, firm, rocklike texture of that breast, and when she had a mastectomy on the other breast, she wanted the reconstructed breast to match the encapsulated one. The plastic surgeon again had a hard time with that—it wasn't what women are supposed to want. If you know what you want and your plastic surgeon argues with you, argue back or change plastic surgeons. It's your body, not the surgeon's, and it's you who will live with that body.

Sometimes an implant can even have a bonus. One of my Facebook friends wrote that she had been "a large 'C,'" and she'd always wanted a reduction. "When I was diagnosed I decided to get what I wanted out of it. I had a reduction on the 'good' side, and expanders put in for my reconstruction during my mastectomy to make me a full 'B.' The expander was removed, and a saline implant was put in after chemo through a small incision under the reconstructed breast before I started radiation. I haven't had any trouble, and the reconstruction looks great."

When the operation works well and the patient's expectations are realistic, implants can make a wonderful difference. As one of my patients says, "I forget it's there—it's a part of me now. It's a little harder than my other breast, but otherwise great. I don't have to worry about what I wear."

One caution: implants don't last forever. Even for the woman who has implants to enlarge her breasts, replacing them can be upsetting. For the mastectomy patient, it can be devastating—like losing the breast all over again. Such patients may require the flap reconstruction described shortly. Having problems with the implant suggests the likelihood of having more problems later on. Even without any problems, implant manufacturers recommend replacing the implants every ten to fifteen years.

The U.S. Food and Drug Administration (FDA) recommends that women with silicone implants be screened for leaks every two years.

Patients need to weigh the comparative ease of the implant surgery against the inconvenience and emotional consequences of possible later surgeries.

To ensure that women are aware of the possible dangers of implants, the FDA has required packaging to include information on the risks and limited duration of the devices. This was prompted by reports linking textured implants, and one brand in particular, to a rare cancer of the immune system called breast-implant-associated anaplastic large cell lymphoma (BIA-ALCL). It is characterized by persistent swelling and the presence of a mass or pain in the area of the implant.[27]

The FDA also mentions an implant-related syndrome called breast implant illness (BII), a cluster of nonspecific symptoms that include joint pain, skin and hair changes, poor concentration, and fatigue. In one of the few studies of patients who reported having BII, researchers found that symptoms did not arise with any particular kind of implant, but chronic infection was found in 36 percent of the fifty patients studied. After the removal of the implants, 84 percent of the patients reported that the symptoms had mostly resolved. Researchers noticed specific cellular changes near the implant in the patients with BII and concluded that the illness was worthy of further study.[28]

Flap Procedures

The breast mound can also be reconstructed using your own tissue. In the myocutaneous flap, a flap of skin, muscle, and fat is taken from another part of your body and moved. It's your own tissue, and because you've got extra skin, it can make a bigger breast and a more natural droop. You may feel more normal since it's real tissue, skin, and fat, though it has little sensation. These flaps can come from the abdomen (transverse rectus abdominis muscle, or TRAM flap), back (latissimus dorsi flap), or buttock (gluteus maximus flap).

There are two different techniques for the myocutaneous flap. One is the pedicle, or attached flap (Figure 13.17). Here the tissue is removed except for its feeding artery and vein, which remain attached, almost like a leash. The site from which the tissue was removed is sewn closed. The new little island of skin and muscle is then tunneled under the skin into the mastectomy wound. Since the blood vessels aren't cut, the blood supply remains.

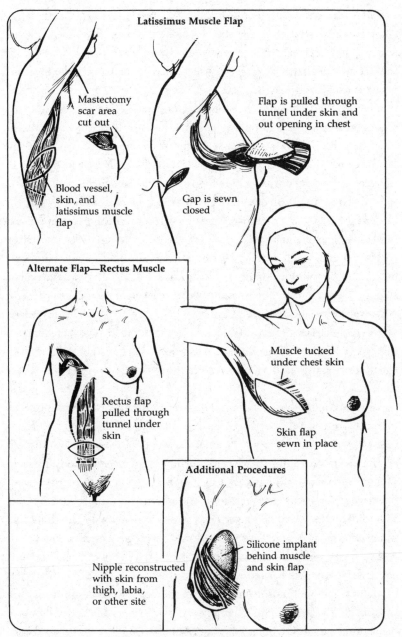

Figure 13.17

The other option is the *free flap*. In this procedure, the tissue is removed and the feeding artery and vein are cut. Then the tissue is moved to a new location and the artery and vein are sewn to an artery or vein in the chest or armpit; the surgeons use a microscope to help them reconnect the tiny blood vessels.

The pedicle flap can only be done from tissue close enough to reach to the breast and so is limited to the abdomen (TRAM) or back (latissimus). The free flap is less limited. The most common free flaps are from the abdomen, either based on the lower blood vessels that feed the skin (inferior epigastric) or from the blood vessels that pass through the muscle into the fat and skin (deep inferior epigastric perforator flap, or DIEP). Other free flaps include those from the infraumbilical area (superficial inferior epigastric artery flap, or SIEA), and the buttocks (SGAP or IGAP, depending on whether it's based on the superior gluteal artery perforator or the inferior one). This means you can have a flap reconstruction even if your abdomen has been scarred and take advantage of whatever abundance nature granted you (Figure 13.18). The advantage of the pedicle flap is that it's easier, so more plastic surgeons can do it. It still involves at least three procedures (reconstruction, nipple, and tattoo) and four if you need something done to the second breast to match.

To recap, a disadvantage is that we can use tissue only from locations that can stretch to the breast—the abdomen or the back. Another disadvantage is that in making the "tunnel" to the breast, we have to disturb all the tissue en route, so we're disturbing a lot of your body surface. This means that you'll have a lot of long-term complications that aren't serious but can be uncomfortable. If we take it from the abdomen, your abdominal muscle will no longer be as strong and you won't be able to do things like sit-ups as well as you used to. One of my patients now has to wear a panty girdle all the time to help support her weakened abdominal muscle. Another has found that since the operation, the area around her upper abdomen is so sensitive that she can't wear anything with a waistband. There is a 25 percent chance of getting a lifetime bulging of the abdomen as well from where the tissue flap was taken. I should add, however, that these problems are relatively unusual, and most patients who have had the procedure have had few problems but much satisfaction. If the tissue is taken from your back, there will be fewer problems, although the muscles may weaken somewhat. This may interfere with

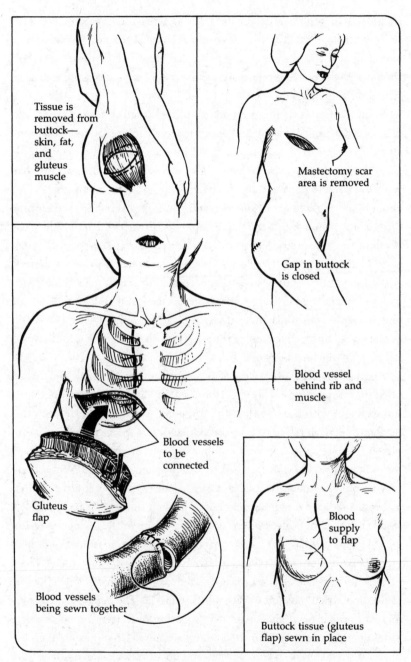

Tissue is removed from buttock—skin, fat, and gluteus muscle

Mastectomy scar area is removed

Gap in buttock is closed

Blood vessel behind rib and muscle

Blood vessels to be connected

Gluteus flap

Blood supply to flap

Blood vessels being sewn together

Buttock tissue (gluteus flap) sewn in place

Figure 13.18

shoulder strength for special sports like mountain climbing or competitive swimming. You also may need more physical therapy. Some women have a lot of stiffness and pain after this flap because it throws their whole shoulder girdle off. In either case, you'll have a long scar on the area from which the flap has been taken.

With the free flap, the surgeon has to be skilled at sewing blood vessels together under the microscope (Figure 13.19) or using a coupler (a staple-like apparatus to connect small blood vessels), and many plastic surgeons aren't. In expert hands, there are fewer complications than with the pedicle flaps because free flaps have a better blood supply. It's about five to eight hours of surgery, and you'll probably be in the hospital for four to seven days. If the blood supply is disturbed, part or all of the flap can die and further surgery will be necessary. The patient I mentioned earlier, who developed an infection from her silicone expanders, was unable to have either the latissimus (back) or rectus (abdominal) procedure because of medical problems in her back and abdomen. The free gluteus flap was the only alternative she had left. Although it was difficult surgery that involved a long healing period, she feels it was well worth the pain and inconvenience.

Another variation of the free flap was introduced by Dr. Robert Allen of New Orleans, the so-called perforator flap, or DIEP. Instead of taking some muscle with the free flap, the surgeon dissects out the arteries that perforate through the muscle to the skin and thus spares the muscle completely. If you have a sufficient number of perforating arteries to support the skin and fat, there is no need to take any muscle at all. While there may be obvious theoretical advantages in not taking any muscle, it does add some additional tedious dissection through the muscle and possibly a small risk of complications related to this portion of the dissection. Also, because one still has to dissect through the muscle, it is uncertain how much benefit there is in trying to save a small amount of muscle. Thus, in the end, it becomes a practical decision as to whether it's worthwhile to do the extra dissection to save a little muscle. The concept of the perforator flap has been very helpful in focusing our attention on the perforating arteries rather than the amount of muscle. As a result, there's a tendency to take less and less muscle and do a "muscle-sparing" free flap. When there are large perforators that make dissection fairly easy, then it is worthwhile to do a perforator flap. This approach usually requires four procedures—the mastectomy with immediate free flap followed by a

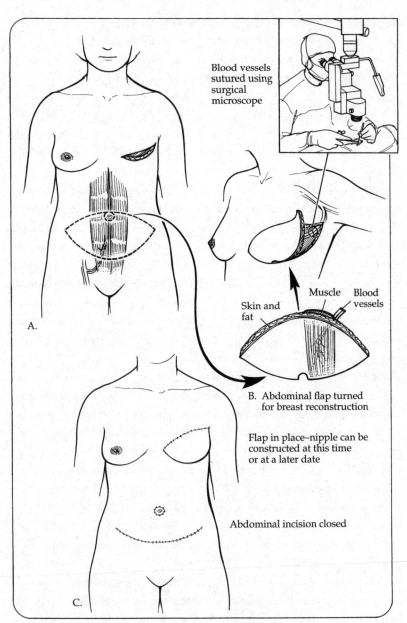

Blood vessels
sutured using
surgical
microscope

Skin and
fat

Muscle   Blood
vessels

A.

B. Abdominal flap turned
for breast reconstruction

Flap in place–nipple can be
constructed at this time
or at a later date

Abdominal incision closed

C.

Figure 13.19

nipple-sparing operation and then a tattoo of the areola. Finally, you may need to have something done to the other breast to match.

More recently the superior gluteal artery perforator flap (SGAP) and the inferior gluteal artery perforator flap (IGAP) have added to the options. Another procedure gaining some popularity is the transverse upper gracilis flap, or TUG flap. This flap takes one of the muscles in the inner thigh (gracilis) with tissue from the upper inner thigh. Sacrificing this muscle usually has no effect on leg function, and the flap can usually supply enough tissue for an A or B cup reconstruction.

As I noted earlier, both versions of the flap procedure require not only highly trained plastic surgeons but also specialized teams. You will want to find a center where they do this a lot and the whole staff is comfortable with the procedure and with its potential risks and complications. Researching and talking to people is important to find the right place. It may be necessary to travel to find the surgeon and team that can best fit your needs.

The advantage of reconstruction with your own tissue includes a softer, more natural-appearing breast mound that will gain weight when you gain and lose weight as you do. The disadvantages include the longer duration of anesthesia, greater blood loss, a longer recovery period, risk of losing part of the flap due to inadequate blood supply, and problems at the donor site. The risk of complications tends to be higher in older and more obese women as well as those with compromised vascular microcirculation, such as smokers or women with diabetes.

Free flap procedures have the advantage that less, if any, muscle is taken and so there are fewer problems at the donor site. They have better blood supply, although there is a small risk of the small blood vessel connections clotting, resulting in partial or complete flap loss. The disadvantages include the increased duration of surgery and the potential risk of clotting in the newly attached blood vessels.

After mastectomy and an immediate flap reconstruction, you come out of anesthesia feeling like a Mack truck just hit you. You've had hours of surgery on both your breast and your abdomen, back, or buttocks. You have continuous pain medication through an IV with a button you can press so that you can control the timing. You're kept in bed rest for one to two days, and you have a catheter so you don't have to go to the bathroom. By about the third or fourth day you start feeling a little better, and you can get out of bed and walk around a bit. You're usually in the hospital for about four to six days. There are drains placed in the abdominal incisions as well as in the chest. You may have pain deep in your chest, which can also feel numb, as well as your abdomen, or the other area the tissue has been taken from. So the double operation is certainly an ordeal. In addition, you'll need further operations for the nipple and the other breast. Sometimes after the operation there is a little too much tissue in one place or another, so the surgeon does some fine-tuning. It won't hurt because the area is now numb.

If a flap procedure is the operation you want, you should take the time to research and locate who in your area can do it. If there's no one in your area and you still want a particular form of reconstruction, you can always wait, have the mastectomy first, and then find the right plastic surgeon when your treatment is done.

Dr. Eric Halvorson is a plastic surgeon from Chapel Hill, North Carolina, who helped with this chapter. He says: "What I tell my patients is that implant reconstruction spreads the risk you take over your lifetime—there is less risk with the initial operation, but living with implants carries the risks of capsular contracture, rupture, infection, malposition, exposure. Tissue flap reconstruction puts all the risk up front—the surgery and recovery are longer, with risks of flap failure, wound healing complications, donor site complications, and so on—but once everything is healed they will rarely have other problems. Also, implant reconstructions tend to look worse with time, whereas tissue flap reconstructions tend to look better with time."

Making a Decision

To decide what's best for you, you should discuss it with your surgeon and, separately, with a plastic surgeon. Make sure you have thought about your goals for reconstruction and share them with both: Do you want to be higher, lower, larger, smaller? Some people assume that their only option is to look the same, but modern techniques have given women the option to change the appearance of their breasts following mastectomy. Some women are even happier with their breasts after mastectomy. Your surgeon will look at you, see how your body hangs together and how your breasts look before your surgery, and tell you what kind of procedure they think would be best for you. Make sure you ask which procedures they are familiar with and perform regularly. Patients have come to me after being told they're not a candidate for a flap when in reality the plastic surgeon they saw just doesn't know how to do the operation. Get a second or even third opinion. Look at websites that discuss reconstruction. My former colleague Dr. Robert Goldwyn, who has done many reconstructions, points out something crucial: you should always be shown pictures of the best and the worst results your plastic surgeon has had. Some doctors will show only the best results—an act comparable to false advertising. It's important for you to know the limits of what the procedure can do for you and the risks you run of having far from ideal results.

You will also need to decide whether you want the reconstruction done immediately or at a later time. When reconstruction is done immediately, you'll have surgery only once. Also, if the surgeon performs a skin-sparing mastectomy, it is easier for the plastic surgeon to close the incision over the implant or flap. In my experience, though, many women don't have immediate reconstruction because they don't want to go through so much surgery at once. Immediate reconstruction involves a longer time in the operating room (usually about six to eight hours) and is harder to schedule. Wound-healing complications also tend to be higher with immediate reconstruction, although the cosmetic result can be better.

Once you have the new breast, you may want a nipple and areola if they were removed at the time of mastectomy. We don't do it right away because the surgeon needs to be sure it's in the right place. There's a lot of swelling after reconstructive surgery, so we need to wait till that goes down and the reconstructed breast has had time to "settle down" due to gravity. The nipple can be created using skin from the breast or flap, but it won't be the same color as your original nipple. It can be tattooed. The areola can be reconstructed with a skin graft or a tattoo.

Sometimes the skin from your inner thigh is used, as it is darker than breast skin. If the skin graft is not dark enough, it can also be tattooed. Some people opt for a 3D tattoo of the nipple and areola. The optical illusion it creates can do wonders for a woman's body image, even if it is only glimpsed out of the corner of the eye while emerging from the shower. Skin grafts tend to have more texture and are thus more realistic, but taking the skin graft will put one more scar on your body unless you take it from someplace where there is already a scar. Whether you want to bother with the nipple depends on why you want the reconstruction. If it's just for convenience to look symmetrical under clothes without having to bother with a prosthesis, you may decide against it. If you want the new breast to look as real as possible, you'll probably want the nipple. Again, it's your decision—you're the one who'll go through the surgery, and you're the one who'll live with the results. I've had a couple of patients who, before they had the nipple put on, showed their reconstruction to anyone who was curious—then once the nipple was on, they didn't want to show it. Somehow it felt more like a real breast, and displaying it seemed immodest.

The Unacceptable Reconstruction

Sometimes reconstruction isn't entirely successful despite the best efforts. It may not give you the look you want, or it may be a source of chronic pain or medical problems. It can cause unpleasant sensations ranging from pins and needles to burning to sharp pain. You may find it hard to adapt to the feel of an implant. An implant may seem solid, even rocklike to the touch. The breast's hardness isn't due to the saline implant but to the scar tissue that has formed around it, encasing it in a tough capsule. One woman described her implant reconstruction like "wearing an iron bra that [she] couldn't take off!"

Sometimes plastic surgeons may focus on crafting the "perfect breast," not on replicating the patient's natural breast. The result is often a breast that is, or feels, too big. Even when the breast with its implant is matched in size to the original breast, the new breast is often heavier because the implant and scar tissue weigh more than breast tissue. Also, the new nipple may be higher or lower than the nipple on the other breast.

Because surgeons see patients lying on an operating table, they see breasts from a different perspective than do the patients, who usually see themselves standing before a mirror or looking down at their breasts. As a result they may misjudge the way a breast will hang when the person is on their feet. If it is a good match for the other breast, which appears flatter when the person is lying on their back, it will probably look smaller when they stand up. Most plastic surgeons are aware of this and will sit you up in the operating room to make sure things look symmetrical.

You don't have to simply resign yourself to such problems. A plastic surgeon can surgically remove the hard scar tissue and replace the implants, exchange an implant for a tissue flap, reduce or enlarge a breast, or lift and reorient nipples. Technology is improving, and so are surgical techniques, as experience with the procedure—and the demand for it— grows. Get a referral to a plastic surgeon from a friend or your breast surgeon, explain your problem, and have the plastic surgeon outline a plan for correcting it. If possible, get a second opinion. Again, ask for pictures of the plastic surgeon's best and worst outcomes.

Occasionally, if the skin has been altered by radiation or is not elastic enough to make additional reconstructive surgery advisable, the best course may be to remove the implant and get a prosthesis instead.

Sometimes you can feel ambivalent about the outcome. One woman on Facebook found the first reconstruction okay and not the second. "In 1996 I had a tram transplant. I was very happy with the end result as it was my own body being used rather than a silicon implant. The second was in 2004. This time we used the latissimus flap. Different result. As it turned out, by the time they wrapped the muscle around my torso there was little left for the breast pocket. The solution was to add an implant. I came within two days of getting on the table when I realized that I had put myself through all of this to avoid an external object in my body and canceled the procedure. So now I look odd to a first time viewer but I'm comfortable in my own skin."

Some don't stop getting things fixed until they have it right. "I had both breasts reconstructed after BC . . . last change I made was to change implants & wanted silicone & try to get my real size back. Before OR asked doc to have 4 size options. Prior to anesthesia I sat up in OR & announced to all present that I wanted all 4 sizes tried out with the Doc sitting me up for all to see which suited me best. Had great ones put in & no bruising."

Today, a reasonably good breast reconstruction can be achieved after mastectomy by any of these techniques, using expanders and implants or your own tissue from the abdomen, buttocks, back, or thighs. Achieving symmetry between the nonmastectomy breast and the reconstructed breast, however, sometimes requires reshaping, reducing, or enlarging the normal breast. A large, droopy breast on the normal side can be reduced to match the reconstructed breast. If the breast volume is satisfactory, then the breast can be reshaped by "mastopexy" techniques to lift the nipple and reshape the breast. A normal breast that is too small may be augmented with an implant behind the muscle. This should be done cautiously because the implant-augmented breast tends to be firmer without the natural droop, thus presenting a potential problem for achieving symmetry if the reconstruction opposite is done with one's own tissue. Also, you should be careful about the potential problems in follow-up of this breast, as this side, unlike the mastectomy side, will still require regular breast exams and annual mammography.

PROSTHESES

Many women don't get reconstruction because they are very comfortable with a prosthesis. It isn't invasive and can be removed at will. A former patient of mine told me of her experience with a Beverly Hills surgeon "who tried to sell me a breast as if he was selling a car." When she said that at the moment all she was looking for was information, and she didn't yet know if she wanted reconstruction, he was appalled and demanded, "Why not?" She explained her reservations about getting additional surgery and said she had come to learn more and discuss the pros and cons of reconstruction. Then he sent her to an office where she was shown the before-and-after photo album.

"It felt like it was a showroom and they were selling. I didn't buy any of it and have been quite satisfied with my prostheses for the past sixteen years. Please remind women that they have choices and some (many?) of us are doing just fine 'au naturel' with prosthetics."

The option of wearing a prosthesis will probably be offered to you in the hospital after your surgery (unless you've had immediate reconstruction and obviously won't need one). In most areas of the United States the hospital arranges for someone to visit you to talk about prostheses while you're still there. Your visitor will be from the American Cancer Society's Reach to Recovery program or a firm that sells prostheses. You can get a temporary prosthesis first and then shop around for a permanent one. The prosthesis fits into a pocket in a postmastectomy bra (Figure 13.1). You can shop for them in person or online, from catalogs, in medical supply houses, or in fancy lingerie stores. Each supplier has its advantages and disadvantages. You may be put off by the implications of disability, the wheelchairs, and the artificial limbs in medical supply outlets. In a lingerie store you may feel painfully reminded of the breast you no longer have. Your doctor or the American Cancer Society can help you find the stores, catalogs, or websites to buy your prosthesis, or you can ask friends who've had mastectomies. Y-ME, a volunteer organization of breast cancer survivors, will send you a prosthesis if they have the size required in stock.

There are suppliers that will make a custom prosthesis for you; it's expensive and your insurance company may not pay for it, but you may want a precise match. (It's a good idea to check with your insurance company before buying your prosthesis anyway; different companies have different quirks, and you may want to be sure of what your own expenses will be.) Medicare pays for prosthesis every year or two—with a prescription. (Why you need a prescription for a prosthesis, I don't know—I've never met anybody who bought one for the fun of it. But the ways of bureaucracies are mysterious.) There are also specific forms for swimming, though most of the better prostheses are made of silicone and are waterproof.

Prostheses come in a range of prices and quality. If you don't have insurance to pay for one, or if you haven't decided between prosthesis or reconstruction, you'll probably want the least expensive form available, at least temporarily. Catalogs and many stores offer forms for as low as $20 and mastectomy bras for around $15.

Prostheses are made in different sizes and for different operations. If you had a radical mastectomy, you can get a fuller prosthesis. If you had a wide excision that's left you noticeably asymmetrical, you can get a small "filler," or shell that fits comfortably in your bra. In the past, prostheses didn't have nipples, which caused problems for women whose remaining breast had a prominent nipple (Betty Rollin in her book *First, You Cry* has a very funny description of her efforts to make her own "nipple" out of cloth buttons.) Fortunately any prosthesis you buy now has a nipple, and you can get a separate nipple to attach to it if your own nipple is more prominent than the one on the prosthesis. There are also groups like Knitted Knockers that make soft, comfortable prosthetics for free. Their website also features patterns if you want to knit your own or make one for a friend.

Some situations may affect what makes a prosthesis right for you. Certain kinds of disabilities, for example, can make a particular form uncomfortable. Judith Rogers, an activist in Breast Health Access for Women with Disabilities, has mild cerebral palsy, and she found that her first prosthesis caused problems. "It was good in terms of matching the size of my remaining breast," she says. "But it was bad for my shoulder: it was too heavy for me. It pulled down, harming my muscles and increasing the effects of lymphedema." When she got a lighter one, she had less pain. You need to take time to consider all the factors involving your body and mind when you choose a prosthesis.

GOING FLAT

Finally there is a third option, which a few people have embraced—not disguising the operation at all. If your lumpectomy doesn't create a dramatic lopsided look, you may decide just to ignore it. Even with the more noticeable change that comes with a larger lumpectomy or a mastectomy, some prefer doing nothing cosmetically. One of my patients early in my career thought about her options, then concluded that "a prosthesis sounded too uncomfortable, and reconstruction hasn't been around long enough to see what long-term effects it can have. And then I decided I was comfortable with the way I looked." She went to work dressed normally, jogged in a loose T-shirt, and felt that it was other people's problem if they were uncomfortable with it. Once in a while, she felt a need to look more "normal"—especially when she had important meetings with new business associates. Her solution was to stuff shoulder pads from her dresses into her bra.

For other people, refusing to create the illusion of a breast is part of their feminist beliefs. Artist Matuschka created photographs of herself in a cutaway gown, showing not her remaining breast but her mastectomy scar. One photograph was on the cover of the August 15, 1993, *New York Times Magazine*. The effect is of harshness and defiance, showing the world what breast cancer does to a woman's body. Writer Deena Metzger, whose book *Tree* addresses her cancer, includes a photograph with a different approach: she softens the effect of the amputation by covering her scar with a beautiful, evocative tattoo of a tree, creating a new beauty where the beauty of her breast once was.[29]

Some people feel too conspicuous in public without a prosthesis, but they still don't like how the form feels. In that case there is another possible alternative: you can have both breasts removed. Although this destroys a healthy breast, it does make it possible to wear loose shirts without self-consciousness. I had only one patient take this route, and she had to fight with her insurance company to get them to pay for the removal of the healthy breast. She told them that since they paid for re-construction for symmetry they should pay for a contralateral mastectomy for symmetry.

Having the self-confidence to feel comfortable without the appearance of a breast shows wonderful courage, but most of us are products of our culture and still need to feel cosmetically acceptable to the outside world. In some cases there are actual penalties for failing to appear "normal." If nonconformity will cost you your job, for example, you're likely to want to have reconstruction or wear a prosthesis at least part of the time.

Over the years businesses have emerged to cater to the fashion needs of breast cancer survivors. One example is Cancer Be Glammed, an on-line site with a range of items from hospital gowns to scarves. If your clothes no longer fit like they used to, use your search engine to see what's out there. You may be surprised.

As more people live and even thrive after a breast cancer diagnosis, more attention has been paid to the results of surgery. As with every-thing, what road you take is your choice. The good news is that there are now lots of options and you can make a choice at the time of your diagno-sis or years later. In a disease where you often feel out of control, this is one area where you can make the choice that works for you.

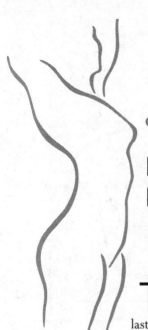

CHAPTER 14

Local Treatment: Radiation Therapy

The idea of radiation therapy may make you nervous. After all, radiation can cause cancer, and the last thing you want is to find yourself in danger of even more cancer. But, as you saw in Chapter 5, the doses given in radiation therapy rarely cause cancer and often cure it. As a form of local control (treatment of an original cancer), radiation is more effective in some forms of cancer than others. Luckily it's been very effective with breast cancer. It can also be used to treat metastatic disease, as I discuss at the end of the chapter.

Radiation is ordinarily used in conjunction with surgery, so you may have had a lumpectomy (or even a mastectomy) before your radiation. It works best when it has comparatively few cells to attack—it's least effective on large chunks of cancer. So we try, if possible, to do the surgery first, getting rid of most of the tumor before cleaning up what's left with radiation.

Radiation is generated by electricity in machines called linear accelerators. The edges of the beam from this type of machine are "sharper," sparing most of the adjacent tissue. Also, the treatment is planned more precisely, with newer planning machines called simulators. Further, it is aimed in tangents (at an angle) to the breast, so that it goes through the breast tissue of one breast and out into the air, with much less getting into the heart or lung (Figure 14.1). Even so, the radiation beam can still be scattered once it enters the body and can affect other spots. Some patients who were treated with radiation for Hodgkin lymphoma ten or fifteen years ago now have breast cancer (see

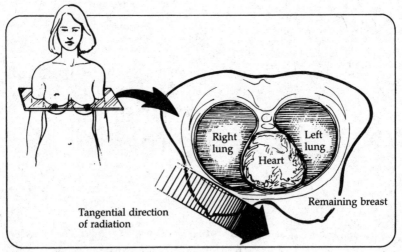

Figure 14.1

Chapter 5). Unfortunate as that may be, radiation therapy is important. If the Hodgkin had gone untreated, those people probably would have died long ago.

Like surgery, radiation is a localized treatment. (Chemotherapy, however, is given by injection or in a pill, and goes through your bloodstream and affects your entire body.) The radiation is aimed at a specific area and affects only that area. The linear accelerator, as you might guess from its name, accelerates charged particles and shoots them at a target that generates photons (forms of electromagnetic radiation). These photons are aimed directly at the body part they're intended for, as a beam. The beam is sharpened in the head of the machine to minimize scatter and aimed at the area where cancer cells are suspected. More recent data, however, suggest that low-dose radiation may also have an immune-enhancing effect, and studies are ongoing to figure out how it works and how to maximize its utility in this regard.

As I explained previously, primary radiation complements lumpectomy as an alternative to mastectomy and may also be used with mastectomy. In the past twenty or twenty-five years, as adjuvant chemotherapy and hormone treatment have improved survival, the role of radiation in reducing the risk of recurrence is even more important. This has also fueled the current trend to do more postmastectomy radiation in certain groups of patients—those most at risk for local recurrence in the scar after mastectomy, such as the ones with positive nodes, inflammatory breast cancer, or large tumors. (See Chapter 11.)

INITIAL CONSULTATION

In every phase of your treatment it is important that you have a team of doctors who are comfortable working together to coordinate your care. Radiation oncologists (who are always medical doctors, MD or DO) like to see patients soon after the biopsy—ideally while they still have the lump—to get a firsthand sense of the tumor. Sometimes the initial consultation is held in the radiation therapy department. The doctor will want to discuss the usual side effects of the treatment and explain plans involving a team approach. The consultation also involves a physical exam.

This first visit doesn't mean you'll necessarily have radiation treatment. The radiation oncologist will talk with you and get your medical history, do an examination, review the breast imaging and slides from your biopsy, and talk with your primary doctor, your surgeon, and, if you have one, your medical oncologist. They will then come up with one or more recommendations. Make sure you are offered options. Ask what your risk of local recurrence is with and without radiation therapy. Ask about different techniques like whole-breast irradiation (WBI) versus accelerated whole-breast irradiation (AWBI), accelerated partial-breast irradiation (APBI), and even intraoperative radiation therapy (IORT) (see Chapter 11) and why they are recommending a specific option. These are not just idle questions as the timing of each approach is quite different. IORT is given while you are on the operating table, so it is the quickest if you are a good candidate. Partial-breast radiation most commonly requires the placement of a catheter or a balloon into the lumpectomy cavity at surgery so that the treatment can be delivered directly to the tumor bed (also known as brachytherapy) twice a day for five days. This can also be done with external-beam radiation therapy but is less often used. The whole-breast option takes six weeks, whereas the accelerated whole-breast approach takes only three to four weeks. These can be decided post-surgery, but it is important to know about the differences in duration.

Also ask how they are going to integrate radiation into your whole treatment plan. Cancer centers usually have multidisciplinary teams who follow recommendations for an integrated treatment plan of surgery, radiation, and systemic therapy. But if you are outside an integrated cancer center, you may have to make sure that all your team is on the same page. Don't be afraid to ask the doctors to talk to one another!

There are other issues that affect the decision to use or not use radiation. First, if you have very large breasts, the available equipment may or may not be able to accommodate them. You may need to find a center that has the correct equipment. Breast size should not be a criterion for excluding radiation.

Second, a bit of the lung and heart (if the tumor is on the left) gets radiated, which can be dangerous if you have chronic lung disease. So with patients who have conditions like chronic obstructive pulmonary disease, chronic asthma or emphysema, and/or risk for cardiac disease, we always have a planning session just to do the measurements. These involve studying how much lung and heart will be affected and how best to minimize any damage. Previous radiation to the chest used to be considered a contraindication to breast radiation; however, there are modern radiation therapy options (such as brachytherapy, proton beam radiation therapy, and intensity-modulated radiation therapy) that may be possible, so make sure you ask. The radiation oncologist should carefully review your previous treatment records to assess whether breast radiation is safe and what approach will be best for you.

THE PLANNING SESSION

If the choice of whole-breast radiation (accelerated or not) is appropriate for you, you'll be sent for a planning session and whatever X-rays are needed. This usually takes place about two to four weeks after surgery (or after chemotherapy, if this was part of your treatment), if any surgery has been done, to make sure everything's healed and you can get your arm over your head comfortably.

A planning session is also called a simulation—sort of a dry run—and takes about an hour. It can be technical and impersonal, unlike your earlier conversation with the radiation oncologist. The goal is to set up—or simulate—the exact position you will be in during your treatment and program this into the computer that delivers the radiation. You put on a hospital gown and lie on a table with your arm lifted and resting on an immobilization device above your head. During your daily treatments this immobilization device is used to make sure that your arm is in the same position each day, ensuring precise radiation treatment. Although we used to use a machine similar to an X-ray machine, called a simulator (see Figure 14.2), most radiation oncology facilities now use CT scan–based simulators for radiation planning, so much more anatomical information is available. In some cases a mold is made for you to hold your arm so that you'll be in the same position every day of your treatment. People with very large breasts are sometimes treated lying on their stomachs or in a special device called a prone breast board.

The CT simulator collects images of your anatomy in the same position you'll keep for treatments. Radiographic information is taken to map where your ribs are in relation to your breast tissue, where your heart is in relation to your ribs, and so on, figuring out precisely how that area of your body looks. Depending on what area of your body is going to be radiated, you may also be sent for other radiographical studies (X-rays, CT scans, PET/CT scan, MRI, bone scan, ultrasound, and so on) to get more information. Then they'll put all the information into a

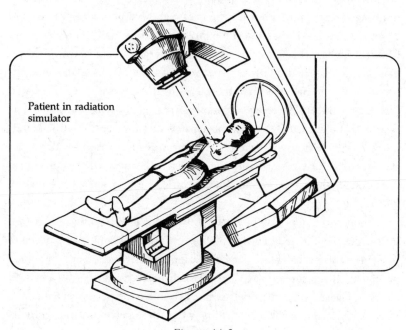

Patient in radiation simulator

Figure 14.2

computer that calculates the angles at which the area of your body should be radiated. This also helps protect your heart and lungs.

Patients often worry about other organs in radiation planning. Remember that most statistics on the risk of damage to the heart and lungs were collected several decades ago when techniques were less sophisticated and literal blocks were used to shoot radiation through the body. Now, as our medical advisor Dr. Stephanie Graff puts it, radiation oncologists "paint by number." They take a complex picture of the tumor with a CT, PET, or MRI and color it yellow in the system. Then they paint other key things they do *not want to radiate* other colors, like the heart red or the lungs blue. A computer calculates the right dose to the yellow cancer zone and also the amount of radiation that may accidentally hit the wrong areas (blue lung or red heart). If this last bit is above the safety limit, they can use the computer to bend and shape the beam in ways to keep the organs safe. The radiation settings for each particular patient are computed together with a physicist and dosimetrist—a whole team behind the scenes protecting your healthy tissue by "painting by number."

Before the planning starts, the radiation oncologist or therapist marks out the area of the body that's going to be treated. In most cases, it is only the breast. Sometimes it's the breast and lymph nodes. You should be aware that the breast and the lymph node areas will be treated from different angles, thus covering a fairly large area of your chest. Most radiation oncologists use tattoos—permanent little blue or black dots (approximately the size of a small freckle)—to mark the area to be radiated (see Figure 14.3). There are a couple of reasons for the markings. The first is to be sure that during the treatment they use the same "landmarks" and position you exactly the same way. The second is to ensure that in the future any radiation oncologist will know where you've had radiation in that area, because often you can have it only once on any given spot.

Although the dots may be unattractive, they're not going to turn you into Lydia the Tattooed Lady. They're tiny and, depending on your skin coloring, can be invisible. One radiation nurse I know says, "I've had patients call me up and say, 'I've washed my tattoos off—I can't find them!'" These days some doctors use henna ink or permanent markers like Sharpies; the problem with this is that the markings can eventually wash off, and you won't have this guidance for the doctors in the future.

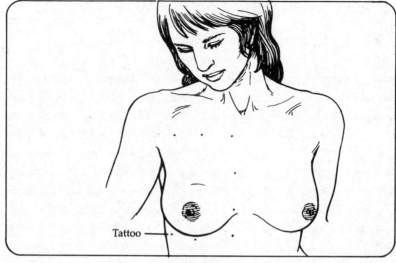

Figure 14.3

Some doctors have also started offering the option of using fluorescent tattoo ink, which may be slightly visible in regular light but is easy to see with a black light.

The tattooing can be somewhat uncomfortable, like pinpricks or bee stings at worst. The other discomfort patients sometimes feel from the planning and tattooing procedure is a stiff arm; especially after recent surgery, it can be awkward to lie with your arm above your head for ten to twenty minutes. Because of this, you may want to practice raising your arm above your head at home beforehand. If you can't get your arm above your head, learning and practicing some shoulder stretching exercises may be recommended so that you can achieve the range of motion you need to get into the proper arm position for your treatments.

Another useful thing to do before the actual treatments start is to visit the area ahead of time where they will take place. This will take the mystery out of the machine, which can look awfully intimidating when you're not familiar with it. Finally, you will set up your appointments with the radiation oncologist. During the treatment you will see your radiation oncologist and/or nurse only weekly, but your radiation therapist or technologist daily. If you have questions or problems, don't be afraid to ask to see or speak to your nurse or radiation oncologist, even if it is not your scheduled weekly appointment day with them.

THE TREATMENTS

Postlumpectomy Radiation

Radiation treatments are scheduled to be spaced out, once or twice per day with Accelerated Partial-Breast Irradiation (APBI), for a given number of weeks. There is always a balance between killing as many of the cancer cells as possible and avoiding as much injury to the normal tissue as we can. The treatment schedule varies from place to place. Usually it's given in two parts. First, the breast as a whole is radiated, from the collarbone to the ribs and the breastbone to the side, making sure the entire area is treated, including, if necessary, lymph nodes. This is the major part of the treatment and lasts about five weeks, often using about 4,500 to 5,000 rads—also known as centigrays—of radiation (a chest X-ray is a fraction of a rad). If there are any microscopic cancer cells in the breast, this should get rid of them. After this, the "boost" (described later) is given. As mentioned in Chapter 11, the value of whole-breast radiation therapy for early-stage breast cancer has been questioned. A long-term Italian study showed that APBI is equally effective but with better cosmetic results and less toxicity.[1]

How soon after the planning session (simulation) the treatment begins varies from hospital to hospital, depending on how many radiation patients there are, how much room there is in the radiation department, and how large the staff is. Typically, the time from simulation to treatment takes from less than one week to two weeks. Sometimes the patient waits two weeks to a month. This may cause the patient to worry that the delay will allow the cancer to spread. It won't in that amount of time, but waiting can be emotionally hard.

Radiation may be delayed for other reasons too. Depending on the status of the lymph nodes, you may get chemotherapy right away, and your doctors may not want you to get them both at the same time. With some drugs, like Adriamycin (doxorubicin), Cytoxan (cyclophosphamide), and Taxol (paclitaxel), you usually have the chemo first and then the radiation.

There are important skin-care guidelines to follow during your treatment. You should use a mild unscented soap, such as Dove, Pears, or Neutrogena. During the course of your treatment don't use soaps with scents or fragrance, deodorants, or any kind of metal. All these can interact with the radiation, and it's important that you avoid them. Don't use antiperspirants on the side receiving treatment; almost all antiperspirants contain lots of aluminum. (You can use one of the "natural" ones, such as Tom's, that have no aluminum and often come unscented. If you do this, read the label very carefully. Not all "natural" products are the same.) Through the course of the treatment, you can also use a light dusting of cornstarch as an antiperspirant; it's generally pretty effective but varies from person to person.

When you go for your first treatment, you may want to bring someone with you for support. You're facing the unknown, and that's scary. Most patients don't need anyone after the first session. On a more practical level, if you've come by car, make sure to request parking accommodations, which most institutions will help you with.

For the treatment itself, you'll change into a hospital gown from the waist up. It's wise to wear something two-piece so you only have to remove your upper clothing. You can wear earrings or bracelets during the treatment, but no neck jewelry. After you've changed, you'll be taken into a waiting room; the wait may be longish and varies from place to place and day to day, so you may want to bring a good book or your music player, or download movies to your tablet. Then you're taken into the treatment room. You're there for ten to twenty minutes, and most of that time is spent with the technologist setting up the machine and getting you ready. There's a table that looks like a regular examining table, and above it is the radiation machine (Figure 14.4). Just as with your planning session, you lie down on the table, on an immobilization device similar to the one you used during your simulation. After you're set up, the technician will position you, leave, and turn on the machine for a little less than a minute. The radiation isn't given all at once but is done a number of times from different angles—twice if only the breast is radiated, more if lymph nodes are also being treated. The technician will then come back in, reposition the machine, and go out again. If you're claustrophobic, you may find lying under the machine a little uncomfortable, but it is open, not like an MRI, and doesn't last long, and the machine never moves toward you.

Radiation therapy units have cameras, so they can see you while you're being treated, and an intercom system so that if you're anxious and need to talk with the technologist, you can. If a friend or family member has come with you, many hospitals allow that person to sit in the room outside the treatment area, watching on the monitor and hearing you

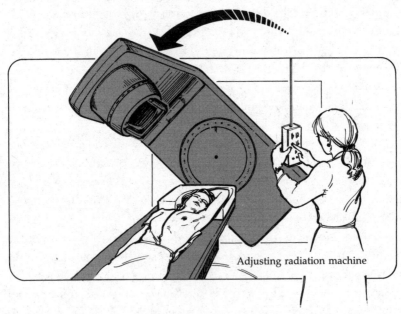

Adjusting radiation machine

Figure 14.4

through the intercom. If your children are old enough to be curious or are scared of not knowing what's going on, you may permit them to wait outside the treatment room so they can communicate with you if the hospital allows. This can demystify the process and alleviate their fears.

The most important thing for you to do during the treatment is to keep still. You can breathe normally, but don't move otherwise. Just close your eyes and think of your favorite place. It will be over before you know it.

Your blood may be drawn during the course of treatment—once at the beginning of the therapy process or maybe once a few weeks later, to make sure there's no drop in your blood count. This is rarely a problem with breast cancer, as there's not much bone marrow treated, but some doctors will check, especially in patients who have had chemotherapy.

What most people find hardest to deal with is the length of treatment—approximately one to seven weeks (depending on the details of the treatment), five days a week. If your workplace and home are near the hospital, you may be able to come in before or after work. Otherwise, you may have to cut into the middle of the workday or take time off from your job. Some parents use babysitters; others bring their children to the hospital along with a friend who stays with them while the parent has their treatment.

The Boost

After a course of radiation to treat your breast, you may be given a boost—extra radiation to the spot where the tumor was. This is delivered by the same radiation machine, but instead of X-rays, it uses an electron beam, in contrast to the rest of the treatment, which delivered photons. Electrons are a special kind of charged particle; they give off energy that doesn't penetrate very deeply, so most of the dose is deposited shallowly in the breast or skin. It's good if the original tumor wasn't very deep. It doesn't require hospitalization. There is some controversy regarding the need for a boost. It was added in the days when we did not demand clean margins from surgery. With the current practice of removing more breast tissue, the boost may not be as important, but it still seems to add a small degree of local control.

Cardiac-Sparing Techniques

Your radiation oncologist may use some modern radiation techniques to reduce the dose to your heart if you are receiving left-sided radiation. These can include using intensity-modulated radiation therapy (IMRT), heart blocks (placed in the tangent fields), prone positioning (laying you on your stomach so that the breast falls away from the chest), or deep-inspiration breath holding (where you take a deep breath and hold it for ten to twenty seconds to keep your chest wall expanded away from your heart). Another breathing technique is respiratory gating, where a device monitors your breathing so it can adjust the radiation beam as needed. All these options are available, and you and your care team will decide which is the most appropriate for you.

Partial-Breast Radiation

As mentioned in Chapter 11, there is increasing interest in confining radiation after lumpectomy to the area of the tumor bed alone. Several different techniques are being studied, all of which attempt to get the same local control in less time. In general, these new techniques reduce the six weeks to four or five days.

The most commonly used form of partial-breast radiation in the United States is catheter-delivered intracavitary brachytherapy. It takes advantage of the fact that after a tumor is removed there is a cavity left behind in the breast that fills up with fluid as the area slowly heals. Because the place where tumor cells are most likely to be left behind will be the lining of that cavity, it makes sense to use the cavity to deliver the radiation.

In this situation, a balloon or catheter can be placed into the biopsy cavity in the operating room, or a week or two after surgery, when the doctors know the margins are clear. A small incision is made under local anesthesia and a catheter device is inserted into the cavity (see Figure 11.2, page 247). The catheter position is examined with the CT scan simulator in the radiation oncologist's office. If all looks well, the radiation oncologist calculates the appropriate dose for the catheter to deliver. The treatments themselves consist of hooking the protruding catheter to a computerized delivery device (called an afterloader) that sends a tiny radioactive pellet into the device. Each treatment typically takes less than ten minutes. This is done twice a day, six hours apart, for five days. At the end of each treatment, the radioactive pellet automatically retracts back into the afterloader, the catheter device is detached from the afterloader, and you are free to go about your business. You are not radioactive. You will not feel the radiation, and the catheter device usually doesn't hurt. Some patients will feel soreness, sensitivity, or pressure, but there should be no pain. The catheter is flexible, so it folds neatly under your clothing.

After the final treatment, the radiation oncologist or surgeon removes the catheter device by collapsing it and slipping it out of the breast. This can hurt a little bit, so patients with low pain thresholds may want to take a pain pill an hour before removing the device.

At present, there are several radiation delivery devices on the market, each with its own benefit. The first one that is still used is the single-lumen MammoSite. This works well unless your tumor is too close to the skin. This happens about 10 percent of the time.[2] The newer, multilumen catheters allow better shaping of the radiation dose so that the skin and chest wall doses can be kept lower when needed. These include the multilumen MammoSite, SAVI, and Contura catheters. The single-lumen Xoft catheter device uses low-energy, short-range X-rays so it does not require shielding. The potential delayed risks (occurring months to years after treatment) with using any of these APBI catheter devices can include thick scars that you can feel in your breast, prominent blood vessel changes in your skin, and fluid or blood filling the cavity. The potential acute side effects (occurring within days to weeks during or after treatment) may include radiation dermatitis (redness of the skin), infection, or bleeding. Most of the time, these acute effects can be prevented by making sure there is adequate clearance of the catheter device from the skin and taking prophylactic antibiotics. We are still in the early days of this approach, and I have no doubt that there will be other variations over the next several years. If you are interested in using this approach, the key is to find an experienced treatment team and go with the device they are most comfortable with using.

Rarely used these days due to the relative simplicity of placing the APBI catheter devices just mentioned, some centers may employ another form of partial-breast radiation called interstitial brachytherapy. It's been around for a while—we used to use it as a boost before the days of the electron beam. Now it has a more primary role. The tubes can be placed while you're in the operating room or as an outpatient process (see Figure 14.5). Thin plastic tubing is hooked like thread into a needle and drawn through a spot on the breast where the biopsy was done. Then the tubing is left in and the needle withdrawn. The number of tubes varies, and they are often inserted in two or more layers. Small radioactive pellets called iridium seeds, which give off high energy for a very short distance, are put into the tubes, treating the immediate area of the biopsy. This implant is left in for thirty-six to forty-eight hours; the time varies depending on how active the seeds are, how big your breast is, and how big the tumor was. Long-term results from this approach have been comparable to those achieved with external-beam radiation therapy.[3] Although this low-dose rate (LDR) approach allows the radiation dose to be given more precisely where it is needed, it is also the most technically difficult way to do partial-breast irradiation and so is used less often.

Because the balloon approach requires special equipment to deliver the radiation and the brachytherapy approach is difficult to get right, there was pressure to develop an approach that uses linear accelerators that are already in place to deliver radiation therapy to just the involved area. This third approach uses external-beam radiotherapy from a linear accelerator and is called conformal or intensity-modulated partial-breast irradiation. This treatment also lasts four or five days.[4]

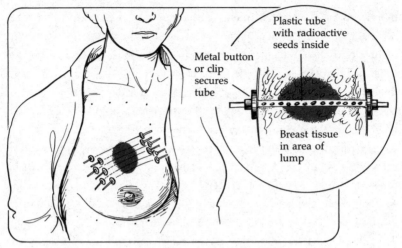

Plastic tube
with radioactive
seeds inside

Metal button
or clip
secures
tube

Breast tissue
in area of
lump

Figure 14.5

Early data using this technique has demonstrated that the cosmetic outcomes (increased skin fibrosis, telangiectasias [spider veins], and so on) may be inferior to intracavitary brachytherapy APBI.

There is also the single-dose intraoperative approach favored in Europe and being used by some centers across the United States. A lumpectomy is done, and then a barrier is placed between the muscle and the breast tissue to protect the chest wall. A mobile linear accelerator made especially for the operating room is used to aim the radiation therapy directly into the bed of the tumor. In a single treatment the breast tissue receives twenty-one grays of radiation. A randomized European clinical trial concluded that intraoperative radiation therapy (IORT) has local control and cancer survival results similar to those of whole-breast therapy.[5] The major benefit of single-dose radiation is that you will not have any subsequent radiation therapy. It may be particularly good for older patients with small hormone-positive tumors. They can be finished after one procedure and not have to travel for treatment.

Postmastectomy Radiation

The procedures for postmastectomy radiation are much the same as those used with breast-conservation surgery. You will have a planning session, be given tattoos, and be treated in the department of radiation therapy.

It usually takes about five to six weeks. Depending on the clinical situation, it may include radiating the lymph nodes behind the breastbone and above the clavicle as well as any remaining ones under the arm. A boost to the scar may or may not be used, depending on the circumstances.

In the setting where a mastectomy is done with immediate reconstruction using an implant (most often, a saline expander), radiation therapy can often be safely used when needed. There is an increased risk of infections and tissue fibrosis when an implant is in place and radiated, but these risks have not been found significant enough to preclude radiation when it is indicated. The plastic surgeon, breast surgeon, and radiation oncologist will need to communicate with one another if this is intended.

SIDE EFFECTS OF RADIATION

As I was writing this I asked my Facebook friends what they wished they had known about radiation therapy and what I should tell you. The consensus was that the whole thing is an exercise in being powerless and scared! The initial planning and mapping seemed to be the hardest as it takes the longest and you don't know what to expect.

That being said, the actual radiation treatments (most had the traditional radiation) were pretty quick. Many felt that chemotherapy was worse, but one respondent found the radiation experience more difficult emotionally because it was so isolating and daunting. Another woman said that she had a great team in radiation therapy that made it all easy, but she still had to ask for advice about skin care. And everyone mentioned fatigue! (See the following discussion.)

The side effects of radiation depend on the part of the body being treated. Your radiation oncologist will tell you about possible side effects before your treatment starts. It's a good idea to ask to talk to someone who has already been treated.

You'll probably have a mild sunburn effect (called *radiation dermatitis*). The severity varies considerably from patient to patient—one person gets a severe skin rash while another is hardly bothered at all. There may or may not be a correlation with skin color and your reaction to the radiation. My Facebook crowd mentioned Aquaphor, aloe, vitamin E, and essential oils as helpful. Calendula cream, made from a natural extract from the marigold flower, has also been shown to be effective in reducing the skin reaction when used during radiation therapy.

The other major symptom virtually every radiation therapy patient experiences is tiredness. I used to attribute this to the length of treatment, but there's more and more evidence that, like anesthesia (see Chapter 13), radiation itself creates fatigue. The body seems to exhaust its resources coping with the radiation and doesn't have much energy for anything else. This is believed to be caused by inflammatory proteins released by the radiated skin that circulate around the body. This tiredness usually gets worse toward the end of the treatment, and its severity depends on what else is going on in your life. Research suggests that the best way to combat this fatigue is with physical activity (such as walking). It seems that physical activity helps to fight off the effects of the inflammatory proteins that make you tired. That said, you don't want to push yourself too hard, and you don't want to do any activities that create friction on the radiated skin. The fatigue may last several weeks to months after the treatment has finished, but most patients will return to their pretreatment baseline.

The extent of the fatigue varies greatly. One of my patients, a lawyer, had no problem working a full day but said she "didn't feel like going out for dinner after work." A Facebook friend didn't even have that much trouble, saying it was "no big deal; I had the radiation over my lunch hour."

For others, fatigue is a bigger problem. One patient compared hers to the effects of infectious hepatitis, which she'd had years before. "The symptoms sound very nondescript," she says. "But I felt really rotten. I was tired all the time—not the tiredness you feel after a hard day's work, which I've always found fairly pleasant. My body just felt wrong—like I was always coming down with the flu. Some days I couldn't function at all—I had to keep a cot at my job." She also experienced peculiar appetite changes. "My body kept craving lemon, spinach, and roast beef—I ate them constantly, and I couldn't make myself eat anything else."

When the breast is being radiated, it may swell and become more sensitive; if you sleep on your stomach, you may feel uncomfortable. As I explained in Chapter 13, one trick is to hold a pillow between your breasts and sleep on the side that hasn't been treated. This sensitivity, like the other side effects, can take months to disappear, and you may find that breast especially sore or sensitive when you're premenstrual. When the treatments are over, the tenderness and soreness in your breast will gradually go away. Some continue to experience sharp, shooting pains from time to time—how often varies greatly from person to person.

Few of my patients would get depressed during radiation, but many got depressed afterward—possibly because, time-consuming as the treatments are, there is a sense of activity, of doing something to fight the cancer. Once treatment ends, there's a sense of letdown. This really isn't surprising. It occurs in other intense situations, like the classical postpartum depression, or the feelings that occur when any time-consuming structure in your life is over—a job you've worked at, the end of a school term, and so on. This may be the time to get involved in a support group if you haven't already done so. You'll have a little more time as you're not going to the treatments, and the company of others who know how you're feeling may help you get through these emotions.

Often the skin feels a little thicker right after radiation, and sometimes it's darker colored. That will gradually resolve itself over time. The nipple may get crusty, but that too will go away as the skin regenerates. This can take up to six months, and in the meantime you'll look like you've been out sunbathing with one breast exposed.

If you have received a lot of radiation to the lymph node areas, it will compound whatever scarring the surgery caused, and the combination can also increase your risk of lymphedema (see Chapter 18). A rare side effect of radiation to the lymph nodes is problems with the nerves that go from the arm to the hand, causing numbness to the fingertips (called neuropathy).

Aside from skin reactions and tiredness, there can be later side effects. Some women get costochondritis, a kind of arthritis that causes inflammation of the space between the breasts where the ribs and breastbone connect (Figure 14.6). The pain can be scary—you wonder if your cancer has spread. It's easy to reassure yourself, though. Push your fingers down right at that junction; if it hurts, it's costochondritis and can be treated with aspirin and antiarthritis medicines. It will go away in a few weeks. Another side effect can occur between three and six months after you've finished your treatment. The muscle that goes above and behind your breast, the pectoralis major muscle, will get extremely sore, and it's worse if you grab it between your fingers. That's because the radiation causes inflammation of the muscle, and as it begins to regenerate, it can get sore and stiff, just as it would if you threw it out during strenuous

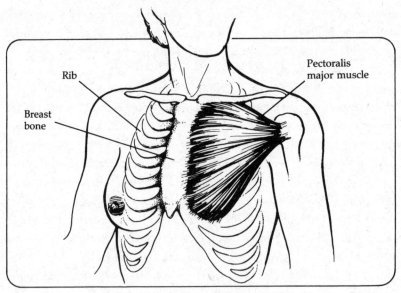

Figure 14.6

exercise. Most people think it's the cancer spreading—especially since the radiation has been over for months and they're not expecting new side effects from it.

If your cancer was in your left breast, there is also a possibility of cardiac side effects from radiation near your heart. This used to happen more often in the past when doses were higher and less precise, but today many procedures are in place to protect the heart as much as possible.

Those who receive radiation to the breast and have soft bones may develop asymptomatic rib fractures years after treatment: you don't feel them but they show up on X-ray. Depending on how your chest is built, a little of the radiation may get to your lung and give you a cough (called *pneumonitis*).

Frequently patients worry that being radioactive can cause them to inadvertently harm other people. They ask, "Can I hug my grandchild? Can I pick up my kids?" Once you leave the treatment room, you can be close to anyone (the LDR implants described earlier are an exception). It's like lying in the sun—once you're out of it, the effects remain, but the sunlight isn't inside you and can't be transmitted to anyone else.

Rarely, radiation can cause second cancers. This is usually a different kind of cancer, a sarcoma, and doesn't occur for at least five years after radiation therapy. Our best guess is that for every one thousand five-year survivors of wide excision and radiation, about two will develop a radiation-induced sarcoma (a cancer of the muscle, bone, or cartilage in the radiated area) over the next ten years.[6]

After your treatment is completed, your radiation oncologist may continue to see you, as will your surgeon. In addition to making certain there are no new tumors, the radiation oncologist is watching for complications from the radiation, and the surgeon is looking for surgical complications. These complications are rare, and radiation remains one of our most valuable tools in the treatment of local breast cancer.

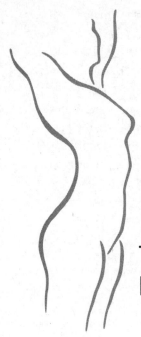

CHAPTER 15

Systemic Therapy: Chemotherapy, Hormones, Targeted Therapies, and Immunotherapy

The hallmark of systemic therapies is their ability to affect the whole body, not just one area. The systemic treatments used for breast cancer include chemotherapy, hormone therapy, targeted therapy, and immunotherapy.

When systemic therapy is given at the time of diagnosis, it is termed "adjuvant therapy" because it started out as an addition to the primary treatment, surgery. If it is given prior to surgery to shrink a tumor it is called "neoadjuvant therapy" (because it's still of secondary importance to the surgery, but it's "added" before the primary treatment is used). If it is given to treat known metastatic disease, it is just called "systemic therapy," since at this stage it is indeed the most important therapy. That being said, the way it is given and the side effects don't change based on when or why you get it. So this discussion covers all three of its applications.

Those of you who have read Chapter 11 about the decisions needed after diagnosis know that often these systemic treatments are combined. You may get chemotherapy and targeted therapy, or hormone therapy, or just one of those. We will probably learn a lot more about each pairing's successes and side effects down the road. Although these treatments are usually given in combination, I will tackle them individually so you can get a better understanding of what they entail.

Chemotherapy has had a lot of bad press, and now that I've experienced it myself, I understand why. Still, it's one of the most powerful weapons against cancer that we have. *Chemotherapy* literally means the use of chemicals to treat disease. As we colloquially use it, however, it usually refers only to the use of chemicals as opposed to hormonal therapy, targeted therapies, or immunotherapy.

How does chemotherapy work? Cells go through several steps in the process of cell division, or reproduction. Chemotherapy drugs interfere with this process so that the cells can't divide and consequently die. Different drugs are used in this process at different points, and often more than one kind of drug is used at a time (Figure 15.1). Unfortunately, this effect on cell division acts on all cells that are rapidly dividing—not just cancer cells but also hair, the lining of the GI tract, and, more importantly, bone marrow cells. Bone marrow produces red blood cells, white blood cells, and platelets continuously (Figure 15.2). This is one of the reasons chemotherapy is given in cycles, with a time lapse between treatments to allow the bone marrow to recover.

Another reason the drugs are given in cycles is that not all the cancer cells are dividing at any one time. The first treatment kills one group of cells; three weeks later a new set of cancer cells is starting to divide, and the drugs knock them out too (Figure 15.3). The idea is to decrease the total cancer cells to a number small enough for your immune system to take care of, without wiping out the immune system while we're at it. When we first started giving adjuvant chemotherapy after breast surgery, we gave the treatments over a two-year period. Later studies showed that six months was as good as a year, which was as

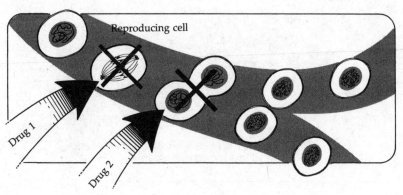

Figure 15.1

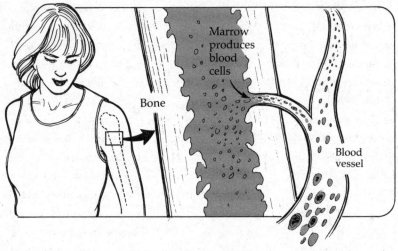

Figure 15.2

good as two.[1] The extra treatment may have actually harmed the immune system without having any additional effect on the cancer. There probably is a certain key dosage or duration beyond which an additional drug is useless, but what it is hasn't been determined yet.

Another kind of systemic therapy is the use of hormones or hormonal manipulations to change the body's own hormonal environment in order to affect the growth of hormonally sensitive tumors. This can include surgical procedures such as oophorectomy (removing the ovaries), radiating the ovaries, using drugs that block hormones, or even using hormones themselves. We don't fully understand all the reasons these

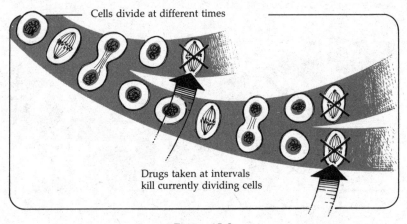

Figure 15.3

hormone treatments work, but there is no question that they do work well in certain patients. Because hormone therapy affects only hormonally sensitive tissues, its side effects are more limited than those of chemotherapy. It doesn't damage other growing cells, such as hair, the lining of the GI tract, and bone marrow. Hormone therapies can kill or control tumor cells by depriving them of the estrogen they require to grow. We prescribe them for five to ten years because hormone-receptive blood cells divide more slowly, so a long, slow exposure is needed to starve any remaining cells, which can hide for years. Without estrogen, some tumor cells will, in effect, commit suicide (apoptosis) while others will go to sleep, in a sort of coma at least for a while.

Certain systemic therapies are more targeted, such as Herceptin (trastuzumab) and Perjeta (pertuzumab), which are being used to treat cancers that overexpress HER2/neu (see Chapter 10), and Tykerb (lapatinib), which blocks tyrosine kinase, an enzyme involved in all the epidermal growth factors. Recently approved was Lynparza (olaparib), a PARP (poly [ADP-ribose] polymerase) inhibitor for BRCA-mutated early-stage HER2-negative breast cancer. Several more are in the pipeline, including others that target epidermal growth factor (EGF; see Chapter 11).

PRETREATMENT CONSULTATION

If you need systemic treatment, you'll meet with a medical oncologist who specializes in it. After talking with you at length and reviewing your records, the doctor will discuss with you the kind of cancer you have and the drugs they feel are appropriate for you and why (see Chapters 9 through 12). They will also tell you about any clinical trials that may be appropriate for you. (As I pointed out in Chapter 11, all our advances in this field have come because patients were willing to participate in clinical trials.) There are also general guidelines for breast cancer treatment, drawn up by a group of nationwide breast cancer specialists. Check the Internet for the latest recommendations (www .nccn.org has patient guidelines, as does the American Society of Clinical Oncology [ASCO]).

Your doctor or medical team will also discuss with you the role of systemic treatment in your overall treatment, the expected toxicity, and the projected management of side effects. Before you make a decision and sign a consent form, all these things must be very clear. (See Chapter 11 for how to pick a good doctor or team.)

Sometimes oncologists spend a lot of time explaining chemotherapy but relatively little time telling you about the side effects, risks, and complications of hormone therapy such as Nolvadex (tamoxifen). Make sure you understand exactly what drugs you are getting, how you will be getting them, what short- and long-term side effects you can expect, and what can be done to prevent or lessen these side effects (see Chapter 18). Also ask exactly how much benefit you can expect in your situation from these drugs—they may or may not be worth it to you. Finally, remember to record your visit or take notes, so that you don't have to worry about forgetting anything. Reach out to other members of your team. As a rule, the nurses, nurse practitioners, and social workers are more than willing to be of support. Don't be shy—the whole team is there for you and just waiting for you to ask for help.

In Chapter 11 I explained the decision-making process and options for adjuvant therapy at length. Now we look at the actual experience of receiving chemotherapy, hormone therapy, targeted therapy, and/or immunotherapy.

ADJUVANT CHEMOTHERAPY

Once you have decided with your doctor to receive adjuvant chemotherapy, you may need some preliminary tests to assess your heart and general health as well as tests for viruses such as hepatitis and HIV because chemotherapy suppresses your immune system, and occult infections (those for which you have no apparent symptoms) can become a problem. In addition, you may want to get a catheter device that will allow for intravenous administration of your medication. They come in a variety of types, including a peripherally inserted central catheter (PICC) line, which is inserted in the side of the body away from the chest, and a port-a-cath, which is placed or tunneled under the skin into a major blood vessel in the upper chest (Figure 15.4).

Needles can go in and out of the device and spare the patient the discomfort of having peripheral veins (the ones close to the surface, which are normally used for needles) stuck. The chest port results in fewer complications than the PICC line and is preferred for chemo, as it is

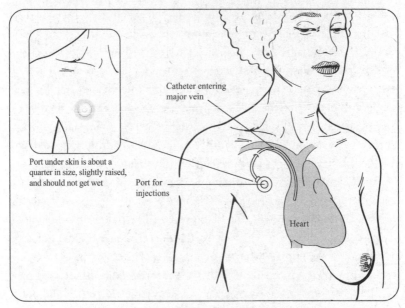

Catheter entering
major vein

Port under skin is about a
quarter in size, slightly raised,
and should not get wet   Port for
injections

Heart

Figure 15.4

much safer to administer centrally. When it's not in use you can treat the quarter-size device like any other part of your skin, and getting it wet is not a problem. It can remain in place until the end of chemo, when it is removed. Although patients like the fact that they don't have to get stuck with a new needle each treatment, having a port under your skin can feel a little strange. The other issue is that the device is a foreign body and on rare occasions can cause an infection. It also needs to be flushed occasionally with a blood thinner to prevent a clot. For most patients, the decision to use a port or not is reasonable either way, but it is essential for a patient who has trouble with their veins. Some chemotherapy can damage skin or soft tissues if an IV doesn't work well, so a port is preferred.

You will probably be evaluated for your level of stress and support systems, so assess how you are doing emotionally and marshal additional support if you need it.

During this preliminary period you also may want to see the chemotherapy room. It may be in a clinic, your doctor's office, or, rarely, a hospital and is usually set up for your comfort and the nurse's convenience. It can reduce your anticipatory fear to see the space where you will be treated, with people reading, writing, watching movies, or sleeping as they receive their drugs.

On the day of treatment you are usually checked in and weighed (at least the first time), and a blood sample is taken to check your blood count. These measurements help determine the dose of drugs you will receive and can serve as a baseline for comparison later. Your initial dose is determined in part by your body surface area (height and weight). This is a good (but not perfect) guess at what the optimally safe and effective dose of chemotherapy is for you. Nonetheless, when giving adjuvant chemotherapy, your oncologist should be reluctant to administer anything but the standard dosage. Dose reduction (lowering) should only be undertaken for severe, life-threatening toxicities, because it is the standard doses that have been shown to be effective.

After the first treatment, the blood test will help determine the bone marrow's recovery rate, which helps the doctor adjust the drug dosage or schedule. Sometimes when the count is too low, you have to wait a week before treatment to allow your bone marrow more time to recover. Think of the bone marrow as a factory churning out red blood cells, white blood cells, and platelets. Chemotherapy injures a portion of the factory's employees, and the factory doesn't work as well until they have recovered. Often you will receive drugs that help accelerate the recovery of the patient's bone marrow—keeping all the workers healthy so the factory can get back on track.

The major drug we have for this is GCSF (granulocyte colony-stimulating factor), a substance you normally have in your blood. It stimulates the bone marrow to make more white blood cells in times of stress or infection, when you need to build up your immune system. Now we've found a way to use it in chemotherapy treatment.[2] It's a natural product made from bacteria through genetic engineering. (Although this may sound unnatural, it's just a way for bacteria to serve as the production factory.) So now when a patient's white blood cell count becomes too low, we give them GCSF in an injection, to hasten the bone marrow's recovery. It's like treating those injured factory workers and getting them back to work.

You may be given this medicine preventively if the risk of low blood counts warrants it, or as a rescue if your counts get unexpectedly low during chemotherapy. GCSF is thus able to reduce the time it takes your bone marrow to recover after chemotherapy. Our initial enthusiasm for GCSF has been dampened as data suggested that bone marrow problems like myelodysplastic syndrome and even acute myeloid leukemia can occur with combined radiation and chemotherapy regimens with anthra-cycline/cyclophosphamide. Although the rate was still low at 2.4 percent, it was still more than double the incidence observed in patients treated with surgery alone.[3] This has led to more caution in its use. People taking a dose-dense schedule of chemotherapy (see Chapter 11) may need GCSF because the abbreviated schedule does not give the bone marrow time to recover on its own.

If your treatment begins the day the blood count is taken, you'll have to wait for fifteen to forty-five minutes for test results before you begin. In any event, you'll probably have to wait while the drugs are being mixed, though again this will depend on the practice in your institution. The wait may be annoying, but it can also be an advantage; often this is an opportunity for patients to talk to one another and find support in being together or for you to catch up on your reading, video watching, or whatever you do to keep yourself entertained.

Standard chemotherapy treatments are given on a variety of sched-ules, including weekly, every two weeks, three weeks, or monthly. The schedules vary depending on the drugs being used. The standard chemo-therapy for primary breast cancer treatment is given every two to three weeks. So it is important to ask your doctor what your schedule will be.

This means, for example, that you'll get them every two to three weeks, in fourteen- or twenty-one-day cycles. If it's a twenty-one-day cycle, you come in for an infusion every three weeks. During this time, your treatment may be all intravenous or a combination of intravenous medicine and a pill you take at home. Antinausea medications are usu-ally given before treatment starts, and you will be given prescriptions for medicines to take at home. Make sure you have written instructions about how and when to take them. Some people find a calendar with the days to take the drugs helpful. Sometimes you may be instructed to take medication the day before treatment to prevent side effects, and that also should be explained in writing.

Treatment areas vary. In the hospital there may be an entire floor for oncology patients or just a separate area of a larger floor. Chemotherapy can also be given in a private doctor's office. Everyone is aware of patient anxiety levels and tries to make the area as comfortable as possible. Be-cause the process doesn't involve machines, the chemo room doesn't look as intimidating as the radiation area. The room is comfortably lit and often has television sets in it. You may have a room to yourself or may sit among several other patients who are getting their treatments. Dress in light layers and a shirt that allows easy access to your port, such as a V-neck or button-down. You'll usually sit in a comfortable lounge chair for the procedure (Figure 15.5). Often patients bring blankets, or the doctor may supply them, as the chemo is cooler than your body temperature and can make you cold. Many patients bring smartphones, tablets, laptops, books, drinks, Kleenex, and anything else that will help pass the time as pleasantly as possible. I must admit that while I always gave great thought to this and laid out all my planned activities, I usually fell right asleep and never touched a thing! If you want to have a friend or family member with you, most hospitals and doctors will permit that. One woman I know would bring her own pillow and blanket from home to help her get through the four hours of her dose-dense treatment while friends came along and kept her entertained.

The length of time a treatment takes and the intervals at which treatments are given will vary depending on the type of drugs, the institution giving you the treatment, and the protocol being used. Several different combinations of drugs may be used, each requiring its own time length

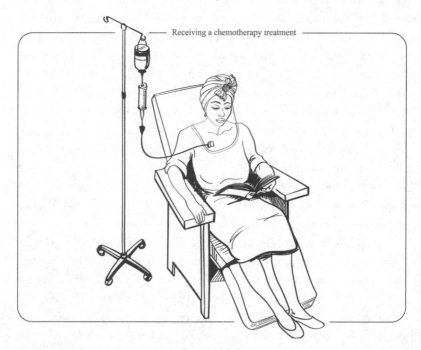

Receiving a chemotherapy treatment

Figure 15.5

for administration. Sometimes a treatment will last ten minutes, sometimes three or four hours. In addition, you will likely be given extra fluid as well as medications to control nausea and vomiting. My Facebook advisors all say that you should always take the nausea medications offered. Once nausea sets in it is much harder to treat than it is to prevent.

There's nothing particularly painful about the treatment, which feels like any IV procedure. The chemicals come in different colors; in breast cancer the drugs we use are usually clear, yellow, and red. One woman I counseled told me that she used to have the nurse give the red doxorubicin under the covers because she did not like the color. If it helps you get through the treatment and doesn't inconvenience the staff, never hesitate to ask for something like this.

You usually don't feel the medications go into your body, though some patients feel cold if the fluids are run very quickly or if they're cold to begin with, or if their bodies are especially sensitive to cold. Cyclophosphamide can cause a weird feeling of pressure in your sinuses, which stops once the infusion is finished. The doctor or nurse will always be around, and they're both highly trained specialists in chemotherapy. Sometimes the drugs irritate veins and cause them to clot off and scar during the course of the treatment. This can make it very hard to get needles into the veins. This is another reason to have some kind of intravascular access device. Ask your clinician to put the device where it will least bother you. There are options!

Eight drugs are commonly given as adjuvant chemotherapy for breast cancer: Cytoxan (cyclophosphamide) (C), Paraplatin (carboplatin, also C), Trexall (methotrexate) (M), Adrucil (5-fluorouracil) (F), Adriamycin (doxorubicin) (A), Ellence (epirubicin) (E), Taxol (paclitaxel) (T), and Taxotere (docetaxel) (T). These drugs are usually given in combinations of two or three.

In addition, drugs based on GCSF are given to maintain your white blood count. Two of these, Neupogen (filgrastim) and Leukine (sargramostim), are given as daily injections for ten to fourteen days. Another, called Neulasta (pegfilgrastim), is a long-acting form that is injected only once a cycle. If your tumor overexpresses HER2/neu, then Herceptin (trastuzumab) or Perjeta (pertuzumab) will be added. For triple-negative breast cancer, sometimes Keytruda (pembrolizumab) will be added.

Other drugs are used for metastatic disease. Some of the most common are Abraxane (nab-paclitaxel), Gemzar (gemcitabine), Navelbine (vinorelbine), and Halaven (eribulin mesylate), which are given by IV; and Xeloda (capecitabine), which can be taken orally (see Chapter 20). Although the side effects vary somewhat from one drug to another, they are basically similar to those of the adjuvant drugs.

While you are on chemotherapy, your immune system will not be functioning at its best. Although your blood cells may be fairly normal (particularly if you are getting GCSF support), the immune system is affected in less obvious ways. This doesn't mean you have to hide in your house and avoid all contact with the human race during therapy. Talk with your oncologist or nurse about your daily activities. Are you a teacher? Do you have young children in the house? Do you own pets? Many oncologists recommend avoiding cat litter or bird droppings. The doctor can give you specific advice about how to minimize your risk of getting an infection. You should make sure you are up-to-date with your vaccinations (seasonal flu, pneumonia, and so on) before you start. You may also want to get a good dental cleaning if there is time (you do not want to do this during chemotherapy, as dental cleanings can introduce bacteria into your bloodstream while your counts are low). Practice good hand-washing and consider investing in a small bottle of alcohol-based sanitizer for when you can't get to a sink. Wear a mask if you are around people with colds or flu.

SIDE EFFECTS OF CHEMOTHERAPY

Here we will talk about the side effects during and right after treatment. The longer-term consequences of therapy will be described in Chapter 18. Side effects vary according to the drugs used. Check with your oncologist about your specific breast cancer regimen. Unusual signs and symptoms should be reported to your doctor as soon as possible. The most immediate potential side effect concerns Adriamycin (doxorubicin), which can leak out of the vein and cause a severe skin burn that could require skin grafting. For this reason it's generally given in a specific way: avoiding weak veins and running in the IV with lots of fluids, so that it can't cause as much harm if it does leak out.

Nausea and Vomiting

A more common side effect with many types of chemotherapy is nausea and vomiting. We've learned that not all chemotherapy-induced nausea is the same; some drugs are worse than others. Unfortunately the ones commonly used for breast cancer, Adriamycin (doxorubicin) and Cytoxan (cyclophosphamide), are in the high-nausea group. Taxanes (Taxol and Taxotere) tend to provoke less nausea.

The timing of nausea differs as well. With Cytoxan, nausea starts about six to eight hours after treatment and lasts eight to twenty-four hours, while with Adriamycin it starts in one to three hours and lasts four to twenty-four hours. Acute vomiting, which usually occurs in the first twenty-four hours after a chemotherapy treatment, seems to be related to serotonin and responds well to serotonin inhibitors like Anzemet (dolasetron), Kytril (granisetron), Zofran (ondansetron), and Aloxi (palonosetron). Maxidex (dexamethasone, a steroid related to but not the same as those used illegally by athletes) is also helpful for acute vomiting. These medicines are usually given intravenously with your chemo.

Delayed nausea and vomiting are caused by something called substance P and occur one to five days after therapy, with a peak effect around forty-eight to seventy-two hours, and respond to a drug called Emend (aprepitant). For treatments with high potential for nausea and vomiting, the National Comprehensive Cancer Network (NCCN) recommends starting drugs before chemotherapy with aprepitant, dexamethasone, and one of the serotonin inhibitors.[4] Once nausea has set in, it is much harder to control. For chemotherapy regimens with the highest risk of nausea, Zyprexa (olanzapine) has been shown effective and may be recommended. The NCCN website is worth checking (www.nccn.org). If these approaches are not enough, dopamine antagonists (metoclopramide, prochlorperazine, domperidone, or metopimazine) can be added to the serotonin inhibitors and steroids. Cannabinoid (dronabinol, marijuana) has also been used for both acute and delayed chemotherapy-induced nausea and vomiting, and studies show that it is very effective. (The woman who brought her blanket and pillow to her dose-dense treatments swore by it.) It is also available as a pill (Marinol), which is legal but not as effective. Obviously using marijuana has all the downsides—both legal and physical—that you are aware of. If you are going to try it, do so under an experienced doctor's supervision and prescription. And of course only if medical marijuana is legal in your area.

The final type of nausea and vomiting is anticipatory and occurs days to hours prior to chemotherapy. This means you have experienced nausea and vomiting in the past and now just thinking about getting chemotherapy next week makes you nauseated today. This type can be controlled with benzodiazepines, starting one or two days prior to treatment, or behavioral techniques. Some people with nausea may actually be experiencing gastritis, an irritation of the stomach lining, and may respond well to medicines traditionally used to treat heartburn. These days most oncologists try to prevent nausea and vomiting before it occurs. Make sure you discuss this aspect of your care with your doctor and nurse so that you understand which drugs are being given to prevent nausea and why. All my Facebook advisors agree that you should not try to tough it out, but take all the drugs offered to you.

Because the thought of chemotherapy can be frightening, it is a good idea to bring someone with you for your first treatment to see how well it goes and drive you home if necessary. Usually, if you start off feeling all right and your antinausea drugs are effective, you'll get through the rest of the treatments with relative comfort. Still, you may well want company or at least a ride, as the antinausea drugs can make you woozy.

In addition to the drugs, many hospitals incorporate antistress mechanisms such as visualization, imagery, and relaxation techniques into their treatment program. These are often very effective. If your hospital or doctor doesn't offer such techniques, you may want to try some of the ones described in Chapter 16. Many of the techniques are simple and easy to learn. In addition, many adult education centers and holistic health institutes in cities and towns all over the United States have visualization programs. Acupuncture and Chinese herbs, discussed in Chapter 16, can also bring nausea relief. There are many options, and if what you are receiving from your doctor does not work, you need to ask for something different. There is no reason for anyone to suffer needlessly.

Weight Gain

Although weight gain can occur in people getting chemotherapy, the causes are multifactorial, including occasional steroid use, early-onset menopause, fluid retention (especially with taxanes), and even comfort eating. Yet one study showed that not all people gain weight.[5] This topic has attracted closer examination because weight gain is linked to more recurrences. Some data suggest that overweight women have a third higher mortality than lean ones, especially if they have ER-positive breast cancer.[6] This has stimulated interest in nutritional and exercise programs for survivors. (See Chapters 16 and 18.)

Effects on Appetite and Sense of Smell

Sometimes chemotherapy causes you to lose your appetite (anorexia, which is different from anorexia nervosa). Food may taste different to you,[7] and some chemicals interact badly with certain foods, though both loss of appetite and chemical interaction are less common with breast cancer drugs than with others. For a long time after my chemotherapy, everything tasted like metal to me.[8] It certainly spoiled my first post-treatment Thanksgiving dinner. Using plasticware instead of silverware can decrease the metallic taste. Play with spices and herbs to find what appeals to your chemo taste buds—you can even infuse water with fruit or herbs. My taste has certainly gotten better but has never completely come back. The National Cancer Institute publishes a helpful recipe booklet for people whose eating is affected by their chemotherapy. You may also experience peculiar odors.

Premature Menopause

More than half of premenopausal people have hot flashes while on adjuvant chemotherapy. One German survey of 1,506 women with an average age of 49 reported that 72 percent of those given adjuvant chemotherapy had hot flashes.[9] The drugs can create a transient or permanent chemically induced menopause, with hormonal changes, hot flashes, mood swings, and no periods.

An article in the *Journal of Clinical Oncology* suggests that the strongest predictors of whether you go through permanent menopause with treatment are age and type of chemotherapy.[10] The closer you are to natural menopause, the higher your risk. The average age of menopause is 51. A 45-year-old woman who receives chemotherapy has an 80 percent likelihood of going into menopause as a result, which is much greater than is the case with Nolvadex (tamoxifen) (note that Nolvadex works just as well regardless of menopausal status). A 35-year-old woman has a 20 percent chance of becoming postmenopausal. Many people don't know this ahead of time and have to deal with something unexpected in the midst of their treatment. (See our discussion later in the chapter on when you want a medically induced menopause.)

Less than 15 percent of women younger than age 40 who receive four cycles of AC (Adriamycin and Cytoxan), and 60 percent of those over age 40, will become menopausal.[11] Overall it is the cumulative dose of Cytoxan that is strongly related to premature menopause. It is not known what effect the recent addition of taxanes to AC has on the ovaries. Although roughly half of the patients younger than age 40 may regain some menstrual function, the percentage is much lower for older patients.

In medicalese we call premature menopause ovarian failure. This is one of my pet peeves. The ovaries did nothing wrong and they certainly did not fail—we poisoned them with chemotherapy! Nonetheless, if you do experience early menopause, you will of course be infertile. In patients with tumors that are not sensitive to hormones (ER-negative and PR-negative), this may not be necessary. A recent study showed that premenopausal patients could take Zoladex (goserelin) to suppress their ovaries during chemotherapy and thus increase the odds of preserving their fertility.[12] If this is of interest to you, be sure you mention it to your doctor before you start treatment.

Of course not everyone is put into permanent menopause. If your period comes back, you can still conceive. It may take a few months to know, so make sure you use mechanical birth control during treatment if you're heterosexually active. Hormone-based contraception may stimulate the tumor, and the chemotherapy drugs could severely injure a first-trimester fetus. (See Chapter 12 for more on fertility options for patients who are about to undergo chemotherapy, and Chapter 18 for a description of treatments for menopausal symptoms.)

Hair Loss

Chemotherapy treatments used in breast cancer, as in many other cancers, often cause partial or total hair loss. This is somewhat predictable according to the drugs used and duration of treatment. Patients who get Adriamycin as part of their treatment almost always lose their hair, usually within two to four weeks after the onset of treatment. If you get Taxol or Taxotere, the hair loss can be quite sudden. You'll wake up one morning and find a large amount of hair on your pillow or in the shower, or you'll be combing your hair and notice a lot in your comb. This is almost always traumatic, so you may want to buy a wig before your treatment starts. You can ask your oncologist to give you a prescription for a "cranial prosthesis" (wig), and often insurance will cover it. It's best to go to a hairdresser or wig salon before starting treatment, so the hairdresser knows what your hair usually looks like and how you like to wear it—it makes for a better match. Many patients end up not using the wig. (You can always donate it to a local breast resource center.) Patients who don't prepare in advance for the hair loss tend to have a difficult time emotionally if it does occur. The Breast Cancer Network of Strength, a national support organization, sends wigs to people with hair loss for a nominal fee.

You can also look into a cold cap to reduce the blood supply to your scalp and potentially decrease the loss of hair. The cold contracts the blood vessels in the scalp, reducing the amount of chemo meds that can get through. The low temperature also slows the activity of cells at the roots of your hair, putting them into a lethargic state like hibernation. Together this reduces the uptake of chemo absorbed by the scalp. In the early days of this technique, the caps were purchased by the patient, who also furnished a cooler of dry ice needed to keep them cool. Because the caps thawed during the procedure, they had to be changed every 30 minutes or so, which required help. Fortunately this system has been eclipsed by more modern scalp cooling systems that use small refrigeration machines to circulate a cold gel through the cap for the duration of the treatment. The catch is that you have to begin the cooling process 30 minutes before the chemo starts and remain, depending on the treatment, another 60 to 180 minutes once it's finished, so visits are longer. Hair loss is a tricky thing to quantify, given the variations in both hair and chemotherapies, but scalp cooling is estimated to be about 50 to 80 percent effective—that is to say you would lose 50 to 20 percent less hair. Unfortunately, insurance coverage for scalp cooling is not yet standard in the United States, so you may want to check the cost before you commit. The good news is that at the time this book was being updated, Medicare and Medicaid covered $1,850 of the cost.

Remember, it isn't only the hair on your head that falls out. Pubic hair, eyelashes and eyebrows, leg and arm hair—some or all of the hair on your body will fall out, although in most patients the eyelashes and eyebrows only thin a bit. The U.S. Food and Drug Administration (FDA) approved the use of a prescription medicine called Latisse that encourages lash growth when they are sparse, so if you are interested, talk to your doctor. Most of the time loss of brows and lashes isn't a big problem cosmetically—you can thicken your eyebrows with pencil, for example, and apply false eyelashes if you feel inclined—but it can be startling if you're not prepared for it.

It may take a while after the treatments have ended for your hair to grow back. A little down will probably appear even before your treatments have ended, and within six weeks you should have some hair growing in, though the time depends on how fast your hair normally grows. Often it comes back with a different texture—curly if it's been straight. Eventually the curl relaxes and your hair returns to normal after several haircuts. It may come back in a different color, most commonly gray or black. Other body hair is variable. Sometimes taxane chemotherapy with Taxotere (docetaxel), and to a lesser extent Abraxane (nab-paclitaxel), can cause permanent hair loss.[13] If you are given these, and your hair is important to you, be sure to enlist in scalp cooling for the duration of your therapy.

Sexual Problems

Some patients experience sexual problems, often related to the vaginal dryness of menopause. You may suddenly encounter problems with your diaphragm or an IUD due to dryness. In addition there are the physical and psychological effects of the treatment. It's hard to feel sexy when you are tired and bald. This is an important time to communicate with your partner about each other's feelings and needs and to try to find a comforting compromise. (See Chapter 18 for a discussion of sexual issues and breast cancer.)

Fatigue

Fatigue is a common side effect (see Chapter 18) that has been noted in 40 to 80 percent of cancer patients.[14] If this is a problem, bring it to the attention of your doctor or nurse. Five factors often associated with fatigue are pain, emotional distress, sleep disturbance, anemia, and low thyroid. All are treatable, so be sure to get them checked out. Other causes can be infection, electrolyte disorders, and cardiac dysfunction. Moderate to severe fatigue is always worth complaining about.

More tolerable fatigue can be considered the "pooped-out syndrome." Your body has been assaulted by surgery, radiation, and chemotherapy and is still trying to heal. It needs longer to get back to normal than we previously understood. One patient says it takes as long to get back to normal as it took to get the treatment: if you have six months of chemotherapy, you have six months of recovery.

There are two ways you can approach this fatigue: drugs and exercise. Several studies show that aerobic exercise decreases fatigue.[15] This may be hard to force on yourself—the last thing you feel like doing when you're exhausted is exercise. But it's worth pushing yourself. Probably it works by increasing endorphins. And it can help prevent another side effect: weight gain.

"Chemo Brain"

There are many aftereffects of chemotherapy that we're just beginning to acknowledge, either because they are subtle or because they take longer to materialize. One of these is the decreased cognitive function that many patients experience and have called "chemo brain." They feel they are not as sharp as they were before their cancer treatment, multitasking is more difficult, and their brain is not functioning as efficiently.[16] This subject is tackled fully in Chapter 18, which explores the longer-term side effects of chemotherapy and cancer treatment that I call "collateral damage."

Other Side Effects

Other common side effects include mouth sores, conjunctivitis, runny eyes and nose, skin and nail changes, diarrhea, and constipation. You may get headaches, which is often from the antinausea medication. Any of these can be mild or severe or anything in between.

Long-Term Side Effects

The long-term side effects of chemotherapy include chronic bone marrow suppression and second cancers, especially leukemias. The risk of leukemia is small—0.5 percent in the NSABP series—and probably worth the benefit of the treatment, but you need to be aware that it exists.[17]

Adriamycin (doxorubicin) in particular can be toxic to the heart. The likelihood of this is related to the cumulative dose of Adriamycin that you get over a lifetime, and it's rare with four to six cycles.[18] We're only beginning to consider this now because in the past we used Adriamycin only for metastatic cancers, and those patients usually died of the cancer within a few years. Now that we're using it more frequently for patients with negative lymph nodes, they may well be alive in twenty or thirty years, and we may see more delayed side effects than we did before. It is important not to assume that a drug or treatment that is relatively safe at the time will be safe over the long haul. We know that Adriamycin causes heart damage by itself, but it also interacts with some other forms of heart disease. Consequently a patient on this drug may have more problems with coronary artery disease years later. Overall the risk of having a heart problem due to Adriamycin is about one in two hundred treated women. One of my former patients developed heart disease many years after being treated with Adriamycin and ended up with a heart transplant.

I'm not suggesting that we abandon Adriamycin for adjuvant treatment. My patient, after all, survived long enough to develop a heart ailment. And as these associations came to light over the years, we have made corrective changes—better left-sided radiation techniques, rarely giving Adriamycin with Herceptin (trastuzumab), and using prevention medications when we do give Adriamycin. So we are likely getting better.

Adriamycin is one of the best drugs we have to treat metastatic breast cancer. If it is indicated, it should certainly be used. But we should not use it indiscriminately in patients who are not at particularly high risk for metastases.

Taxol (paclitaxel) can cause a dose-dependent, cumulative neuropathy.[19] This is a pins-and-needles sensation, often in the hands and feet, which can get worse with each dose but is generally at least partially reversible. Taxol can also cause hand-foot syndrome, an itchy rash on the palms of the hands and the soles of the feet. In about 5 to 15 percent of women a syndrome of muscle and joint aches and pains can occur, starting about twenty-four to seventy-two hours after the infusion and lasting two to four days. It ranges from mild, requiring only occasional nonnarcotic pain relievers, to incapacitating. A woman I counseled through her treatment experienced this and required narcotics to deal with it; the narcotics led to nausea and vomiting. Once you know that you react this way, you can be treated with dexamethasone for several days to prevent the pain. Taxotere (docetaxel) also causes neuropathy, though it is generally milder than Taxol. Taxotere can cause a unique syndrome of swelling and fluid retention; some fluid retention is fairly common, but occasionally it can be severe. Fortunately this is reversible, but it takes a long time. A newer form of Taxol, Abraxane (nab-paclitaxel), has been shown to be at least as effective as and possibly more effective than Taxol and is used for metastatic breast cancer. Although it generally has fewer side effects than Taxol, the one side effect that is worse than Taxol's is neuropathy. There are drugs that can be used for peripheral neuropathy that are discussed in Chapter 18.

Though there's no way to know in advance how you'll react to your treatments, your doctor or nurse can tell you how other people treated with the drugs you're on have done in the past. Ways to deal with each of these side effects are discussed in Chapter 18.

Getting Through Chemotherapy

Although it's important to be prepared for possible side effects, it's equally important not to assume you'll have all or even any of them. This assumption can intensify and sometimes even create the symptoms. Sometimes people see the side effects as a sign that their illness is getting worse and consequently contribute to their own negative feelings. Dr. Bernie Siegel, who has worked intensively with mental techniques to reduce pain and help heal diseases, reports in his book *Love, Medicine and Miracles* on a study done in England in which men were given a placebo and told it was a chemotherapy treatment.[20] Thirty percent of the men lost their hair! Positive thinking and—importantly—exercise, as well as keeping up your normal activities, can significantly reduce the side effects of chemotherapy.

Most chemotherapy treatments are given on an outpatient basis. You will soon know whether you are going to feel sick and, if so, on which day the nausea hits and how bad it is. Most people are able to continue their normal lives and maintain their jobs with minor adjustments while receiving treatment. You won't feel great, but you'll be functional. Currently up-to-date chemotherapy treatments should be tolerable, and you should be able to function well. Generally you should have one to two days of feeling lousy for each dose. If there are severe or persistent symptoms beyond that, ask your doctor or nurse for strategies to reduce the side effects. Many options are available.

Most of my Facebook advisors said that maintaining a healthy diet and exercise program were critical to getting through things. Not only is exercise anti-inflammatory and good for you, but you will feel morally superior! And don't just give up if you can't run six miles as you used to—do what you can. Maybe it is time to use a stationary bike, swim, or just go for a walk! The key is to keep moving.

This may be a good time to take up your friends' offers of help. A ride to your treatment can be wonderful, both for the company and the release from worry about traffic and parking. Child care may well give you a breather in a stressful time, as can offers to cook dinner or clean the house. Most friends and family members really do want to help, and this may be the best time to use their support. The key is to tell them what you need. It may not be a casserole but rather an invitation out to dinner or company on a walk.

Don't expect to feel perfect the minute your last treatment is over. Your body has been under great stress and needs time to recuperate. As mentioned, it often takes six months or even a year to feel normal again. It will happen, however, so don't despair. (See Chapter 18 for a discussion of rehabilitation after breast cancer.)

ADJUVANT HORMONE THERAPY

Hormone therapies are generally presented as having fewer side effects than chemotherapy. Of course, nothing is ever that simple. Chemotherapy can be likened to a sprint—that is, it is given intravenously for a period of months—while hormone therapies are more like a marathon, pills that you generally take for ten years. They both have significant side effects. In premenopausal people one of the options is Nolvadex (tamoxifen), a drug that blocks hormones from getting into the estrogen receptor in the tumor while sometimes acting like estrogen in other organs. Post-menopausal people have less circulating estrogen, so they do better with aromatase inhibitors. In terms of administration, these common hormone therapies are the simplest of the breast cancer treatments. You don't need to go anywhere or have anything done to you—you simply take a pill.

In the case of adjuvant hormone therapy, side effects can include phlebitis (blood clots), pulmonary emboli, visual problems, depression, nausea (but very rarely vomiting), vaginal discharge, joint stiffness, muscular aches and pains, and hot flashes. All of these are rare except for the hot flashes and muscle pains. A lot of patients who have these symptoms ask me if they could be caused by their medication. When I say yes, they say, "Thank God—I thought I was going crazy because my doctor said I wouldn't have side effects."

Nolvadex (Tamoxifen)

The most common side effects in both pre- and postmenopausal people are hot flashes, which occur in about 50 percent of patients on Nolvadex (tamoxifen). Like all hot flashes, they can be severe or mild. They eventually go away but "eventually" may mean years. Drugs like Effexor (venlafaxine) or Neurontin (gabapentin) can reduce the number and intensity of these hot flashes.[21] Alternative choices are discussed in Chapter 18.

About 30 percent of women on Nolvadex (tamoxifen) experience major gynecological discomforts—anything from vaginal discharge to severe vaginal dryness.

There's some evidence that Nolvadex (tamoxifen) may, in unusual cases, increase *thrombophlebitis*, a form of phlebitis in the leg in which the vein gets irritated and forms clots.[22] It is rare but very dangerous, as the blood clot can travel to the lung, causing pulmonary embolus. It can even be fatal. In a reanalysis of a study on Nolvadex, the National Surgical Adjuvant Breast and Bowel Project (NSABP) found this to occur even less frequently than initially thought—in under 1 per 1,000 patients.[23] Although this side effect is rare, it is important to let your doctor know right away if you develop leg swelling and pain.

The most serious side effect of Nolvadex (tamoxifen) is a slight risk of uterine cancer. In the same NSABP study (see Chapter 6), researchers found the risk of endometrial cancer to be higher than they initially thought, but the 0.3 percent risk at five years is statistically insignificant within the framework of the study. It occurs almost entirely in women over age 50. This is reassuring because postmenopausal patients now have an alternative option to aromatase inhibitors (see the following discussion), and premenopausal patients can take this drug without worrying about getting uterine cancer.

Premenopausal people have an increased risk of benign gynecological problems, including uterine polyps, fibroids, endometriosis, and ovarian cysts.[24] (See Chapter 12 on the use of Nolvadex (tamoxifen) to induce ovulation for in vitro fertilization [IVF].) If you are premenopausal on Nolvadex, be aware that new gynecological complaints may be related to it.

As with chemotherapy, a heterosexually active woman should use some type of effective mechanical contraceptive while taking the drug. Because Nolvadex (tamoxifen) can damage a fetus, it's very important not to get pregnant while you're taking it.

Some patients have elevated liver blood enzymes, which go away once they stop taking Nolvadex (tamoxifen). Many patients on Nolvadex experience eye problems, including blurry vision and, uncommonly, cataracts.

Nonetheless, there are several benefits with Nolvadex (tamoxifen). It raises your high-density lipoproteins and lowers your low-density lipoproteins, which may make you less likely to get heart disease.[25] Nolvadex often improves or at least stabilizes bone loss in postmenopausal women, much like Evista (raloxifene).[26]

The most important thing about Nolvadex (tamoxifen) is that it treats the cancer you have and reduces your chance of getting cancer in the opposite breast by 50 percent—that is, from 15 to 20 percent to 7.5 to 10 percent. So considering all these pros and cons, it is worth taking unless you have had problems with blood clots in the past.

As I explained in Chapter 11, the current data suggest you take Nolvadex (tamoxifen) for at least five years. Much to everyone's surprise, the benefits of decreasing the chance of relapse and of second cancers continue even after you stop taking the drug. Nolvadex therefore probably kills cancer cells or, likely, puts them into a long-lasting dormant state. But women with ER-positive disease may want to consider taking Nolvadex a few years longer, according to a large clinical trial called ATLAS. Nolvadex taken for a full ten years in these cases can roughly halve breast cancer mortality in the second decade after diagnosis.[27] It takes six weeks for Nolvadex to clear from your system after you stop. So if you miss a pill one day, it isn't the end of the world. Just resume taking it the next day.

Although Nolvadex (tamoxifen) is the drug most commonly used, Fareston (toremifene) is a drug that has been approved by the FDA for treatment of metastatic disease and is sometimes used in place of Nolvadex, especially for patients who do not tolerate it. Evista (raloxifene), another drug sometimes used, is a SERM (selective estrogen receptor modulator; see Chapter 6) that has been shown to decrease breast cancer when given to postmenopausal patients with low bone density; however, it is primarily used in women at risk for breast cancer. One study of fourteen patients with metastatic breast cancer showed no effect from Evista.[28] A second study showed an 18 percent response rate in metastatic disease.[29] At this time it is definitely not an alternative to Nolvadex as an adjuvant treatment of breast cancer.

Aromatase Inhibitors

Aromatase inhibitors (AIs) are now being used rather than Nolvadex (tamoxifen) in postmenopausal patients (see Chapter 11). Like Nolvadex, they are taken in pill form. Three drugs commonly used are Arimidex (anastrozole), Femara (letrozole), and Aromasin (exemestane). The postmenopausal ovary and adrenal glands produce the precursors of estrogen, which are converted in particular organs into estrogen by the enzyme aromatase. These drugs block this conversion, reducing the amount of estrogen in most organs. Because they block estrogen production and have no estrogenic effects, it is not surprising that some of the side effects are similar to those of Nolvadex; others are quite different. The main complaint with the aromatase inhibitors seems to be joint pain; this can be quite disabling for some patients. Furthermore, the lack of estrogen increases bone loss and resulting fractures, as well as higher cholesterol and the resulting increase in heart disease. Because Nolvadex lowers cholesterol, it could be better in someone with known high lipids. In general, when compared to Nolvadex, aromatase inhibitors have a lower incidence of stroke, blood clots, hot flashes, and vaginal bleeding.

We started using these drugs about a decade ago. Now we have several studies investigating the best way to use them. They can be used in a variety of schedules: up front for five years, switching after two to three years of Nolvadex (tamoxifen), or as extended therapy after five years of Nolvadex. The approach that makes the most sense for you will depend on your age, how many years it's been since you began menopause, risk of recurrence, bone health, history of blood clots, menopausal symptoms, and sexual activity. People who are not sure whether they are menopausal, are within a year of their last period, or have chemotherapy-induced menopause are best started on Nolvadex with monitoring of blood hormone levels. If they have no periods for two years and show a menopausal hormone pattern, they can be switched to an AI. In fact, a study showed that premenopausal people who took Nolvadex and then subsequently went into menopause benefited from taking an AI for an additional five years even if it was not started until up to six years after they become menopausal. The benefit in this case was similar in patients who were up to six years past concluding a regimen of five years of Nolvadex.[30] Why not just use an AI from the beginning? Because they do not work in premenopausal people who are still producing hormones, as they have estrogen from their ovaries and don't need to use aromatase to make it from testosterone.

Two studies have explored a way around this by testing aromatase inhibitors together with drugs that suppress ovarian function, thus sidelining the estrogen production that can cause cancer growth. Large international trials called SOFT and TEXT found that five years of ovarian suppression does decrease breast cancer recurrence when added to Nolvadex (tamoxifen) or Aromasin (exemestane). Among premenopausal patients, the addition of ovarian suppression to aromatase inhibitors resulted in a significantly higher eight-year rate of disease-free survival. This rate was 76 percent in patients taking Nolvadex and an ovarian function suppressor, 80.5 percent for those taking Aromasin with an ovarian function suppressor, and 71 percent for those taking Nolvadex alone.[31]

Researchers also checked whether postmenopausal people with hormone-positive cancer who already had five years of AI would benefit from another five years. They found that only the first two years of the extension were beneficial, and the remaining three years only resulted in a greater risk of bone fractures.[32]

Other ongoing trials are looking to confirm optimal length of therapy for AI or for patients who switch from Nolvadex to AI.

When you ask patients or oncology nurses for the biggest complaint about aromatase inhibitors, they specify bone pain and musculoskeletal stiffness, but these symptoms may not last. Follow-up of the trial that confirmed the safety and efficacy of AI Aridimex (anastrozole) for hormone-sensitive early breast cancer suggested that in approximately one-third of women, joint symptoms improved, usually within six months of continuing on therapy.[33]

Although all three AIs cause symptoms, studies show that switching from one to another will often lessen the symptoms.[34] Usually these symptoms go away after about three months, but getting through that time period takes patience and endurance. In addition, exercise has been shown to decrease stiffness in the joints, as counterintuitive as that may seem. Anti-inflammatories (NSAIDs) seem to help some patients, as do warm baths, acupuncture, and massage. Because many patients are also coming off hormone replacement therapy (HRT), it is sometimes difficult to know which of the side effects are from withdrawal from HRT and which from the new drugs. A nurse friend of mine says that bioflavonoids help both bone pain and hot flashes in some patients. Vaginal dryness and pain with intercourse are also side effects of the lack of estrogen in some patients and can be managed with lubricants and vaginal moisturizers (see Chapter 18).

GnRH Agonists: Blocking Hormones Produced by Ovaries

GnRH agonists aim to slow the growth of hormone-positive breast cancer by curbing the body's own production of estrogen. There are currently three GnRH agonists: Zoladex (goserelin), Lupron (leuprolide), and Trelstar (triptorelin). They work by telling the brain to block the manufacture of hormones that stimulate the ovary, placing patients into a reversible menopause. By eliminating this natural source of estrogen, you also eliminate the fuel that allows ER-positive breast cancer to grow. These drugs are given by a monthly injection under the skin of the abdomen. As you might expect, they produce many of the side effects of normal menopause. First, your periods will stop. This is not a contraceptive, however, so you should be sure to use another means of contraception as well if you are heterosexually active. Hot flashes, lower sex drive, joint pain, and weight gain are common side effects. Most of the time your period will return when you complete your course of treatment, although in some patients close to menopause it may not. Zoladex has been combined with Nolvadex (tamoxifen) or an aromatase inhibitor in a randomized controlled trial, with a small improvement when the latter is added. Although this sounds good, it is important to remember that this small improvement is accompanied by side effects, with 88.7 percent of the patients who received ovarian suppression plus exemestane reporting musculoskeletal symptoms compared to 76 percent of patients treated with Nolvadex and ovarian function supression.[35] Obviously we need to better refine who really benefits and who does not.

Other Hormonal Therapies

More than a dozen new drugs are being developed and tested with the goal of altering and degrading estrogen receptors on cancer cells. These will be particularly useful in cases where there is resistance to aromatase inhibitors or Nolvadex (tamoxifen).

Faslodex (fulvestrant) is a steroidal antiestrogen. Unlike Nolvadex (tamoxifen) and Evista (raloxifene), it has no estrogenic effects, and when given to women with metastatic breast cancer, it appears to be as good as Arimidex (anastrozole) and causes fewer joint problems (see the following discussion). It is given by intramuscular injection once a month rather than orally. Faslodex is what is known as a selective estrogen receptor degrader (SERD) and is the first drug in this class to be approved for hormone-positive breast cancer by the FDA. It can be used both as an initial treatment, in combination, and as an alternative if there is resistance to other therapies. Many oral SERDs are currently in development.

SIDE EFFECTS OF HORMONE THERAPY

Bone Loss and Bisphosphonates

Women with breast cancer tend to have high bone density due to their higher estrogen levels. The problem is that chemotherapy (by putting some people into premature menopause) and some of the current hormone therapies accelerate the normal bone loss that occurs with aging. But others, notably Nolvadex and, to a lesser extent, Fareston (toremifene), help maintain bone by preventing its loss. They have about the same effect as Evista (raloxifene), improving bone density by 2 to 3 percent and preventing vertebral fractures.

In women on aromatase inhibitors the issues are more complicated. At a minimum, women who have had breast cancer should follow the general recommendation from the National Osteoporosis Foundation: first bone density test at age 65 or, at the latest, when the therapy is finished. It is not clear that the decrease in bone density resulting from treatment will last indefinitely. A study of two years of treatment with the aromatase inhibitor Aromasin (exemestane) showed that after the drug was stopped, the bone density of the lumbar spine improved and that of the hip stabilized, suggesting that the effects of these drugs are not permanent.[36] Overall the bone densities after treatment were greater in the treatment group than the placebo group, a reminder that all women lose some bone. Bone does not change quickly, and the test itself is not that precise, so the current recommendations are to repeat a bone density test only after a minimum of two years.

In an attempt to prevent bone loss and subsequent fractures altogether, it has become clinical practice to put women taking aromatase inhibitors (AIs) on drugs to try to maintain their bone. This usually involves Zometa (zoledronic acid). Interestingly, bone density is maintained,[37] and a recent study suggested a survival benefit as well, but a recent meta-analysis did not show that the number of fractures decreased.[38] Most of the time intravenous bisphosphonates have been used in cancer patients. They do not have the gastrointestinal problems seen with oral drugs such as Fosamax but can be associated with flu-like symptoms such as bone pain, transient joint and muscle pain, nausea, and fever. These symptoms usually occur after the first or second infusion and last about forty-eight hours. They respond well to aspirin or an NSAID. Because low calcium can be seen with these drugs, women are encouraged to take vitamin D and calcium and are monitored for their calcium blood levels. Kidney toxicity is also possible with these drugs, especially in women who already have diminished renal function. The other side effect is necrosis (tissue death) in the jaw bone. This can be a serious problem that consists of an area of exposed nonhealing bone, following dental work. For this reason any woman considering taking one of these drugs should have a good dental exam first.

Premature Menopause

The most common long-term side effect of hormonal therapies is premature menopause and the resulting infertility. We describe this in Chapters 12 and 18.

TARGETED THERAPIES

HER2/neu Targeted Therapy

Herceptin (trastuzumab) has been used extensively to treat patients with HER2/neu-overexpressing cancers. Although it is pretty safe when given alone, it has shown an increased risk of heart failure in women who also take or have taken Adriamycin (doxorubicin). This possibility is usually monitored, particularly in women taking it as adjuvant treatment as opposed to treatment of metastatic disease. Monitoring typically involves a multigated acquisition (MUGA) scan or echocardiogram (echo) to evaluate how well your heart is pumping prior to treatment. The test is then checked every three months during Herceptin therapy and every six months for at least two years following the completion of the one-year course. If your heart's ability to pump blood decreases, the drug will be suspended for at least four weeks to see if the situation improves. If it doesn't improve in eight weeks, then the drug is stopped permanently.

Herceptin (trastuzumab) is given by injection weekly or every three weeks. The side effects are most common with the first treatment and include fever and/or chills in about 40 percent of women. They are easily managed with acetaminophen or aspirin. Other possible but less likely side effects include nausea, vomiting, diarrhea, headaches, difficult breathing, and rashes. Herceptin is usually given with chemotherapy, at least in the initial cycles, and thus all the usual chemotherapy side effects are present.

Another drug that has an effect in HER2/neu-positive cancers is Tykerb (lapatinib). It is a tyrosine kinase inhibitor and has been shown to be beneficial in women who are resistant to Herceptin. Though it is often used in metastatic disease, it is not yet used as an adjuvant therapy.

We also have Perjeta (pertuzumab) for women with HER2/neu-positive cancers. Perjeta also blocks HER2 but at a different point than Herceptin; however, it too may have cardiac effects.

Enhertu (trastuzumab deruxtecan) is a newer addition to the toolbox and has proved effective in patients with HER2-positive metastatic cancer who have received numerous previous treatments. Enhertu has also had a notable effect on patients with treated brain metastasis. The average duration of progression-free survival with Enhertu was 16.4 months in all patients and 18 months for those with brain metastasis. Side effects can include nausea, bone marrow suppression, and inflammation in the lungs.[39]

Enhertu has also proved to work well in the first ever trial focused on a potentially new cancer subtype called HER2-low. For years there has been a group of HER2-negative patients that never responded as well as expected from treatment, and now studies are beginning to tease out why. When pathologists first look at biopsy tissue under a microscope, they score the number of HER2 receptors from zero to three. Three was considered HER2-positive, and anything below was considered HER2-negative. To confirm that, a fluorescence in situ hybridization (FISH) test was usually done to see if the gene was amplified. If that was negative, then HER2-negative status was confirmed. But patients whose HER2 score is 1+ or 2+ still express HER2 to some degree and tend to be hormone-positive. Although traditionally treated the same as all HER2-negative patients, these patients still have HER2 expression that can be targeted for treatment. HER2-positive breast cancer comprises about 20 percent of newly diagnosed breast cancer cases, while an estimated 40 to 60 percent have breast cancer that is now considered HER2-low.[40]

Not only do we now have a middle category of HER2 expression, but also the first successful clinical trial aimed specifically at HER2-low metastatic breast cancer. The DESTINY-Breast04 trial tested Enhertu versus any choice of chemo (the standard treatment for HER2-negative cancers) and found it to improve overall survival. The median progression-free survival was 9.9 months in the Enhertu group and 5.1 months in the physician's choice of chemotherapy. Overall survival with Enhertu was 23.4 months versus 16.8 months, respectively.[41]

Nerlynx (neratinib) has shown a modest improvement in early-stage HER2-positive breast cancer in patients who have received up to two years of chemotherapy with Herceptin. In a trial testing Nerlynx against a placebo, the two-year invasive disease-free survival rate was 94 percent in the Neratinib group compared to 92 percent in those taking a placebo. Unfortunately the 2 percent benefit often came with a side effect of severe diarrhea, which should be taken into account.[42] However, as tends to happen in research, Nerlynx may be effective in a different setting—as a part of a combination of drugs for patients with heavily treated HER2-positive metastatic breast cancer.[43]

Kadcyla (trastuzumab emtansine) had once been the standard of treatment for patients with HER2-positive metastatic cancer but has recently been eclipsed by Enhertu (trastuzumab deruxtecan). In a multicenter randomized trial comparing the two, Enhertu had a greater impact. Among 524 randomly assigned patients, those alive without disease progression at one year with Enhertu was 75.8 percent compared to 34.1 percent with Kadcyla.[44]

Tukysa (tucatinib) has also been found to be effective in brain metastases when combined with Herceptin (trastuzumab) and Xeloda (capecitabine). This drug works in patients with limited options whose cancer progresses after two or more anti-HER2 treatments. In a recent trial, progression-free survival at one year with the Tukysa-combination group was 29 percent compared to 14 percent in the placebo-combination group. Those enrolled in the trial included patients with brain metastases.[45] These survival outcomes are particularly encouraging as up to 50 percent of patients with HER2-positive metastatic breast cancer will develop brain metastases at some point, according to the study. An ongoing clinical trial is now exploring the use of Tukysa as part of the initial treatment of breast cancer, together with Herceptin (trastuzumab) and Perjeta (pertuzumab).

Cyclin-Dependent Kinase Inhibitors

Researchers are continuing to explore the potential of a new class of drug for the metastatic treatment of women with ER-positive tumors. Called cyclin-dependent kinase (CDK) inhibitors, these drugs target enzymes involved in cell division and Nolvadex (tamoxifen) resistance. Three of these CDK inhibitors have been approved for breast cancer since the last edition of this book, expanding treatment options for patients with advanced or metastatic hormone-positive, HER2-negative disease. Studies are also looking into their effectiveness with other drug combinations and subtypes.

At this writing, however, studies have shown some tumor resistance to CDK inhibitors after initial treatment, and eventually, after several months, there is disease progression.[46]

The three CDK inhibitors currently in use for breast cancer treatment in combination with hormone therapy are Ibrance (palbociclib), Kisqali (ribociclib), and Verzenio (abemaciclib).

Each of these three CDK inhibitors improved outcomes with patients with hormone-positive metastatic breast cancer, but only Verzenio had an effect as well in early-stage, high-risk, hormone-positive breast cancer.[47] When Ibrance (palbociclib) was tested in the same patient subset there was no benefit to adding it to the standard hormone therapy,[48] and a trial with Kisqali is still waiting to report out. Researchers speculate that the differences may be due to length of time taking the medication, subtle differences in the stage or risk of breast cancer patients who enrolled in the trials, or possibly drug potency. One trial found a biomarker for reduced response to Ibrance and Femara (letrozole), opening the door to debate on the value of biomarkers in treatment decisions.[49]

IMMUNOTHERAPY

The whole field of immunotherapy has flourished since the last edition of this book (see Chapter 11). We now have two FDA-approved checkpoint inhibitors and several targeted immunotherapy drugs for specific subsets of breast cancer.

A trend is developing in immunotherapy to base treatment not so much on the location of cancer (breast, uterus, skin) as on molecular markers and results of gene sequencing. It is taking targeted immuno-therapies in the direction of individualized medicine, and leading the way are trials by the American Society of Clinical Oncology (ASCO) and the federal government's National Cancer Institute. Both trials match pa-tients to treatments by way of genetic mutations. So far, drugs used in breast cancer have elicited some response in head and neck cancer, skin cancer, and uterine cancer. But as of yet few drugs for other cancers have enhanced breast cancer treatment.

Targeted antibodies and immunotherapy drugs use synthetic versions of immune system antibodies (proteins) to bind to targets like the HER2 protein on breast cancer cells to stop their growth. But to succeed, there has to be at least some activity from the body's own immune cells, a rarity in most breast cancers. That's why they're sometimes called immunologically "cold"—because tumors are surrounded by cells that shut down the body's natural immune response.

Personalized Immunotherapy with TILs

Researchers are now testing a way of jump-starting your own immune cells to fight metastatic breast cancer. Still in clinical trials, it involves extracting and turbo-charging your immune cells, then putting them back in your body. The TILs (tumor-infiltrating lymphocytes—a kind of white blood cell) are taken from your biopsied tumor tissue, multiplied, and then reprogrammed to fight cancer, instead of ignoring it. They are reinserted via blood transfusion after chemotherapy. Unfortunately, TILs can't always be found in biopsied breast tissue, but they have been located in patients with hormone-positive cancers—previously thought incapable of an immune response and thus not responsive to immunotherapy.

Checkpoint Inhibitors

Although there are two checkpoint inhibitors for breast cancer treatment, one is tailored for a particular and rare cancer. The main checkpoint inhibitor for breast cancer is Keytruda (pembrolizumab). In combination with chemotherapy, it can be used to treat inoperable, locally advanced, or metastatic triple-negative, PD-L1-positive breast cancer.

When a cancer is described as PD-L1-positive, it is because it has been oozing this subversive PD-L1 protein to turn off the immune system. The immune system's T cells have a receptor, PD-1, that must bind with the tumor to trigger an immune response. But tumors dodge this by secreting the PD-L1 protein that neutralizes the T cell receptor, like a bank robber shutting down the surveillance cameras. Checkpoint inhibitors like Keytruda block either PD-L1 or PD-1 and alert the immune system that the cancer is a threat. These drugs have a completely different profile than we are used to. For example, the PD-1/PD-L1 inhibitors can show a flare response or a temporary worsening of disease, such as progression in TILs, before the tumor stabilizes or regresses.[50]

The second checkpoint inhibitor is Jemperli (dostarlimab) and is used to treat a rare advanced breast cancer known as mismatch repair deficient (dMMR). It is indicated if the cancer has grown during or after treatment and if no other treatments are available. Less than 1 percent of breast cancer has the dMMR marker.[51]

Vaccines

Another approach to immunotherapy to watch out for is the use of vaccines to prevent recurrence. A surge of research on their use for different cancers has followed the success of COVID-19 vaccines using mRNA (the messenger molecule that carries a cell's instructions for making proteins). Currently there are several potential vaccines being studied alone or in combination with other drugs, including ones focused on HER2,[52] mammoglobin,[53] MUC1,[54] and α-lactalbumin[55] (see Chapter 11). Clinical trials in several different stages are underway to explore their effectiveness, but so far antitumor immunity has not lasted long enough to make any difference in survival.[56] You may want to investigate them once your primary treatment is done.

SURVIVORSHIP CARE PLAN

At the end of your treatment, both local and systemic, you should receive a succinct summary of the technical details (diagnosis, stage, drugs given/doses, radiation and doses, hormone therapy, recommendation for follow-up such as mammograms, and testing). It should include who will be following you, where, and when. You should review this carefully with your doctor or nurse so that you fully understand what you have been through. In addition, make sure that a copy is sent to your primary care physician so they have a record and can coordinate your care and what screening you may need five to ten years later when, hopefully, you will have forgotten all the details.

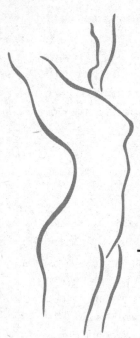

CHAPTER 16

Systemic Therapy: Lifestyle Changes and Complementary Treatments

Patients often ask me what they can do to boost their treatment and decrease the chance of recurrence. Frequently, they are thinking about such complementary treatments as acupuncture, meditation, or a particular diet or herb. These have their place in the overall healing, but there are other, equally important and better studied complementary tools: lifestyle changes. These can range from exercise, a wholesome diet, reduction of alcohol consumption, and a healthy weight. The only prerequisite is willpower. We use the word "complementary" here to highlight that these steps do not replace traditional treatments but improve upon them.

Most of the treatments discussed in the previous chapters are aimed at killing breast cancer cells. But as I explained in Chapter 3, we also have other tools to treat this disease. We can change the environment of the body or the neighborhood the cells live in. We are starting to understand what some of the more toxic environments look like, and how they can be changed. This knowledge is beginning to give scientific underpinnings to some of the lifestyle changes and complementary treatments that may have been dismissed in the past. Most have few or no side effects, and they often improve the quality of your life and prevent other diseases. I encourage all who have had breast cancer to consider these techniques and try to find ways to incorporate them into their new lives. Usually the lifestyle changes and complementary treatments can be combined with your medical treatments and then continued long afterward. Complementary medicine is often confused with so-called alternative medicine, but the two are very different. The Office of Cancer Complementary and Alternative Medicine (OCCAM) defines complementary medicine as any medical system, practice, or product not thought of as standard care but used along with standard medicine. Alternative medicine is a system, practice, or product that is used in place of standard treatments.

I think it's very important to be looking at lifestyle changes and complementary (not alternative) treatments if you have breast cancer. For all its limitations, Western medicine is still an important component of any successful effort to cure cancer or to put it into significant remission. At the same time, lifestyle changes are gaining more support as we find evidence of their ability to further improve outcomes.

LIFESTYLE CHANGES

There are many theories as to how lifestyle changes may affect breast cancer recurrence. In the past, most of the research has focused on hormone levels. Fat has aromatase and can make estrogen, so it was thought to feed many tumors.[1] Thus, weight loss can help by decreasing that excess estrogen. While this may well be true, the fact that obesity and physical inactivity also seem to be harmful in nonhormonal cancers like triple-negative suggests that an additional mechanism may be playing a role.

In an effort to find another explanation, Dr. Pamela Goodwin from Toronto has been exploring the relationship between insulin resistance and breast cancer. "Insulin resistance syndrome" is the term we use to talk about the condition in which the body makes high levels of insulin in an attempt to overcome the fact that the muscle and fat seem to be less sensitive to it than normal. This syndrome is associated with obesity, hypertension, and type 2 diabetes. In our overweight society it is thought to be present in 20 to 30 percent of the general population and 60 percent of obese individuals. Goodwin's study has been interesting for those of us concerned with breast cancer because it shows that nondiabetic women with high insulin levels (reflecting insulin resistance syndrome) have twice the risk of recurrence and three times the risk of death compared with women with low levels.[2] This may be one factor in the connection between obesity and breast cancer. Goodwin's clinical trial to see whether an insulin-lowering drug could improve outcomes in early breast cancer when added to chemotherapy recently concluded it could not.[3] Of course, insulin resistance can also be modified through weight loss.

The third related area that is attracting attention is chronic inflammation, which is increasingly seen as a component in the development of many cancers. Note I said inflammation, not infection. Infection is caused by an outside pathogen, while inflammation is a reaction in the body itself against harmful stimuli. This is a reflection of the immune system being in a hyperalert state all the time. It could be considered another factor in a destructive neighborhood, urging the mutated cancer cell on (see Chapter 3). Chronic inflammation has been shown to promote breast cancer cells in a petri dish in the lab. And blood markers of inflammation at the time of diagnosis have been linked to reduced survival in breast cancer patients.[4] We are studying whether we can detect evidence of chronic inflammation in ductal fluid from the breast before people get cancer.

Let's cut to the chase. What does this mean for you, the individual with breast cancer? What can you do with this information? To start with, there are a lot of observational data suggesting that obesity, low physical activity, a Western diet, and alcohol consumption may worsen breast cancer prognosis.[5]

Weight

Weight is a sore topic for most women, and as someone who struggled most of my life to maintain my weight, I am very sensitive to it. However, I have to tell you that the data increasingly indicate that being overweight increases the incidence both of postmenopausal hormone-positive breast cancer and premenopausal triple-negative breast cancer. In addition, overall, women who are obese when diagnosed with breast cancer have a third higher mortality than women of normal weight with comparable cancers and treatments, particularly if they were pre- and perimenopausal.[6] That doesn't mean that their mortality was 30 percent but rather that if, for example, the mortality of one group was 15 percent, then the obese individuals would have a mortality of 5 percent more, or

20 percent. This was demonstrated in one randomized controlled trial of women with positive nodes receiving chemotherapy, which showed that obese women had a 5 percent lower overall survival rate than others. This was true for both premenopausal and postmenopausal participants.[7] Amazing though it may seem, this difference is similar to the difference we see in many chemotherapy trials comparing different drugs, or comparing drugs to placebo, but weight loss has much more tolerable side effects than chemo. Whether this is related to hormone levels (fat can make estrogen after menopause), insulin resistance, or low-grade chronic inflammation is not clear.

"Gee, thanks," you say bitterly. But here you are with breast cancer now, and unless they've come up with a method of time travel, you can't go back and lose weight before you were diagnosed.

So the question arises, can weight loss—or gain—*now* make a difference? One study showed that in early-stage breast cancer, women who gained about seventeen pounds during their treatment had a higher risk of breast cancer recurrence, breast cancer death, and all causes of early mortality than did women who did not gain weight.[8] A few small studies have shown that increased physical activity and mild calorie restriction can help prevent weight gain during and after breast cancer treatment.[9]

"Great," you mutter, unpacified. Like many people, you've already gained weight from your medical treatments. Well, that doesn't have to continue. Dropping extra pounds can still make a difference in the long-term. Two large weight loss studies, LISA and SUCCESS-C, confirmed the beneficial effect of weight loss in disease-free survival and breast cancer outcomes. It is worth a try; you have nothing to lose but weight.

It doesn't actually matter what approach you take. It can be a commercial program or you can just cut back on high-calorie foods and increase exercise. It is probably better to begin slowly and team up with a buddy, but make it your goal to get your weight to a healthy level.

Physical Activity

Apart from helping with weight loss, physical activity has been shown to decrease the risk of developing breast cancer, decrease the side effects of treatment, and decrease the chance of recurrence! Several studies showed that consistently higher levels of physical activity before and after breast cancer diagnosis were linked to a lower risk of mortality from breast cancer.[10] One study lends even more support to this approach, showing that walking three to five hours a week at an average pace reduced the participants' recurrence risk by 6 percent. In another study,[11] an additional five metabolic equivalents (METs) an hour each week resulted in a 15 percent decrease in breast cancer mortality. (Five METs is what you'd get walking at 4 mph for an hour.) Most intervention trials of physical activity have been relatively short, with endpoints of quality of life, improved fitness, and increased weight loss rather than improved survival. Still, they have shown that physical activity is certainly feasible during and after breast cancer treatment and is associated with an improved quality of life, including decreased fatigue.[12]

This area of research is now focused on determining why exercise plays such a positive role. Interesting data is emerging that it has an effect on reducing inflammation and insulin resistance even when it does not cause weight loss. This is another area that is likely to yield new information over the next few years.[13]

There are many ways you can ramp up your physical activity, and a number of these can be fun. You can start a walking group with friends, dance, swim, or skate. If there's a sport you've thought of starting, this is a good time to do it. The key is to find something you will do and enjoy (or at the very least can tolerate) for a longer, healthier, and happier life.

You can even combine exercise and activism by participating in walks and other activities to promote breast cancer awareness. You can join a dragon boat team and train to participate with other survivors rowing a dragon boat. These are very popular in Canada, and they're catching on in the United States. In Boston there is a yearly swim against breast cancer. Further, and most relevant here, increased physical activity has been shown to decrease the symptoms of menopause and improve brain function.[14]

Diet

The effects of dietary change have been more difficult to prove, but there is some evidence that it can help. Two randomized clinical trials have explored the effects of certain diets after breast cancer diagnosis. The Women's Intervention Nutrition Study (WINS)[15] and Women's Healthy

Eating and Living (WHEL)[16] study looked at different populations and investigated different dietary patterns, both including the potential role of fat reduction. The WINS results were updated in late 2018 and showed that the deaths of women with hormone-negative breast cancers were reduced by up to 56 percent[17] when they followed a program to reduce their dietary fat intake. This suggests a lifestyle effect for those of you who are triple-negative. After a median of five-year follow-up, researchers saw a 9.2 percent reduction in fat calories and a six-pound reduction in weight. Recurrence was 24 percent lower in the group that changed their diet compared to the control group (9.8 percent versus 12.4 percent). It is not clear whether it was the weight loss (see the previous discussion) or the diet, but either way it is good news. The WHEL study, however, focused on vegetable and fruit intake, with either five or eight servings per day, and a reduction in dietary fat. The estrogen levels were lower in the eight-a-day group, probably due to the increased fiber. This study showed the positive effects of a diet high in fruits and vegetables with regular exercise—but proved that eight servings were no better than five.[18]

At this point we have the most data on the Mediterranean diet, which encourages an abundance of food from plants, moderate amounts of cheese and yogurt, weekly consumption of small to moderate amounts of fish and poultry, limited sweets and red meat, and low to moderate consumption of wine. This diet not only will help you lose or maintain your weight but has been shown to decrease mortality from many causes, of which breast cancer is only one.

The low-glycemic diet, or diabetes risk reduction diet, shares a lot of the same principles with the Mediterranean one. Crafted initially for breast cancer patients with type 2 diabetes, it entails lots of cereal fiber, coffee, nuts and fruit, and very few sugary drinks and juices, trans fats, and red meat. A study recently scored a cohort of 8,482 nurses on how many approved foods on the diet they consumed (vegetables were not included as part of the study because they were not associated with the risk of type 2 diabetes). Women who more strictly adhered to the low-glycemic diet had a 20 percent lower risk of breast cancer death and a 34 percent lower risk of death from any other cause compared to women who did not follow the diet.[19]

Whether or not you embrace either of these regimes, look for serious diets rather than any of the current trendy diet fads out there. A diet high in any fat or sugar—the usual baddies—is never "best for you," no matter how good it tastes. You don't need to give up all the goodies you enjoy, but you do need to limit their place in whatever food plan you embrace.[20]

If you decide to include a nutritional approach to your healing, you should work very closely with a nutritionist and your physician to create your particular diet and to coordinate it with your other treatments. Certain foods may be better to avoid or to consume during specific aspects of your medical treatments.

Overall I think that this is the simplest decision regarding breast cancer treatment. These are two things *you* can do to make a worthwhile difference that lies in your power. Not surprisingly, these recommendations are the same ones also suggested to improve the quality of your life and decrease the chronic diseases of aging.

Lately, I have been speaking out more in public forums about the need to increase physical activity. A Women of Color luncheon in Los Angeles gave me a great boost when an elderly woman, who had already been established as a forty-year survivor, stood up and testified that after her diagnosis she had gotten off the couch and started walking—and had not stopped yet!

Alcohol Consumption

The link between alcohol consumption and cancer has often been overlooked. I know, I've already warned you off sugar and fat and now I'm going after your wine. The American Society of Clinical Oncology has warned in an official statement that alcohol consumption is an established risk factor for several malignancies, among them breast cancer.[21] The increase of blood alcohol concentrations from drinking can affect biological and metabolical processes, and binge drinking also increases inflammation levels and insulin resistance—both believed to be key for the development of breast cancer.[22] Clinical studies so far, however, have been uneven when testing the connections between prediagnosis drinking and breast cancer, showing increases in risk, decreases in risk, and no effect. Researchers speculate that the type of alcohol imbibed as well as quantity may play a part in the mixed results, prompting a call for further investigation. In a global population-based study, the International Agency for

Research on Cancer placed breast cancer among alcohol-related cancers with the largest global numbers of new cases in 2020, at 98,000.[23] An older epidemiological study placed the increased breast cancer risk of even one daily drink at 7 percent,[24] which supports the American Cancer Society's updated stance that there is not truly any safe amount of alcohol. You can also approach alcohol as the Alcohol Research Group suggests in a recent campaign, "Drink less for your breasts."

COMPLEMENTARY THERAPIES

The Society for Integrative Oncology Guidelines Working Group updated their "Clinical Practice Guidelines on the Use of Integrative Therapies as Supportive Care in Patients Treated for Breast Cancer" in 2017.[25] They recommended music therapy, meditation, stress management, and yoga for anxiety and stress reduction. For depression and mood disorders they also include relaxation and massage. Meditation and yoga also are suggested to improve quality of life. Acupressure and acupuncture are recommended for reducing chemotherapy-induced nausea and vomiting. While many other interventions had weak or no research evidence for benefit, only one was likely to be harmful: acetyl-L-carnitine for the prevention of taxane-induced neuropathy. This set of guidelines is a milestone in integrative medicine and should encourage more research in the future.

Placebo Effect

Many techniques seem to work because of the placebo effect: your mind tells your body that it's getting a certain healing substance, and your body responds as though it were true. As Norman Cousins pointed out years ago in *Anatomy of an Illness*, the effect has worked throughout history— doctors once had some success with such "treatments" as bloodletting and administering powdered "unicorn horns." He calls the placebo "the doctor who resides within," who "translates the will to live into a physical reality."[26]

The application of this concept to cancer treatments was examined when Gisele Chvetzoff and Ian Tannock reviewed all the studies in oncology that included a placebo arm.[27] They found that placebos some-times help control symptoms such as pain and appetite but rarely bring about positive tumor response.

Although most of the following therapies have not been studied or have shown no effect on the survival in women with breast cancer, many have been shown to improve quality of life. For example, in 1989 Dr. David Spiegel from Stanford ran a support group for eighty-six patients with newly diagnosed metastatic breast cancer. For a year, the groups met weekly for ninety-minute sessions, focusing on enhancing social sup-port and encouraging the expression of disease-related emotion.[28] Much to everyone's surprise, the study showed an improvement in survival. However, it was a small study, which means that the result could well have been due to chance. Since then a large multicenter randomized study was done that demonstrated no survival benefit, although the dis-tress of many patients did lessen.[29] This study found that some patients, even in the placebo arm of the study, were helped with the control of symptoms such as pain and appetite that result from medical treatments, but their tumors were not affected. Although this was disappointing to the believers in the mind-body approach, it certainly does not discredit its ability to improve the quality of life, if not to lengthen it. There was one very promising study by investigators at Ohio State University, ex-amining whether stress reduction training has any effect on survival after breast cancer. The researchers randomized 227 breast cancer survivors to either a stress reduction program (three hours per month for twelve months) or to a usual care arm. After an eleven-year follow-up, they dis-covered that the participants who received the stress reduction training had 59 percent fewer breast-cancer-related deaths than those who only got usual care.[30] This was a small study, but the results are certainly in-triguing. Regardless of whether these results can be repeated in a larger randomized trial, there is certainly no downside in learning techniques or practicing lifestyle interventions that make you feel less stress.

Prayer

For centuries, people of all religions have believed in the power of prayer—and for some of them it seems to have worked. Estelle Disch, a Boston-area therapist and PhD who has worked with many cancer

patients, says: "If you're praying for health, on some level you're seeing yourself as healthy, and I believe that makes a difference." Faith in a
power that can make you well—whether that's God, your surgeon, or
your own will—can help you to get well. I often pray for my patients,
hoping to harness whatever forces I can to help them achieve the result
that is best for them. As with Spiegel's group, the initial small studies[31]
suggested a benefit for patients with various conditions, whereas a larger
study of patients undergoing coronary artery bypass surgery in six hospitals found that intercessory prayer had no effect on complication-free
recovery.[32] Does this mean those of you who believe in it should abandon
it? Absolutely not. In a time of crisis such as breast cancer, we all reach
for familiar approaches that may help. If prayer or having someone pray
for you gives you comfort and support, you should not let research findings stop you. If you don't find this approach helpful, the research suggests you don't need to start.

Meditation, Visualization, and Mindfulness

Meditation, visualization, and mindfulness are tools that have been very
helpful to survivors in dealing with stress, pain, and anxiety. But again,
they have not been shown to make a difference in survival. Meditation
has been an important part of almost every major religion in history.
Although there are many forms, the ones most commonly used in conjunction with healing work are variants of a very simple, basic one in which
the person sits in a comfortable position, eyes closed, focusing on the in-
haling and exhaling of breath, and chanting a mantra, a particular word
or phrase. The Eastern "om" is fine, but you can also use different language—"peace" or "health," for example, or a brief phrase from a prayer.

Dr. Herbert Benson, who has extensively studied various forms
of nonmedical healing, describes this particular form of meditation as
"the relaxation response," and it is the basis of his work as director of
the Benson-Henry Institute for Mind Body Medicine in Boston. He and
his colleagues run a number of groups for people with various diseases.
The technique creates physiological responses that contribute to stress
reduction.

Most programs that use meditation combine it with visualization,
or imagery. This too is an ancient technique, based on the belief that if

you create strong mental pictures of what you want, while affirming to yourself that you can and will get it, you can make virtually anything happen.

The pioneers of visualization in disease treatment were Carl and Stephanie Simonton, an oncologist and a psychologist. Their book *Getting Well Again* recounts their experiences with "exceptional cancer patients"— those who recover in spite of a negative prognosis—and maintains that their visualization techniques have significantly extended patients' lives.[33] However, no controlled studies have proved this. Studies *have* proved that visualization and meditation combined can reduce pain and the uncomfortable side effects of cancer treatments, which certainly makes them worth trying.[34]

Affirmations are similar to visualization and are often used in conjunction with it. They are statements affirming one's value and intentions, recited aloud if possible, mentally if not. One of my patients had a list of her favorites, which included "I am now renewing my body's ability to heal itself" and "I now let the light from above heal me with love." Others prefer to frame their affirmations in terms of choice: "I choose health." They should always be used positively rather than negatively— not "I will not stay sick" but "I am growing healthier each day." Affirmations can be repeated regularly and frequently. You can say them while taking your shower, walking to your car, or unloading your groceries. Dr. Susan Troyan, one of my surgical colleagues in Boston, has patients bring in positive sayings, which are then read during their surgery. She says that whether or not it helps healing, it gives patients a much-needed sense of control.

Mindfulness has been championed by my friend Ellen Langer, a psychology professor at Harvard, in her classic book *Mindfulness*. Several recent studies have supported the benefits of mindfulness stress reduction on side effects of treatment that lasted at least twelve months.[35]

Another study randomized "distressed" survivors of stage I–III breast cancer to either a mindfulness-based cancer recovery program or supportive expressive therapy (talking about your problems). Not surprisingly, the patients who received their preferred form of support between the two types did better than those who were randomized to their nonpreferred type of support. Most (55 percent) preferred the mindfulness cancer recovery program over the traditional support group.[36]

Laughter

Even simple laughter can be a healing tool. When Norman Cousins set about to cure himself of his neurological illness, he "discovered that ten minutes of genuine belly laughter had an anesthetic effect and would give me at least two hours of pain-free sleep."[37] There appears to be some medical basis for this: laughter can stimulate endorphins, chemicals that act like narcotics in the brain.

One of my patients with inflammatory breast cancer said, "I told people I wanted to laugh. Friends send me funny books, cut out cartoons, call me and say funny things." Though she eventually died from her cancer, her multileveled approach to fighting it gave her the strength she needed to live her life fully to the end—including helping launch the breast cancer political movement.

During my time in the hospital recovering from chemotherapy for my leukemia I enjoyed watching old *I Love Lucy* TV shows with my siblings. They really are funny!

Giving yourself time when you are not thinking about your cancer, just escaping into zany humor, can be emotionally healing. Be sure to pick the things that make you laugh heartily, whether it's a P. G. Wodehouse novel or the Marx Brothers or reruns of *Friends*.

Vitamins and Herbs

The increase in the use of vitamins and herbs, which are essentially unregulated by the U.S. Food and Drug Administration (FDA), has led to concern about safety and interactions with chemotherapy.[38] A 2019 review of supplements that should be *avoided* include garlic, ginseng, milk thistle, and St. John's wort. Grapefruit juice has also been found to interfere with some chemo drugs.[39] Other lists also include ginkgo, echinacea, soy, valerian, and kava. You can still eat garlic, soybeans, and grapefruit but avoid them in supplements while you're on chemotherapy.

A 2020 study on dietary supplements during chemotherapy found an increased risk of recurrence, and to a lesser extent death, with any antioxidant supplement before or during treatment. These include vitamins A, C, and E, α-carotene and β-carotene, and the antioxidant coenzyme Q10. Vitamin B12 used both before and during chemotherapy was significantly associated with poorer disease-free survival, and the use of iron was associated with recurrence.[40]

As a rule be wary of the claims of dietary supplements, as they do not always contain what they say. The National Center for Complementary and Integrative Health notes that the FDA has found prescription drugs, including anticoagulants and anticonvulsants, in products sold as dietary supplements. They also warn that "natural" does not always mean safe. The kava plant is a member of the pepper family, but taking kava supplements can cause liver disease. A 2018 investigation found that between 2007 and 2016 the FDA identified 746 supplements adulterated with pharmaceuticals such as steroids and erectile dysfunction drugs.[41]

Memorial Sloan Kettering's Cancer Center has a useful app called About Herbs that allows you to check on any herbal supplement you may be unsure about. It is compatible with most touch devices and provides comprehensive, objective information about herbs, botanicals, supplements, and complementary therapies.

A 2015 review[42] of complementary and alternative medicines (CAM) on cancer symptoms of women with breast cancer found ten studies that met their criteria. They found some support for the use of guarana (which is high in caffeine) and *Ganoderma lucidum* (reishi mushroom) to improve fatigue, and for the use of glutamine (an amino acid) to improve mouth sores. If you are going to try CAM, find a reliable practitioner to guide you, and check any specific herb or vitamin against the National Cancer Institute's listing and with your oncologist.

Acupuncture and Chinese Medicine

Some branches of complementary healing involve treatments such as the ancient Chinese science of acupuncture, which sees healing in terms of energy channels that run through the body. Special needles are inserted along these "meridians." Acupuncturists have worked with breast cancer patients, usually in conjunction with Western medical treatments. Numerous randomized trials have found that acupuncture can help to reduce hot flashes and muscle/joint aches in breast cancer survivors who take antiestrogen drugs, as well as fatigue, chemotherapy-induced nausea and vomiting, and postoperative pain. It can also improve psychoemotional quality of life (lower stress, anxiety, and depression scores) and lymphedema and chemotherapy-induced neuropathy. If you decide to try acupuncture, make sure to ask if the acupuncture practitioner is experienced in working with oncology patients and survivors. There are certain precautions that they need to be aware of before inserting needles into you. Experienced and oncology-trained acupuncturists are aware of these issues.

There have been several good studies on the benefits of Chinese medicinal herbs for the treatment of side effects from chemotherapy in breast cancer patients. The Cochrane Collaboration (a voluntary group that reviews the evidence behind many common treatments and procedures; see www.cochrane.org/reviews) found seven randomized studies involving 542 breast cancer patients addressing this question. These studies used six different herbal remedies to treat the side effects of chemotherapy. The studies compared the Chinese medicinal herbs in conjunction with chemotherapy versus chemotherapy alone. The results suggest that using Chinese herbs may improve blood counts, immune system functioning, and the overall quality of life.[43]

As with the use of any supplements, you need to find a practitioner who is not only knowledgeable in the use of these compounds but experienced in working with oncology patients and survivors. You'll want to ask them about their education and experience before you decide to work with them.

Homeopathy

A popular area of alternative medicine is homeopathy, a method of self-healing stimulated by very small doses of drugs that produce symptoms like those of the disease being treated.

Eight controlled trials (seven placebo controlled and one trial against an active treatment) with a total of 664 participants were reviewed by the Cochrane Collaboration. Three studies concerned the side effects of chemotherapy, three studied the side effects of radiation therapy, and two focused on menopausal symptoms associated with breast cancer treatment. Of these, two well-designed studies have shown that homeopathy can work better than standard therapy for the side effects of radiation or chemotherapy. One involved 254 participants and demonstrated benefits from calendula ointment in the prevention of radiotherapy-induced dermatitis (red, sore skin),[44] while the other, with 32 participants, demonstrated benefits from Traumeel S (a complex homeopathic medicine) over placebo as a mouthwash for chemotherapy-induced mouth soreness (stomatitis).[45] Other studies showed no benefit from the homeopathic remedy. One used Hyland's Menopause or a placebo and showed no difference in the hot flash score between the two.[46] Another hot flash study from Scotland showed no difference between individualized homeopathic remedies and placebo, although both groups saw some relief of symptoms.[47]

It is very encouraging seeing these randomized studies of homeopathy in the literature. Only through studies like these on both traditional and complementary therapies will we be able to figure out what works, what does not, and what can harm patients.

Mistletoe (Iscador)

Preparations from the European mistletoe are among the most prescribed drugs in cancer patients in several European countries.[48] Proponents claim that mistletoe extracts stimulate the immune system, improve survival, enhance quality of life, and reduce adverse effects of chemo and radiotherapy in cancer patients. The Cochrane Collaboration review found that there was not enough evidence to reach clear conclusions about the effects of mistletoe on any of these outcomes. Nevertheless, there is some evidence from two well-done studies that mistletoe extracts may offer benefits to quality of life during chemotherapy for breast cancer.

ALTERNATIVE TREATMENTS

Some therapies have been proposed to take the place of medical treatments, and several have gained more notoriety in popular books. Most of them have not been studied in any scientifically rigorous way, and their risks and complications are largely unknown. I mention them to be complete, but I don't endorse their use.

The best known is laetrile. It hasn't been shown to work in any randomized, controlled studies,[49] but it has a fair amount of nonscientific support. It's illegal in the United States and is currently being used in clinics in Mexico. It contains cyanide, and there have been reports of deaths from cyanide poisoning in patients taking laetrile.[50]

Stanislaw Burzynski has developed antineoplaston therapy, which is available at his clinic in Houston, Texas. Although there have been anecdotal reports on its efficacy on cancer, there is no scientific proof.[51]

Shark cartilage was very popular for a time as a cancer treatment, based on its antiangiogenic properties, but a study showed no benefit.[52]

CanCell is a remedy developed by James Sheridan in 1936, composed of common chemicals and apparently nontoxic. It has not been tested in a clinical trial.[53] Essiac, another popular herbal cancer alternative, is made up of burdock, turkey rhubarb, sorrel, and slippery elm. A retrospective study done in Canada showed no improvement in quality of life or mood in women with breast cancer who took this herbal remedy. Data[54] supporting its anticancer effects are lacking; it is illegal in Canada but available in health food stores in the United States. A study in 2004 used Flor-Essence (a variant of Essiac) in a rat model and showed that it promoted mammary tumor development.[55]

Because cancer is scary, there are always con artists looking to profit on that fear. If you have to pay large amounts of cash for a treatment not covered by insurance or travel outside the United States to receive it, your scam radar should be on high alert. Insurance does not like to cover treatments without high-level data confirming that they work, and centers outside the United States offering such treatments are probably not regulated.

RESEARCH

In researching this chapter, I have been impressed by how many good studies have been done on complementary and even alternative therapies. With the National Institute of Health's National Center for Complementary and Alternative Medicine up and running, there is financial support as well as interest in exploring these avenues of treatment. Many time-tested herbal and diet-based therapies are being studied for their abilities to induce or extend remission. For now, however, the absence of government regulation of supplements means that scores of unproved remedies or inadequate dosages of proved ones are on the shelves of pharmacies and grocery stores.

Many people go online for information on alternative and complementary healing as well as traditional medicine. This can be a good tool, but you need to know how to use it. Check a few things. Is the organization that is giving the information well-known? Can you tell who's sponsoring the site, and what their qualifications are? Is it for profit or not for profit? Is the information dated and referenced? Is there data for safety and efficacy, or just anecdotes? Remember that anyone can have a website. The website of the National Center for Complementary and Integrative Health at http://nccih.nih.gov is a good place to start. You can also check your local American Cancer Society division office, http://quackwatch.org, and https://integrativeoncology-essentials.com. They keep statements on these treatments that describe exactly what is involved, as well as discussing known risks, side effects, the opinion of the medical establishment, and any lawsuits that have been filed. Make sure you are really informed.

Though I am leery of using treatments that lack a medical component, this is a highly personal decision. What risks any of us will take for what reasons depends very much on who we are and what our values are.

When a particular cancer or stage of cancer has a bad prognosis, refusing traditional treatment isn't really much of a risk. When chemotherapy isn't likely to extend your life for any length of time, the discomfort may not be worth the slight chance of cure, and an alternative treatment may offer hope of survival and more comfort during the remainder of your life.

Having work that one is passionate about and wants to complete has kept many people alive longer and fully alive until the end. One of my patients, a forty-six-year-old woman whose cancer metastasized to her bone marrow, also did remarkably well for a time. A devout Catholic, she cherished the advice of a nun who told her to "work as though everything depended on you, and pray as though everything depended on God." She had surgery and hormone therapy, went on a macrobiotic diet, took a mind-body course at Beth Israel, and continued a regular meditation and visualization program. Whenever any church had a healing service, she went to it. She carried a rosary made of healing stones. She went to Lourdes. Though she ultimately died from her cancer, her health improved for a while. In spite of the cancer in her bones, she went mountain climbing and cross-country skiing—and dancing.

PART SIX

After Treatment

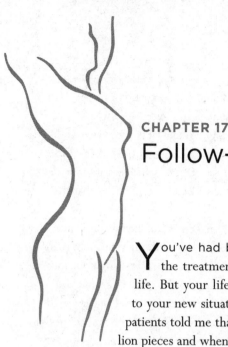

CHAPTER 17
Follow-Up

You've had breast cancer and you've finished the treatment; now it's time to get on with your life. But your life has changed, and you have to adjust to your new situation on a number of levels. One of my patients told me that "it's like your life breaks into a million pieces and when you put the pieces back together they don't quite fit exactly the same."

NEW FEELINGS, NEW FEARS

When you go back to your normal activities, you look fine and you expect to feel fine. Everybody's relieved that things are back to normal again—everybody but you. Physical problems that wouldn't have bothered you before now seem ominous. The slight headache that two years ago you would have dismissed as stress now leaves you wondering—has the cancer metastasized to your brain? And does the bruise on your arm mean you have leukemia? You're now in the "I can't trust my body" stage. Well, why should you trust your body? It betrayed you once, and you know it can do it again. Every time you go for a checkup and every time you get a blood test, you're terrified. As our medical advisor Dr. Stephanie Graff puts it, "Every broken fingernail feels like a cancer recurrence." In previous editions I said this "stage" lasts two to three years, but based on my own experience, a collection of Facebook posts, and people I've talked to, I no longer think that's accurate. Although cancer may not be at the top of your mind at every moment, it is always on your radar when a new ache or pain arises. This is normal. Now I believe that it becomes a part of you like every big experience in your life, but it no longer defines you.

However, if a fear of recurrence is taking over your life, don't be afraid to seek professional help. Many therapists specialize in people who have been treated for cancer, and you should ask your doctor or team for a referral. Sometimes the whole experience can't even be processed for a couple of years. Your reaction is not wrong or right; it is your own, and it usually changes over time. Like any trauma, processing the entire cancer experience tends to happen in starts and stops. Be gentle with yourself. The important thing to remember is that cancer is something that happened to you but it is not who you are.

Most people celebrate the end of treatment. You have been dealing with your cancer for six months or more, and although you may still need to take medicine (Herceptin or hormone blockers) for a lot longer, the main act is over. In fact, many treatment centers award you a diploma at the end of chemotherapy to mark the special occasion. It is thrilling to be done with treatment, but the finality of the occasion also tends to spark new and sometimes surprising fears. Your support network is there for you, but they too are getting on with life now that your treatment is over, and they aren't as intensely there as they were when your needs were primary parts of their lives. New worries arise: Will the cancer come back now that I am no longer being treated? (In this regard, taking Herceptin, Nolvadex, or an aromatase inhibitor may be reassuring—you're still in a treatment process for a while.) Whom do I call if something comes up? What symptoms should I look for? Who is going to follow my health now? Eventually you begin to get used to this new set of feelings, and your life begins to seem a little like it used to be.

And then, just when you are settling down and starting to forget about it, something pops up on Facebook, in the paper, or on the news about a risk factor or new treatment, and it all comes back. You start wondering if it was the alcohol you drank or the birth control pills you took (or whatever happens to be on today's "hit list") that caused your cancer. Or you regret the decisions you made, thinking, "If I'd known this back then, I might have done things differently."

But you need to remind yourself that what's past is past. You can't change the way you lived your life in the past based on new information just coming to light today. Accept that you probably got the best treatment that was available at the time you were diagnosed and that your decision was the right one at the time. If there are improved treatments now, that's wonderful—but you can't waste your energy on what might have been. Read the newspapers and keep informed if you're interested, but don't use it to torture yourself. Gradually you will regain your perspective.

Life will never be completely the same as it was before, but most people eventually stop living in terms of cancer. The fears and memories will come back occasionally—maybe at your checkups, maybe on the anniversary of your diagnosis, maybe when a friend has a recurrence. But they'll be part of your life, not the center of it.

As I was writing a previous edition, I posted a query on my Facebook page asking for comments about what to expect when you are living with a diagnosis of breast cancer. I expected that people would respond about specific symptoms, but most spoke to the emotional pressures and gave some excellent advice: "Expect the unexpected!" wrote one reader. "Every survivor I have met has such different experiences [that] it's so hard to prepare anybody for what to expect. For me the range of emotions I had surprised me . . . expect to discover new things about yourself physically and emotionally throughout the journey. Expect to be tired!!! I'm four years out and still tired."

Another wrote wryly, "I'd say expect to do battle at least internally with those dear folks who say things they think are helpful but are actually blaming the survivor for his or her breast cancer. Case in point— 'just be positive' or 'just have faith' sound supportive to one who hasn't faced the beast, but to the survivor this says 'If I'm not positive enough, or if I don't have enough faith, I'll fail myself and my loved ones.' Then there's, 'What did you do to yourself?' Implying it's your fault."

LONG-TERM FOLLOW-UP

A diagnosis of breast cancer means, for one thing, being medically followed for the rest of your life. Therefore the first thing you should do when you complete therapy is to ask your oncologist for a summary of your cancer and treatment to keep for your records. ASCO (American Society of Clinical Oncology) has templates you can use if you want. As fresh as everything is in your mind now, it will soon fade as you become used to life after your diagnosis of breast cancer. The care summary plus copies of your pathology report, a summary of your radiation therapy treatment if relevant, chemotherapy drugs and doses, and a copy of your operative note should then go into a file and be put in the safe or wherever you keep your important papers. Survivors need to have knowledge about what they were treated with, so they can remind their family doctor or tell any new doctor about it, and have medical records to show them. Further, these records can make a big difference to your own peace of mind. If you read that new long-term complications of treatment have been discovered or new research can predict certain outcomes—Did I get that drug? Was my tumor sensitive to estrogen?—you can quickly access the answer and either call your doctor if the answer suggests possible problems, or go back to not worrying.

While you are asking your oncologist for your care summary, ask also for a guide to your follow-up (ASCO has templates for this) so you know exactly what they plan in terms of scans and tests over the next few years. There is a great website, www.journeyforward.org, that helps survivors ask their physicians for a survivorship care plan and has online templates (following ASCO content) that can allow the provider to easily complete the treatment summary and survivorship care plan.

Current recommendations from the American Society of Clinical Oncology and American Cancer Society are as follows:[1]

1. Regular evaluations with a physical exam by someone experienced in monitoring people who have undergone breast cancer treatment and yearly mammography. Physical exams should be performed every three to six months for the first three years, and every six to twelve months for the next two years and then every year thereafter.
2. Genetic counseling referrals for women at high risk for familial breast cancer syndromes.
3. Annual mammograms for people who have undergone breast conservation, and on the intact breast for those who have had unilateral mastectomies.
4. Annual gynecological examinations for postmenopausal people on selective hormone therapies.
5. Follow-up for women with early-stage breast cancer (tumor smaller than five centimeters and fewer than four positive nodes), which can be transferred to a primary care doctor after

the first year, and allowing them to coordinate with the oncology team if needed.

6. Primary care clinicians should screen for other cancers as they would for patients in the general population.

Most importantly, they recommend against the use of blood tests, bone scans, chest X-rays, liver ultrasounds, pelvic ultrasounds, CT scans, PET scans, MRI, and/or tumor markers (CEA, CA 15-3, CA 27.29) in patients who do not have symptoms or findings on a physical exam. In other words, looking for recurrence on tests and finding it before there are symptoms has not been shown to make any difference in the outcome of the treatment. In this situation early detection does not change the treatment or the sensitivity of the disease to the treatment. And the best quality of life comes with thinking you are okay. So resist any doctors' efforts to scan and test you unless you have symptoms.

Although I agree with these recommendations, they focus only on finding cancer recurrences and new cancers. I think it is also important that those who have undergone treatment for breast cancer consult about the collateral damage of treatment (see Chapter 18). This can be trickier because it is neither in the purview of the primary care doctor nor that of the oncologist. As more and more people are surviving longer with breast cancers, it is becoming impossible and impractical for everyone to be followed by medical oncologists, surgeons, and radiation therapists. I certainly agree that your primary care doctor can most likely perform as well, but you should ask them first whether they are comfortable with that role.

Some cancer centers have follow-up programs in which patients are seen every three to six months for the first two to three years and every year after that. The program includes not just exams and mammograms but also physical therapy, nutritional counseling, psychosocial support, and involvement in research. Usually the oncologist and/or surgeon who did your primary treatment will follow your health at regular intervals for a period of time, but you may need to ask for referrals for help with the collateral damage from other palliative care specialists who focus on symptom management.

This care should involve addressing chronic treatment-related results of your therapy (such as fatigue, sexual dysfunction, "chemo brain," and pain syndromes) and monitoring for potential late treatment effects such as heart disease, lymphedema, and non–breast cancer malignancies (see Chapter 18). This collateral damage from treatment is not always acknowledged, and the treating doctors are often not the best ones to deal with this. Surgeons and radiation therapists, for example, are looking for lumps in the breast, mastectomy scar, or other breast. They check your neck and the area above the collarbone for lumps that may indicate an affected lymph node, and they feel under both arms. Medical oncologists are looking for recurrences elsewhere in your body. They will question you about how you're feeling. They ask to see whether you've had persistent and unusual pain in your legs or back, a persistent dry cough, or any of the other symptoms described at length in Chapter 19. None of these specialists is likely to have extensive experience in managing the chronic side effects of treatment.

And you yourself should be vigilant. If you have a new symptom that doesn't go away in a week or two, tell your doctor about it. Usually that's what most patients do anyway. One study found that a third of recurrences were manifested by the symptoms, a third were detected by physical exam, and a sixth were found by mammogram (for those of you mathematically inclined, the other one-sixth covers everything else).[2]

Patients are often surprised when their doctor doesn't find anything on their follow-up exam; they've been waiting for the cancer to pop up again and tend to be anxious about examinations. Some people start getting nervous days before these visits, and the visits themselves often trigger fears of recurrence. This is normal and is often referred to as "scanxiety" on social media and in support groups. However, if worry creeps in weeks before, further evaluation of how you are coping may be useful. You may want to consider seeing a counselor or getting some antianxiety medications. And certainly you should consider sharing your feelings with others in the same boat in a support group, in an online chat, or even just casually with a friend who has been through it.

Sometimes patients think their cancer doctors are also following their cholesterol and high blood pressure. This is usually not the case. In our segmented health care system, the oncologists are usually focused only on cancer. So don't neglect the rest of your health. Keep getting regular checkups from your primary care physician so any other health problems that emerge independent of your cancer can be dealt with.

Studies of a large group of breast cancer survivors by my oncologist colleague Dr. Patricia Ganz found that the age of the patient when they are followed up and the fact of having received adjuvant chemotherapy (versus other treatments) increased worry about a recurrence.[3] Younger people perceive themselves as having more to lose, and most people consider the use of chemotherapy a marker of more aggressive disease. Interestingly, the type of surgery did not seem to affect worry: people who underwent a mastectomy worried no more or less than those who had lumpectomy and radiation. This is surprising since many people say they have a mastectomy so that they won't worry!

Unfortunately the post-treatment worry seldom disappears. Although some people worry less as they put their treatment behind them, others experience constant concern. As one woman said, "Worry just comes with the territory." Unless it is disrupting your daily life and plans, this recurrence anxiety need not be treated with psychotherapy or antianxiety medication.

Not all symptoms that you will find over time mean your cancer has spread. Breast cancer treatment decreases the risk of breast cancer, but not colon or cervical cancer, so we still do screening. People who have had cancer are as likely as anyone else to get other diseases as they age. Having had cancer doesn't make one immune to arthritis or diabetes, for example. Furthermore, aside from ordinary, nonrelated problems as mentioned, patients may experience conditions that result from the cancer treatment, such as heart disease, leukemia, and osteoporosis (see Chapter 18). Your body also experiences physical changes as a direct result of your therapy. For instance, a breast that's been radiated undergoes a lot of changes. There will be a lumpy area under the scar and perhaps some skin firmness and/or puckering. By keeping track of this on a regular basis, the doctor can assure you that the changes you're experiencing are related to the treatment, not the disease itself—and if there's a different, more ominous change, the doctor can distinguish it from these others.

In addition to monitoring the treated breast, the doctor will examine your other breast yearly for the possible development of a new cancer, as women with cancer in one breast have an increased risk of getting it in the other. (See Chapter 12 for a discussion of the second primary cancer.) This is particularly important if you are a carrier of the BRCA 1 or BRCA 2 gene (see Chapter 4), and you may want to have an MRI in addition to your mammogram (see Chapter 7). High-risk MRI screening may also be indicated if you have dense breasts, were diagnosed before age 50, or have other conditions to bring your life-time risk to over 20 percent. In people who do not carry the gene, breast cancer in the other breast is less likely; the risk is about 1 percent per year, or an average of 15 percent over a lifetime.[4] In this latter situation an MRI is usually not done. Some types of breast cancer indicate a greater propensity for a second breast cancer to develop. Cancers with a lot of lobular carcinoma in situ (see Chapters 10 and 12) have been thought to fit into this category.[5] Even in this situation, however, the increased risk to the second breast is just 2 percent per year, a cumulative lifetime risk of 30 percent. And remember that women who take Nolvadex (tamoxifen) or an aromatase inhibitor have the added benefit of reducing their risk of contralateral breast cancers by 50 percent. Obviously the younger you are and the longer you live, the greater your chance of developing a second cancer.

In addition to your surgeon, your whole team may follow you; your radiation oncologist and/or your medical oncologist may also want to check on you regularly. Some patients find this overwhelming and don't want to spend all that time trekking back and forth to doctors. More typically, you'll be followed up by one of the members of the team, or even by your local family doctor, if they have experience with breast cancer. In a 1996 study, participants were randomized to be followed up by either their primary care doctor or a specialist. Interestingly, specialist care did not lead to earlier diagnosis of a recurrence, improved quality of life, or even lower anxiety levels.[6] Your HMO or insurance company may pay for only certain kinds of follow-up. But basically the choice is yours: don't worry about hurting your doctor's feelings. It's your feelings that matter now. Pick the doctor with whom you have the greatest rapport or in whom you have the greatest confidence. You can even find a new doctor after treatment if you have not been happy with your medical oncologist. You were probably in a hurry to get treatment underway when first diagnosed, but now you are picking someone for a long-term relationship and may want to shop around.

RECURRENCE

Of course what we are following up with you for is recurrence, which I discuss in Chapter 19. If you are looking at the statistical possibilities, it is important to remember that whatever happens to you is 100 percent. So if you read that 80 percent of people like you die at five years and you are alive at year six, you are still alive. That being said, since my own diagnosis with leukemia, I know I often sneak a peek at the statistics now and again just to see where I stand. The breast cancer statistics are a moving target as we identify the molecular subtypes, develop new therapies, and improve our abilities to treat metastatic disease.

Unlike some other cancers, with breast cancer we can't be sure that if it hasn't recurred within five years, it won't. However, as I mentioned in Chapter 11, recent studies show that women who have triple-negative breast cancers have their peak rate of recurrence at three years, while those with ER-positive tumors have theirs at four years. This means that if you make it to five years you have only a 2 to 3 percent per year chance of recurrence thereafter. The ER-positive cancers are usually slow growing, and some people with such cancers have had recurrences ten or even twenty years after the original diagnosis. It is likely that these later recurrences are related to the fact that those people have stopped taking hormone blockers, as well as changed their diet or other things that affect the local environment (neighborhood) around dormant cancer cells, causing them to wake up. In some ways this is similar to a chronic disease. You are never quite sure if or when it will come back. Time can affect the likelihood of recurrence—the longer you go without a recurrence, the less likely you are to have one. So going ten years without the cancer coming back should give you reason for optimism, if not certainty.

A paper from British Columbia[7] demonstrated this well. They compared the rates of recurrence in women with stage I–III breast cancer treated at two different times: 1986–1992 and 2004–2008. (See Figure 17.1.) Note that in Canada they have a single-party government-run health care system that allows them to easily access data. This is close to comparing the outcomes when the first edition of this book was written in 1990 with those in the last edition, published in 2015. They measured "relapse-free survival," which means the number of women who are still alive without any signs of recurrence of breast cancer at that time. As has been known, in the early group the women with HER2/neu breast cancer did the worst, regardless of whether they were ER-positive or ER-negative. It is important to point out that Herceptin did not exist at this time. In fact, the risk of relapse was highest in the first year or two

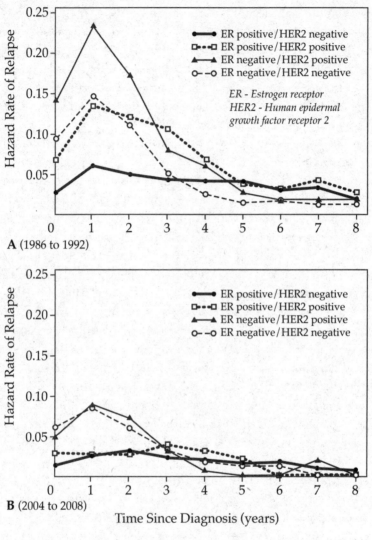

Figure 17.1

for both the HER2-positive women and the triple-negative women. Although there still is a higher risk of recurrence in the first two years, for these women in the second time period, it is now much lower. And the hormone-positive women are also doing better. It is not good enough but still an improvement.

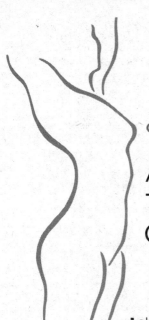

CHAPTER 18

After Breast Cancer Treatment: Living with Collateral Damage

I always knew intellectually that there were side effects from cancer treatment, but it took my own experience with the disease (leukemia) to fully understand what I call the collateral damage. You cannot undergo surgery, radiation, chemotherapy, hormone therapy, and targeted treatments and not pay a physical price. Yet when acting in the capacity of a physician, I often downplayed the extent of the collateral damage. My great revelation was that the doctors who treat you are comparing you to the people who died and are patting themselves on the back, metaphorically, because you are still alive. But patients like us are comparing ourselves to how we were before and we are acutely aware of the price we paid, both physically and emotionally.

Researchers and clinicians have become more and more aware of the issues of "survivors." I purposely put the term in quotation marks as I don't like using that word any more than I like the warrior or battle imagery used for those dealing with a cancer diagnosis. It implies that we have more control than we actually do. Yes, we can make the best decisions and get the best medical team we can, but we can't will a cure, and those who die of the disease are no less worthy than those who survived. Rather than a battle, it is more like surviving a natural disaster like an earthquake. You did not cause it, but you may have contributed to the collapse of your house by not having built it to code. And you then fix it as well as you can but it is never the same. I am not sure if my metaphor works, but it feels more accurate to me than the war one. The medical profession has to take ownership of the collateral damage that its treatments cause if we are ever going to reduce it.

When I got back to work after my own treatment, I decided we needed to document the collateral damage from the patient's perspective. There is increasing research on what is termed "patient-reported outcomes." Most of these studies report on how patients responded to questionnaires developed by physicians and researchers. Therefore, the questions focus on side effects and collateral damage that the researchers anticipate patients will have. Although these studies are not without merit, they risk missing some of the consequences of treatment experienced by patients that have escaped the doctor's notice. At the Dr. Susan Love Research Foundation, we decided to go straight to the people who received the treatment. We put out a call to survivors to visit a specific web page and tell us about the collateral damage of their treatment. We were overwhelmed with over three thousand responses in forty-eight hours. Not unexpectedly, some of the complaints and queries were about known consequences of treatment, whereas others were totally new.

This kind of research is critical because it is the first step to figuring out why some people experience certain problems after treatment such as "chemo brain" whereas others do not. Could it be that people with restless leg syndrome have more peripheral neuropathy? We won't know until we look at the whole person and not just the cancer.

In this chapter I hope to acknowledge some of the consequences of treatment that you may or may not experience and how best to manage them. I hope we will see more and more research in this area so stay tuned.

PHYSICAL ADJUSTMENTS

Long-Term Side Effects of Surgery and Radiation

In previous chapters I discussed some of the possible side effects of surgery including scarring, cellulitis, and pain, and I will talk further about the more chronic ones in this chapter. The most serious long-term effect of surgery on the lymph nodes is lymphedema, a swelling of the arm. Luckily this is much less common as physicians are moving to less axillary surgery (see Chapter 13), but it still can happen. Furthermore, it can appear years after the original surgery.

Unfortunately your body doesn't always feel the way it did before your cancer began. Radiation can cause delayed problems. A certain side effect can occur between three and six months after you've finished your treatment. The muscle that goes above and behind your breast, the pectoralis major muscle (see Figure 18.1), will get extremely sore, and it's worse if you grab it between your fingers. That's because the radiation caused inflammation of the muscle, and as it begins to regenerate, it can get sore and stiff, just as it would if you threw it out during strenuous exercise. Most people think it's the cancer spreading, especially since the radiation has been over for months and they're not expecting new side effects from it.

Other long-term problems may also result from the surgery. Although most people experience some pain in the weeks after surgery, especially after mastectomy, many will have pain for years. It can even begin years after the operation. Forty-nine percent of patients who have operations for breast cancer say they have some sort of ongoing pain or change in sensation, and 10 percent say it interferes with their daily lives.[1] The biggest complaint is "aching," but "stabbing," "shooting," "sharp," "tiring," and "throbbing" are other descriptions. They feel the pain in the

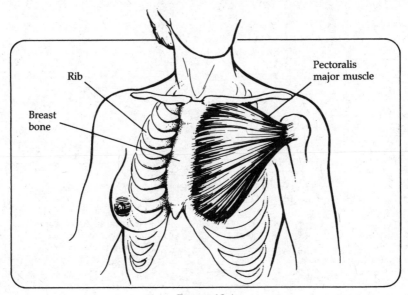

Figure 18.1

mastectomy scar, the arm, even the muscle under the breast. I've known a number of people with this problem, and it affects their lives. Approximately half of all patients undergoing mastectomy and breast reconstruction experience postoperative pain syndromes. There are treatments that can help. One option is myofascial release, a form of massage.[2] Another option recommended by some of my patients is acupuncture.

Lymphedema

As mentioned, the most serious long-term effect of surgery on the lymph nodes is lymphedema. As physicians move to less axillary surgery (see Chapter 13), it happens less, but it still occurs, sometimes years after the original surgery. Swelling of the arm and sometimes even the breast— lymphedema—results from lymph node removal (see Chapter 13). It can be so slight that you notice it only because your rings begin to feel too tight on your fingers, or so severe that your arm becomes huge, even

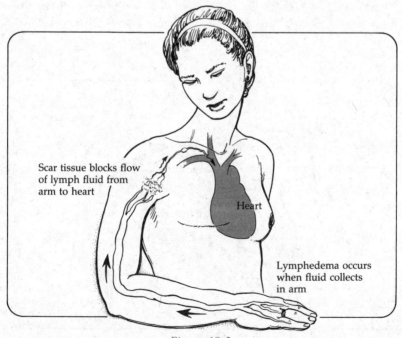

Scar tissue blocks flow of lymph fluid from arm to heart

Heart

Lymphedema occurs when fluid collects in arm

Figure 18.2

elephantine (Figure 18.2). It can be temporary or permanent. It can set in immediately or years after your operation. What causes it? Basically lymphedema—sometimes called milk arm—is a plumbing problem. Normally the lymph fluid is carried through the lymph vessels, passes through the lymph nodes, and is returned to the bloodstream near the heart. The lymph nodes act like a strainer, removing foreign material and bacteria. They also house specialized immune cells (see Chapter 3) that respond to any threats that arrive in the waste they cleanse.

So if you have surgery in the area and it scars over, some of the holes are blocked. The fluid doesn't drain as well as it needs to, and everything backs up and swells. Protein leaks into the tissue and then it scars, causing the condition to be chronic.

As I mentioned, the move to sentinel node surgery has decreased this problem. This condition used to be much more common—we'd see it in about 30 percent of cases—because more extensive surgery was done. In the past the treatment of choice had been the more intrusive axillary dissection, but studies revealed a higher rate of lymphedema with this approach than with the more limited sentinel node dissection. This fueled a transition to the latter option with less surgery. In addition to the amount of surgery, other studies noted age and obesity as the two biggest factors leading to more lymphedema.[3]

Most patients are cautioned about hand and arm care after surgery to help them prevent lymphedema from happening in the first place. These recommendations are hypothetical and are based on trying to prevent the production of excess lymph and blocked flow. In a twenty-year study[4] done by the late Dr. Jane Petrek, the only factors other than treatment that correlated with lymphedema were weight gain after surgery and arm/hand infection or injury. This is yet another reason to try to avoid weight gain. It's a good idea to watch out for infections in the affected arm and have them treated sooner rather than later.

One study showed that having women lift weights under supervision not only didn't cause an increase in lymphedema but actually decreased swelling, reduced symptoms, and increased strength.[5] Another study contradicted the common recommendation that all women who have had axillary surgery wear a compression garment in airplanes. In this study 145 of 287 breast cancer survivors without lymphedema were exposed to air travel, and there was no difference in the rates of either chronic or temporary lymphedema.[6] The blood pressure cuffs and syringes for blood samples used in routine medical care do not affect lymphedema, according to the American Society of Breast Surgeons. A review[7] of thirty so-called "risky" behaviors found sauna use to be the only one that held up as risky. In particular, aerobic exercise was found to be okay.

If you think you have swelling, find a lymphedema center or a physical therapist or doctor who has been trained in lymphedema treatment. The National Lymphedema Network (www.lymphnet.org) can help you locate one in your neighborhood. Physical therapy and exercise[8] can help in early cases. Complex decongestive therapy remains the standard of care for long-term treatment and has variable results.[9] Long support gloves, similar to the stockings used for varicose veins, although unattractive, can reduce the swelling. (Ask for class 2 [30–40 mmHg] or class 3 [40–50 mmHg] support.) And compression pumps that exert intermittent pressure have been used with some success.[10]

A newer surgical approach to bypass blockages is by microsurgery[11] as well as low-level laser therapy.[12] So far results have been encouraging, but the decrease in the extent of axillary surgery since the first edition of this book will surely do more to reduce the incidence of lymphedema than any of these treatments.

Frozen Shoulder

Many patients have a stiff or frozen shoulder a month after breast surgery. These arm and shoulder problems result from not moving your arm rather than anything done in the surgery. When your armpit hurts, it's natural to try to protect it by keeping your arm immobilized. But when you don't use your arm, your shoulder muscles grow weak and the tendons and ligaments tighten. You may have difficulty reaching and feel pain when you raise your hand above your head. Not using your arm for a long time may lead to frozen shoulder—the joint becomes locked. Frozen shoulder can be more difficult to treat than a stiff shoulder, and it sometimes requires surgery. Bear in mind, however, that arm and shoulder problems are not an inescapable consequence of the procedure. They can be prevented or reversed. Start with gentle exercises, like climbing the wall with your fingers and circling your arms as soon as you feel able (see Figure 13.14, page 368). The YWCA has a wonderful exercise program, Encore, that focuses on helping people recover. Swimming is also good because it doesn't put weight on the arm. Over time, you can resume any exercise routine you enjoyed in the past.

If exercising on your own isn't successful, a physical therapist can assess what you are capable of doing and where you need help and then devise a program to increase your strength and flexibility. The therapist will train you to do exercises properly so that you don't get hurt when you do them. Insurance plans often cover physical therapy after breast surgery, so be sure to ask.

Massage has effects similar to those of exercise. It can help relax tight tendons to get your shoulder back in commission. Acupuncture is another possibility. Although it has been tested for only a few applications in Western medicine, acupuncture hasn't been demonstrated to cause harm or cause lymphedema. There is some evidence it can help relieve lower back pain, so it may also help shoulder stiffness. However, there is no scientific data about this.

Scars

Scarring is an inevitable consequence of breast surgery, as it is for any type of surgery. Initially, many people are so intent on saving their lives that they don't think about how their bodies will look after therapy. Of course, the appearance of the scar depends not only on the extent of surgery but on your skin, your body type, the size of your breast, and the type of surgery you had. To avoid being surprised by your body's appearance after surgery, ask your doctor to show you pictures of people who have had a similar operation, do a little image research online, or read books on the subject. There are several things you can do to make the scar more acceptable to you, from working with the surgeon to prevent surprises to having plastic surgery.

After mastectomy, the incision can take more than a year to heal completely. It may be difficult to know whether a problem that arises is temporary or will be with you long-term. Either way, you should discuss problems that seem significant or unusual with your surgeon. It's also important to remember that you don't need to wait a year to have additional surgery or procedures to correct the problems.

The scar may be raised, seemingly filled with extra skin. This is a keloid scar and results from an overly aggressive effort by the body's immune system to heal the wound. The body keeps filling the scar with collagen long after the wound has closed. The tendency to form keloid scars is probably inherited and can't be prevented. If you know you have a tendency to get them, discuss surgery strategies with your team to minimize keloid formation. A plastic surgeon may be able to improve the scar's appearance. There is nothing wrong with being concerned about how you look. You've been through a very unpleasant and life-changing experience; you're entitled to do what you can to make its aftermath as comfortable as possible for yourself. Talk to a plastic surgeon about all the possibilities and decide what's best for you.

A mastectomy leaves a fairly large wound. When the surgeon pulls the skin and underlying tissue together to close it, the surface of the chest is drawn taut. In contrast, the surrounding tissue under the arm may seem baggy and excessive and hang over your bra. If fat is a major component of the extra tissue under the arm, it can be removed through liposuction. Excess skin can also be eliminated without increasing scarring.

Even a lumpectomy can change the appearance of the breast you've saved. It may look foreign and disturbing to you; it may have a dent, look shrunken, or appear to be pulled to one side.

If you are still troubled by the appearance of your breast months or years after surgery, you can always have a reconstructive procedure. A plastic surgeon can discuss various techniques to realign nipples, reshape breasts, and make the breasts more symmetrical (see Chapter 13).

Pain

Radiation and surgery can cause pain in the chest and arm. A meta-analysis of thirty studies found that women who underwent axillary lymph node dissection experienced a 21 percent increase in risk of chronic postoperative pain. This kind of pain tends to affect younger women who had radiation therapy and preoperative pain.[13]

Various long-term problems may also result from the surgery. Although most people experience some pain in the weeks after surgery, especially after mastectomy, many will have pain for years, which can even begin years after the operation.

A study from Helsinki reported that one year after breast cancer surgery, 50 percent of patients had mild pain and 16 percent had moderate to severe pain. The key predictors of pain at twelve months were chronic preoperative pain, preoperative pain in the area of the surgery, preoperative depression, lymph node dissection, chemotherapy, and radiotherapy.[14]

Pain can also be experienced in the arm after surgery. There are several causes for this. One is what has been termed an "axillary web." This consists of a visible web of axillary skin over a taut palpable cord of tissue, like a string, under the skin that can stretch to the inner elbow or even the wrist. It usually occurs within three months of axillary surgery. It is probably related to an inflamed lymphatic or vein.[15] Pain could also be related to nerve damage. A third cause of pain can be traced to shoulder mobility. It is best treated by a physical therapist, particularly one experienced with breast cancer patients.

From these studies it is clear that chronic pain is not unusual. It can include sensory loss or change, phantom sensations from a breast or nipple that is no longer present, or odd sensations and even pain in the absent breast. You can have pain and numbness in the axilla from damage to the intercostal brachial nerve as a result of an axillary dissection or, less commonly, a sentinel node biopsy (see Chapter 13). Finally, you can have neuroma pain, which occurs when a nerve is cut or injured. This pain may often be treated with an injection of long-acting local anesthetic.

This kind of pain isn't common and, as mentioned, has been treated with myofascial release, a form of massage.[16] Also my patients report that acupuncture has helped. Another study suggests that if the pain is caused by damaged nerves, antidepressants can relieve it; this has no relation to the patient's frame of mind but to the specific way such drugs work on nerves.[17] Most large hospitals have pain specialists on staff to consult with patients who experience long-term problems with treatment-related pain.

Cellulitis

Cellulitis is a skin infection occurring in places that have diminished access to the immune system, such as areas of swelling or areas that have been radiated. It can start from any small infection and rapidly spread, often with a red streak up the arm or redness of the arm and/or breast. Sometimes it can be accompanied by lymphedema. There is usually a fever as well. Although this type of infection can sometimes be treated with oral antibiotics, usually it requires hospitalization for intravenous drugs. Some people who are prone to recurrent attacks of cellulitis ask the doctor for a standing antibiotic prescription so they can start taking it at the first sign of impending infection.

OTHER LONG-TERM EFFECTS

In rare cases, as mentioned in Chapter 14, radiation can cause second cancers. This is usually a different kind of cancer, a sarcoma, and doesn't occur for at least five years after radiation therapy. Less than 5 percent of sarcomas are due to radiation exposure, according to the American Cancer Society. Our best guess is that for every one thousand five-year survivors of wide excision and radiation, about two will develop a radiation-induced sarcoma over the next ten years.

Lung cancer after radiation therapy for breast cancer is also a rare long-term effect and is associated with the dose received and a history of smoking.[18]

Another infrequent consequence of radiation is heart disease. In the old days, when radiation was less sophisticated, this was a possibility especially in people who had left-sided breast cancers. A long-term follow-up study demonstrated an increase in coronary events with increasing doses regardless of whether the participants had risks for heart disease.[19] Yet women who have received modern radiation therapy for breast conservation have shown a lower-than-expected (2.7 percent) increase in heart attack or coronary artery disease after ten years.[20] Newer techniques may have you lie on your stomach for radiation, allowing gravity to cause the breast to hang away from the heart.[21]

A large analysis of all the randomized studies of surgery and axillary dissection with and without radiation has shown a small increase in mortality in the radiated patients. Most of the studies were older, including women who received postmastectomy radiation that included the nodes under the breastbone. It was observed mostly in women surviving more than five to ten years from treatment, and particularly in women who were treated with less attention to sparing the heart. I am not surprised. My aunt was treated in the 1960s for a left-sided breast cancer with four positive nodes. She had the standard treatment of the day: a mastectomy and cobalt radiation therapy. She suffered acutely from difficulties swallowing that I now know were from treating the nodes under the breastbone. Years later she developed significant heart disease, requiring bypass surgery and ultimately left-sided lung cancer, from which she died in the early 1990s. She was also a smoker, which I am sure contributed; however, I am also sure that these problems stemmed in part from the radiation therapy. The real question is whether we would have had her around for the additional thirty years without it—and that we will never know.

LONG-TERM SIDE EFFECTS OF CHEMOTHERAPY

In the past, chemotherapy was used only to treat metastasis. Oncologists at that time weren't thinking about long-term effects; they hoped to keep patients living a few years longer than they would without the treatment. If they lived long enough to be concerned with long-term effects, they and their doctors were happy. Because we now do adjuvant chemotherapy in patients who we think have a higher chance of having undetectable microscopic spread of the disease, we are becoming more aware of the damage to healthy parts of the body that this toxic treatment causes. A person treated with chemotherapy may now live for many years if not a full lifetime, and the issues surrounding their long-term well-being are more important. Since my own experience with chemotherapy for my leukemia, I have been acutely aware of the price we pay for the cure.

"Chemo Brain"

In any group of breast cancer survivors someone is bound to mention "chemo brain," followed by the knowing smiles of their audience. Numerous people have shared this feeling that their brains just weren't working the same way as before their cancer and ensuing treatments. This change in memory, attention and focus, and ability to multitask has now been documented on cognitive tests as well as functional MRIs (MRI imaging done while the person performs certain mental tests or actions). This disconcerting collateral damage is not a product of our imagination and is finally getting researchers' attention.

At this point there seem to be more questions than answers. A recent study looked at patients after they'd had surgery but before they went through chemotherapy or hormone therapy. The researchers found that a small subgroup performed lower than expected as compared to healthy people in the control group and patients with noninvasive breast cancer. And, yes, they did also test participants for depression, anxiety, and fatigue, finding that these feelings were more common among the cancer patients than among the healthy people in the control group.[22] This brought up some interesting hypotheses about possible associations between low-grade inflammation and DNA repair problems (see Chapter 6), both of which are associated with the development of cancer as well as the development of neurocognitive disorders after surgery (see Chapter 13). However, in another study, one of my colleagues at UCLA, Dr. Patricia Ganz,[23] has shown that there was an increase in a pro-inflammatory marker in some patients, and this correlated with increased memory complaints and changes in brain metabolism. Throughout the year following chemotherapy, the levels of the cytokine decreased along with the memory complaints. This suggests an inflammatory cause of some of the brain problems. The question is which came first: Does the inflammatory environment stimulate cancer growth, and does brain dysfunction improve with treatment, or does the chemotherapy cause an inflammatory environment that manifests in part as "chemo brain"? These kinds of intriguing biological questions will help us understand not only what is going on but also how to prevent or treat it.

The fact that we can't identify the exact cause of "chemo brain" doesn't mean it isn't real. A meta-analysis[24] of studies on the subject concluded that cognitive impairment occurs reliably in women who have undergone adjuvant chemotherapy but that the degree of impairment tends to be mild. These impairments usually occur in attention, concentration, verbal and visual memory, and processing. A review of the studies, however, showed how different designs result in different degrees of cognitive impairment, depending on factors such as whether the researchers compared test results from before and after treatment, used tests that participants can improve on with practice or repeat application, and included women taking hormone therapies. In one study, for example, they compared the survivors as a group to healthy people in a control group. Although on the surface this may seem a good thing to do, it may miss subtle differences: Is this the result of the chemotherapy or of the premature menopause brought on by chemotherapy in younger patients? How do Nolvadex (tamoxifen) or aromatase inhibitors contribute to the changes? Is it because of depression over having breast cancer in the first place or the hot flashes and night sweats that prevent sleep and result from the premature menopause? Obviously this is an area that needs a lot more work.

Over the last decade "chemo brain" has been acknowledged as real and a lot more research is being devoted to studying it. Timothy Ahles[25] from Memorial Sloan Kettering suggests that there may be different patterns in different people. In some it is like fast-forwarding aging for a few years and then stabilizing the pace, while for others it accelerates aging but does not stabilize, and then for still others there is no immediate decline but evidence of decline years later.

Imaging studies revealed changes in the brain with decreases in white matter and gray matter.[26] Most importantly, two studies did functional MRIs before and after chemotherapy and demonstrated changes after treatment.[27]

Not surprisingly, "chemo brain" is related to the dose as demonstrated by a group in the Netherlands. They compared functional MRI and neurocognitive tests on patients who were, on average, eleven years from their chemotherapy. Some had received high-dose chemotherapy in the era when we thought that might be better, while the rest had a standard dose. They demonstrated that there was sustained cognitive decline in 10 percent of the patients who received high-dose chemotherapy, 8.3 percent of those who received the regular dose, and 6.7 percent of those who only got radiation therapy.[28]

Many doctors say "chemo brain" improves with time. I don't agree. As Ahles suggests, it probably varies in different people. Mostly I think you just get used to it and stop complaining. A long-term follow-up study from Germany looked at people who received the earliest chemotherapy used with breast cancer, CMF, more than twenty years earlier. And, indeed, when their performance on neuropsychological tests was compared to a random control group, they showed the same deficits that are described in patients immediately following treatment.[29]

This same group published a companion report of these patients that showed that among those who had received chemotherapy twenty years previously, the microstructural integrity of the brain's white matter had deteriorated with accumulating time since treatment.[30] And none of this even starts to address the consequences of being put into menopause either by chemotherapy or by the subsequent hormonal therapies.

What about patients who just take hormone therapy? We now have data on them as well. A study from China shows that premenopausal people who were taking Nolvadex (tamoxifen) had impairments in their decision-making function as well as in verbal memory tests and executive function.[31]

In another study from the United States, patients were studied six months after starting hormonal therapy with either Nolvadex (tamoxifen) or an aromatase inhibitor (see Chapter 15). The hormonal therapy affected language communication, as suggested by their answers to questions like "How often do you have difficulty thinking of the names of things?" and "How often do you have difficulty thinking of the words (other than names) for what you want to say?" This was most marked in patients who had been on hormone replacement therapy before their diagnosis.[32]

This should not come as a surprise to anyone who has gone through menopause or any large hormonal shift. Does anyone's brain work right during puberty or postpartum, much less during perimenopause? Mine certainly didn't! Sudden menopause brings on hot flashes, night sweats, and difficulty in sleeping, all of which can affect your brain.

With all this data for why those who undergo chemotherapy experience chemo brain—or cancer-associated cognitive dysfunction—there is no question that it is real. Although most of the research on "chemo and/or hormone brain" has been to describe it, a few studies are looking at how to make it better. One that we recruited participants for through our Research Army suggests that the use of a computerized cognitive training program would improve cognitive function even in long-term survivors.[33] Certainly tools to help cue your memory are helpful, as are electronic devices to remind you of appointments and important dates, help you avoid losing things, and enable you to make lists.

Other studies have shown that cognitive behavioral therapy as well as meditation, yoga, and exercise can help with these symptoms.[34] A study[35] from Dr. Patricia Ganz at UCLA showed that an immediate cognitive rehabilitation program improved both self-reported cognitive complaints and objective memory tests that persisted for at least two months. This area of cognitive rehab is in its infancy, but at least researchers are paying attention and starting to focus on this issue, which plagues many people after breast cancer treatment.

In addition, there is a suggestion that drugs used for attention deficit disorder (ADD) (methylphenidate; brand names are Concerta and Ritalin), Alzheimer's (donepezil; brand name Aricept), and sleep disorders (Modafinil; brand name Provigil)[36] may help, although I haven't found any direct scientific trials demonstrating their benefits.

Luckily this is an area of increasing research and more information will not be long in coming.

Heart Disease

Almost all the treatments used for breast cancer have the potential to damage the heart. As we mentioned earlier in this chapter, local therapy with radiation therapy (particularly on the left side) can increase the incidence of heart disease. Chemotherapy as well as targeted treatments like Herceptin can also cause heart disease, as does drug-induced menopause; Nolvadex, however, lowers cholesterol and may help reduce heart disease.

The anthracyclines (doxorubicin, epirubicin) used in chemotherapy have been shown to increase heart failure or cardiomyopathy. It can start as soon as a year after treatment or much later. Although it is particularly related to the dose, other risk factors are also important, such as age, risk factors for heart disease, prior radiation dose, and coexisting drug therapy.[37]

Herceptin (trastuzumab), which is given to women with HER2/neu-positive cancers, is also associated with cardiac problems, especially when given with anthracyclines like Adriamycin (doxorubicin). Although this sounds ominous, one large Danish study comparing long-term effects on women who had chemotherapy plus Herceptin (trastuzumab) to those on a group with only chemotherapy found the difference was small. After nine years of follow-up, the cumulative incidence of heart failure in the Herceptin group was 3.3 percent, compared to 1.3 percent in the group with chemotherapy alone.[38] Now that oncologists are using fewer anthracyclines in combination with Herceptin, this difference is expected to be smaller still. The newer anti-HER2 drugs such as Tykerb (lapatinib) have not shown cardiac toxicity, and a review of seven studies on Perjeta (pertuzumab) revealed a low rate of heart problems: eight patients in one thousand with Perjeta compared to four in the placebo group.[39]

Second Cancers

Chemotherapy such as Adriamycin (doxorubicin) or Cytoxan (cyclophosphamide) have been shown to increase the chances of getting leukemia, although the rates are low—0.21 to 1.01 percent.[40]

We had worried that giving granulocyte colony-stimulating factor (GCSF) to boost blood counts during chemotherapy would increase leukemia, but so far the data has not supported that fear.[41]

Ultimately it seems that, compared to the normal population, there is an increased rate of MDS (myelodysplastic syndrome, or pre-leukemia) and AML (acute myeloid leukemia) in breast cancer patients under age 65, those treated with radiation, and those treated with radiation and chemotherapy, but the incidence is low.[42]

Finally, there are the second cancers from hormonal therapy, principally Nolvadex (tamoxifen), which increases the risk of uterine cancer for at least five years.[43]

Fatigue

Many cancer survivors identify fatigue as the most frequent and distressing cancer-related symptom.[44] A subset of breast cancer survivors experience moderate to severe symptoms years after cancer treatment has ended.[45] For example, large prospective studies have found that 30 to 41 percent of breast cancer survivors report fatigue one to five years post-diagnosis.[46]

This fatigue is related to radiation therapy (see Chapters 14 and 16) as well as chemotherapy. The studies mentioned earlier linking both cancer and cancer treatment with inflammatory reactions show that these reactions could be responsible for some of the collateral damage, including fatigue. These interesting studies have found that there is an increase in blood markers of low-grade inflammation, which could be related to fatigue.[47] Another study from this group has shown a blunted hormonal stress reaction in survivors with chronic fatigue[48] as well as variations in the expression of inflammatory markers.[49] It is exciting to at last see biological explanations for many survivors' experiences.

With all this data on inflammation it's not surprising that several studies show that aerobic exercise decreases fatigue.[50] One large prospective study noted that participants who exercised four or more hours per week had 50 percent less fatigue. This may be easier said than done—the last thing you feel like doing when you're exhausted is exercise! But it's worth pushing yourself. Other interventions[51] that have been shown to help are psychosocial support and mindfulness[52] and mind-body practices including acupuncture,[53] meditation, and yoga.[54] All these have anti-inflammatory benefits and are a proven way to decrease all those inflammatory markers and decrease recurrence as well. What hasn't been shown to work are drugs that just mask the symptoms.[55]

Neuropathy and Other Pain

Having gone through chemotherapy myself, I am all too aware of the short- and long-term consequences of these drugs. They can cause painful peripheral neuropathies, most often described as symmetrical pain in your hands or feet, experienced as tingling, burning, and a painful numbness. However, they can also cause weakness and balance problems, which can disturb your gait. The taxanes (Taxotere, Abraxane), platinum-based drugs (Paraplatin, Platinol, Eloxatin), and Halaven have all been shown to cause temporary and sometimes permanent effects.[56]

There are a number of approaches[57] to treating this symptom, and the trick is to find the one that works for you with the least side effects. They include anticonvulsants (Neurontin, Pregabalin), antidepressants (Amitriptyline, Nortriptyline, Duloxetine), topical drugs (lidocaine patches or creams), narcotics, and acupuncture. If you suffer from persistent neuropathy and need treatment, ask to see either a neurologist or palliative care doctor. The latter are no longer only treating people at the end of life but moving up to be the experts in improving a patient's quality of life by managing pain and other distressing symptoms of a serious illness. Palliative care should be provided along with other medical treatments, giving symptom relief for people who will live a long time with the collateral damage of treatment.[58]

Arthralgias

Pain in the joints, or arthralgia, is the result of the increasing long-term use of aromatase inhibitors. Prime complaints are joint stiffness and pain in the hands (including fingers and wrists), arms, knees, ankles, hips, and back. In one study of women taking an aromatase inhibitor for at least three months, 47 percent reported joint pain and 44 percent reported joint stiffness.[59] Many people stop taking their drugs because of this pain, but it is important that you think about this step first. If you are suffering, my first suggestion is to ask your doctor how much benefit you are getting from taking the drugs. The benefit is directly related to your risk of recurrence (see Chapter 11). If your risk is low, the benefit will also be low, and the side effects may not be worth it. If, however, your risk is significant, then you might ask if you can switch to a different drug. There are several aromatase inhibitors including Arimidex (anastrozole), Femara (letrozole), and Aromasin (exemestane). Sometimes switching can help with the side effects. And you can always switch to Nolvadex (tamoxifen). Although the aromatase inhibitors have been shown to work a bit better, there is not a huge difference, and Nolvadex has a completely different mechanism of action and, therefore, different side effects.

The best way to deal with arthralgias is an exercise program. Again, it is counterintuitive, but exercising is anti-inflammatory and can actually improve the pain and stiffness.[60] Find something you actually enjoy and will do. The list of possibilities is long: water aerobics, swimming, yoga, or biking can give you a workout without pounding your joints. The key is to find something you will stick with. The local YMCA often has some good programs. Nonsteroidal anti-inflammatories work for some women, as does acupuncture.

Weight Gain

Although weight gain resulting from breast cancer treatment is less of a problem with modern therapies than it was in 1978 when first described, it still can be a problem.[61] It's more common in people who receive chemotherapy or ovarian suppression and are put into menopause. Most patients gain five to ten pounds, but some gain as much as fifty! Not surprisingly, weight gain seems to be higher in premenopausal patients who receive chemotherapy and are put into menopause.

Obviously it represents in part a change in metabolism; however, another culprit is decreased exercise.[62] Because data suggest that overweight people have a higher mortality than lean ones, this is another reason to take up exercise. We discussed the increasing data (see Chapter 16) on the effects of weight and physical inactivity, whether by increasing diabetes and insulin resistance, or by causing a state conducive to low-grade inflammation. All this makes me strongly suggest maintaining your weight at a healthy level after a breast cancer diagnosis. It is probably the most important thing you can do.

Bone Loss

Women with breast cancer tend to have low bone density. The problem is that the normal bone loss that occurs with aging is accelerated by chemotherapy and some of the current hormone therapies (by putting some patients into premature menopause), but others, notably Nolvadex (tamoxifen), help maintain bone by preventing its loss. At a minimum, women who have had breast cancer should follow the general recommendation from the National Osteoporosis Foundation: first bone density test at age 65 or at the end of therapy, and then again two years later to see whether the decrease in bone density is permanent. Bone does not change quickly, and the test itself is not that precise, so the current recommendations are to repeat a bone density test only after a minimum of two years.

Most fractures occur late in life, and there is no evidence that treating osteopenia (low bone density short of osteoporosis) reduces your chances of having one. The thinking is that by the time you reach age 65 we know whether your bone density has stabilized, and we can treat you if you indeed have osteoporosis. Although women who have been treated for breast cancer may accelerate this process and have a fracture at an earlier age, this has not been proved.

Some oncologists give bisphosphonates to postmenopausal patients who are taking adjuvant hormonal therapy or are in premature menopause. If you have bone loss, you may as well be taking a drug that improves breast cancer outcomes, however modestly. If you have a very high-risk disease it may be offered even without bone loss. Also remember that vitamin D and exercise are also great for bones, and you can combine them by a brisk fifteen-minute walk in the sunshine without sunscreen. Bisphosphonates may prevent bone loss, but there is no evidence suggesting that they help prevent fractures in women who do not already have osteoporosis.[63] If you decide to have a bone density test, be careful of falling into the trap of thinking that you should take a bisphosphonate if you have osteopenia; don't confuse bone density with fractures. These drugs are meant to treat fractures, not bone density. The trend is not to give drugs to women to prevent bone loss but to reserve them for those at high risk of fracture (5 to 10 percent) in the next five to ten years. All women should be taking calcium and vitamin D and getting enough weight-bearing exercise and weight training. Randomized clinical trial evidence supports the use of vitamin D supplements (400–800 IU/day) plus calcium to reduce fracture risk in older postmenopausal patients and those with low bone mineral density.[64] Some data suggest that bisphosphonates may reduce the risk of bone metastasis in patients who are past menopause or on ovarian suppression. The ZO-FAST study supported giving women on Femara (letrozole) an aromatase inhibitor, Zometa, which both preserved their bone density and improved disease-free survival.[65]

As mentioned in Chapter 15, one risk of bisphosphonates is the rare side effect of osteoporosis of the jaw.[66] This occurs when a woman has dental work while on these drugs. It is not yet known whether their use is worth it in patients whose ovaries are suppressed. The American Society of Clinical Oncologists does not recommend adjuvant Prolia (denosumab), a drug with a different mechanism but still with the potential for jaw problems, to prevent breast cancer recurrence.[67]

Menopausal Symptoms

Someone who has had a mastectomy but not/chemotherapy or Nolvadex (tamoxifen) may go into natural menopause right on cue. Or they could be thrown into menopause by a hysterectomy that includes oophorectomy (removal of ovaries) for bleeding or some other problem unrelated to their cancer. In these situations they will have the same symptoms as those who have not had breast cancer (which means symptoms can range from nonexistent to severe). The only difference is that the estrogen question looms larger for this patient than for someone who is not at any particular risk of breast cancer or recurrence.

A person also can be thrown into menopause by chemotherapy or ovarian suppression, or they may have been taking hormone replacement therapy only to have it abruptly discontinued. The symptoms that arise in these situations will be doubly hard to sort out, since chemotherapy, Nolvadex (tamoxifen), and aromatase inhibitors add their own side effects to the mix. Similarly, a patient may be prescribed Zoladex (goserelin), which creates a state of reversible menopause.

With natural menopause, the ovaries continue to produce hormones, albeit at a much lower level than before. Obviously a person who has gone through surgical menopause—removal of the ovaries—has no ovarian hormone production afterward, although the adrenal glands may produce some very small level of estrogen as well as testosterone and androstenedione, which are converted by fat, muscle, and breast tissue into estrogen by aromatase. With people who have chemical menopause, however, we don't know what happens: Does the chemotherapy destroy the ovaries so they never produce estrogen again? Or does it simply throw the person into regular menopause, so they get postmenopausal levels of hormone production? We do know that people around thirty who receive chemotherapy often go into temporary menopause and then get their periods back (see Chapters 11 and 15). This may mean that the chemicals don't totally wipe out the ovaries' capacity to produce hormones. But in a middle-aged person the chemicals simply push them in the direction they're already heading. Thus patients who are apparently thrown into permanent menopause may still have some ovarian hormone production. Or maybe some of them do and some don't. This is an area we still need to study more.

There are two aspects of menopause a person needs to consider. The first is that symptoms can come with a sudden or an erratic change in hormones. These symptoms, as I explained in Chapter 1, are usually transient, lasting for two to three years on average. If they occur, they need to be treated specifically, and there is a large menu of options.

The second is the way menopause is often portrayed by the media and the pharmaceutical companies—as the cause of diseases that occur in later life, such as dementia and osteoporosis. There are several global approaches to these problems, and there are specific remedies for specific symptoms and preventing specific diseases. Before I launch into an analysis of the pros and cons of the options, however, I think it is important to point out that doing nothing is an acceptable choice. Unless you have symptoms that bother you, you don't have to "treat" or "manage" menopause, which is a natural phase of every woman's life.

Hormone Replacement Risk

As I explained at length in Chapter 6, the data are pretty compelling that taking hormone replacement therapy (HRT) increases the risk of breast cancer. This alone should be enough to cross it off the list as an option for someone who already has the disease.[68] Studies have added further data leading to the conclusion that such patients should never use HRT. The HABITS trial began in 1997 to recruit volunteers willing to help investigate whether a two-year HRT treatment for menopausal symptoms was safe in patients with a previously treated breast cancer.[69] Participants with in situ breast cancer up to stage II were eligible if they had menopausal symptoms for which they felt they needed treatment, whether or not they were on Nolvadex (tamoxifen) (21 percent). A total of 434 participants were randomized, and 345 had at least one follow-up. After a mean follow-up of 2.1 years, 26 participants in the HRT group and 7 in the non-HRT group had a new breast cancer. Because of this, the researchers stopped the trial and announced that HRT posed an unacceptable risk to people with breast cancer. Of the participants with a new cancer in the non-HRT group, two had been taking HRT on their own. (This, by the way, was unfair: if you are part of a study group and decide not to abide by its rules, you should always let them know and leave the study.)

A more recent treatment for menopausal symptoms is bioidentical hormones—hormones identical to the ones your own body makes when it is premenopausal. Since the last edition, the U.S. Food and Drug Administration (FDA) has approved a drug called estradiol and a combination of estradiol/progesterone for treatment of hormonal symptoms.

But be aware that if a product is labeled as a *compounded* bioidentical hormone, it is not the same thing. At this writing, the FDA has warned against these compounded hormones, which have not been tested in rigorous clinical trials, are not subject to government regulations, and may have dangerous side effects.

A large 2019 meta-analysis of menopausal hormone therapy concluded that every type of this kind of therapy, except vaginal estrogens, was associated with some breast cancer risk, which increased steadily with use. In comparing patients taking five years of hormone therapy with estrogen alone and five years with estrogen and progestogen (a synthetic progesterone), researchers found increased risk with the latter group. The addition of a daily progestogen increases the risk of breast cancer from one in two hundred users to one in fifty users.[70]

As we saw in Chapter 5, women with high levels of their own hormones—estrogen and testosterone—are at greater breast cancer risk. An abstract by a group at Northwestern indirectly implicated the body's own progesterone.[71] Researchers measured salivary levels of progesterone and breast tissue density (a strong risk factor for breast cancer mentioned in Chapter 6) over six months. Only the women on Nolvadex (tamoxifen) who had an increase in progesterone had an increase in breast density. I should point out that the PEPI study on the effects of estrogen and progestin on heart disease in postmenopausal people also showed increased breast density in the women on natural progesterone.[72] Indeed, the mere fact that people who go through menopause late have a higher risk of breast cancer should suggest that even your own hormones are not all that good for you after a while. So the fact that we don't yet have any extensive data on bioidentical hormones does not mean they are safe. A review of early versions of these hormones, with estriol and bioidentical formulations of estrogen (Triest), confirmed that estriol causes endometrial stimulation, just as HRT does, and that it stimulates breast cancers to grow (6 of 24 women).[73] In 2017 the FDA approved a reformulated version with progesterone as the first bioidentical hormone therapy.[74] It is very likely not the type of hormones that you are taking but the fact that you are taking "replacement" hormones at all that puts you back in premenopausal range.

In 2022 the U.S. Preventive Services Task Force reviewed the evidence once again regarding the use of menopausal hormonal therapy to prevent chronic diseases and found no benefit.[75]

Finally there is Livial (tibolone). This is a nonestrogenic drug available only outside the United States. Studies are investigating its use in breast cancer patients, but the Million Women Study, which looked at people in England on various forms of HRT, found that it too increased breast cancer risk as well as endometrial cancer.[76] A large randomized study of 2004 breast cancer patients reported that although the drug reduced bone loss and hot flashes, it also increased breast cancer recurrence.[77]

TREATMENT FOR SYMPTOMS

If HRT is out, what can you do for the menopausal symptoms brought prematurely by cancer therapy? As with normal menopause, most of the symptoms that cause discomfort come in the transition when your body is experiencing shifts in hormones. So treatments may not be needed for a long time.

Hot Flashes

A behavioral approach can help some people. For one thing, you can avoid triggers. These vary greatly among individual women, but you can soon figure out what yours are by keeping a daily hot flash diary. Spicy foods, alcohol, caffeine, stressful situations, and hot drinks are among the more common triggers. Once you've identified them, you can avoid them. Sleep in a cool room, wear wick-away pajamas, or use wick-away sheets so that the soggy sheets from night sweats don't wake you up. There are also cooling blankets, pillows, and mattress pads that help. Dress in cotton and in layers; practice paced-respiration exercises (deep, slow abdominal breathing); try acupuncture; or walk, swim, dance, or ride a bike every day for at least thirty minutes. If none of this helps, try vitamin E (800 milligrams)[78] or the herb black cohosh (Remifemin). If nothing helps symptoms, you can join or create a support group to help you deal with them. (See also "Healing the Mind" later in this chapter.)

The North Center Cancer Treatment Group (NCCTG) at the Mayo Clinic is at the forefront of research on menopausal symptom relief in people who have had breast cancer.[79] It has studied more than 650 women with breast cancer and reported a number of findings. First, researchers found that a placebo alone appeared to cause a 20 to 25 percent reduction of symptoms in four weeks. This may show a psychological component to hot flashes or it may reflect the nature of hot flashes: they tend to come and go on their own. My own example is fairly common and serves to illustrate the capricious nature of hot flashes. I had ten and a half weeks of horrible hot flashes and no period. "This is it," I thought. "These things will go on for a few years, my periods will stop, and—if I don't end up in an insane asylum first—so will the hot flashes." All of a sudden, on a Sunday while I was at a medical convention in Atlanta, the hot flashes stopped, and I found myself wondering what had happened. I'm sure if I had been started on a new treatment or had been on a placebo in a study, I would have thought happily, "I'm not in the placebo group, and this blessed treatment works!" Because this wasn't the case, I just whispered a prayer of devout gratitude to my guardian angel. Four weeks later, my period was back, and of course that was why the flashes had stopped.

A review of all nonhormonal therapies for hot flashes found data supporting the efficacy of antidepressants (SSRIs and SNRIs), clonidine (an antihypertensive drug), and gabapentin (an antiseizure drug) in reducing the frequency and severity of hot flashes.[80] Of the antidepressants, Effexor (venlafaxine) is the most promising while Paxil (paroxetine) and Prozac (fluoxetine) interfere with Nolvadex (tamoxifen). These are all drugs with the potential of side effects; however, they also often work on pain from peripheral neuropathy and so may be worth trying. It may take a few tries to figure out what works for you. Another option is Ditropan XL (oxybutynin), a drug initially approved for overactive bladders that patients discovered reduced their sweating considerably. A subsequent clinical trial proved its effectiveness with hot flashes, even among breast cancer survivors on antiestrogens.[81] If hot flashes are a serious problem for you, you should talk to your doctor, who will help you sort through the options to find something that works.

Libido and Vaginal Dryness

Sexual problems are very common in women who have been treated for breast cancer. In one study when participants were questioned, 96 percent reported at least one problem. Study participants reported decreased libido (64 percent), pain on intercourse (38 percent), lack of orgasm (44 percent), and problems with lubrication (42 percent).[82] And most of the participants did not discuss these issues with their doctors. Needless to say, the type of treatment you have received also makes a difference. People who have undergone chemotherapy are 5.7 times as likely to report vaginal dryness, 5.5 times as likely to have pain during intercourse, 3 times as likely to have decreased libido, and 7.1 times as likely to have difficulty achieving orgasm than those who have not undergone such treatment. Although younger patients are more likely to have problems initially, they tend to get better over the next ten years.

Hormonal therapy with Nolvadex (tamoxifen) does not cause as many difficulties with sexuality, while the aromatase inhibitors increased vaginal dryness, pain on intercourse, and decreased libido.

The biggest culprit for sexual problems seems to be vaginal dryness, which leads to pain during intercourse and decrease in orgasms. There are a couple of initial options: vaginal moisturizers and vaginal lubricants. The moisturizers, like Replens, are better suited for dealing with chronic dryness or itching and are meant to be used on a daily basis. Lubricants, like Astroglide, are good to use prior to sex or the use of sex toys, and also before exercises like pelvic floor strengthening.

If these options don't work, then there are stronger treatments. The American College of Obstetricians and Gynecologists prefers to err on the side of caution in women with a history of breast cancer, suggesting nonhormonal approaches first. A nonestrogen vaginal tablet that helps is DHEA (prasterone; brand name Intrarosa), designed for postmenopausal people with severe vulvo-vaginal symptoms. A 2019 study examined its effects in participants with a history of breast cancer and found that although hormone concentrations did increase with use, they were still in the lower half of the postmenopausal range. Estrogen concentrations in participants taking aromatase inhibitors remained unchanged.[83]

Vaginal estrogens should be tried last, and only if you are unresponsive to nonhormonal remedies. The decision to use vaginal estrogen ought to be made in coordination with your oncologist so you can consider the risks and benefits. Vaginal estrogens require a prescription and may have some risk. The creams are absorbed into the bloodstream, especially if your vaginal tissues are inflamed. The safest are probably the slow-release type such as Estring, which lasts twelve weeks, or the tablet Vagifem.

If you have not had intercourse for a while, you may find that, along with dryness, your vagina can become tighter as it loses elasticity. A dilator can help with this by stretching things out again. Testosterone improves sexual desire only when combined with estrogen, and so is not an option.

Physical therapy, specifically pelvic floor physical therapy, has also proved to be effective in improved sexual function by restoring the tone and elasticity of vaginal muscles. Pelvic floor exercises can eliminate tension and strengthen atrophied muscles, and even improve bladder and bowel function.

The first step in getting help for sexual problems after breast cancer treatment is to ask! Some breast centers actually have specialists in sexual issues while others have clinics specifically to address these problems.

Insomnia and Mood Swings

Although insomnia is often related to night sweats, it is also true that you don't sleep as well when your hormones are awry. Some easy measures can help. Keep your bedroom cool, exercise (but earlier in the day; exercising right before going to bed will keep you awake), avoid caffeine and liquor, take warm baths or showers, and have cereal and milk products at bedtime. Also avoid screens at bedtime—phones and tablets emit a blue light that curbs the production of melatonin, the hormone that controls your sleep cycle. There is a link between insomnia and depression, so if you feel tired during the day and find it hard to fall asleep and stay asleep at night, you may want to speak to your doctor.

To counter mood swings and anxiety, which can also be brought on by hormonal changes, try using the relaxation response (see Chapter 16), exercising (including yoga), eating a plant-based rather than a meat-based diet, and some of the techniques of calming emotions described in the following section.

HEALING THE MIND

The experience of being treated for a potentially life-threatening disease is different for everyone. Having been there myself, I now understand how recovery is a process that continues for the rest of your life. What works for one person may well not be the best option for someone else. Here are some ideas, but the best healer of all is time.

Psychotherapy can be a tremendous tool at this time as it is whenever you experience great emotional stress. An experience like breast cancer can be the catalyst to encourage you to work on other issues that you have swept under the rug. Sometimes brief one-on-one counseling helps, particularly if you are finding it difficult to move on from the aftermath of your illness. About a quarter to a third of patients have post-treatment symptoms that warrant evaluation. Persistent feelings of sadness, loss of self-esteem, and lack of interest in things that brought you pleasure before you had cancer are *not* typical and should be followed up.

This may be the time to try a support group, especially if you were too overwhelmed to do it during therapy. Or you can join an online chat group, bulletin board, or mailing list. Check out www.breastcancer .org, Living Beyond Breast Cancer (www.lbbc.org), or the Young Survival Coalition (www.youngsurvival.org). If updating everyone on your progress is overwhelming, there is also CaringBridge (www.caringbridge .org/breast-cancer-support), a free online tool to streamline updates to family and friends and also to request help when needed—be it groceries, supplies, or moral support.

Many people keep a journal of their experiences to refer to later and to help them cope with their feelings. Or you can join others on Twitter at #bcsm (breast cancer social media) to connect with people who share your struggles and triumphs. Some people take their healing beyond themselves—reaching out to others who are going through what they've been through. Writer and poet Anne Boyer penned a 2020 Pulitzer Prize–winning book, *The Undying*, to chronicle her treatment for a highly aggressive triple-negative breast cancer. Authors Audre Lorde, Linda Ellerbee, Katherine Russell Rich, and Joan Lunden as well as performers like singer Melissa Etheridge and skater Peggy Fleming have spoken out or written about their experience. Indeed, much of the success we've had in battling the stigma attached to breast cancer comes from early pioneers such as Shirley Temple Black, Happy Rockefeller, and Rose Kushner, who fought publicly for greater recognition of and attention to the disease.

Often the need to "give back" and find a positive side to this experience can be channeled to helping other people with breast cancer. Sometimes this can be done through your work. Two of my patients are psychotherapists who now specialize in breast cancer therapy. Another did breast cancer workshops at her corporation. If you're a salesclerk, you may want to work in a store selling prostheses, since you now have a special understanding that may help your customers.

If your profession isn't one that can be adapted to some form of working with breast cancer, or if you don't feel drawn toward spending your work life dealing with the disease, you can still help other people—and thus yourself—on a volunteer basis. For example, you may want to get involved with Reach to Recovery or a similar group that works with breast cancer patients. You know how frightened you were when you were first diagnosed. The presence of someone who's survived the disease can be enormously reassuring to a newly diagnosed person.

You can also become involved in political action, possibly with the National Breast Cancer Coalition (www.stopbreastcancer.org). You can define the level of your participation according to your own energy, time constraints, and degree of commitment: anything from writing an occasional letter to your congressperson to organizing demonstrations and fund-raising events. Jane Reese-Coulbourne, a former NBCC vice president, found that in her own experience political activism was "a very good way to channel anger at the fact that you've had this disease. For me, it was the next step after a support group. Talking about it with other women was important, but I wanted to do something about it."

You may want to run or walk in one of the many athletic events that take place to fund breast cancer research and support. Although I think the "pinking" of October may be overdone, it has achieved enormous awareness of the disease.

And you can join us at the Dr. Susan Love Research Foundation (www.drsusanloveresearch.org) in our research to document the collateral damage of treatment and find the causes of the disease. Our Love Research Army (formerly the Army of Women and 375,000 strong) consists of people with and without breast cancer who are willing to participate in research. Scientists come to us with their studies and we review them and make sure they are worthy of your attention. Then we email out to all the members of the Research Army the details of the study, encouraging them to spread it as widely as possible. We have successfully recruited for many studies and are accelerating research. The Health of Women Study (www.healthofwomenstudy .org) is our online cohort that asks participants to fill out periodic questionnaires to try to figure out what causes breast cancer as well as to document the collateral damage of treatment. And we do our own research in areas that others have ignored, such as whether bacteria or viruses could be involved in causing breast cancer development or mapping the anatomy of the breast ducts. If you want to be involved in research to end this disease, then we want you!

Finally, make sure you don't feel ashamed of what you've been through. Cancer still carries a stigma in some parts of our culture, and breast cancer can have especially difficult associations. You need to demystify it to yourself and to others. You don't have to dwell on it, but it's not a good idea to repress it either. You need to have friends you can talk freely to about your disease and your feelings about it; you need to know you can include it in casual conversation, that you don't have to avoid saying, "Oh, yes, that was around the time I was in the hospital for my mastectomy."

One of the newest areas of survivorship research is called *benefit finding*. As usual, it takes doctors and researchers a while to catch up to what the patients have known all along—that there are many positive things that you can take from this experience. I often hear people say that while they would not wish cancer on anyone, they find themselves living more fully: they "don't sweat the small stuff," they cherish their families, and they truly value each day.

RELATIONSHIPS AND SEX

As noted earlier in the section on libido, one of the least discussed subjects about life after breast cancer is sexuality. From your surgeon to your physician, they won't bring it up if you don't; in fact, most caregivers will assume that if you're not complaining, everything must be fine. Yet most people find sex hard to talk about—especially when it concerns feelings, perhaps only half recognized, about losing both their sexual attractiveness and their libido when they lose a part of their bodies so strongly associated with sexuality. Doctors need to learn how to open the subject delicately, in a way that doesn't feel intrusive to the patient but communicates that they have a safe place to discuss sexuality concerns. I remember one surgeon who had referred a patient to me on his retirement. He said that after her mastectomy she had surprised everyone with her rapid recovery and exclaimed over how well she had "dealt with it." I took over the case, and in my first conversation with her I found out that, however well adjusted she seemed on the surface, she had not yet looked at her scar—and this was five years after the operation. She had never resumed sex with her husband and even dressed and undressed in the closet so he couldn't see her.

Many people have difficulties with sex and intimacy following a breast cancer diagnosis. Aside from feeling that your body has betrayed you, there can be a feeling of invasion from the treatments. All these strangers have been poking and prodding you for weeks, you may almost feel violated, and you forget that your body can provide you with pleasure. It takes a while to feel good and in control of your body again. You need to communicate these feelings to your partner so they can help you in your healing.

Some people find that after surgery, whether mastectomy or lumpectomy, a sexual relationship becomes even more important in helping them regain their sense of worth and wholeness. There may, however, be changes. One patient of mine who had had bilateral mastectomies felt that all the erotic sensations she had formerly had in her breasts had "moved south," and that her orgasms were doubly good. Other people miss the stimulation from a lost breast so much that they don't want their other breast touched during sex. Dr. Patricia Ganz, who has both worked with and studied the problems of women with breast cancer, talks about the problems people who have had lumpectomy and radiation may experience: "Especially with women who had radiation a number of years ago, they often find the breast isn't as soft and beautiful as it was before the radiation." These changes in the conserved breast can carry over into their sexual relationships.

Some of the changes may be more practical than emotional. Your arm or shoulder may not be as strong on the side of your surgery, and this can make certain positions more difficult during intercourse, such as kneeling above your partner. You may feel uncomfortable lying on the side of the surgery for many months. You should let your physician know so you can be referred to physical and exercise therapy. It is equally important that you communicate with your partner so that together you can explore new ways of lovemaking that you both enjoy.

Dr. Ganz adds that it's difficult to separate out the physiological and emotional aspects of libido loss. "Sex is at least partly in the brain," she says, "and the hormones circulating in the body affect the brain and thus sexual arousal. Psychological distress can affect hormones; we've found in our work that women who have a lot of psychological distress have more sexual dysfunction." This was demonstrated by a recent study from the Mayo Clinic using transdermal testosterone or placebo in breast cancer survivors experiencing low libido.[84] Interestingly both groups, those with and those without the testosterone, showed equal improvement in all the measures. This suggests a large placebo effect as well as the fact that sexual desire is complicated, with many factors involved.[85]

There are no aspects of sexual intimacy that cause cancer or increase the chance of recurrence. Nor can cancer be "caught" by sucking on a nipple. Barbara Kalinowski, clinical nurse specialist, who once co-led support groups with me at the Faulkner Breast Center in Boston, finds that "sometimes women who have had lumpectomy and radiation have a fantasy that the breast still has cancer in it, and don't want it fondled because they fear it will shake things up and send the cancer cells through the rest of the body." Even when your intellect knows such fears are groundless, your emotions may not, and that's bound to affect both partners' sexual pleasure.

Sheila Kitzinger in her book *Woman's Experience of Sex* writes that for some women, having a brief affair was an important part of their healing process.[86] They said it was all well and good for a partner of thirty-five years to still love them without a breast, but they needed confirmation of their sexual attractiveness to feel whole again. That may work for you, though it could also put a severe strain on your relationship. At the very least, however, you'll want to be in touch with whatever feelings you're having about sex and decide which ones to act on and which ones simply to fantasize about.

This brings up another issue. If you are single and dating, should you tell or not? Again, this is an individual decision. Some people will tell a prospective lover way in advance, preferring to have it out in the open before the moment of passion. Others will wait until the last instant when there is no turning back to disclose their secret (never a good idea). For the person who has had a small lumpectomy or has had mastectomy with a natural-looking reconstruction, the need to tell a casual lover about their situation may or may not arise. However, in a long-term relationship, it's important to be honest. For the person whose surgery leaves visible alteration, dating can be a matter of concern. Yet it doesn't mean you have to resign yourself to a life of celibacy. Barbara Kalinowski found that several women in her support groups were able to form new romantic relationships shortly after surgery. She recalls one woman who had never married and had a mastectomy with reconstruction in her fifties. "I got a call from her a couple of years ago. She was as giggly and happy as a teenager. 'Guess what!' she told me. 'I'm getting married!' They were planning a honeymoon in Paris and she was ecstatic." Another woman from one of Kalinowski's groups was happily married to a man who was wonderful to her during treatment. Two years later he died of a heart attack. Soon after his death she met a widower and they fell in love. "They decided not to wait," Kalinowski says, "because they both knew how chancy life was. She told me, 'We both learned that we don't want to wait for anything anymore.'"

Many people worry that their partner will be turned off by their condition and new body. There are many horror stories of partners who opt out of having sex or even walk out entirely. The impact of cancer can be as devastating to the partner as to the patient. Partners may feel angry, ashamed, and vulnerable to illness themselves. Their lives and dreams have been changed, but they typically get less support. They feel guilty complaining when they are not the ones undergoing treatment. Some people have problems dealing with serious illness, and others may use it as an excuse to get out of a relationship they thought was not working anyway. Most important is the quality of the relationship and the level of communication. Work by David Wellisch at UCLA indicates that the partner's involvement in the decision-making process, hospital visitation, early viewing of scars, and early resumption of sexual activity are important for couples to function optimally.[87] Open dialogue is critical in this process for couples of every sexual orientation and marital status.

Another study found that patients' and partners' levels of adjustment were significantly related; when one partner was experiencing difficulties in adjustment, the other was also likely to be having problems.[88] Difficulties in communication and sex need to be addressed promptly. Dr. Ganz found that most sexual issues were resolved by one year; if not, they were never resolved.[89] She conducted a randomized, controlled trial comparing a six-week psychological education group versus printed material for people who reported moderately severe problems in body image, sexual function, or partner communication. They found that the participants randomized to the education group had more improvements in relationship adjustment and increased satisfaction with sex than those in the group given only written material.[90]

Counseling or a group—where you can talk about your feelings in a protective environment—can be important in preventing serious problems. Hoping a situation will get better on its own rarely works and usually causes the problem to become chronic. You should request help for such problems as decreased libido and vaginal dryness; you may even consider seeing a sex therapist.

PREGNANCY

If you are still menstruating, a question that nearly always comes up is whether you should risk getting pregnant once you've had breast cancer. There are two areas to consider—the ethical implications and the health-related implications.

In the past doctors (usually male) tended to impose their own value judgments on patients and told them not to get pregnant for at least five years after having breast cancer. If you survived five years, they reasoned, there was a good chance you'd won your bout with breast cancer; otherwise, they didn't want you bringing a child you couldn't raise into the world.

This is a moral decision for the patient to make, not the doctor, and there are two equally valid ways of looking at it. Some people do not want to have a child they're not reasonably sure they'll be around to raise. Others feel that even if they do die in a few years, they'll still be able to give a child the love and care needed in the early years, and they want to pass on their genes before they die. Considerations of a partner's ability to nurture a child and support from family and friends will weigh on the decision as well.

Having a child is never a decision anyone can make lightly, and a life-threatening illness complicates it further. Think it through carefully and get the thoughts of people whose opinions you respect—and then make your decision.

The other question is medical. Can getting pregnant decrease your chances of surviving breast cancer? A large international review and analysis of thirty-nine studies on pregnancy after breast cancer showed that childbirth has no effect on long-term survival. Women who have had breast cancer are 60 percent less likely to get pregnant and tend to have smaller babies, but childbirth does not adversely affect their overall health. In addition, the review found that a pregnancy two to five years after chemotherapy was not associated with any additional risk of complications.[91]

If you have a tumor that is sensitive to hormones you may want to consider a "holiday" from your estrogen blockers in order to have a pregnancy. We have no data on whether this is safe or not. Again this is a conversation you need to have with your doctor and your partner.

If you get pregnant, how will your breasts react? If you've had a mastectomy, obviously nothing will happen on the chest area where your breast was, but your other breast will go through all the usual pregnancy changes I described in Chapter 1. If you've had lumpectomy and radiation, the nonradiated breast will probably go through the normal changes. Radiation damages some of the milk-producing parts of the breast, so the radiated breast, while it will grow somewhat larger, won't keep pace with the other breast and will produce little or no milk. You can nurse on only one side if you want. The problem with that is increased asymmetry, the milk-producing breast will grow and may stay larger after you finish breastfeeding. If you wish, you can have the larger breast reduced later through plastic surgery (see Chapter 1). One of my patients got pregnant shortly after finishing radiation treatments and successfully breastfed the baby. But one breast ended up twice as large as the other. Knowing she wanted another child, she decided to wait till after her next pregnancy to get the breast reduced.

It's probably a good idea to wait till a year or so after your treatment to get pregnant. It's a stressful process and you won't want to add morning sickness to the nausea you're likely to get from the chemicals.

However, I had a patient who inadvertently got pregnant right after finishing chemotherapy. After talking it over with her husband and her caregivers, she decided to have the baby; last I heard, mother and daughter were both doing fine.

We have been talking about having a child after breast cancer when you are still fertile, of course. I discussed this at length in Chapter 12, including newer research on transplanting ovarian tissue and using Nolvadex (tamoxifen) and Femara (letrozole) for in vitro fertilization (IVF). But the fact that we *can* do it does not mean it is safe to do. As the numbers of young people who are breast cancer survivors increase, we need more studies to answer these questions. (Two good places to research the latest information on this are www.livestrong.org and www.youngsurvival.org.)

The decision is up to you. If the stress of dealing with cancer and its uncertainties is too great, you may not want to have a child. However, if you do want to have a child and feel prepared for it, perhaps creating a new life can help you cope with the knowledge of mortality that a life-threatening illness carries with it—a reminder that death isn't the end.

INSURANCE AND GETTING A JOB

Unfortunately, medical and emotional problems aren't the only ones you'll have to face. A survey[92] of 1,592 cancer survivors indicated that one-third experienced financial and work-related difficulties. People with cancer often experience what amounts to discrimination, and there are some precautions you need to take.

First, of course, you don't want to let your insurance lapse. Your company can't drop your policy because of your illness, so you're safe on that score. But many insurance companies won't take on someone who's had a life-threatening illness, and others will take you on but exclude coverage in the area of your illness. If you change jobs and go from one company's coverage to another, you'll probably be all right (but make certain of this before you accept the new job). If you quit for a while, make sure you keep up your insurance on your own. It's costly, but not nearly as costly as having no coverage if you get a recurrence. Unfortunately, having insurance may not be enough as insured patients are paying more out of pocket for cancer care because of increased cost sharing.[93] Treatment decisions are not made with considerations of these expenses, which often lead people to skip medications or just not take them. If you are experiencing "financial toxicity," make sure you tell your health care team so they can help you navigate the options. In addition, investigate potential sources of assistance by nonprofits such as the Pink Fund (https://pink fund.org). Life insurance and disability insurance are also harder to get if you've had breast cancer. More and more cancer survivors are fighting to get this changed, and it should get better in the future. But for now, be very alert.

One of the hardest questions is whether to tell employers and coworkers about your cancer. There are pros and cons either way. Federal law prohibits federal employers, or employers who get federal grants or federal financial assistance, from discriminating against people with disabilities or anyone mistakenly thought to have a disability. The Americans with Disabilities Act (ADA), which was passed in 1992 and amended in 1994, extends this concept to the private sector. Any employer with fifteen or more employees is prohibited from discriminating against qualified applicants and employees because of any disability. Cancer and other diseases are considered disabilities under the terms of this legislation. The employer must also make reasonable accommodations to the disability; for example, if you have trouble reaching a high shelf because of pain from your mastectomy, your employer must make material accessible on a lower shelf, or even build you a lower shelf if feasible. However, a 2014 follow-up study showed that unemployment among survivors of breast cancer four years after diagnosis was both not voluntary and more likely if they had received chemotherapy.[94]

Many people fear that employers will find subtle ways to discriminate against them if their cancer is discovered. One of my fellow breast cancer activists tells a great story of how she handled the loss of her job after her mastectomy, before the ADA was passed. Furious, she stormed into her boss's office, reached into her dress, pulled out her prosthesis, and slapped it on his desk. As he gaped at her in horror, she snapped, "Sir, you are confused—I had a mastectomy, not a lobotomy!" Then she calmly walked out, leaving her boss to buzz his secretary and ask her to remove the prosthesis.

The other possibility is that your boss and coworkers will offer you increased support if you are open with them. More and more attention is being given to cancer survivors in the workplace, and you may find a career counseling center that can give you good advice.

If you are looking for a new job, there can be even more difficulty. Some companies are reluctant to hire a person with cancer. This too is illegal under the ADA, but there is always the fear that an employer will find some excuse not to hire you. You may want to be open about your cancer because you don't want to work for someone with that attitude. However, you may need the job too much to risk being turned down. But if you don't tell and then end up missing a lot of time for medical appointments or sickness, you could run into problems that might have been avoided if you'd been frank in the beginning. It's a tough dilemma, and there are no easy answers. (A good place for information is the National Coalition for Cancer Survivors, https://canceradvocacy.org.)

To quote one of my Facebook friends again: "All I can say is a new door opens and the old one closes. So expect a new perspective on life and living."

PART SEVEN

Recurrence of Breast Cancer

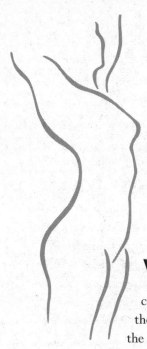

CHAPTER 19

When Cancer Comes Back

When I sat down to tackle this chapter I posted on one of the restricted metastatic breast cancer Facebook pages and asked what the members wished they had known or wanted to see in future editions of the book. I was overwhelmed! First there were the women who felt that it was important for the public to realize that "early detection" of an invasive cancer through screening does not guarantee that you will not get metastatic disease. The celebratory pink haze of "survivorship" denies the fact that the unfortunate people who develop metastatic disease and die of breast cancer "battled" just as hard, were just as worthy, and almost always got just as good care as the ones who lived. As I realized when I was diagnosed with leukemia, there has got to be some room for bad luck. We all need to be careful in our own desire to convince ourselves that we will be okay because we were diagnosed early, we exercise, we have a great doctor, or whatever other magical thinking we use for ourselves, when in fact sometimes nothing you do is going to change the outcome; you were just not very lucky and got a particularly bad kind of breast cancer.

That being said, there is some good news. We can cure some local recurrences, and although we still may not know how to cure metastatic breast cancer, the survival is much, much longer than it was when I wrote the first edition of this book more than thirty years ago. The new targeted therapies, hormonal drugs, and immunotherapies are keeping many women with recurrences alive for years rather than months. A Swedish study compared trends in survival from 1979 to 2004 and showed significant improvement, particularly in women under age 60.[1] And that is before many of the treatments that have come online in the last nineteen years. So read on to better understand what we know, whether for yourself or in solidarity with your fellow survivors who may be living with metastatic disease.

THE SHOCK OF RECURRENCE

It is always a shock when breast cancer cells reappear, whether it is in the area around the breast (local or regional recurrence), in the scar after a mastectomy, or elsewhere in your body. How could this be? You thought it was gone. For the most part, these are those microscopic tumor cells that presumably got out before your diagnosis and hid, somehow protected from the systemic therapies you received. Then after a long while conditions change and these cells wake up from their hibernation and begin doubling again. Another possibility is that the surviving cells were put to sleep by Nolvadex (tamoxifen) or chemical menopause and then randomly develop a mutation that makes them wake up or become resistant. (Figure 19.1). (If we could figure out what puts these cells to sleep and then what wakes them up, we'd be a long way toward eliminating breast cancer or controlling it for a much longer time—maybe a normal lifetime.) Or perhaps the local environment controlled the cells for

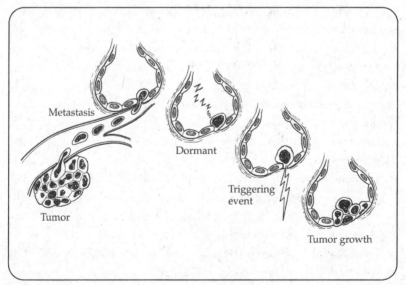

Figure 19.1

a time, and then something changed to stimulate them. Finally, it could be that the environment of your whole body changed—for instance, you increased the inflammatory cells through a different illness, surgery, or stress, causing them to wake up. The answer to this would be big news, but so far we have only hypotheses based on observations and conjecture.

Being diagnosed with a recurrence can be devastating. The process of psychosocial adjustment starts all over again; learning to trust your body may take longer when you've been doubly betrayed by it. The feelings you experienced the first time around are intensified because now you not only don't trust your body but begin to second-guess your doctors and treatment in general. Should I have gone somewhere else for treatment? Was it the fact that I was too stressed? Should I have had a mastectomy or chemotherapy, exercised more, or drunk that special tea my cousin told me about?

These are common feelings, but it is important to remember that a recurrence is almost never your fault or your doctor's fault; it's the result of factors that we do not understand and cannot control. And no matter how much you second-guess your treatment, you can't change it now. If you get stuck in these kinds of feelings, you should mention them to your caregivers. In addition, you'll want to get support and help from friends and family, counselors, therapists, support groups, and even social media.

When I wrote the first edition of this book back in 1989, the only support available was in person and varied widely, depending on where you were geographically. These days, through the Internet, you can find groups online specifically formed for people with metastatic breast cancer. There are many sites and advocacy groups focused on this disease (METAvivor, www.mbcbrainmets.org, and the Metastatic Breast Cancer Alliance). Within these, there are also particular subgroups such as the Young Survival Coalition, Latinas Contra Cancer, and Sisters Network. If you don't like the first group you encounter, keep looking. The mere fact that we have many different groups focused on metastatic breast cancer is testimony to the fact that we have made progress—there are now enough people living with breast cancer to participate in all this advocacy and support.

In order to better deal with your recurrence, you need to know more about the nature of breast cancer recurrences. In the rest of this chapter we'll examine the types of recurrences, their symptoms, and their treatments. In describing these situations I will use statistics to help you get a sense of how often they occur. As with all statistics in breast cancer (see Chapter 3), it is important to remember once again that whatever happens to you is happening 100 percent—no matter how often it does or doesn't happen to other people. Statistics are good only for giving you an overall idea of what can happen. Current data about the risk of recurrence is largely collected from clinical trials. However, trials historically only track five or ten years of recurrence data, thus underreporting late recurrences. Furthermore, with only about 5 percent of patients diagnosed with breast cancer being treated on a clinical trial, the data overall lacks diversity.

Statistics can't tell you what will happen with your particular cancer in your particular body with your particular treatment. Nonetheless, it is important to know how serious your particular situation is. Some types of breast cancer have a long survival post-recurrence; others do not. You are an adult and you get to decide what you want to do with your life, should it be foreshortened. When my wife's cousin had a scan showing asymptomatic metastases from her lung cancer, I encouraged her to take that cruise to Alaska she had always wanted to do and another in the Caribbean while she was still feeling well. Although she ultimately died of her disease, she did not regret having experienced those trips.

And you also may want to get your legal affairs in order. I know when I was diagnosed with acute myelogenous leukemia, the numbers were not promising. I made time to talk with my siblings and my family and let them know how important they were to me, and also got my will in order. As you can tell, I am still here. I don't regret taking the time to express my feelings, asking my loved ones to forgive me for anything I had done to hurt them, forgiving them for anything they had done or said to hurt me, and telling them I loved them. These are always good conversations to have, even if your disease doesn't kill you.

Local and Regional Recurrence

Local recurrence means the cancer has come back in the remaining breast tissue or, in the case of mastectomy, in the scar. Regional recurrence means it has come back in the nodes in the armpit, or around the collarbone.

Local and regional recurrences may feel just as devastating as distant disease, but depending on the circumstances, they may represent a different situation with a somewhat better prognosis. First, it is important that the type of breast cancer that has recurred is identified. If the recurrence is noninvasive cancer or DCIS (see Chapter 12), it's most likely left over from the original cancer and just needs to be cleaned up with further surgery. However, if the recurrence is invasive, it may have had a second opportunity to spread.

As I mentioned, the recurrence may not match the subtype of the original tumor, and with new technologies that map the molecular types of breast cancer, we have discovered that the tumors are often heterogeneous with several different subtypes of cells. In this setting, knocking off one type may allow other types to become dominant. In other words, you may have had a hormone-positive tumor initially and have been religiously taking your hormone blockers, but then develop a recurrence in the mastectomy scar that is no longer hormone-positive. It is always worth biopsying a local recurrence to determine which type it represents. Sometimes it is hard to distinguish between an entirely new cancer, called a second primary, and a local recurrence. People who develop invasive local recurrences generally have more aggressive disease to start with. In addition we base our decisions in part on the initial therapy because a local recurrence in the breast after radiation has a different significance than a local recurrence in a mastectomy scar.

As physicians, we tend to downplay local and regional recurrences because they are not as life-threatening as metastatic disease can be. Nonetheless, for the patient they can be devastating. When a person gets a local recurrence, they find it much harder than they did the first time not to think of themself as doomed. They gave it their best shot and it didn't work—how can they trust any treatment again? This became obvious to me years ago when we first set up our support group for women with metastatic disease at the Faulkner Breast Center in Massachusetts. I wanted to exclude women with local recurrences because I thought their situation wasn't serious enough for this group. My coworkers and patients convinced me that this was not true, and they turned out to be right. The desperate feelings are the same. Barbara Kalinowski, one of the oncology nurses there, describes the difficulties women with recurrences have, even around other women with breast cancer. "They find themselves being 'polite' in mixed groups. One woman was talking about having just had her sixth chemotherapy treatment, and the woman next to her said, 'Oh, good, you're almost through!' And she didn't have the heart to tell her this was her second time around." A woman who has gone through the tough round of surgery, radiation, and chemotherapy and thinks she has put it behind her can feel overwhelmed to find out that she has to go through it all over again. (I discuss ways to cope with this situation later in this chapter.)

Local Recurrence After Breast Conservation

Although local recurrences after breast conservation are unusual, when they do occur it is usually in the area of the original tumor, an average of three to four years after the initial therapy.[2] The first sign of a local recurrence can be a change in how your breast looks or feels. Changes in the physical exam that occur more than one to two years after the completion of radiation therapy should always be looked into immediately with mammograms and MRI. Retrospective studies show that the patients themselves detect 76 to 86 percent of local recurrences, just as they detected the original tumor.[3] Less commonly, a mammogram reveals something suspicious. Although MRI can be used to try to distinguish between a local recurrence and scar tissue, only a biopsy can show for certain. Usually a core needle biopsy is sufficient, though sometimes further surgery is necessary.

Once a local recurrence has been diagnosed, we do tests to see whether there are signs of cancer elsewhere in the body. These may include a chest X-ray, CT scan, MRI or PET scan, and blood tests (some of the latter are looking for tumor markers [see Chapter 10]). If the tests are normal (only 5 to 10 percent of women with local recurrence have signs of disease elsewhere), then we have to figure out how best to treat the tumor in the breast. Usually in these cases we do a mastectomy, since the less drastic surgery and radiation didn't take care of it. If the lesion is small and your breast is generous, then you can often preserve your breast with additional limited surgery and partial-breast re-irradiation. Research has shown this to be an effective alternative to mastectomy.[4]

Overall, the prognosis is better in women who are older, have smaller tumors, and have gone a long time between the initial treatment and the recurrence. After mastectomy for a local recurrence, the prognosis is still pretty good, with a five-year disease-free survival rate of 55 to 73 percent.[5] A recent study suggests that local recurrences that occur more than five years after your initial treatment may have an even better prognosis. The role of systemic therapy after a local recurrence in the breast is still not clear, but it is often considered in high-risk patients. If your tumor is still sensitive to estrogen and you were on Nolvadex (tamoxifen), it is reasonable to switch to an aromatase inhibitor, or vice versa. The role of chemotherapy, especially if you were previously treated with it, is not clear and is still being studied.

There's something else we call a "local recurrence" that actually isn't a local recurrence at all—it's a new cancer in the breast (often referred to as a new primary). This typically occurs many years after the original cancer and in an entirely different area of the breast. Its pathology is often different—lobular instead of ductal, for example. These second cancers appear 15 to 23 percent of the time in the large-scale studies that have followed patients after their first diagnosis.[6] But they are possible as long as you have your breast. Though they are often counted as recurrences in the statistics for breast conservation, they should be treated as completely new cancers, much as with new cancers in the opposite breast (see Chapter 12). In the past the local treatment would most often be a mastectomy as it was believed you could receive radiation therapy only once to any area. However, the newer approaches of partial-breast radiation (see Chapter 14) are changing this, and a number of studies have proved its effectiveness. The addition of chemotherapy and/or Nolvadex (tamoxifen) will depend on the size and biomarkers of the tumor (see Chapter 10).

Local Recurrence After Mastectomy

Local recurrence after mastectomy usually shows up as one or more pea-size nodules on or under the skin near the scar. It may appear on the scar itself.[7] After reconstruction a recurrence can appear at the suture line of the flap or in front of the implant. When it's in the skin itself, it is red and raised. It's usually so subtle the surgeon is likely to think at first that it's just a stitch that got left in after the operation. Then it gets bigger and needs to be biopsied. That can be done under local anesthesia, since the area is numb. Reconstruction rarely if ever hides a recurrence. With implants, the recurrences are in front of the implant. With a flap, the recurrences are not in the flap itself (tissue from the abdomen) but alongside the edge of the old breast skin.[8]

Some people are told they have a local recurrence in the chest wall, which is inaccurate because it implies that the cancer is in the muscle or bone. But usually such a recurrence appears in the skin and fat where the breast was before; only rarely does it include the muscle (see Figure 19.2). The risk of this happening after a mastectomy and no radiation is about 8.5 percent.[9] Ninety percent of these recurrences happen within the first five years after the mastectomy. Approximately 20 to 30 percent of patients with local recurrences after mastectomy have already been diagnosed with metastatic disease, and another 20 to 30 percent will develop it within a few months of diagnosis. Therefore, just as with local recurrences after breast conservation, tests should be done to look for distant disease.

The treatments for a local recurrence are also local. Most commonly the lesion is removed surgically and followed by radiation to the chest wall if the person has not previously had radiation. Occasionally larger areas are surgically removed, including sections of rib and breastbone. Although this approach has not been shown to increase survival, it can

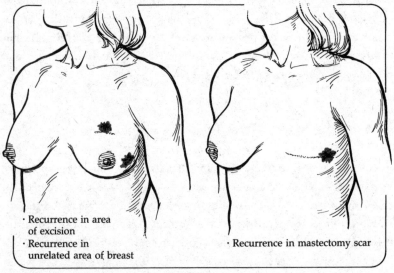

· Recurrence in area
  of excision
· Recurrence in
  unrelated area of breast

· Recurrence in mastectomy scar

Figure 19.2

improve the quality of life by preventing farther local spread, which can be difficult to manage.

Despite aggressive local treatment, 80 to 85 percent of patients with an isolated local recurrence following mastectomy eventually develop distant metastases. This is not because the local recurrence spreads, but rather because it is an obvious sign that things have changed and dormant cells in other organs may also be waking up. Studies, both randomized and nonrandomized, have suggested, however, that if the recurrence can be removed and radiation given, the addition of systemic therapy such as Nolvadex (tamoxifen) or chemotherapy can lead to five-year remissions in 36 to 52 percent of such patients.[10] The current recommendation is similar to that for a recurrence within the breast, described earlier. The biggest predictor of overall survival is the length of time between the original therapy and the recurrence—that is, the disease-free interval: the later the recurrence, the better. If you can join a clinical trial testing therapies for local recurrence, you will help us answer the questions about chemotherapy.

In rare cases a person has extensive local recurrence after mastectomy, with many nodules in the skin. They merge and act almost like a coat of armor across the chest and even into the back and the other breast. At this point we call it "en cuirasse," a French term meaning "in casing." This is because the tumor, which can be fairly limited, may block lymph vessels in this area and these, in turn, become scarred. Some patients have large tumor masses on the chest wall that weep and bleed. Both of these situations are rare, but they're very distressing because you are watching the cancer grow on the outside. We believe there must be a different genetic mutation for this type of local recurrence than for distant metastasis because these patients usually do not have extensive disease in the rest of their body for a long time. Unfortunately, we lack a good therapy for it. Surgery cannot cut out enough tissue to clear it, and radiation therapy is limited in extent as well. Some have tried hyperthermia (very high heat) in an attempt to burn off the tumor, but its effect has also been limited. Sometimes chemotherapy gives some relief but not always. There are reports of success in using both heat and chemotherapy, especially Doxil, a form of doxorubicin (Adriamycin) that tends to concentrate in the skin. These cases are very upsetting for the doctor and patient, and we are still searching for the right treatment approach.

Regional Recurrence

A regional recurrence is one in the lymph nodes under the arm or above the collarbone. Now that we are taking out fewer lymph nodes from the axilla (see Chapter 13), a cancerous one can be left behind. This is rare, occurring in only about 2 percent of breast cancers. Further treatment to this area with either surgery or radiation often takes care of the problem, although systemic therapy may also be used. My cousin had a mastectomy in 1985 with a local recurrence in 1988 and another recurrence under her arm in 1994. She was already taking Nolvadex (tamoxifen) and so had the lump removed, with clean margins, followed by radiation for three weeks. She has been disease-free since. This disease is full of surprises, so please don't ever write yourself off!

Regional recurrence in lymph nodes elsewhere, such as in the neck or above the collarbone, is more likely to reflect spread of the tumor through the bloodstream. Akin to local recurrence following mastectomy, it usually warrants a more aggressive approach.[11]

DISTANT RECURRENCE (METASTATIC DISEASE)

When a cancer spreads to a different organ, it's known as a distant recurrence, or a metastasis. If a metastasis is detectable at the time of first diagnosis, the patient is described as being in stage IV (see Chapter 10). We are just starting to understand the biology of metastases. I noted in Chapter 11 that cancer cells can get out of the breast tumor early on either via the lymph nodes to the bloodstream or directly. It is those cells that sometimes take up residence in other organs, and it is those cells that we are trying to treat with our systemic therapies such as chemotherapy, hormone therapy, and targeted therapy (HER2/ neu-blocking drugs). If and when cancer comes back, the cancer cells that escaped the breast are to blame. Obviously if your recurrence is ten years after your diagnosis, we assume that the cells have been dormant (sleeping)[12] all that time and missed the treatments aimed at dividing cells.[13] In the past few years tests have been developed to identify these errant cancer cells while they are in the bloodstream (circulating tumor cells or CTCs)[14] and even map out their genetic mutations (circulating tumor DNA).[15] The surprising thing is that they are more ubiquitous than we thought. Given this, what's amazing is the relative lack of metastatic disease.

All this new technology has allowed us to better understand recurrences as well as start to refine the ways we treat them. For example, we have always assumed that recurrences stem from the initial tumor and, therefore, match its markers. But studies now have demonstrated that tumors are not composed of just one kind of cell and that a metastasis may not be the same type as the original.[16] We are still trying to figure out how to use this information. What is obvious even now is that we need to keep biopsying and testing the tumor cells at each decision point to be sure of what we are dealing with. I keep thinking it is like fighting terrorists: Just when we get good at screening for the "shoe bomber," the "underwear bomber" appears. If you are reading this because you have a recurrence, you should ask about having it biopsied if possible, so that it is clear exactly what "flavor" of breast cancer you are dealing with.

As hard as it is to face a local recurrence, metastatic disease can be even more devastating. It causes the same feelings that go with any recurrence, compounded by the knowledge that the chance of cure is slim. Here you need to face the fact that you are not immortal and create the best quality of life for yourself in the time you have, all the while maintaining hope. Contrary to common belief, metastatic breast cancer is rarely an immediate death sentence, and these days, with good treatment, people with metastasis often live for quite a number of years, with a reasonable quality of life. The prognosis for metastatic disease depends on which molecular subtype your tumor or recurrence belongs to. People with hormone-positive breast cancers tend to have recurrences much later than those with hormone-negative ones. This may be in part because they take hormone therapy for five to ten years that may keep things under control, and also because these cancers tend to be less aggressive. They also tend to respond better to treatments for their metastatic disease. HER2/neu-positive tumors used to be the most aggressive, but now with the use of Herceptin at the time of diagnosis and new anti-HER2 drugs at the time of recurrence, they have a much better outcome. And even people with triple-negative metastatic disease, who generally have the worst prognosis, can use a menu of new and old drugs to keep the tumor guessing for a couple of years. Finally, not to be too optimistic, new drugs such as immunotherapy are also changing the scene (see Chapter 15). To quote Dr. Andrew Seidman, a medical oncologist from Memorial Sloan Kettering Cancer Center in New York, you need to remember that "metastatic breast cancer often behaves biologically . . . like a novel with many chapters, fortunately, rather than a short story."[17]

We have always known that some types of breast cancers—the hormonal ones—like to spread to the bones and skin, whereas the hormone-negative ones are more likely to go to the lungs, liver, and brain. Throughout this book we have emphasized that breast cancer is not just one disease, and this indeed remains true with metastases. Luminal A breast cancer, which is usually ER-positive and PR-positive and HER2-negative, is most likely to go to the bones and skin, whereas triple-negative likes the lungs and HER2-positive the liver and brain.[18] Just like some of us prefer to live in the city while others like small towns, the tumor cells have certain environments that are more compatible. This analysis certainly suggests we may need to be thinking about how to prevent and treat metastatic disease differently, focusing on tailored surveillance and maybe even specific approaches to make these destination organs less appealing. Maybe it is time to change the local neighborhood rather than focusing just on the bad cells!

Researchers are studying the question and perhaps one day will give us a better understanding of it. The cancer cell may be responding to some sort of propensity to spread to a particular organ, or perhaps the environment of certain organs is more conducive to growth for this type of cancer cell. Bone is overwhelmingly the most common organ that breast cancer cells go to, and there are data that the niche that metastatic cells hide in may well be in the bone marrow.[19]

As I mentioned in Chapter 10, when breast cancer shows up in your lungs, liver, or bones, it's still breast cancer—not lung, liver, or bone cancer. As with local recurrence, the metastatic cancer cells often—but certainly not always—are the same molecular type as those of the primary tumor. We can test a biopsy in the same way we can test the original tumor. This can prove difficult, however, depending on which organ the metastases are located in. Some subtypes of breast cancers, the hormonal ones, spread to the bones and skin; the hormone-negative ones are more likely to go to the lungs, liver, and brain. It may also be true that the ER-negative ones also go to bone first but show up first in other organs, so we discount the one, focusing on the more life-threatening disease in the liver, lungs, and brain. Research in the basic biology of metastatic disease has blossomed. There are now data in mice suggesting that the local neighborhood of the tumor can determine where and whether the metastatic cells will be able to survive.

At the moment, nothing we know of can offer a cure for metastatic breast cancer. However, as new therapies are continuously being developed, we have reason to hope that, as with AIDS, we can one day convert metastatic breast cancer into a chronic disease. Recent studies suggest that in certain situations where the recurrence is limited and the patient can be rendered disease-free with multidisciplinary treatments, 3 to 30 percent of patients with metastatic breast cancer can be put into remission for over twenty years.[20] Is that a cure? I suspect it doesn't matter to those patients what you call it—what matters is that they are alive and well.

Alternatively, occasional long survival may occur because the cancer is just very slow growing, which has little or nothing to do with the therapy. Some people may think of it as a miracle—and until or unless we can prove otherwise, it's as good an explanation as any.

Many factors can help predict who will live a long time, but they're not absolute. As stated earlier, one is the length of time between the original diagnosis and metastasis. If the metastasis shows up six months after the diagnosis, it suggests that the cancer is much more aggressive than if it's six years after the diagnosis. However, patients with metastases at the time of initial diagnosis often do quite well. This is probably because their cancer has been growing slowly below the surface for some time, unlike the person whose cancers may have grown quickly for a short time.

Still another factor is whether the tumor is sensitive to hormones. We also look at how many places it's metastasized to—if there's only one or if there are multiple organs involved. Where it recurs is also a consideration. Metastasis to the bone or the skin is less serious than metastasis to the lung or liver.

This is all just so many statistics, however, and as noted earlier, what happens to an individual may or may not conform to the norm. I've had patients with metastatic disease who have far outlived the most optimistic prognosis. One patient developed lung metastasis while she was getting her adjuvant chemotherapy. So she had hardly any disease-free interval, and the cancer seemed resistant to chemotherapy. Statistically, she should have been dead within a year or two. She was treated with hormones and the cancer disappeared for two years. It came back, and another treatment made it disappear for another two years. When it came back that time, we gave another hormone. Ten years after her initial diagnosis, she died of breast cancer. When she was diagnosed she had an eight-year-old son, and she was able to raise him almost into adulthood. So we can't accurately predict the course of any individual's illness. This is true of initial disease, and metastatic disease is even more unpredictable.

Studies have shown that all cancer patients want to know their prognosis, treatment options, curability, and probable length of survival. Most want to know this when they are first diagnosed, although there may be some variability about how much, when, and by whom.[21] Having had a cancer diagnosis myself, I get angry with doctors who paternalistically say that their patient can't handle such information! I think they are the ones who can't handle it. Adults deserve to have the information they need to make decisions about their lives, how long they may be around, and how they want to spend the time they have.

Usually I find that people who have just finished breast cancer treatments don't want to think about the possibility of spread. But my own experience revealed to me that sometimes you want to know the worst-case scenario, even if only to reassure yourself that it hasn't happened to you. It becomes up to us to guide our caregivers about what we want to know and when. There's nothing particularly brave about toughing it out when you're worried. Every person's pace is different. This may be one of those times when you bring that family member or friend to the appointment who will ask for you. And take a printout of the information you found online that scared you to death. That way you can check to see if it actually relates to your situation.

That being said, studies have shown that doctors are afraid to mention the symptoms of metastatic disease. In medical school, we were taught that we shouldn't tell people who had been treated for cancer what to look for if they were worried about recurrences, because they'd start imagining that they had every symptom we told them about. I've never liked that idea. It doesn't soothe people at all; it just means they'll be afraid of everything, instead of a few specific things. When you've had cancer, you're acutely aware of your body, and any symptom that's new—or that you never noticed before—can take on terrifying significance as you worry that your cancer may be back. Inevitably this will mean a lot of fear over symptoms that turn out to be harmless.

But if you know that the symptoms of breast cancer metastasis are usually bone pain, shortness of breath, lack of appetite, and weight loss, and neurological symptoms like pain or weakness or headaches, there are at least limits to your fear. You'll probably be frightened when anything resembling those symptoms comes up, even if it turns out to be nothing but a tension headache or a mild flu. But at least you won't be terrified by a sore spot on your big toe or an unexpected weight gain. Knowing what symptoms to look for reduces fear; it doesn't increase it. Dr. Daniel Hayes, the clinical director of the breast cancer oncology program at the University of Michigan and an old friend of mine, puts it this way: "I tell patients it is common sense: if you stub your toe, and it hurts just like it did before your diagnosis of breast cancer, it is normal. If you have a new symptom that is particularly unusual, severe, and lasts longer than you expect, then you should see your caregiver. And be sure he or she remembers you had breast cancer, even ten or twenty years ago. (I frequently see late metastases that get missed because doctors forget the patient had breast cancer once a long time ago.)"

As I pointed out earlier, most recurrences are diagnosed because of symptoms the person noticed. Although scans used to be done to look for early metastases, that approach has been found to make no difference in the outcome (see Chapter 11). Diagnosing metastatic disease early on a scan or blood test does not make the treatment easier or more effective. This means you do not have to kick yourself for not complaining sooner. If you have a symptom that feels abnormal, get it checked out, but don't feel it is an emergency.

Symptoms of Metastatic Spread

Symptoms appear differently in different areas of the body. So now we'll consider some of the most common sites of metastasis.

Bone

Bone, as I mentioned earlier, is the most common site of metastases in people with breast cancer. This is true partly because it's more obvious there than in other places, and partly because it creates definite symptoms. Even if it first appears elsewhere, as the disease progresses, it usually reaches the bone at some stage.

Metastasis to the bone is generally diagnosed when the patient experiences pain. Sometimes it's hard to know whether the pain is ordinary low back pain or some other condition, like arthritis. Usually the pain you get with breast cancer in the bones is fairly constant and doesn't improve over time, but it may wax and wane and it may move around. With arthritis, you wake up in the morning and feel stiff but get better as you move around during the day. Also the location is important. Pain in the feet, ankle, and hands is usually caused by arthritis or even by your treatment: Nolvadex (tamoxifen) and especially the aromatase inhibitors can cause muscle and joint pain. With some muscular problems that cause bone pain, the more you do, the worse the pain gets. But the pain from cancer is steady and usually persists during the night when you're not doing anything. Sometimes, however, it is more erratic. Oncologist Dr. Craig Henderson tells me he has been "impressed with how often the cancer pain would decrease substantially or even disappear for weeks or months on end and then reappear without any treatment at all. I think bone pain is sometimes overlooked as bone metastasis because it is not steady." The pain is probably caused by the cancer taking up room in the bone and pressing on it, and it can be worse in different positions and under different conditions. If you have pain that lasts for more than a week or two with no sign that it's going away, and it isn't like whatever pains have become familiar to you, you should get it checked out.

We usually check bone pain by doing an X-ray and then a bone scan, PET scan, or even CT scan, depending on the situation. The X-ray can show one of two things: either lytic lesions (holes where the cancer has eaten away the bones) or blastic lesions (an increase of bone where the growth factor of the cancer has caused the bone to get more dense). CT scans and MRI, described in Chapter 10, can be used to confirm a diagnosis of cancer in specific bones.[22] PET-CT scanning (two in one) is also being done more, although its accuracy is unproved. However, there may be a lag in time between the first evidence of cancer on a bone scan and the appearance of metastases on an X-ray or even a CT scan.

A woman I know told me her experience with discovering bone metastasis. She felt generalized pain around her rib cage and groin and called her internist. He was out of town and so she was seen by a nurse practitioner, who attributed the pain to tendonitis and ordered an anti-inflammatory drug, which relieved the pain. Later when she saw her surgeon, he suggested it could be bone metastasis and ordered a PET scan (a bone scan could have been done). But she was feeling better and did not follow through until four weeks later, when she was hiking and experienced severe pain. She was found to have bone metastasis and was started on a hormonal therapy and an intravenous bisphosphonate. She has been feeling well since but now wishes that she had followed up on the scan sooner. The result would not have been different, but she would have had pain relief earlier.

When patients have cancer in their bones, we worry about the possibility of fractures. If the cancer eats away enough bone, it will no longer be strong enough to hold you up. Then you can get what's called a *pathological fracture*, which is caused by something wrong in the bone itself, not by a blow from outside (Figure 19.3). It's similar to osteoporosis in that it doesn't take much to cause this fracture because the bone is so weakened. A slight pressure that usually wouldn't even cause a bruise triggers the fracture. (It's different from osteoporosis, however, in that it doesn't affect all your bones.)

The American College of Clinical Oncologists has come out with guidelines for the use of drugs focused on increasing bone metabolism, which suggest that they be given to patients with metastatic breast cancer

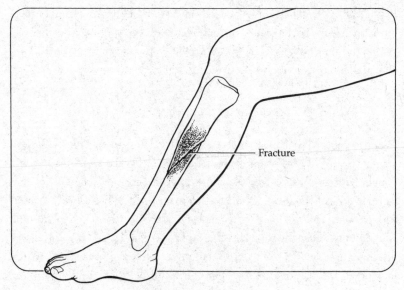

Figure 19.3

to bone, thus slowing bone destruction. They don't list these in any order of preference or effectiveness. The list includes Prolia (denosumab) injected subcutaneously every four weeks, bisphosphonates, Aredia (pamidronate) given by IV every three to four weeks, or Zometa (zolendronic acid) given by IV every three to four weeks for a year and then every three months for the same benefit. The use of these drugs has dramatically lowered the risk of bone fractures.[23] However, they also come with a risk of complications such as osteonecrosis of the jaw (described in Chapter 11), so prior to starting, everyone needs to have a dental exam and routine preventive dental work.

We try to make sure that the key bones are not at risk. The ones to worry most about are the ones that hold you up—your leg or hip bones and spine. The upper arm can also fracture, but it's less likely because you don't put as much constant pressure on it. If X-rays show that a bone in a critical place has metastatic disease that puts it at risk for a fracture, we can do surgery or radiation ahead of time to pin the hip or stabilize the bone. Again, the idea is to keep you stabilized and functional, with as high a quality of life as possible for as long a time as possible. More often the patient has both radiotherapy and systemic therapy (chemotherapy or hormone therapy). These therapies may kill the tumor in the bone without, however, relieving the pain, leading you to think that the therapy hasn't worked. In these cases it may be that there are residual fractures that haven't healed and can't be managed with radiotherapy or systemic therapy alone. Some sort of brace or, in some cases, the surgical insertion of a pin or rod may be necessary to relieve the pain and stabilize the fracture so you don't keep refracturing that area.

Lung

We also see breast cancer metastasis fairly often in the lungs (Figure 19.4). Usually the symptoms are shortness of breath and/or a chronic cough. Among patients who die of breast cancer, 60 to 70 percent have it in their lungs. The lungs are the only obvious site of metastasis in about 21 percent of cases. There are a couple of different ways it can form. One is in nodules—usually several—that show up on a chest X-ray. If it shows only one nodule, we can't tell if it's lung cancer or a breast cancer that has spread. So we do a needle biopsy or a full biopsy to find out. (Lung cancer usually starts in just one spot, but a cancer that has spread to the

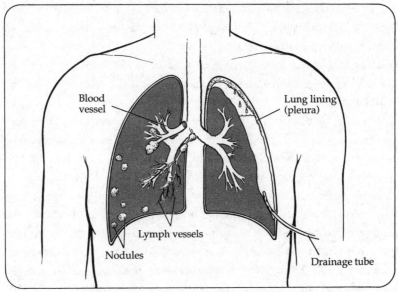

Figure 19.4

lung through the bloodstream or lymphatic channels is likely to hit multiple spots in the lung.)

If your breast cancer has spread to your lungs, you may experience shortness of breath on less-than-normal exertion. It can be fairly subtle. It comes on slowly, since the cancer has to use up a lot of your lungs before it compromises your breathing.

Another form of metastasis in the lung is called lymphangitic spread. Here the cancer spreads along the lymphatics. Instead of forming nodules, it occurs in a fine pattern throughout the lung. This isn't all cancer because, like the *en cuirasse* of the skin described earlier, some of the changes in lung are due to lack of lymphatic drainage and fibrosis of these lymph channels. It's subtler and harder to detect on a chest X-ray. It ultimately causes shortness of breath, since it takes up room and scars the lungs, making them less able to expand and contract and bring oxygen into your bloodstream.

The third way it can show is through fluid in the pleura, the lining of the lung. (The pleura is a sac with a smooth lining around it; the lung sits in it so that it can move without sticking to the chest wall.) This usually indicates that the spread is in there rather than in the lung itself. The cancer creates fluid around the lung (effusion), and the fluid causes the lung to collapse partially (see Figure 19.4). Here again, you'll experience shortness of breath. Usually breast cancer in the lungs doesn't cause pain.

If we think your cancer may have metastasized to your lung and the chest X-ray doesn't show nodules, fluid, or any of the other signs, we can still do a CT scan.

For lung metastases the treatment is usually systemic—that is, chemotherapy. However, fluid in pleura can be treated by sticking a needle into the chest and draining the fluid. This works immediately but frequently for only a short time. Often the fluid comes back right away. In order to prevent the reaccumulation, we fasten the pleura to the lung itself. When I was in medical school we used to open up the chest, take a piece of gauze, and rub it against the lung to irritate the spot. That got it red and raw and so it stuck together and created a scar, leaving no room for fluid. A less invasive approach is to drain the fluid through a tube and then put in material that will scar up the lining of the sac. Talc powder irritates the pleural surfaces and causes them to scar together so that fluid can't accumulate between them. However, often an effective hormonal therapy or chemotherapy will keep the fluid in the lung from reaccumulating, at least for a while. Eventually many people with recurrent pleural effusions do receive the scarring procedure with talc and chest tube drainage. Occasionally people with recurring fluid will have a catheter left in so that they can be drained as needed. However, many people with such fluid in the pleura will get permanent relief by a combination of local drainage, scarring of the pleura (using any one of the methods just described), and a systemic therapy.

Liver

The liver is the third most common site for metastasis. Again, this can be subtle. The symptoms occur because the cancer takes up a lot of room in the liver, and that takes some time to happen. About two-thirds of women who die of breast cancer have it in their liver, and about a quarter have it there initially. The symptoms are common—weight loss, anorexia (loss of appetite), nausea, gastrointestinal symptoms, and pain or discomfort under your right rib cage. You may have some pain in the right upper quadrant of your abdomen, which occurs when the liver's covering tissue is stretched out.

A diagnosis of liver metastasis is often suspected from blood tests and confirmed by CT, MRI, PET scanning, or, on occasion, ultrasound. The major treatment for extensive liver disease is chemotherapy, especially if your liver function blood tests are elevated. Hormone therapy can work well on hormone-positive and slower-growing liver metastases, and the decision to use it usually depends on the extent of damage present in the liver. In certain kinds of cancer, like colon cancer, liver metastasis can be a single lesion or just a few and thus on rare occasions can be cut out. But with breast cancer there is usually more than one spot involved and surgery becomes impossible. In the uncommon exception when there is only one spot, we can surgically remove part of the liver to relieve symptoms or use X-ray therapy, but this is really a last resort when the patient has a large and painful liver that is not responding to chemotherapy.

There are also new techniques for a small number of liver metastases that involve putting hot (hyperthermia) or cold (cryosurgery) probes into the tumors and burning or freezing them. In addition, there are interventional radiology techniques such as radiofrequency ablation, chemoembolization, and bland embolization of liver tumors. These can help the obvious spots but must be followed with systemic therapy to control the rest of the micrometastatic liver disease.

Sometimes when patients have a lot of pain, we radiate the liver to shrink it. But we do this only for particularly severe symptoms that are not responding to systemic therapy or for the rare case of a patient whose only apparent disease is in the liver. Sometimes we put chemotherapy directly into the liver through a catheter in the artery leading into the organ, to achieve a more direct treatment of the metastasis if we can't get a good response with less drastic and more comfortable forms of chemotherapy. Liver transplants do not work in this situation because the disease is usually more extensive, not just in the liver.

Brain and Spinal Cord

Neurological metastases are less common but very serious. Breast cancer can spread to the brain and the spinal cord. It's still fairly uncommon— less than 5 to 15 percent of women with breast cancer will ever experience them. However, women with triple-negative[24] and HER2-positive cancers[25] have a higher incidence of brain recurrence, between 33 and 45 percent or so. Adjuvant chemotherapy does not get into the brain as effectively as it does into the rest of the body. Because of this, we are seeing brain metastases with somewhat greater frequency, as systemic adjuvant therapies have become better at eradicating disease outside the brain. The most common symptoms are headache, visual changes, and/ or persistent nausea. I almost hate to say that, since most people get a lot of headaches during their lives, and I'm afraid any reader with breast cancer who gets a tension headache or the flu will be terrified. But if the headache doesn't go away in a reasonable time, check it out. In some patients it's the kind of headache that occurs with a brain tumor. It begins early in the morning before you get out of bed, improves as the day goes on, but then gets worse and worse over time.

Behavior or mental changes are sometimes, though rarely, caused by the tumor. You can have weakness or unsteadiness in walking, or seizures. It can resemble a stroke: you suddenly can't talk, part of your body is abruptly very weak, or you can't see out of one eye. Those kinds of symptoms occur when a portion of your brain is blocked, which the cancer growth can cause. The best way to diagnose it is through MRI or CT scan. About half of patients have one lesion; the rest have several. Another kind of brain metastasis you can get is a form of meningitis called *carcinomatosis meningitis*. This affects the lining of the brain rather than the brain itself. It causes weakness in the eye and mouth muscles, headaches, stiff neck, and sometimes confusion, the way any form of meningitis does.

Surgery can be used for treating metastases if there are one or a few lesions that can be easily removed, or if a tumor is larger than four centimeters and near critical structures like the eyes. Stereotactic surgery is now commonly used for patients with one to five lesions, but research has shown it can be effective with up to ten tumors and possibly more.[26] It is a noninvasive procedure that uses multiple focused radiation beams that intersect to target the cancer and little else. Whole-brain radiation therapy can be used to treat the entire brain if there are more than a few areas of cancer. Although it can help shrink the tumors, side effects include problems with thought and memory.

You'll also probably be put on steroids (dexamethasone) right away to reduce the brain swelling, although when brain metastases are very small, detected on screening by MRI—something increasingly done on high-risk metastasis patients—there may be no brain swelling or other symptoms and steroids may not be needed. Because the skull in which the brain sits is a hard, bony shell, there isn't much room for swelling before important structures are injured. If you're having seizures, you'll also be put on antiseizure medication. Unfortunately chemotherapy and hormone therapies don't work well on brain metastasis, although responses can occur with both.

Metastasis to the spinal cord is also very serious. This is the one area where early detection makes a big difference. The tumor can push on the cord and cause paralysis. Sometimes this happens because the bone metastasis is in the vertebrae and pushes against the spinal cord as it grows out of the bone into the spinal canal (Figure 19.5). Sometimes the tumor grows directly in the spinal cord itself. Before the paralysis, however, there are earlier symptoms—pain, weakness, sensory loss, and bowel or bladder disturbances. Pain is the most common—85 to 90 percent of patients with spinal cord metastasis have pain. It may be the only symptom for months. The problem is that if you have cancer only in the bones and the back, you'll also have pain. So we have to be able to differentiate, or at least be extremely alert, to be certain that the patient with bone metastasis in their back isn't on the verge of spinal cord compression.

Most of the pain is aching and continuous. Its onset is gradual and it gets worse over time; it often becomes severe as it pushes on the spinal cord. And it's very localized: you feel it exactly on the spot where

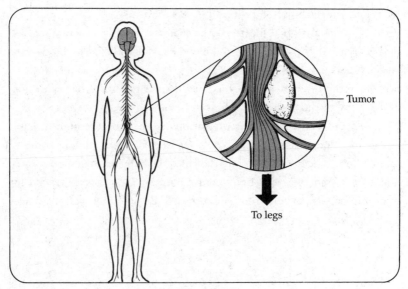

Tumor

To legs

Figure 19.5

the tumor is. There is another kind of pain that goes downward the way sciatica does, when a disk compresses the nerves and goes down your leg, getting worse if you cough or sneeze. You may also feel pain in your shoulder or back from spinal cord compression. Seventy-five percent of patients with metastasis to the spinal cord have weakness in their muscles from the tumor pushing against the nerves, and about 5 percent have spots of numbness. Anyone with metastatic breast cancer who has unrelenting pain in one spot and any neurological symptoms should be concerned. If you have no other signs of metastasis, it probably isn't spinal cord compression as that's rarely the first sign of metastatic disease, although it can be. We diagnose it with CT scan or MRI. The treatment is generally emergency surgery if there is any evidence of nerve damage, muscle weakness, or a large tumor pressing on the spinal cord. If it's one spot, we may be able to remove the tumor and decompress the spinal cord. Surgery, if performed, is then followed by radiation therapy. Alternatively, the treatment could be emergency radiation alone; it is one of the few instances in which radiation is used as an emergency treatment. The radiation shrinks the tumor, and steroids prevent the spinal cord from swelling.

Breast cancer can also metastasize to the eye, though again it's rarely the first place such spread occurs. The initial symptoms are double or blurred vision. It's diagnosed by CT scan or MRI. It's also treated with radiation, which can often prevent loss of vision.

Another area is bone marrow. The main symptom is anemia, caused by a decrease in the number of red blood cells, and the white blood cells and platelets can also decrease. Though it sounds grim, metastasis to bone marrow often responds very well to treatment, either with hormones or with chemotherapy. This remission can last for several years.

Breast cancer in all its manifestations is an unpredictable disease. These are general descriptions. As I write this, many people come to mind whose cancer didn't follow the rules. Use this information to help understand your own situation and ask questions, not as a blueprint for what will happen to you. Your situation will be unique to you no matter what happens.

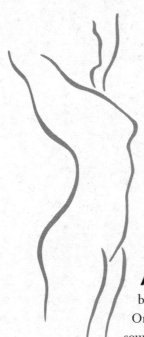

CHAPTER 20

Living with Recurrence

As I mentioned before, more and more people are living for years with metastatic breast cancer because of a range of new treatments that are available. Once you are diagnosed with metastatic disease, a major source of stress is having no clear idea of what to expect— how long you will live and how much you may suffer from pain and other problems. There are two important considerations here. One is dealing with your own emotions through counseling, a support group, religion—whatever works best for you. The other is to get as much information as your doctor has about the probable progress of your illness and what it entails. Sometimes doctors deal with a patient's fear by using every kind of therapy as rapidly and in as great a dose as possible, in an attempt to ward off the inevitable. Often the patient also goes along with this approach. But it's as dangerous as the opposite extreme of shying away from any treatment at all.

Our deeper understanding of the many kinds of breast cancer has improved effectiveness and survival rates over the past decade. According to the National Cancer Institute, the highest five-year survival rate was seen in hormone-positive, HER2-positive cancers at 44 percent, and the lowest was for hormone-negative HER2-negative at 12 percent.[1] Yet even these numbers may not show the whole picture as newer treatments and approaches are approved on a regular basis. Statistics may vary according to each study's focus, approach, and cancer subtype, ranging from a worst-case scenario of six months to an encouraging ten years. I know when I was diagnosed with leukemia I spent a lot of time looking for the paper or study that said what was going to happen to me! I didn't find it, however, and the two-year numbers were not good. But a decade later I am still here! I didn't do anything other than the standard of care, but I have been lucky so far!

Several years ago a PBS special on cancer called *The Emperor of All Maladies* aired. While the whole show is good, I was most struck by the people who should have died and didn't because they tried something new (one of the first women to get Herceptin) and were lucky.

In the rest of this chapter I'll explain the treatments specific to metastatic disease, and what you can reasonably expect from them. As my friend and mentor Dr. Craig Henderson put it: "Most patients with metastases will receive multiple forms of therapy both in combination and sequentially. At each decision point the potential for a therapy to relieve symptoms, restore organ function, and prolong survival must be balanced against the toxicity of the treatment and the patients' net quality of life. In general, more toxic therapies are associated with a higher likelihood of response but not necessarily with a greater survival benefit or quality of life." The key is to figure out whether the symptomatic problem is local. If so, surgery or radiation may be more effective, or should at least be considered.

PALLIATIVE CARE AND TREATMENT

As I have mentioned before in this book, palliative care should not be saved for the last few weeks of life. This growing specialty focuses on symptom management and control. It is important to ask to see the palliative care specialist or team when you are diagnosed with metastatic disease. This will ensure that you will benefit from the latest of symptom control—you want to maximize the quality of your life, no matter how many years it is.

The first goal in treating disease at this stage is to prolong your survival by keeping the cancer well under control. Hormone therapy, radiation, chemotherapy, targeted therapy, and immunotherapy can induce remissions that last about one year on average but can last as long as ten years. Some of the newer treatments for metastatic breast cancer are being shown to improve the time before the cancer begins to progress more effectively than some of the older chemotherapy and hormone options. Remember, however, that increased time to progression does not necessarily mean increased survival. It means that you have more symptom-free time before the cancer recurs. In this case, you live comfortably for a longer time and spend less time actually ill.

Several newer drugs and treatment combinations have opened the door for a host of options for metastatic breast cancer since the last edition. Faslodex (fulvestrant) is effective in treating HER2-negative advanced breast cancer alone or with other hormonal or targeted therapies.[2] And the U.S. Food and Drug Administration (FDA) approved four cyclin-dependent kinase (CDK) inhibitors for breast cancer, which function by curbing the cyclins in cancer cell division. They also approved a biomarker test to determine in which cancers these agents will be most effective. There are also additional targeted treatments for advanced disease, such as Tukysa (tucatinib)[3] and Enhertu (trastuzumab deruxtecan)[4] for patients who have already been treated with one or more previous anti-HER2 regimes. And immune therapy with Keytruda (pembrolizumab)[5] has been approved in combination with chemo for triple-negative metastatic disease.

Older drugs like Herceptin (trastuzumab) and the taxanes Taxol (paclitaxel), Taxotere (docetaxel), and Abraxane (nab-paclitaxel) have also been shown to substantially help some patients live longer than do the even older chemotherapy regimens.[6]

No one knows how long someone with metastatic breast cancer will live. Therefore our second, main, and achievable goal is called palliation—keeping you feeling as good as you can for as long as you can. This is often thought to mean "end of life" therapy, but actually palliation means finding ways to deal with the symptoms of your disease and the collateral damage secondary to your treatment. Palliation is achieved by choosing the therapies with both the best chance of working and the fewest side effects. What the term "working" means depends on the situation. If the metastases involve a major organ such as the liver or lungs and are significantly interfering with its function (major organ dysfunction), then you will need something that shrinks the tumor and stabilizes the situation. If your disease is stable, keeping the tumor from spreading farther is the best achievable outcome of treatment. Although it is sometimes assumed that chemotherapy works faster than hormonal therapy, this isn't always the case, and immunotherapy may be slower yet.

Dr. Daniel Hayes, clinical director of the breast cancer oncology program at the University of Michigan, tells his patients that "there is bad news and good news. The bad news is you have metastatic breast cancer, meaning that it is unlikely that you will be cured with any therapy, no matter how aggressive." He stresses that both the doctor and the patient must understand this, or the patient can become disillusioned and distrustful. It is too easy for someone with a frightening disease to hear what they would prefer to hear, and for a caring doctor to allow them to. "But," Dr. Hayes continues, "the good news is you have metastatic breast cancer." He explains that there are numerous therapies available to achieve palliation and they are growing yearly. They include local treatments such as surgery, radiation, cryotherapy, radiofrequency knife, breast ablation, chemoembolization, and phototherapy. Systemic therapies include, at last count, at least fifteen chemotherapy drugs (both IV and oral) as well as at least ten hormonal therapies and now six biologic or targeted therapies (see www.cancer.gov for an up-to-date list). It is important to recognize that treatment for a person with metastatic breast cancer is pretty much continuous throughout their life, with short breaks, rather than one term of therapy and no more. The goal is to stay ahead of the cancer, which becomes resistant to one treatment but will often still respond to another.

In addition there are new supportive therapies such as bisphosphonates (which treat bone metastasis), erythropoietin (which combats anemia), antinausea drugs, white blood cell growth factors (which prevent infection), and better pain medications. "The challenge," says Dr. Hayes, "is judicious application in sequence of these treatments, which will optimize the patient's feeling as good as she can for as long as she can."

HORMONE TREATMENTS IN METASTATIC BREAST CANCER

We've known for a long time that breast cancer in women is often an endocrine disease—the endocrine glands are the ones that make hormones. We can test the cancer when the tumor is first removed and tell if it's sensitive to hormones by doing the estrogen receptor test described in Chapter 10.

In women who have metastatic disease and a tumor that's sensitive to hormones, using endocrine treatments first often makes more sense than chemotherapy, at least in the beginning, while the tumor is still sensitive to this approach. When a patient has responded to one hormone therapy, we know they are likely to respond to a second and possibly a third one—or, occasionally, more—so we use them in sequence.

With the recent introduction of targeted cyclin dependent kinase inhibitors (CDKs), hormonal therapy can get an extra boost. As you may recall, CDK inhibitors interrupt or slow the growth of cancer cells by targeting proteins involved in cell division. There are three CDK inhibitors approved for use in hormone-positive, HER2-negative, metastatic breast cancer, which are given with standard hormone therapy. Typically, a diagnostic test is done on your biopsy tissue or blood first to check that you are a good candidate for this kind of therapy. One of these drugs, Verzenio (abemaciclib), can also be given alone as an initial therapy. The other two are Ibrance (palbociclib) and Kisqali (ribociclib).

But this is only one of the newer classes of drugs on the scene since the last edition of this book. Sparking excitement on the research front are selective estrogen receptor degraders (SERDs), which decrease the number of estrogen receptors on tumor cells and alter them so they no longer work properly. These drugs could follow CDK inhibitor therapy once resistance begins to develop. At the time of writing, Faslodex (fulvestrant) is the only SERD with approval for treatment of hormone-resistant breast cancers. But it is administered by injection, which necessitates inconvenient doctor visits, so another ten different oral SERDs are now in development for use in metastatic breast cancer and may be available by the time this book is published.

Newer treatments are encouraging, but they should not completely sideline older but still effective approaches. Historically, the first hormone treatment consisted of oophorectomy—surgically removing the ovaries in premenopausal patients. Now we can either do this or use drugs (ablation) that achieve the same aim. In menstruating patients whose tumors are ER-positive, the response to oophorectomy is 35 percent. This means their obvious disease will temporarily disappear. An additional 25 percent will have improved symptoms and a prolonged period of stable disease.

Removing your ovaries puts you into menopause right away, complete with mood swings and hot flashes (see Chapter 18). But it can also relieve your metastatic breast cancer symptoms almost immediately, often by the time you leave the hospital. In fact, patients with painful bone metastasis have been reported to wake up from the anesthesia post-oophorectomy pain-free and with calcium levels under control.

This approach went out of fashion with the introduction of chemotherapy, but it has resumed an important place in the treatment of metastatic disease with the introduction of several drugs that can turn off the ovaries' ability to make estrogen. Such an approach can be just the right treatment for a person with bone metastasis and an ER-positive tumor. Whether we remove the ovaries or inactivate them with drugs, the treatment is effective. Reversible menopause can be induced by using GnRH agonists such as Zoladex (goserelin), Lupron (leuprolide), or Trelstar (triptorelin) (see Chapter 15), which block the body's own production of hormones and stop your periods.

Another standard way to treat breast cancer is to use drugs that can change the local hormonal milieu. This is the way antiestrogens such as Nolvadex (tamoxifen) and Fareston (toremifene) work. They can be used in both premenopausal and postmenopausal people whose tumors are sensitive to estrogen. If you were on Nolvadex in the past and then stopped, it's worth trying it again to treat your metastatic disease. However, if the metastasis became apparent while you were on Nolvadex (tamoxifen), your tumor is probably resistant and you should try something else. Note that Fareston (toremifene) and Evista (raloxifene) work the same way that Nolvadex does. Consequently if you are on one of these and your cancer comes back or grows, it is useless to switch to the other one.

In people who are postmenopausal (whether by chemotherapy or naturally), estrogen is principally made by the enzyme aromatase, which converts testosterone and androstenedione to estrogen. This enzyme is found in the adrenal glands, fat, muscle, and breast tissue. Therefore it was thought that blocking this conversion could starve the tumor of estrogen. The first aromatase inhibitor used was aminoglutethimide, but it isn't very potent. In addition, it causes other symptoms by blocking the adrenal glands' production of other hormones. The most recent aromatase inhibitors—Arimidex (anastrozole), Femara (letrozole), and Aromasin (exemestane)—are more potent. They are also specific blockers of aromatase and are therefore much less toxic than aminoglutethimide and have very good response rates. They are currently the drugs of choice once a tumor becomes resistant to Nolvadex (tamoxifen) or even if a patient has never received Nolvadex or stopped it years ago.

The aromatase inhibitors have been shown to improve patients' overall survival better than Nolvadex (tamoxifen) or Megace (megestrol acetate), discussed shortly. The common side effects are hot flashes (30 percent) and weight gain (20 percent) as with Nolvadex; musculoskeletal pain (40 percent); and gastrointestinal complaints (5 percent). But the aromatase inhibitors work only in postmenopausal people. For premenopausal people they are ineffectual and potentially dangerous.

Faslodex (fulvestrant) is an estrogen receptor blocker that does not have the estrogenic effects of Nolvadex (tamoxifen). It benefits 20 to 30 percent of patients when used after an aromatase inhibitor. Its effects are equivalent to Nolvadex and Arimidex.[7] It will often work in patients with tumors that have become resistant to Nolvadex and other forms of endocrine therapy. It is usually given as an intramuscular injection once monthly.

Another interesting choice for patients who are resistant to aromatase inhibitors is estrogen itself, surprising though that may be.[8] One hypothesis is that cancer cells subjected to the estrogen deprivation of aromatase inhibitors become more sensitive and are thus inhibited by low-dose estrogen therapy. It seems you have to keep the cancer cells guessing.

You may think that if all these hormones work separately, they'd work even better together. As I mentioned in Chapter 15, the study on Aridimex (anastrozole) and Nolvadex alone and in combination did not show a synergistic effect between the two in the adjuvant setting. Several studies of combination hormone therapy versus single agents have shown increased likelihood of response but no increase in overall survival, except perhaps in premenopausal people, for whom the combination of ovarian ablation and tamoxifen may be beneficial. A more recent exception is the combination of Faslodex (fulvestrant) combined with Arimidex compared to Arimidex alone. In a recent clinical trial the median overall survival of the Arimidex group alone was 42 months compared to 50 months in the combination therapy group.[9] But sequential use is an approach situation: patients who respond to one therapy are more likely to respond to the next one when the first treatment fails.

Similarly, combinations of hormones and chemotherapy have no long-term advantage over either therapy alone. Patients whose tumors are ER-positive but still only marginally sensitive to hormones are more likely to have a response, but for those who respond to hormone therapy alone, the response from adding chemotherapy will not be longer and there will be no better survival. Moreover, the combination of hormones and chemotherapy will be much more toxic than hormone therapy alone.

If a patient's tumor is ER-positive, it is better for their doctor to wait to give chemotherapy if they do not respond to hormones or after they have had a response (or series of responses) and then stop responding. At that point they are very likely to benefit from the chemotherapy alone.

Some patients experience a phenomenon called "flare" with hormone treatment of metastatic breast cancer (and this can sometimes occur with chemotherapy too): within the first month of therapy there is an exacerbation of the patient's disease. It actually indicates a good prognosis. Typically it occurs with someone who has bone metastasis and is put on Nolvadex (tamoxifen). Suddenly their pain is worse than ever. But then they're back to normal soon after. We think this happens because Nolvadex actually works initially as a weak estrogen in some people, stimulating their cancer, before it starts to function as an antiestrogen. But you need to be aware of this because a flare can be very scary. We also can see a flare in the tumor markers. This is important to know because your doctor, seeing a rise in the markers, may assume that the treatment is not working, instead of recognizing the flare as a sign that it is working. Even if you don't have a flare, markers such as CEA or CA15-3 may rise for a while before they begin to fall, and you may continue to have symptoms such as bone pain (see Chapter 19 regarding microfractures or compression fractures), so be sure to give any therapy—hormones or chemotherapy—a chance to work before changing treatment. Generally you want to stay on any treatment for at least three months unless there is unequivocal evidence that your disease is growing rapidly in spite of the treatment.

The overall effectiveness of all the hormone treatments is about 40 percent. That means in slightly less than half of such cases symptoms are alleviated for a significant period of time. But it doesn't work out equally for everyone. If your tumor is strongly ER- and PR-positive, you'll have a 60 percent chance of responding. People with lower levels of estrogen (ER) and progesterone (PR) have a lower response rate, but it is still significant. In most patients the effects of endocrine treatments last for about twelve to eighteen months, but many stay in remission (with their disease under control) for two to five years, and some are free of disease for as long as ten years. The twenty-four-year survivor mentioned earlier was treated with hormone therapies only. A widely held belief among medical oncologists is that chemotherapy works faster than hormone therapy in reversing symptoms. One reason for this belief may be that chemotherapy often results in faster tumor shrinkage, as seen on

X-rays. Another reason may be that patients who respond to endocrine therapy are usually those with the more slowly growing disease. There is probably a relationship between the rate at which the disease grows and the rate at which it disappears. When the tumor does show up again, especially if the patient is on Nolvadex (tamoxifen), sometimes just stopping the drug can give a secondary response. We think this is because the antiestrogen Nolvadex can, after long periods of treatment, sometimes become estrogenic and eventually stimulate tumor growth; therefore, stopping Nolvadex can halt the growth of the tumor cells again. This "withdrawal" therapy has not been reported for the aromatase inhibitors or Faslodex (fulvestrant), and it is rarely used anymore because there are so many effective, low-toxicity agents to use after stopping Nolvadex.

To sum up, for premenopausal patients, we usually start by trying ovarian ablation by either surgical or chemical means. If the patient has a response, we stay with it until the symptoms recur and then go on to one of the other hormone agents not used the first time (Nolvadex or an aromatase inhibitor, depending on whether the patient is still menstruating). Then, if they have had their ovaries removed, we may try Faslodex (fulvestrant) with or without an aromatase inhibitor—Femara (letrozole) with Ibrance (palbociclib) or Afinitor (everolimus) with Aromasin (exemestane)—or one of the other hormone treatments.

With postmenopausal patients we start with an aromatase inhibitor (because ablating the ovaries of a postmenopausal person doesn't change much). In 25 to 30 percent of cases, when one kind of aromatase inhibitor fails (steroidal or nonsteroidal), changing to the other type can produce a further response.

When the tumor seems resistant to the aromatase inhibitors, estradiol, a form of estrogen, may be tried before moving further down the list, which includes Faslodex (fulvestrant, an estrogen blocker), Nolvadex (tamoxifen), or Halotestin (fluoxymesterone). If a patient was on Nolvadex adjuvant therapy at the time of their metastasis, we would start with Arimidex (anastrozole) for postmenopausal patients and Zoladex (goserelin) or oophorectomy for premenopausal patients. With metastatic breast cancer, only when a patient stops responding to hormones do we go on to chemotherapy. It is important to remember that this may not be a matter of extending life but of maintaining the best quality of life for the longest time. Sometimes oncologists, especially if there is a tumor in the liver or lungs, may lead off with combination chemotherapy for a number of cycles to try to get a quick response before backing off to hormonal treatment to maintain it. As hormonal options are increasing rapidly, we suggest you check the practice guidelines of the NCCN for up-to-date information (www.nccn.org).

A person with metastatic breast cancer whose tumor is sensitive to hormones is comparatively lucky, since they have more avenues of treatment that are less toxic than does someone whose tumor is resistant to hormonal influence. As I noted earlier, however, even a person with hormone-negative tumors occasionally responds to hormone therapy. This may be because the older methods of measuring estrogen and progesterone receptors were somewhat inaccurate and people whose cancer was called negative were actually low positive. Most oncologists feel that a patient with any degree of estrogen or progesterone positivity, however small, should be given treatment with hormone therapy at some time during the course of their metastatic disease. Everyone with metastasis should question their medical oncologist about the possibility of hormone treatment. It may not occur to them to try a hormone maneuver first (or at all) unless you bring it up. The best quality of life is associated with less toxic but successful hormone treatments. It is always a discussion worth having, although chemotherapy is probably the better choice if you have moderate to severe symptoms or life-threatening organ dysfunction.

CHEMOTHERAPY IN METASTATIC BREAST CANCER

The good news about breast cancer is that it responds to many different kinds of chemotherapy drugs. Indeed, chemotherapy is the best choice for people whose tumors are not responsive to hormone therapy or for those whose ER-positive tumors have become resistant to hormone treatment. In those who also have HER2-positive tumors, targeted therapies (see the following discussion) should also be considered. Only sometimes does chemotherapy cause a remission—the disappearance of the signs or symptoms of cancer—but it certainly can reduce symptoms from metastatic disease even better than narcotics. If you have not received chemotherapy for metastatic disease before, or it's been at least a year since you received it, the likelihood of the disease reacting to this first line chemotherapy is between 35 and 55 percent. In one study pooling all the data, the median survival was 21 months, but the 10 percent of participants with the worst survival rate lived an average of 6.3 months and the 10 percent with the best survival lived almost five years!

These drugs are usually used in patients with ER- and PR-negative tumors and patients who need a rapid response because the metastases are causing organ dysfunction. The median time to respond is around two to three months, which means that only half of all patients who eventually go on to respond will have evidence of it within two to three months. This is important because both patients and doctors often get impatient and don't give the treatment enough time. In addition, the scans and markers are not that accurate. Sometimes a 25 percent increase in the size of a lesion (which is within the error margins of the test) will prompt a shift in treatment. Dr. Craig Henderson points out that in the original Herceptin trial, "the earliest that any patient was evaluated was eleven weeks (the protocol called for twelve weeks), and I think it is one reason why we found the 11.3 percent responders that we did find—in someone else's hands the drug would have been abandoned."[10]

Symptoms generally improve within a few weeks; the average duration of the response is 5 to 13 months on the drug, but individual patients' responses can last longer. The maximum duration that we've so far found is over 180 months—over fifteen years—and thus could be called a cure. (Unfortunately this length of survival is very rare.) The average survival of the responders is 15 to 42 months. It is generally less for patients whose cancers are resistant to chemotherapy. So chemotherapy, like hormone therapy, can help you live with symptom improvement for anywhere between one and four years, and there's a small chance it can give you ten or more years with a high quality of life.

More than eighty cytotoxic drugs—drugs that kill cells—have been tested. Thirteen are used commonly in breast cancer treatment. Interestingly, breast cancer creates the kind of tumor that is responsive to the greatest array of drugs. Most other cancers don't respond to as many chemicals (hence, Dr. Hayes's "good news" observation cited earlier). The standard drugs are the same ones I discussed in Chapter 15 in terms of adjuvant treatment: cyclophosphamide (Cytoxan) (C), methotrexate (Trexall) (M), 5-fluorouracil (Adrucil) (F), doxorubicin (Adriamycin) (A), epirubicin (Ellence) (E), paclitaxel (Taxol) (T), docetaxel (Taxotere) (D), eribulin mesylate (Halaven), and carboplatin (Paraplatin). These drugs have the highest antitumor activity among all the patients studied. They also have only limited cross-resistance, meaning that if the cancer becomes resistant to one, it is not likely to be resistant to another.

What is used depends on what was used at the time the disease was diagnosed. If you already had CMF, then Adriamycin (doxorubicin or pegylated liposomal doxorubicin, Doxil) may be tried. If you had Adriamycin when you were diagnosed, paclitaxel (Taxol) or docetaxel (Taxotere) or nab-paclitaxel (Abraxane) may be the next choice. Fortunately there are other drugs as well. These include capecitabine (Xeloda), mitoxantrone (Novantrone), vinorelbine (Navelbine), gemcitabine (Gemzar), and, less commonly, irinotecan (Camptosar), cisplatin (Platinol) or carboplatin (Paraplatin) (especially in patients with triple-negative cancer or who are BRCA positive), and mutamycin (Mitomycin-C), all of which have documented antitumor activity in breast cancer. Both Ixempra (ixabepilone) and Doxil (liposomal doxorubicin) are usually given alone rather than in the combinations we use for adjuvant therapy (see Chapter 15) because single-agent therapy simplifies treatment planning, has less toxicity, and does not appear to compromise length of survival.

There are always new drugs being tested in clinical trials, so make sure you check out www.clinicaltrials.gov or www.breastcancertrials .org to find out if there is a study you can participate in. All the current effective therapies started out as clinical trial drugs.

Each drug has limitations. With Adriamycin (doxorubicin), we can give only a certain dosage, and then it becomes toxic to the heart. Once you reach that point you can't ever use it again. Some of the other drugs you can take indefinitely.

Many chemotherapy drugs produce the standard side effects (vomiting, bone marrow suppression, and so on). As I mentioned in Chapter 15, there are now terrific antinausea drugs that have almost eliminated this problem. When the drugs are combined they tend to be worse. For this reason, giving one chemotherapy drug at a time can significantly reduce side effects. At this point a sensible approach may be to use single agents sequentially in situations in which there is no organ dysfunction and mild to moderate symptoms, saving the combinations for cases with organ dysfunction and severe symptoms.

Most chemotherapy drugs involve some hair loss. Several have a very low potential to cause leukemia down the road. Because you're dealing with metastatic breast cancer, though, that risk is not a reason to eliminate them. Most will decrease your white cell count. Attempts have been made to test the tumor cells against a variety of drugs in a test tube to predict the right drug or combination of drugs. Although it sounds like a great idea, it hasn't worked in practice as well as we would like.

Although cancer cells can build resistance to a particular drug, they don't always do so. Sometimes we treat metastatic cancer with a drug and get a response; then the disease recurs and we are able to use the same drug again, and again it works. It always amazes me how often we find a drug that doesn't work for the majority of patients but turns out to be exactly what one particular person needs. I had a patient with horrible lumps all over her chest. We treated her with just about everything, including experimental drugs, and nothing seemed to work. Then we went back and tried straight 5-fluorouracil, which usually works only modestly in breast cancer—and everything disappeared. So we sometimes can't predict what the right drug is for a particular person, and if you have metastatic disease, you need to keep that in mind. You may feel discouraged if particular drugs don't seem to be working, especially if they're the standard breast cancer drugs. But you never know when we'll hit on the one that will alleviate your symptoms.

Once we've found a drug that works, we generally continue it for a long time. How long is something on which doctors disagree. There are two philosophies. One is that we'll get as much response as we're going to get in about six months, so we should give the chemo for six months and then stop. The other is to give it continuously until the patient becomes resistant to it, and then move on to something else. There are arguments for both schools. Most of the studies suggest improved quality of life and better symptom control with continuous therapy, but again this may not be best for every person. It's something you should discuss with your doctor and be clear about before you start treatments.

Dr. Hayes tells his patients that four things can happen with treatment for metastatic disease:

1. Terrible toxicity: it is the wrong drug and should be stopped and something else tried.
2. Obvious disease progression: it is the wrong drug or the cancer has become resistant and it is time to stop that drug and try something else.

3. A stable situation: it is not clear whether the drug is holding the disease in check; continue the drug with monitoring of disease and side effects.

4. Improvement with little toxicity: it is the right drug and should be continued.

It is not hard to figure out which of the four categories you are in—you know how you feel and what your physical exam and data from X-rays and markers reveal. Often people have symptoms that are not really associated with their disease but frighten them nonetheless, leading them to assume their disease is getting worse when it is not. Oncologists too tend to assume that everything that happens is due to cancer. Both need to be sure that the tumor really is getting worse before changing drugs. For this reason many oncologists monitor the patient about every twelve weeks of chemotherapy with the same tests you had in the beginning—comparing apples to apples. In addition they do routine blood tests for liver function and tumor markers (CA 15-3, CA 27.29, and CEA) every three months. Some studies have shown that we can measure specific tumor cells known as circulating tumor cells (CTCs) in the blood of people with metastatic disease.[11] If there is an increase in circulating tumor cells, you probably are on the wrong drug and should switch. A study that examined whether this change improved survival, however, found it did not make a difference and that more treatment was needed beyond the standard chemotherapy.[12]

It may seem that combining chemotherapy and hormone therapy would work better than either one alone. But it doesn't. In people with hormone-sensitive tumors, adding chemotherapy to hormones doesn't increase the disease-free or overall survival, and they get unpleasant side effects. However, after hormone therapy has been used as it would in the first place, chemotherapies work just as well as they would if used earlier.

Anyone with metastatic disease needs to investigate the available clinical trials. But the sooner this is done the better, as many trial organizers tend to have strict requirements, and one of them, ironically, is basic good health (other than the cancer, of course). Eligibility criteria often reject older patients or those with other diseases as well, like diabetes and heart disease. The FDA recently issued rules to change this, so trials can better represent the people who will be taking the clinical trial drug. Either way, the effort to get into a trial is worth it. New drugs and/or new combinations of drugs and biologic agents are being tested continuously and may be the best choice for someone with metastatic disease. It's important to talk with your doctor and get clear, precise information about what drugs may be best for you, how long and in what sequence you can take them, and what their side effects are.

For a while we thought that giving higher doses of chemotherapy would be better. These required harvesting and storing some of your own bone marrow and then giving the drugs at doses that destroyed what was left. The preserved cells were then transplanted back (autologous transplant). Although we showed we could safely give these high doses, six randomized controlled studies examining its use in women with metastasis showed that they had no benefit over standard doses of chemotherapy.[13] Although there's always a temptation to go for what appears to be the most aggressive therapy, in this case there was no benefit to compensate for the increased side effects for most patients.

TARGETED THERAPY IN METASTATIC BREAST CANCER

We have always dreamed of finding something distinctive about the cancer cell and developing a therapy specific to it. We would then give the antibody, kill or control all the cancer cells, and do little or no harm to the rest of the body. Several drugs have been developed in the past decade to target molecules that may be specific to, or overexpressed by, the cancer cells. The most successful are specific antibodies to target HER2 (Herceptin [trastuzumab]).[14] About 20 percent of women with breast cancer have too many copies of the HER2/neu oncogene. This particular oncogene tells the cell to grow: harder, stronger, and longer. Herceptin is an antibody to that oncogene, which blocks it in its tracks. With each passing year we get more drugs of this targeted type: Kadcyla (ado-trastuzumab emtasine), Perjeta (pertuzumab), Tykerb (lapatinib), Tukysa (tucatinib), Enhertu (trastuzumab deruxtecan), and Zeno (zenocutuzumab). They are all being used in combination and in addition to chemotherapy.

There are now several trials suggesting that Herceptin (trastuzumab), in combination with Perjeta (pertuzumab) with chemotherapy, is very effective in HER2/neu-overexpressing metastatic breast cancer. In one large study called, amusingly enough, the Cleopatra (Clinical Evaluation of Pertuzumab and Trastuzumab) randomized controlled trial, women who received chemotherapy plus Herceptin and Perjeta had increased progression-free survival and overall survival without an increase in heart problems.[15] So all women with HER2/neu-overexpressing metastatic breast cancer should receive Herceptin either alone or with chemotherapy unless they have preexisting heart failure. When or if breast cancer progresses on Herceptin, it is not clear that this antibody should be continued. This has been examined in a small German study, which suggested that continuing Herceptin after the disease grows is still worthwhile.[16] Another option is to doubly block HER2 with both Herceptin and Tykerb with or without chemotherapy. This whole area is changing quickly, and I encourage you to search out a clinical trial whenever possible.[17]

Kadcyla (ado-trastuzumab emtansine) is part of a relatively new class of drugs in that it combines a targeted antibody to HER2/neu with a chemotherapy drug, emtansine.[18] The idea is that it will deliver the chemotherapy just to the targeted cells (those that are overexpressing HER2/neu). This allows these very toxic chemotherapy drugs to be given in much slower doses, making it tolerable. Another of these newer drugs, Enhertu (trastuzumab deruxtecan), is particularly effective in women with low HER2 expression, of +1 or +2. Administering Enhertu instead of standard chemo in these cases may help delay disease progression and extend survival.

As I mentioned in Chapter 15, cyclin-dependent kinase (CDK) inhibitors have been shown to be effective in metastatic hormone-positive HER2-negative tumors. Ibrance (palbociclib) is the first approved drug of this type[19] and has since been followed by Kisqali (ribociclib) and Verzenio (abemaciclib). In what one medical review glowingly called a "renaissance" of this therapy, there are about forty CDK inhibitors aimed at preventing cancer cells from multiplying in various stages of development. Two that show promise for breast cancer are dinaciclib, which demonstrated an antitumor effect, and Seliciclib (roscovitine), which hinders the tumor cell's ability to repair itself and thus makes it more vulnerable to chemotherapy. Although these drugs all use the same mechanism, there are differences among them in effectiveness and safety.

People with triple-negative, PD-L1-positive breast cancer will be heartened to hear there is now an immunotherapy for them. Keytruda (pembrolizumab) is a checkpoint inhibitor that helps the immune system recognize and attack cancer cells. When a cancer is described as PD-L1-positive, it is because it has been releasing that specific protein to turn off the immune system so it can grow uninterrupted. Keytruda is used in combination with chemotherapy to treat inoperable, locally advanced or metastatic, triple-negative, PD-L1-positive breast cancer.[20] About 10 to 20 percent of breast cancers are triple-negative and are not sensitive to hormones, so this offers another option.

At least three new targeted drugs have recently received approval against different checkpoint inhibitors: Piqray (alpelisib), which focuses on the PIK3CA mutation, found in 30 to 40 percent of breast cancers; Afinitor (everolimus), which targets mTOR kinase, a protein that frequently mutates in cancer cells; and Lynparza (olaparib), which targets heat shock proteins (HSPs) that are overexpressed in many cancers.

There are other new targeted drugs in development. One works against insulin-like growth factor 1 (IGF-1), which is involved in different types of solid tumors; another acts against histone deacetylase inhibitors (HDACs); and a third targets the fibroblast growth factor receptor 4 (FGFR4). Someday, one of these strings of initials may be as familiar as HER2 and we will have new treatments. It continues to be important to keep asking your doctor about new options and monitoring the available clinical trials.

Testing Personalized Immunotherapy with CAR-T

A personalized immunotherapy made from a patient's own white blood cells is currently being tested on breast cancer in at least three different clinical trials. White blood cells are removed from the patient and then modified with chimeric antigen receptors (CARs) so they can better recognize and attack cancer cells. The white cells used for this are the T cells, which you may recall from Chapter 3 are the ones that keep a database of previous threats to the body. If they recognize a threat they've seen before, they fight it with specific antibodies or killer T cells. This is why this particular immunotherapy is called CAR-T. One trial is focused on metastatic breast cancer that has spread to the brain, a second is targeting triple-negative breast cancer, and a third is aimed at using CAR-T for preventing metastatic breast cancer and avoiding chemotherapy. In addition, the process of altering immune T cells for reinsertion has been shortened in a preclinical study from almost two weeks to a mere twenty-four hours.

Vaccines

Vaccines against breast cancer are being studied with new enthusiasm after the success of COVID-19 vaccines. Although we commonly think of a vaccine as prevention, such as the ones used for polio or measles, it can also be used in treatment. These vaccines are made by training immune cells to home in on a certain target found on breast cancer cells.[21] It sounds great, but as we've said throughout the book, not every cancer cell is the same. This means that several vaccines will be needed against the many types of breast cancer. Vaccines for metastatic breast cancer are being tested in clinical trials and may be useful in the near future.

Bisphosphonates

Most of the treatments we have considered involve killing or controlling the cancer cell. The other approach is to alter the tissue that the cancer is trying to grow in. A bisphosphonate is a drug that blocks the resorption (breakdown) of bone. Another drug, denosumab, prevents the formation and activation of osteoclasts. Overactivity of these cells that serve in normal bone remodeling are what leads to osteoporosis as we age.

Bisphosphonates will reduce pain in 60 percent of patients with painful bone metastases, and these agents significantly reduce the frequency of fractures and other bone symptoms. They have been shown to be very effective in treating bone metastasis. When there is cancer in the bone, the bone is resorbed—one of the reasons the bone gets weaker and often fractures. Several studies have shown that women who take pamidronate (Aredia) or zoledronic acid (Zometa) every four weeks will have a decrease not only in the resorption of the bone but also in the number of new bone metastases that develop as well as the incidence of bone fractures and bone pain.[22] After the first year, women with bone metastases taking Zometa can reduce the dose to every three months and get the same benefit. Prolia (denosumab)[23] is given subcutaneously every four weeks with fewer side effects than those of the bisphosphonates. However, these drugs, excluding Prolia, can cause complications in the jaw, as described in Chapter 15, so it is important that you have your teeth checked before starting on the drug. A bisphosphonate or Prolia is started as soon as bone metastases are diagnosed and continued indefinitely.

LOCAL TREATMENTS FOR METASTATIC BREAST CANCER

I've been discussing systemic therapies so far, but sometimes local treatment is called for. Certain kinds of metastatic disease respond best to local treatments because they're local problems.

Radiation, for example, works best if the cancer has spread to your eye. Spinal cord compression involvement with impending bone fracture (in which your bone is so weakened that it is about to break) also lends itself well to radiation, as it too is a local problem and there is only one spot to be treated. This may also require surgical treatment to stabilize the bone before radiation.

Radiation for metastatic cancer is the same as for initial breast cancer, but its purpose is different—to alleviate pain or other symptoms. A couple of weeks usually pass before the pain noticeably lessens. After any treatment of any organ and, especially, bone, healing of damage from the cancer must occur before fully normal function returns. Thus, just as it takes months after you break a bone for normal tensile strength to return, it takes months after the treatment with radiotherapy to have normal bone strength again. During this time it is easy to fracture the bone, and in some cases you'll never regain full strength because the therapy (especially radiotherapy) may reduce the bone's capacity to fully heal.

The timing is somewhat different too. There are usually ten to fifteen treatments spread over two and a half to four weeks. A smaller dose of radiation is used. Although a primary radiation treatment to your breast might use 6,000 centigrays of radiation over six and a half weeks, with 180 centigrays per treatment, the treatment for someone with, for example, bone metastasis in the hip might use 3,000 centigrays over ten treatments of 300 centigrays each.

Surgery, as I mentioned earlier, can be helpful if there is one spot in the lung or brain, for example, in someone who has had a reasonably long interval between primary diagnosis and development of metastatic disease. If the cancer has recurred in several places, however, systemic treatment is best.

PAIN CONTROL

In terms of palliation—getting rid of symptoms so that you feel better— treatments of the cancer itself aren't the only options. We've come an enormous way in pain control. If, for example, you're in severe pain because of bone metastasis, radiation can be very effective as mentioned earlier. In addition, we now have ways of putting a catheter in the space along the spinal cord and dripping continuous low-dose morphine to get rid of all the pain. Administered this way, it won't affect your mind the way it would if administered systemically. This won't cure you, but in your last three or four months of life, when systemic therapy is no longer working, it can give you time to enjoy others and activities that are most important to you and reduce or eliminate suffering.

There's now a whole specialty of pain management that includes psychiatrists, anesthesiologists, and internists. Drugs, nerve blocks, and even nerve stimulation can be useful. Because a thorough discussion of all the options is outside the scope of this book, suffice it to say that we have acquired a lot of knowledge about chronic pain and how to deal with it. Anybody who has chronic pain because of metastatic cancer and isn't getting relief should ask to be referred to a specialized pain unit.

Sometimes oncologists and people who work on cancer are so focused on treating and curing the disease that they forget about these ancillary things that can make an enormous difference in a patient's life. So ask to see a pain specialist; even if it means having to travel to the local medical school, it can make a big difference to you.

EXPERIMENTAL TREATMENTS

This is a perfect time for people to participate in phase 3 clinical trials (see Chapter 10)—trials of promising drugs or treatments that have been tested in earlier phases and shown not to harm the patient. The timing is not only right medically but also historically, as a major shift is underway to make clinical trials more equitable and accessible. But your more immediate concern is whether to opt for phase 1 or phase 2 trials. These are earlier stages in the testing of a drug, designed to determine first the toxicity of a possibly useful drug and then whether it works.

Because traditional treatments, which were so helpful with your first diagnosis, may offer only a slim chance of cure, an experimental treatment may be worth considering. Generally with metastatic breast cancer, there is no harm in trying an innovative new therapy and postponing treatment with other standard therapies. Again, check www.breastcancer trials.org to see what trials you may be eligible for and then tell your doctor about them; doctors don't always know what is in the pipeline and so you have to be your own advocate. As I've mentioned before, one of my favorite documentaries is an older PBS special by Ken Burns, *The Emperor of All Maladies*, depicting the history of cancer research and clinical advances over the years. One woman's story related that in the early 1990s she had metastatic breast cancer and refused chemotherapy. She looked for options and found out that Dr. Dennis Slamon at UCLA was trying something new, a targeted drug. She had her tumor tested and indeed she overexpressed HER2. She was on an early trial of Herceptin (trastuzumab) and last I heard lived more than two decades with no sign of disease. Not everyone gets that kind of miracle, but if you don't consider these clinical trials, you will not have even the opportunity to be the lucky one.

As I've noted earlier, in the past, clinical trials have not always been easy to get into. The criteria used to select participants tended to exclude older patients and those with additional health conditions like diabetes and heart ailments—more prevalent in Black, Latino, and Indigenous populations. Over time, restrictions such as these prompted criticism and protests from caregivers, patients, and advocates. Dr. Kelly Shanahan, a retired OB-GYN and metastatic breast cancer patient advocate, wrote on Twitter: "We should not limit #clinicaltrial enrollment to the cancer olympians—trials need to reflect the population who will be eventually using the drugs, comorbidities, brain mets and all."[24] In response to these concerns, in 2022 the FDA launched Project Equity to ensure that data from clinical trials adequately reflects the patients for whom the drugs are ultimately intended. The goal is to improve access to clinical trials among racial and ethnic minorities, rural residents, sexual and gender minorities, and individuals with economic, linguistic, or cultural barriers to health care services. To this end, researchers and their sponsors are expected to submit a Race and Ethnicity Diversity Plan early in the clinical development of a product.

When is the best time to join an experimental trial? Classically, people do it when nothing else has helped and they've run out of options. However, by the time you run out of options, you're least likely to be able to respond to the new treatment: you have no resources left. So the best time may be when you have been diagnosed with metastatic disease but are feeling well. You have a chest X-ray or bone scan that shows a lesion, but you actually have modest symptoms. At this stage, there's no rush to use chemotherapy or hormone therapy because, as I noted before, there's no evidence that treating with chemo earlier will give you better survival odds than waiting until you have symptoms. If you now try something experimental, you have an opportunity to see if it works; if it doesn't you can still get the usual chemotherapy if symptoms worsen.

Only a doctor who is working on the particular experiments is likely to offer such treatments routinely. The best way to find out about them is to go to your local cancer center and see what they're involved in, and you can also go to www.clinicaltrials.gov. You can obtain a list of every clinical trial you're eligible for, either in your own geographical area or in the whole United States if you're willing and able to travel. You can also register at www.breastcancertrials.org to be notified regarding trials you may be eligible for.

I think this is really worthwhile. It's a gamble, but sometimes the gamble pays off. For example, some of the patients who first participated in the tests for Taxotere (docetaxel) had remarkable responses that lasted between eighteen and twenty-four months. Another good example is one of the patients on the first Herceptin (trastuzumab) trial. This was one of my Boston patients who had a recurrence on the chest wall shortly after having had Adriamycin (doxorubicin). We knew both from her HER2 status and the rapidity of the disease recurrence that her prognosis wasn't good. She flew to Los Angeles and was enrolled in the first trial I mentioned earlier. The disease in her chest wall disappeared completely, and the last I heard she was still tumor-free more than a decade after going on the study. This dramatic, long-lasting response and the one featured in the documentary are uncommon in phase 1 and phase 2 trials, but every so often they do happen, making it worthwhile for the individual patient to participate in these studies.

While they may help you, these trials can involve side effects as well. But only you can decide what price in toxicity you are willing to pay. Some people want to try everything new, but others don't. Don't let your doctor or family push you. Decide in your own heart what the best approach is for you.

During and after your treatment for metastatic disease you'll be followed with the staging tests—bone scan, chest X-ray, and blood tests— as well as a few other tests such as CT scans, PET scans, or MRI. These can help determine whether you're indeed responding to treatment, although your symptoms are the best test of effectiveness.

TAKING CARE OF YOURSELF EMOTIONALLY

Women with metastatic disease often feel very isolated. Other survivors, finding their stories too scary, may not want to listen to them, and family and friends may not be able to deal with the seriousness of the situation. Luckily there are many people living with breast cancer recurrences and metastatic disease willing to help you at a click of a browser. I suggest checking out METAvivor.org, the Metastatic Breast Cancer Network (www.mbcn.org), the Dr. Susan Love Research Foundation (www.drsusanloveresearch.org), and the National Breast Cancer Coalition (www.stopbreastcancer.org). If you like Twitter, check out breast cancer social media at #bcsm. I strongly recommend sites such as these. People with metastatic breast cancer are now living long enough to have advocacy groups working toward better treatments and more research.

David Spiegel[25] tells the story of a woman who had always wanted to write poetry and started after her diagnosis of metastatic disease. She had a book of her poems published before her death. One of my own patients, years ago, Susan Shapiro, was very distressed with the lack of analysis of breast cancer from a feminist political perspective. She wrote an article in the local feminist paper and called a meeting. From this she started the Women's Community Cancer Project in Boston a few months before she died. I'm certain she would be happy to know her work sparked a national movement that continues today.

A diagnosis of recurrence or metastasis will remind you that you do not have control over your body, but you certainly do have control over your mind, emotions, and spirit. This is a good time to revisit some of the complementary treatments such as visualization, self-hypnosis, and imagery (see Chapter 16). And find a doctor you can talk to and who will listen to you. Shop around if you have to. If you are in a small town and/or have an insurance plan with limited choice, then schedule an appointment with your oncologist so that you can talk about what you need as well as what they expect from you. You need to know as accurately as possible what to expect from your condition and your treatments so that you can plan. Ask for the information you need, and tell your doctor if there are things you would rather not know. As in any relationship, frank communication about your needs will go far toward having them met.

A diagnosis of recurrent breast cancer often brings fear of increasing pain. As I discussed earlier in this chapter, pain is certainly not inevitable. Pain control has finally gone mainstream in the United States. There are pain centers, and many methods have been developed to deal with pain without clouding your mind and ruining your life. And the field of palliative care—or treatment of side effects or "collateral damage" as I like to call it—is blossoming. The problem is that often oncologists get so tied up in treating the disease they don't pay attention to these potentially life-disrupting side effects. Ask to see someone from palliative care; they are not just for the end of life and may have a lot of good ideas of how you can deal with your symptoms. In fact, insist on it!

Not everyone dies from a recurrence or metastatic breast cancer, but it is certainly a possibility. Atul Gawande's book *Being Mortal* and Spiegel's book *Living Beyond Limits* are invaluable in addressing the needs of the heart and soul in confronting terminal illness.[26] You may not be able to avoid death, but you can control how you want to handle it. One of my patients was a great denier. From the first moment of her diagnosis she refused to let her cancer interfere with her life. When she developed metastatic disease, this pattern continued. She continued to hurl herself through life: sailing, traveling, and enjoying herself. My first reaction was to be a little critical of her inability to face the reality of the situation—until I realized that she had faced it. She knew exactly what she was doing and was determined to take control of whatever time she had left. She slipped into a coma on her sailboat among friends and died as she wanted, where she wanted, in control to the end.

HOW LONG DO I HAVE?

My own feelings have evolved on this issue since my own experience with acute myelogenous leukemia in 2012. When a patient would ask me, "How long do I have to live?" I used to dodge the question—not because I wanted to withhold information from my patient but because I simply don't know what will happen to each individual. There are patients who, according to the statistics, should die in four months but live four years; there are others who should last four years but die in four months. I'm always amazed at the variations. One of my patients had a small cancer and negative nodes with what should have been a good prognosis, but when she finished her radiation we discovered the cancer had metastasized to her lungs, and she died in three months. Another patient, a Chinese woman who spoke no English, had a cancer that was very aggressive, and I privately thought she wouldn't live very long. I had to talk to her through her sons, who kept trying to get me to say how long she had. I wouldn't tell them. It's a good thing, because she was still alive seven years later. Sometimes I think she lived so long because she didn't know she was supposed to die.

It's important for your doctor to be honest with you. I think it's sensible to say to a patient who has asked for a frank response, "This is serious, but we don't know how long you'll live until we see how you respond to treatment. You'll probably eventually die of breast cancer, and you probably won't live another forty years, so you may want to plan your life with that in mind." If you insist on more specific predictions, a doctor may quote statistics, but you should always be reminded that there are exceptions to statistics. If 99 out of 100 patients in your condition die within a year, 1 out of 100 doesn't—and there's no reason to assume you won't be that one. You should know that this is a hard task for your doctor, who really wants to "get it right" for you, neither denying you a chance of extra life in which you might accomplish things you want to get done, or putting you through needless treatment that only makes the last days more miserable. This is something the doctor can only learn by experience. They don't teach it in medical school, and this is a situation in which a doctor who has been through this many times before may have an advantage.

I certainly dealt with this with my own cancer experience. I had the advantage—or maybe disadvantage—of having access and the ability to understand the medical literature, so I knew the statistics were not good. I spent many nights reading articles trying to find the one that described "Susan Love's leukemia" and what to expect. Not surprisingly I never found it! At some point, I realized that it didn't matter what the literature said; my experience was my experience and I was going to go with that!

Still, I welcomed the opportunity to talk from the heart to the people dearest to me and make sure that nothing was left unsaid. I also updated all my legal papers and end-of-life wishes prior to starting treatment. I am very happy that I had the chance to do all that even if it did prove to be unnecessary. I now think that it is important for you to know what the situation is so that you can live your life accordingly. You may have some quality time left to take the trip you have been dreaming of or do something memorable with your kids or grandkids.

So if you want to know, ask, but remember that statistical odds can only tell you what will happen in general. What happens to you is what matters!

WHEN SHOULD I STOP TREATMENT?

This is always a difficult and very personal question. We talk a lot about not wanting heroic care at the end, but it is very hard for a patient or doctor to know exactly when that point has been reached. It is very important to have ongoing discussions with your doctor on this issue. My wife's cousin was diagnosed with lung cancer and initially was treated with chemotherapy when a lesion was found in her adrenal gland. This meant the disease was in fact incurable with modern medicine. Her doctor did not tell her this, however. I had a conversation with her and reviewed the situation honestly. She was not symptomatic but the doctor wanted to give her chemotherapy to treat the lesion. I said to him, "You cannot cure her, correct?" He agreed. "All you can do is potentially make her symptoms better with your treatments, correct?" He agreed. "She has no symptoms right now, correct?" Again he agreed. "So," I asked, "why are you giving her chemotherapy? Why not let her go to the mountains for the summer, where her soul thrives, and when she develops symptoms she can call you?" He thought about it and said, "That makes sense," and indeed left her to have a terrific summer before going back for chemotherapy when she became symptomatic. She died several months later. He was not a bad doctor, but sometimes doctors think we always want treatment even when it is not going to be lifesaving. You need to think about how *you* feel about it and make sure that you and your doctor are on the same page.

END-OF-LIFE PLANNING: MAKING YOUR WISHES KNOWN

Eventually, however, there comes the hardest part. We've tried all the available treatments, and we know that you don't have much longer. Even then, we don't know if it's days or weeks, and there is still the possibility of a miracle. But there's a point at which you're clearly dying, and you have a right to know that. The prevailing belief used to be that it was better not to tell patients they were dying. But this sets up an unhealthy climate of denial. It's likely you'll sense it yourself, but since no one wants to talk about it you pretend it's okay in order to spare them, and they pretend it's okay in order to spare you. Such denial can keep you from finishing your business—clearing up relationships, saying goodbye, saying the things you won't get another chance to say to the people you love, giving them the chance to say those things to you. Atul Gawande addresses this well in his 2014 book *Being Mortal.*[27] I think doctors make a great error in denying death: we tend to look at it too much as a defeat and get caught up in our own wishful thinking at the patient's expense.

While you're still feeling fairly well, it is important to talk with your doctor, and with your family members or friends about how you want to die when the time comes. Do you want to be kept alive at all costs, or not? Do you want to die at home, or in the hospital? And, I hate to add: investigate your insurance to see what they will cover.

Often people die in a hospital or a nursing home, and many think of that as an inevitability. But it isn't, and it's important to consider whether it may be better for you to die in your own home or in the home of a loved one. For many people this is the best option, particularly if a loved one is able to stay with you full time. Dying at home offers more control over your surroundings and a greater likelihood that you will die with loved ones around you. If this is an option you want to explore, there are many hospice programs that can help you. They are experienced in caring for both the patient and the family in a way that can make all the difference. I had firsthand experience when my cousin was dying of bile duct cancer, and I cannot say enough about how terrific they are.

For some people and their families, this is not possible. If it makes more sense for you to die in a hospital, there is much you and your loved ones can do to ensure that the environment is as comfortable as possible. Many hospitals have hospice rooms for dying patients, and even those that don't can make a regular room more homelike. You will want to discuss your wishes with the caregivers there to be sure they are willing and prepared to follow them.

There are other issues you'll want to look into—perhaps even before you have decided that it's time to stop fighting your illness. When the time comes—whether in months or years—do you want to be heavily medicated or as alert as possible? No way is universally better, but one way may be better for you. If your wishes are clearly known—especially if they can be documented in a living will—you may be able to prevent those tragic situations in which doctors and family members are fighting over whether to keep you on a life support system.

A living will is only part of an advance directive—a set of written instructions that also include a health care proxy. The living will spells out what medical treatment you do and don't want if the time arrives when you are unable to verbalize your own decisions. A health care proxy specifies a particular person you authorize to make decisions about your care when you no longer can.

Living wills vary from state to state, and in some cases you may need to add information to yours. As Dr. Daniel Tobin writes in *Peaceful Dying*, the language of the typical living will may not be specific enough.[28] If the document merely says you don't want life-prolonging measures if you have an "incurable or irreversible condition," your doctor may define such a condition differently than you do. So you may want to add a specific "do not resuscitate" to your living will, and other additions concerning artificial nutrition and hydration. You need to spend some time thinking about what you do want when the time comes. Do you want to be tube-fed? Do you want to be given antibiotics to fight infections? Or do you prefer to die from the infection rather than to continue for a short time and die of your cancer? These things may not be fun to think about, but they're important.

If you are in a state that allows physician-assisted dying (eleven as of this writing), you may want to see if your situation makes you eligible for such help. For information about this option, look up www.compassion indying.org or www.deathwithdignity.org.

Dr. Betsy Carpenter, a speaker and activist around issues of advance directives, emphasizes that it's important to make those decisions before you reach the point at which you can no longer speak for yourself. You may or may not want life-extending treatment at some point, and you have a right to decide. Like Dr. Tobin, Carpenter stresses the importance of talking with your family and friends in advance, discussing the options open to you and how you feel about them, and listening respectfully to your loved ones' feelings. Your illness and your ultimate death will affect those who love you deeply, and it's important to involve them in your decision-making process. Understanding your feelings and sharing theirs with you will make it far less likely that they'll go against your wishes when the time comes.

In deciding what you do and don't want, think about your fears in particular. Most people fear pain, loss of control, inappropriate prolongation of life, and becoming a burden to loved ones. And of course some fear death itself. Each of these fears should be explored fully, in terms of what is reasonable to think may happen and in terms of your own emotions.

Pick your health care proxy carefully, Dr. Carpenter says, and spell out whom you don't want involved in making health care decisions for you as well. "This doesn't have to be hostile," she says. "You can write, 'although I dearly love my son Jim, I don't wish him to have any part in decision making around my care.'" The agent you choose should be someone you love and fully trust to honor your wishes, who knows you well enough to make decisions that you haven't spelled out, in ways that you'd want. "For example," she says, "my husband is my proxy agent, and he knows that I wouldn't want my life artificially prolonged. But suppose my daughter, who lives in London, wasn't here when I went into a coma. He might be certain that it was important for her to see me living and breathing one last time. So he might decide to keep me on life support for twenty-four hours until she could get back home. And he would know that, loving her, I would also want this for her." Because of such contingencies, she adds, although your living will should be specific, it shouldn't be so specific that it precludes your agent from making judgments in such unforeseen circumstances. You may want to write out a declaration of precedence: "If a conflict arises between my list and my agent's decision, I give precedence to my agent over my own written word."

If there is someone you don't want visiting you when you're dying, this too should be spelled out, says Carpenter, in a priority-of-visitation statement. Such documents are important even for those not facing imminent death, she says. Healthy people are sometimes injured in accidents and lose the ability to verbalize their wishes.

And remember that there is no universally right choice. You may want to be allowed to die if, for example, you're in an irreversible coma. However, you may decide that no one can know absolutely if a coma is irreversible and you want to have whatever chance there is to go on living, even if that chance is minute. One woman I know tells of how she was walking with her friend, and they passed an old-age home where a very elderly, frail man in a wheelchair sat staring in front of him, seemingly completely unaware of his surroundings. Her friend shuddered and said, "I wouldn't want to live if it had to be like that." My friend shook her head. "Maybe he's looking at the trees and feeling the breeze on his face, and maybe that's worth living for." Neither woman was right or wrong.

These scenarios are important for every one of us to consider, since none of us is immortal, and death can come for anyone anytime. Of course, you may live another ten to twenty years, but you lose nothing by having those discussions, and you may even gain some peace of mind.

We all need to live our lives with the knowledge that time is limited. Those of us who have had to face squarely the possibility of death for whatever reason are in some odd way lucky. We certainly grow from the experience and learn that life is precious.

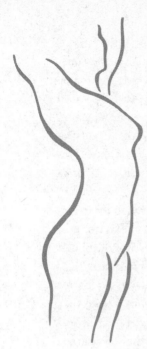

Eradicating Breast Cancer: Politics and Research

THE POLITICS OF BREAST CANCER

Breast cancer has certainly come a long way in the thirty-three years since the first edition of this book. In fact, you could say this book helped to start a political movement.

The first edition of this book made no mention of the politics of the disease: there were none. The second edition chronicled its birth. And someday soon we will be able to rest on our laurels because politics will not be necessary. Until that day I think it is very important that we continue to remember and record our recent history. For those of you who have been a part of it, read it with pride. For those who are just joining the club, know that many strong people stood here before you.

The politics of breast cancer had its forerunners more than fifty years ago. In 1952 the American Cancer Society started Reach to Recovery; all its members had had mastectomies and would visit patients in the hospital and reassure them that there was life after mastectomy. They are now part of the American Cancer Society and continue to be a wonderful resource for people with breast cancer.

All this underlined the fact that there was little psychological support from the medical profession—you had to get it elsewhere. And because breast cancer continued to be hidden from public view, it retained an aura of something shameful and disreputable.

The next big step came in the 1970s when famous people such as one-time child actor Shirley Temple Black, first lady Betty Ford, and Happy Rockefeller, the wife of the then governor of New York, told the world they had breast cancer. Their openness began to create an environment in which breast cancer could be seen as a dangerous disease that needed to be addressed by public institutions rather than a private and shameful secret. There was a dramatic increase in the number of people in America who got mammograms and in the number of breast cancers diagnosed.

Those were the days of the one-step procedure. You'd go in for the biopsy, it would be done under general anesthetic, and if the lump was positive, your breast would be immediately removed. In 1977 Rose Kushner, a writer with breast cancer, penned a groundbreaking book titled *Why Me?* It ushered in the two-step procedure. Kushner saw no reason for someone to have to decide whether to have a mastectomy before they even knew they had breast cancer. She argued passionately that it was important for the patient to have a biopsy, learn whether they had cancer, and then, if they did, decide what avenue to pursue. Doctors were still working on the erroneous assumption that time was everything: if they didn't get the cancer out the instant they found it, it would spread and kill the patient. Kushner had done enough research to realize that wasn't the case, that a few weeks between diagnosis and treatment wouldn't do any medical harm and would do a great deal of emotional good. She pushed for the two-step procedure, and her book influenced large numbers of people to demand it as well.

By the 1980s the "second wave" of feminism had emerged, demanding that all the inequities against women be redressed. They adopted the old Marxist expression "The personal is political," and many social realities began to be defined in a larger context: rape, battered wives, the need for child care. A large component of the movement worked on issues of women's health, urging women to demand control of their own health issues and to learn all they could about their own bodies. Doctors would no longer be seen as omniscient father figures and would become medical specialists who worked with their patients to help them determine individually what was best for them.

New organizations, including the Susan G. Komen Breast Cancer Foundation, began to raise money for awareness, research, and care. Then, in the late 1980s, almost spontaneously in different parts of the United States, a number of political women's cancer groups sprang up.

One was in the Boston area, started by a patient of mine mentioned earlier, a feminist writer named Susan Shapiro. She and others formed the Women's Community Cancer Project. Their scope was fairly broad. It included all cancer that women got and also the role of women as caregivers for children, spouses, and parents with cancer. Inevitably much of the focus was on breast cancer. Shapiro died in January 1990 but the project continues to flourish.

Around the time the Women's Community Cancer Project was beginning, so were the Women's Cancer Resource Center in Oakland, California; Breast Cancer Action in the Bay Area; and the Mautner Project in Washington, D.C. All these groups were aware of the work the AIDS movement had been doing. It marked the first time we were seeing people with a killer disease aggressively demanding more money for research, changes in insurance bias, and job protection. Women with breast cancer took note—particularly those women who had been part of the feminist movement. They were geared, as were the gay activists with AIDS, to the idea of identifying oppression and confronting it politically.

At the time these groups were emerging, I was finishing work on the first edition of the book. As I went on my book tour, talking with women, I began to realize how deep women's anger was and how ready they were to do something. The key moment for me was in Salt Lake City in June 1990 when I gave a talk to six hundred women. It was in the middle of the afternoon on a weekday, and the audience was mostly older women. It was a pretty long talk, and at the end I said, "We don't know the answers, and I don't know what we have to do to make President Bush wake up and do something about breast cancer. Maybe we should march topless to the White House." I was making a wisecrack, hoping to end a somber talk with a little light humor.

I got a great response, and afterward women came up to me asking when the march was, how could they sign up for it, and what they could do to organize it. I realized that throughout the United States this issue touched all kinds of women and that they were all fed up with the fact that this virtual epidemic was being ignored. I saw that it wasn't just the big centers like San Francisco and Boston and Washington, D.C., where I had expected to see political movement springing up. It was everywhere—everywhere women were ready to fight for attention to breast cancer.

I felt we needed to have some sort of national organization to give these women the hook they needed to begin organizing. I spoke to Susan Hester of the Mautner Project, Amy Langer of NABCO (the National Alliance of Breast Cancer Organizations), and Nancy Brinker of the Komen Foundation. We were all enthusiastic, and the result was a planning meeting. The initial groups included Y-ME (Y-ME National Breast Cancer Organization), the Women's Community Cancer Project, Breast Cancer Action, Cancer Care, and CanAct from New York. Then we called an open meeting to be held in Washington and wrote to every women's group we knew of.

We had no idea who'd show up. On the day of the meeting the room was packed. There were representatives from all kinds of groups: the American Cancer Society and the American Jewish Congress were there. So was the Human Rights Campaign Fund, a big gay and lesbian group. There were members of breast cancer support groups from all around the United States, such as Arm in Arm from Baltimore, the Linda Creed group from Philadelphia, and SHARE from New York. Overall there were about a hundred or so individuals representing seventy-five organizations. We were overwhelmed, and we started the National Breast Cancer Coalition on the spot. Out of that meeting came the first board of the coalition.

Amy Langer of NABCO chaired the initial meetings until the bylaws and officers could be chosen. A year later, Fran Visco, a lawyer from Philadelphia who had had breast cancer in her late thirties, became the first elected president and remains the president today. Our first action, in the fall of 1991, was a project called Do the Write Thing. We wanted to collect and deliver to Washington 175,000 letters representing the 175,000 women who would be diagnosed with breast cancer that year. In October we ended up with 600,000 letters—it was an enormous response. We delivered them to the White House. The guards just stood there; nobody would help us lift the boxes. So all these women who'd had mastectomies were lifting heavy boxes of letters onto the conveyor belt.

We were all certain that the letters had just been dumped into the shredder, that our first action had been a flop. But in reality we had succeeded on a number of levels. For one thing, we had organized in such a way that we had a group in every state. That meant a large and potentially powerful organization. For another, even if the White House ignored us, the members of Congress didn't. When we started lobbying for increased research money, they granted us $43 million more, raising the 1993 appropriation to $132 million. That was a small triumph.

We held hearings run by Kay Dickersin, PhD, to determine how much research money was really needed, and it was one of the first times scientists and activists interested in breast cancer had met together. This created an interesting coalition. As a result of the hearings, we decided we needed $433 million for breast cancer research. The total budget was $93 million. So we started lobbying for $300 million more, armed with our report based on scientists' testimony.

At first the reaction was overwhelmingly negative. We testified at the Senate and at the House. We lobbied, we sent faxes, and we called. But despite support from many Congress members, we couldn't figure out how to get enough money. Then Senator Tom Harkin noticed that, amazingly, in the past there had been some money for breast cancer in the Department of Defense (DOD)—$25 million spent on mammogram machines for the army. At our urging, he tried to increase that to $210 million, which, added to an increase in the National Cancer Institute (NCI) funding, would bring the total to $300 million. At this point the DOD people were so worried that the firewall between the domestic budget and the defense budget might be breached, they agreed to have a breast cancer research program within the DOD!

So there was $210 million in the DOD budget and the extra $100 million in the NCI budget. That was $10 million over the $300 million we had gone after. Against all odds, we had succeeded. Part of it was being in the right place at the right time. But most of it was the enormous amount of work all the women in the coalition and around the United States had put in.

We started lobbying, and our next major project was to deliver 2.6 million signatures to the White House in October 1993 to represent the 2.6 million women living with breast cancer at the time—1.6 million who knew they had breast cancer, and 1 million who had yet to be diagnosed. We mobilized around the country collecting signatures and delivered them to President Bill Clinton on October 18. As a measure of how far we'd come from October 1991, this time we were welcomed in the East Room, where Fran Visco and I shared the stage with both Hillary and Bill Clinton along with Secretary of Health and Human Services Donna Shalala. The room was filled with two hundred of our people. It was an awesome moment.

And President Clinton, whose mother died in 1994 of breast cancer complications, followed up. In December we had a meeting to set national strategy—a meeting of activists, politicians, scientists, doctors, laypeople, and businesspeople. We came up with a National Action Plan. Meeting, talking, and working with scientists taught the activists that the answers weren't always easy, that researchers have to work months and years to come up with one useful discovery. The scientists, meanwhile, saw that the activists weren't shrill, uninformed troublemakers but rather intelligent, concerned people fighting to save their own and others' lives.

The DOD program has thrived over these years, although we still have to fight for the money each year in Congress. The National Breast Cancer Coalition also continues to do the difficult work of challenging the status quo and representing real change in breast cancer. One big win was the enactment of the Breast and Cervical Cancer Prevention and Treatment Act. After four years of an intense and aggressive grassroots lobbying campaign, this legislation was signed into law, guaranteeing treatment to low-income, uninsured women screened and diagnosed with breast and cervical cancer through the Centers for Disease Control and Prevention (CDC) National Breast and Cervical Cancer Early Detection Program.

I've learned through this that you really can affect how the government acts. A small group of committed people can do a lot. So few people let their feelings be known that the people who do it and do it vociferously get an undue amount of power. We didn't have any money—but we were organized.

The National Breast Cancer Coalition's goal is to know how to end breast cancer! They are focused on whether a vaccine can be developed to prevent breast cancer and the prevention or cure of metastases. They hold meetings with scientists and advocates once a year in the Artemis Project and are modeling a new approach to eradicating breast cancer. The Komen Foundation continues to fund research as well as support care and awareness.

Breast cancer politics have matured beyond pink ribbons and self-examination shower cards!

PUSHING THE ENVELOPE: THE DR. SUSAN LOVE FOUNDATION FOR BREAST CANCER RESEARCH

While documenting the changes in the diagnosis and treatment of breast cancer, over seven editions of the *Breast Book* have also chronicled over twenty years of my career, from clinical practice and the birth of advocacy, through academics and work on the multidisciplinary delivery of breast cancer treatment, to research in my own foundation on what causes the breast to get cancer in the first place.

Throughout this book I have told you what the studies show and what has not been studied. I am amazed as I write this new edition of this book how much our understanding of the biology of the disease has, over every five years or so, led to new targeted treatments and better outcomes. At the same time, I have become increasingly frustrated that we have not made equal progress in finding the cause of breast cancer. I keep thinking about cancer of the cervix. When I was training as a surgeon in the late 1970s, an abnormal Pap smear meant you had a total hysterectomy. Many young people lost their fertility because we really did not know what else to do. Then, over time, we figured out that local therapies worked as well as hysterectomy and were much less invasive. If this concept sounds familiar to you, it's because we later applied it to breast cancer. In most cases lumpectomy does as well as mastectomies when it's combined with radiation, and it preserves the breast itself.

The parallels, however, stop there. Research on cervical cancer uncovered the fact that it was sexually transmitted and was caused by the human papillomavirus (HPV). Now we have a vaccine against cervical cancer. One of my cousins had a hysterectomy many years ago for an abnormal Pap smear, and more recently my sister had a partial hysterectomy for HPV. But my daughter doesn't have to worry about that—she's been vaccinated. All this happened within thirty years—and with much less money and no pink ribbons, walks, or art exhibits. So why have we been able to do this with cancer of the cervix and not with cancer of the breast? Why had we not learned either the causes of breast cancer or how to prevent it? Ironically, one reason may be that less money was raised for cervical cancer. Are we victims of our own success? Lots of money makes it possible to study interesting molecular biology without addressing the human disease. In addition, cancer of the cervix, until recently, did not have an animal model that could be used for research. This meant the studies had to be done on humans. Although we have learned a lot from rats and mice, it doesn't always translate to humans in any clinically useful way.

I went to some scientists I know and asked them why they did not do breast cancer research on women. The response floored me: "Women are too messy! I can control rats and mice from their genes to their every activity, leading to nice, pretty science!" one of them said to me. "And besides," he added lamely, "I don't know where to find the women." Well, that was something I could solve.

With a generous grant from the Avon Foundation for Women, the Dr. Susan Love Research Foundation (now the Dr. Susan Love Foundation for Breast Cancer Research) launched the Army of Women (now the Love Research Army) in 2008. The goal is to recruit one million people who are willing to participate in research. It is not a matching service or a study, but rather an email list of those willing to consider participating in research to find the cause of breast cancer and to prevent it. You can sign up online (www.drsusanloveresearch.org/love-research-army/). In the first year over 320,000 people joined, 80 percent of whom neither had breast cancer nor were at high risk. Our members came from every state and range from eighteen to a hundred years old. Researchers from all around the United States and potentially even internationally submit their studies for our review, and if approved, we e-blast a description out to everyone in the Army. The ones who fit the study and are interested RSVP, whereas the others do not. We then screen them again and, if they still fit, pass their name on to the scientist. In the first year we launched fifteen studies, and thirteen thousand people participated in the research process. Many studies were closed within twenty-four to forty-eight hours, having recruited all the participants they needed and saving them years of work and lots of money. So they were able to bring their lab findings into the real world far sooner than they would have without our volunteers.

Our biggest problem with the Army is not with the participants: they get it right away! The problem is with the scientists who take longer to try a new way of doing things. This, plus my frustration that there is little original research on finding the cause of breast cancer, led us to start the first large online cohort study, the Health of Women Study (HOW). This group of dedicated people is committed to answering short online surveys on different topics periodically (the study is now closed).

Since my own diagnosis with leukemia, I have realized that if we are going to get anything done, we need to collaborate. We have all been doing this work for twenty-five years, and although women are living longer, they are still being diagnosed with this disease. We launched the Collateral Damage Project with Komen and the Young Survival Coalition and then reached out to all the advocacy groups we knew to use the HOW study volunteers to document the cost of the cure. My goal is to show that the cure is not a good enough goal when it comes with so much collateral damage and still fails many; we need to find the cause and end it for once and for all! If we can find a vaccine for cancer of the cervix, we certainly can find something similar for cancer of the breast.

Our foundation's mission is to achieve a future without breast cancer by engaging the public and scientific communities in innovative research to find the cause and prevent breast cancer. We do this through performing and facilitating innovative and collaborative research, translating science to engage the public as informed partners, and inspiring novel research. Some of the interesting work we are doing has been mentioned in the book. It includes studying whether a bacterium could be involved in causing or preventing breast cancer, accessing breast ducts to better understand where the disease starts, and figuring out a way to map the extent of DCIS in the duct so we can use less aggressive treatments to prevent it from progressing. We are also working on developing a "self-reading ultrasound" that can determine which palpable breast lumps need further evaluation and which are clearly benign. This is particularly important in low- and middle-income countries where resources are limited. The foundation continues to push the envelope, asking the questions and doing the research that no one else will do in an effort to figure out how we can end this disease for once and for all.

As I continue to speak across the country, I often finish my talks with an anecdote about my daughter, Katie. Although she is no longer four years old and her future aspirations have changed, this old story has become a symbol to many women of what this movement is all about.

In 1993, at the Los Angeles Breast Cancer Coalition *War Mammorial*, created by artist Melanie Winter, thirteen hundred white plastic casts of women's torsos were set on a hill. From a distance they looked like graves, but up close they showed the variety of women's bodies: large breasts, small breasts, some with mastectomies, some with implants. Katie was walking around, trying to figure out which breasts she wanted when she grew up. Then she turned serious.

"Are these the graves of the women with breast cancer?" she asked.

"No, these women are all alive," I told her. "But some women do die from breast cancer."

"Well, you're going to stop that, aren't you, Mommy?"

"Yes, Katie, I would like to stop breast cancer before you grow up."

She thought about that a minute. "What if you die first?" she asked.

"I'd like to stop breast cancer before I die," I replied.

She thought again, then turned to me and said, "If there is breast cancer left after you die, it's a big problem. Because I'm not going to be a breast surgeon. I'm going to be a ballerina."

Well, Katie is now thirty-four and is neither a breast surgeon nor a ballerina. But I still have great hopes that neither her future children nor any others will be haunted, as so many of us are now, by the fear of getting breast cancer. As long as we keep fighting, the discoveries we're making, buttressed by the political activism that lets the scientists and the government know we won't let up until we've ended breast cancer, will bring about her wish. And maybe her children won't even have to ask the question. That's what keeps me going.

APPENDIX A

Resources

In past editions we have listed resources, references, and books that may be of help. Because the Internet is so much more extensive and up-to-date than anything we can present here, we are limiting our recommendations to what we feel are the best websites for you to use. For those of you not adept at searching the web, remember that your local library will be happy to help.

WEBSITES

General Information and Research

www.drsusanloveresearch.org (Dr. Susan Love Foundation for Breast Cancer Research): Obviously we feel this is your best resource. We keep it up-to-date as new research data come along.

www.cancer.gov (National Cancer Institute): This is a very comprehensive site, with data for both doctors and patients. It lists clinical trials and is a good source of accurate, unbiased information.

www.cancer.gov/research/infrastructure/cancer-centers/find: This site lists the National Cancer Institute's Designated Cancer Centers listed by state.

www.cancer.org (American Cancer Society): This is also a good resource for the general public.

www.cancer.net (American Society of Clinical Oncology): Comprehensive information for people with cancer and their caregivers.

www.nccn.org (National Comprehensive Cancer Network): Here is where you can find the practice guidelines quoted throughout this book.

www.breastcancer.org (Breastcancer.org): This site is another good overall resource. It was created by Dr. Marisa Weiss, a radiation oncologist.

www.breastcancer.org/drugs (Drugs for Treatment and Risk Reduction): Best list and descriptions of drugs used to treat breast cancer and reduce risk, including side effects.

www.nccam.nih.gov (National Center for Complementary and Integrative Health): Good starting place for scientific information on complementary and alternative therapies.

www.mskcc.org/cancer-care/diagnosis-treatment/symptom-management /integrative-medicine/herbs/search (search About Herbs): Memorial Sloan Kettering Cancer Center searchable database on herbs, supplements, and complementary therapies.

Support and Breast Cancer Subgroups

www.youngsurvival.org (Young Survival Coalition): Focused on the unique needs of young adults facing breast cancer, including fertility preservation and limited research on their age group.

www.tigerlilyfoundation.org (Tigerlily Foundation): Provides education, awareness, advocacy, and support to people ages 15 to 45 before, during, and after breast cancer.

www.stopbreastcancer.org (National Breast Cancer Coalition): The best national organization focused on political and policy issues to end breast cancer.

www.facingourrisk.org (FORCE): Website to support and inform people at high risk for breast cancer due to inherited mutations.

www.lymphnet.org (National Lymphedema Network): Support for all kinds of lymphedema, including that caused by breast cancer.

Clinical Trials

www.drsusanloveresearch.org/love-research-army (Love Research Army): Register for the Love Research Army to receive emails about new research studies as part of my effort to find the cause of breast cancer.

breastcancertrials.org (BreastCancerTrials.org [BCT]): A nonprofit service that encourages individuals with breast cancer to consider clinical trials as a routine option for care.

https://clinicaltrials.gov (ClinicalTrials.gov): A registry and results database of publicly and privately supported clinical studies of human participants conducted around the world.

Metastatic Trial Search (MTS): Part of BreastCancerTrials.org and a tool specifically designed for people with metastatic breast cancer. It was developed with breast cancer advocacy groups and is available on a dozen advocacy sites.

Pathology Checklist

Your name_____

Your age_____

YOUR MENOPAUSAL STATUS:

    Premenopausal _____

    Postmenopausal _____

Your hospital number _____

Your hospital_____

YOUR DOCTORS

    Primary care _____

    Surgeon _____

    Medical oncologist _____

    Radiation oncologist _____

    Date of biopsy/surgery _____

    Place of biopsy/surgery _____

    Name of doctor doing procedure _____

    Place of pathological reading _____

    Name of pathologist _____

    Pathology reference number _____

SPECIMEN TYPE

Biopsy

    Core (needle) _____

    Surgical _____

    Lumpectomy _____

    Mastectomy _____

Lymph node sampling

Axillary node dissection _____

Sentinel node biopsy _____

SPECIMEN SIZE (FOR EXCISIONS LESS THAN TOTAL MASTECTOMY)

Greatest dimension (cm) _____

Additional dimensions _____

SIDE OF TUMOR

Right _____

Left _____

TUMOR SITE

Upper outer quadrant _____

Lower outer quadrant _____

Upper inner quadrant _____

Lower inner quadrant _____

Central _____

MICROSCOPIC

INVASIVE OR IN SITU

In situ

Ductal carcinoma in situ (DCIS) _____

Lobular carcinoma in situ (LCIS) _____

Ductal and lobular in situ _____

Paget's disease in the nipple _____

Invasive/infiltrating

Ductal _____

Tubular _____

Mucinous _____

Adenoid cystic _____

Inflammatory _____

Secretory _____

Medullary _____

Papillary _____

Undifferentiated _____

Not otherwise specified (NOS) _____

Lobular _____

Size of invasive tumor in greatest dimension
Less than 2 cm _____

Less than 0.1 cm (microinvasion) _____

Between 0.1 cm–0.5 cm _____

Between 0.5 cm–1 cm _____

Between 1 cm–2 cm _____

Between 2 cm–5 cm _____

Greater than 5 cm _____

Any size with direct extension to
Chest wall _____

Edema (swelling) _____

Both chest wall and edema _____

Inflammatory carcinoma _____

HISTOLOGY
Grade of tumor
Low _____

Moderate _____

High _____

Differentiation
Low _____

Moderate _____

High_____

Mitosis
Low _____

High _____

Lympho/vascular invasion
Positive _____

Negative _____

Extent of DCIS associated with the tumor (EIC) _____

MARGINS
Negative
No tumor within 1 cm or no residual tumor _____

No tumor within 1 mm of margin _____

Tumor focally (at one spot) next to a margin _____

Positive

Invasive tumor involving inked margin _____

In situ tumor involving inked margin _____

MARKERS

Hormones

Estrogen receptor positive/progesterone receptor positive _____

Estrogen receptor positive/progesterone receptor negative _____

Estrogen receptor negative/progesterone receptor positive _____

Estrogen receptor negative/progesterone receptor negative _____

Her-2/neu

Negative _____

Positive _____

By IHC _____

By FISH _____

Others

P 53 positive _____

Axillary lymph nodes

No lymph nodes _____

Lymph nodes negative _____

Negative on histology but positive on IHC _____

Negative on histology but positive on RTPCR _____

Lymph nodes positive

1–3 nodes positive _____

4–9 nodes positive _____

10 or more positive _____

Notes

CHAPTER 1. THE BREAST

1. Susan M. Love and Sanford H. Barsky, "Anatomy of the Nipple and Breast Ducts Revisited," *Cancer* 101, no. 9 (2004): 1947–1957.

2. Astley Cooper, *On the Anatomy of the Breast* (London: Longman, Orme, Green, Brown, and Longmans, 1840).

3. Michel Teboul and Michael Halliwell, *Atlas of Ultrasound and Ductal Echography of the Breast* (Oxford: Blackwell Science, 1995); D. T. Ramsay, J. C. Kent, R. A. Hartmann, et al., "Anatomy of the Lactating Human Breast Refined with Ultrasound Imaging," *Journal of Anatomy* 206, no. 6 (2005): 525–534.

4. James J. Going and David F. Moffat, "Escaping from Flatland: Clinical and Biological Aspects of Human Mammary Duct Anatomy in Three Dimensions," *Journal of Pathology* 203, no. 1 (2004): 538–544; Jennifer E. Rusby, Elena F. Brachtel, Alphonse Taghian, et al., "Microscopic Anatomy Within the Nipple: Implications for Nipple-Sparing Mastectomy," *American Journal of Surgery* 194, no. 4 (2007): 433–437.

5. A. V. Sluijmer, M. J. Heineman, F. H. DeJong, et al., "Endocrine Activity of the Postmenopausal Ovary: The Effects of Pituitary Down-Regulation and Oophorectomy," *Journal of Clinical Endocrinology and Metabolism* 80, no. 7 (1995): 2163–2167; Takahisa Ushiroyama and Osamu Sugimoto, "Endocrine Function of the Peri- and Postmenopausal Ovary," *Hormone Research* 44, no. 2 (1995): 64–68.

6. M. M. Hreshchyshyn, A. Hopkins, S. Zylstra, et al., "Effects of Natural Menopause, Hysterectomy, and Oophorectomy on Lumbar Spine and Femoral Neck Bone Densities," *Obstetrics and Gynecology* 72, no. 4 (1988): 631–638.

7. W. H. Parker, M. S. Broder, E. Chang, et al., "Ovarian Conservation at the Time of Hysterectomy and Long-Term Health Outcomes in the Nurse's Health Study," *Obstetrics and Gynecology* 113, no. 5 (2009): 1027–1037.

8. Jeffrey A. Tice, Steven R. Cummings, Rebecca Smith-Bindman, et al., "Using Clinical Factors and Mammographic Breast Density to Estimate Breast Cancer Risk: Development and Validation of a New Predictive Model," *Annals of Internal Medicine* 148, no. 5 (2008): 337–347.

CHAPTER 2. COMMON BREAST PROBLEMS

1. Julian B. Herrmann, "Mammary Cancer Subsequent to Aspiration of Cysts in the Breast," *Annals of Surgery* 173, no. 1 (1971): 40.

2. Ron Greenberg, Yehuda Skornick, and Ofer Kaplan, "Management of Breast Fibroadenomas," *Journal of General Internal Medicine* 13, no. 9 (September 1998): 640–645.

3. Cary S. Kaufman, Peter J. Littrup, Laurie A. Freeman-Gibb, et al., "Office-Based Cryoablation of Breast Fibroadenomas with Long-Term Follow-Up," *Breast Journal* 11, no. 5 (2005): 344–350.

4. D. N. Ader, C. D. Shriver, and M. W. Browne, "Cyclical Mastalgia: Premenstrual Syndrome or Recurrent Pain Disorder?," *Journal of Psychosomatic Obstetrics and Gynecology* 20, no. 4 (1999): 198–202.

5. P. E. Preece, L. E. Hughes, R. E. Mansel, et al., "Clinical Syndromes of Mastalgia," *Lancet* 2, no. 7987 (1976): 670–673.

6. R. E. Mansel, "Breast Pain," *British Medical Journal* 309 (1994): 866–868.

7. Alfredo Carlos Barros, Juvenal Mottola, Carlos Alberto Ruiz, et al., "Reassurance in the Treatment of Mastalgia," *Breast Journal* 5, no. 3 (1999): 162–165.

8. K. Kataria, A. Dhar, A. Srivastava, et al., "A Systematic Review of Current Understanding and Management of Mastalgia," *Indian Journal of Surgery* 76, no. 3 (June 2014): 217–222; V. Rosolowich, Society of Obstetricians and Gynecologists of Canada, E. Saettler, et al., "Mastalgia," *Journal of Obstetrics and Gynaecology Canada* 28, no. 1 (January 2006): 49–71.

9. I. S. Fentiman, M. Calef, K. Brame, et al., "Double-Blind Controlled Trial of Tamoxifen Therapy for Mastalgia," *Lancet* 1, no. 8476 (1986): 287–288.

10. Barbara Schmidt Steinbrunn, Richard T. Zera, and Jorge L. Rodriguez, "Mastalgia: Tailoring Treatment to Type of Breast Pain," *Postgraduate Medicine* 102, no. 5 (1997): 183–198.

11. M. M. LeBan, J. R. Meerscharet, and R. S. Taylor, "Breast Pain: A Symptom of Cervical Radiculopathy," *Archives of Physical Medicine and Rehabilitation* 60, no. 7 (1979): 315–317.

12. J. K. Pye, R. E. Mansel, and L. E. Hughes, "Clinical Experience of Drug Treatments for Mastalgia," *Lancet* 2, no. 8451 (1985): 373–377.

13. P. R. Maddox, B. J. Harrison, R. E. Mansel, et al., "Non-Cyclical Mastalgia: An Improved Classification and Treatment," *British Journal of Surgery* 76, no. 9 (1989): 901–904.

14. A. C. Thomsen, M. D. Espersen, and S. Maigaard, "Course and Treatment of Milk Stasis, Noninfectious Inflammation of the Breast and Infectious Mastitis in Nursing Women," *American Journal of Obstetrics and Gynecology* 149, no. 5 (1984): 492–495.

15. Michael M. Meguid, Albert Oler, Patricia J. Numann, et al., "Pathogenesis-Based Treatment of Recurring Subareolar Breast Abscesses," *Surgery* 118, no. 4 (1995): 775–782.

16. Willis P. Maier, Alan Berger, and Bruce M. Derrick, "Periareolar Abscess in the Nonlactating Breast," *American Journal of Surgery* 144, no. 3 (1982): 359–361; Otto Sartorius, personal communication.

17. S. Watt-Boolsen, R. Ryegaard, and M. Blichert-Toft, "Primary Periareolar Abscess in the Nonlactating Breast: Risk of Recurrence," *American Journal of Surgery* 153, no. 6 (1987): 571–573.

18. Verity Livingstone and L. Stringer, "The Treatment of Staphylococcus Aureus Infected Sore Nipples: A Randomized Comparative Study (Letter)," *Journal of Human Lactation* 17 (2001): 116–117.

19. Susan M. Love, Stuart J. Schnitt, James L. Connolly, et al., "Benign Breast Diseases," in *Breast Diseases*, ed. Jay R. Harris, Samuel Hellman, I. Craig Henderson, et al., 15–53 (Philadelphia: Lippincott, 1987), 22.

20. M. H. Seltzer, L. J. Perloff, R. I. Kelley, et al., "Significance of Age in Patients with Nipple Discharge," *Surgical Gynecology and Obstetrics* 131, no. 3 (1970): 519.

21. Bobbi Pritt, Yijun Pang, Marybeth Kellogg, et al., "Diagnostic Value of Nipple Cytology: Study of 466 Cases," *Cancer Cytopathology* 102, no. 4 (2004): 233–238.

22. Neslihan Cabioglu, Kelly K. Hunt, S. Eva Singletary, et al., "Surgical Decision Making and Factors Determining a Diagnosis of Breast Carcinoma in Women Presenting with Nipple Discharge," *Journal of the American College of Surgeons* 196, no. 3 (2003): 354–364.

23. Bernadette Pereira and Kefah Mokbel, "Mammary Ductoscopy: Past, Present, and Future," *International Journal of Clinical Oncology* 10, no. 2 (2005): 112–116.

CHAPTER 3. BIOLOGY OF CANCER

1. D. Hanahan and R. A. Weinberg, "The Hallmarks of Cancer," *Cell* 100, no. 1 (2000): 57–70.

2. Celeste M. Nelson and Mina J. Bissell, "Of Extracellular Matrix, Scaffolds, and Signaling: Tissue Architecture Regulates Development, Homeostasis, and Cancer," *Annual Review of Cell and Developmental Biology* 22 (2006): 287–309.

3. Rodrigo Goncalves, Wayne A. Warner, Jingqin Luo, et al., "New Concepts in Breast Cancer Genomics and Genetics," *Breast Cancer Research* 16 (2014): 460.

4. I. A. Rodriguez-Brenes, N. L. Komarova, and D. Wodarz, "Cancer-Associated Mutations in Healthy Individuals: Assessing the Risk of Carcinogenesis," *Cancer Research* 74, no. 6 (2014): 1661–1669.

5. P. J. O'Donovan and D. M. Livingston, "BRCA1 and BRCA2: Breast/Ovarian Cancer Susceptibility Gene Products and Participants in DNA Double-Strand Break Repair," *Carcinogenesis* 31, no. 6 (June 2010): 961–967.

6. Mahlon Hoagland, Bert Dodson, and Judith Hauck, *The Way Life Works: The Science of Biology* (New York: Times Books, 1998).

7. M. E. Robson et al., "OlympiAD Final Overall Survival and Tolerability Results: Olaparib Versus Chemotherapy Treatment of Physician's Choice in Patients with a Germline BRCA Mutation and HER2-Negative Metastatic Breast Cancer," *Annals of Oncology* 30, no. 4 (2019): 558–566, doi:10.1093/annonc/mdz012.

8. Andrew N. J. Tutt et al., "Adjuvant Olaparib for Patients with BRCA1- or BRCA2- Mutated Breast Cancer," *New England Journal of Medicine* 384, no. 25 (2021): 2394–2405, doi:10.1056/NEJMoa2105215.

9. Kornelia Polyak, "Heterogeneity in Breast Cancer," *Journal of Clinical Investigation* 121, no. 10 (2011): 3786–3788.

10. M. Jamal-Hanjani, S. A. Quezada, J. Larkin, et al., "Translation Implications of Tumor Heterogeneity," *Clinical Cancer Research* 21, no. 6 (2015): 1258–1266.

11. C. R. Holst, G. J. Nuovo, M. Esteller, et al., "Methylation of p16(INK4a) Promoters Occurs In Vivo in Histologically Normal Human Mammary Epithelia," *Cancer Research* 63, no. 7 (April 2003): 1596–1601.

12. V. M. Weaver, O. W. Peterson, F. Wang, et al., "Reversion of the Malignant Phenotype of Human Breast Cells in Three-Dimensional Culture and In Vivo by Integrin Blocking Antibodies," *Journal of Cell Biology* 137, no. 1 (1997): 231–245.

13. J. Bickels, Y. Kollender, O. Merinsky, et al., "Coley's Toxin: Historical Perspective," *Israel Medical Association Journal* 4, no. 6 (2002): 471–472.

CHAPTER 4. HEREDITARY BREAST CANCER

1. The Collaborative Group on Hormonal Factors in Breast Cancer, "Familial Breast Cancer: Collaborative Reanalysis of Individual Data from 52 Epidemiological Studies Including 58,209 Women with Breast Cancer and 101,986 Women Without the Disease," *Lancet* 358, no. 9291 (2001): 1389–1399.

2. K. Michailidou, S. Lindström, J. Dennis, et al., "Association Analysis Identifies 65 New Breast Cancer Risk Loci," *Nature* 551, 92–94 (2017), doi:10.1038 /nature24284; Roger L. Milne et al., "Identification of Ten Variants Associated with Risk of Estrogen-Receptor-Negative Breast Cancer," *Nature Genetics* 49, no. 12 (2017): 1767–1778, doi:10.1038/ng.3785.

3. Chunling Hu et al., "A Population-Based Study of Genes Previously Implicated in Breast Cancer," *New England Journal of Medicine* 384, no. 5 (2021): 440–451, doi:10.1056/NEJMoa2005936.

4. Ruth I. Tennen et al., "Identifying Ashkenazi Jewish BRCA1/2 Founder Variants in Individuals Who Do Not Self-Report Jewish Ancestry," *Scientific Reports* 10, no. 1 (May 6, 2020): 7669, doi:10.1038/s41598-020-63466-x.

5. D. F. Easton, D. T. Bishop, D. Ford, et al., "Genetic Linkage Analysis in Familial Breast and Ovarian Cancer: Results from 214 Families," *American Journal of Human Genetics* 52, no. 4 (1993): 678.

6. D. Shattuck-Eidens, A. Oliphant, M. McClure, et al., "BRCA 1 Sequence Analysis in Women at High Risk for Susceptibility Mutations: Risk Factor Analysis and Implications for Genetic Testing," *Journal of the American Medical Association* 278 (1997): 1242.

7. A. Liede, B. Y. Karlan, and S. A. Narod, "Cancer Risks for Male Carriers of Germline Mutations in BRCA1 or BRCA2: A Review of the Literature," *Journal of Clinical Oncology* 22, no. 4 (2004): 735–742.

8. S. A. Narod, "Modifiers of Risk of Hereditary Breast Cancer," *Oncogene* 25 (2006): 5832–5836.

9. Steven A. Narod and William D. Foulkes, "BRCA1 and BRCA2: 1994 and Beyond," *Nature Reviews Cancer* 4, no. 9 (2004): 665–676.

10. Olufunmilayo I. Olopade and Grazia Artioli, "Efficacy of Risk-Reducing Salpingo-Oophorectomy in Women with BRCA 1/2 Mutations," *Breast Journal* 10, supp. 1 (2004): S5–S9.

11. M. S. Brose, T. R. Rebbeck, K. A. Calzone, et al., "Cancer Risk Estimates for BRCA1 Mutation Carriers Identified in a Risk Evaluation Program," *Journal of the National Cancer Institute* 94, no. 18 (September 2002): 1365–1372.

12. J. T. Bergthorsson, J. Johannsdottir, A. Jonasdottir, et al., "Chromosome Imbalance at the 3p14 Region in Human Breast Tumors: High Frequency in Patients with Inherited Predisposition Due to BRCA 2," *European Journal of Cancer* 34, no. 1 (1998): 1544.

13. A. Dorum, P. Moller, E. J. Kamsteeg, et al., "A BRCA1 Founder Mutation, Identified with Haplotype Analysis, Allowing Genotype/Phenotype Determination and Predictive Testing," *European Journal of Cancer* 33, no. 14 (1997): 2390–2392.

14. J. N. Weitzel, V. Lagos, K. R. Blazer, et al., "Prevalence of BRCA Mutations and Founder Effect in High-Risk Hispanic Families," *Cancer Epidemiology, Biomarkers and Prevention* 14, no. 7 (July 2005): 1666–1671.

15. J. N. Weitzel, J. Clague, A. Martir-Negron, et al., "Prevalence and Type of BRCA Mutations in Hispanics Undergoing Genetic Cancer Risk Assessment in the

Southwestern United States: A Report from the Clinical Cancer Genetics Community Research Network," *Journal of Clinical Oncology* 31, no. 2 (2013): 210–216.

16. Ansari-Pour, Naser et al. "Whole-genome analysis of Nigerian patients with breast cancer reveals ethnic-driven somatic evolution and distinct genomic subtypes." *Nature Communications* vol. 12,1 6946. 26 Nov. 2021, doi:10.1038/s41467-021-27079-w.

17. E. Mocci, R. L. Milne, E. Yuste Mendez-Villamil, et al., "Risk of Pancreatic Cancer in Breast Cancer Families from the Breast Cancer Family Registry," *Cancer Epidemiology, Biomarkers and Prevention* 22, no. 5 (2013): 803–811; J. Iqbal, A. Ragone, J. Lubinski, et al., "The Incidence of Pancreatic Cancer in BRCA1 and BRCA2 Mutation Carriers," *British Journal of Cancer* 107, no. 12 (2012): 2005–2009; Jacqueline Mersch et al., "Cancers Associated with BRCA1 and BRCA2 Mutations Other Than Breast and Ovarian," *Cancer* 121, no. 2 (2015): 269–275, doi:10.1002/cncr.29041.

18. M. Weischer, B. G. Nordestgaard, P. Pharoah, et al., "CHEK2*1100delC Heterozygosity in Women with Breast Cancer Associated with Early Death, Breast Cancer-Specific Death and Increased Risk of a Second Breast Cancer," *Journal of Clinical Oncology* 30, no. 35 (December 2012): 4308–4316.

19. A. C. Antoniou, S. Casadei, T. Heikkinem, et al., "Breast-Cancer Risk in Families with Mutations in PALB2," *New England Journal of Medicine* 371, no. 6 (2014): 497–506.

20. J. D. Iglehart, A. Miron, B. K. Rimer, et al., "Overestimation of Hereditary Breast Cancer Risk," *Annals of Surgery* 228, no. 3 (1998): 375–384.

21. B. Newman, H. Mu, L. M. Butler, et al., "Frequency of Breast Cancer Attributable to BRCA 1 in a Population-Based Series of American Women," *Journal of the American Medical Association* 279 (1998): 915–921.

22. E. Gabai-Kapara, A. Lahad, B. Kaufman, et al., "Population-Based Screening for Breast and Ovarian Cancer Risk Due to BRCA1 and BRCA2," *Proceedings of the National Academy of Sciences of the USA* 111, no. 39 (2014): 14205–14210.

23. C. A. Bellcross, K. Kolor, K. A. Goddard, et al., "Awareness and Utilization of BRCA1/2 Testing Among U.S. Primary Care Physicians," *American Journal of Preventive Medicine* 40, no. 1 (2011): 61–66.

24. J. Peto, N. Collins, R. Barfoot, et al., "Prevalence of BRCA 1 and BRCA 2 Gene Mutations in Patients with Early-Onset Breast Cancer," *Journal of the National Cancer Institute* 91, no. 11 (1999): 943–949.

25. K. A. Metcalfe, A. Finch, A. Poll, et al., "Breast Cancer Risks in Women with a Family History of Breast or Ovarian Cancer Who Have Tested Negative for a BRCA1 or BRCA2 Mutation," *British Journal of Cancer* 100, no. 2 (2009): 421–425.

26. T. S. Frank, A. M. Ceffenbaugh, J. E. Reid, et al., "Clinical Characteristics of Individuals with Germline Mutations in BRCA 1 and BRCA2: Analysis of 10,000 Individuals," *Journal of Clinical Oncology* 20 (2002): 1480–1490.

27. R. Nanda, L. P. Schumm, S. Cummings, et al., "Genetic Testing in an Ethnically Diverse Cohort of High-Risk Women: A Comparative Analysis of BRCA 1 and BRCA2 Mutations in American Families of European and African Ancestry," *Journal of the American Medical Association* 294 (2005): 1925–1933.

28. S. Domchek and B. L. Weber, "Genetic Variants of Uncertain Significance: Flies in the Ointment," *Journal of Clinical Oncology* 26, no. 1 (2008): 16–17.

29. T. Judkins, E. Rosenthal, C. Arnell, et al., "Clinical Significance of Large Rearrangements in BRCA 1 and BRCA 2," *Cancer* 118 (2012): 5210–5216; J. N. Weitzel, V. Lagos, K. R. Blazer, et al., "Prevalence of BRCA Mutations and Founder Effect in High-Risk Hispanic Families," *Cancer Epidemiology, Biomarkers and Prevention* 14 (2005): 1666–1671.

30. National Comprehensive Cancer Network (NCCN), "Genetic/Familial High-Risk Assessment: Breast, Ovarian, and Pancreatic," NCCN.org, Clinical Practice Guidelines in Oncology, March 9, 2022, https://www.nccn.org/professionals/physician _gls/pdf/genetics_bop.pdf.

31. Peter D. Beitsch, Pat W. Whitworth, Kevin Hughes, et al., "Underdiagnosis of Hereditary Breast Cancer: Are Genetic Testing Guidelines a Tool or an Obstacle?," *Journal of Clinical Oncology* 37, no. 6 (2019): 453–460.

32. Eric R. Manahan et al., "Consensus Guidelines on Genetic Testing for Hereditary Breast Cancer from the American Society of Breast Surgeons," *Annals of Surgical Oncology* 26, no. 10 (2019): 3025–3031, doi:10.1245/s10434-019-07549-8.

33. T. S. Frank, S. A. Manley, O. I. Olopade, et al., "Sequence Analysis of BRCA 1/2: Correlation of Mutations with Family History and Ovarian Cancer Risk," *Journal of Clinical Oncology* 16 (1998): 2417.

34. C. T. M. Brekelmans, C. Seynaeve, C. C. M. Bartels, et al., "Effectiveness of Breast Cancer Surveillance in BRCA 1/2 Gene Mutation Carriers and Women with High Familial Risk," *Journal of Clinical Oncology* 19 (2001): 924–930.

35. H. Meijers-Heijboer, B. van Greel, W. L. van Putten, et al., "Breast Cancer After Prophylactic Mastectomy in Women with a BRCA 1 or BRCA 2 Mutation," *New England Journal of Medicine* 345 (2001): 159–164.

36. M. Kriege, C. T. M. Brekelmans, C. Boetes, et al., "Efficacy of MRI and Mammography for Breast Cancer Screening in Women with a Familial or Genetic Predisposition," *New England Journal of Medicine* 351 (2004): 427–437; S. K. Plevritis, A. W. Kurian, B. M. Sigal, et al., "Cost-Effectiveness of Screening BRCA1/2 Mutation Carriers with Breast Magnetic Resonance Imaging," *Journal of the American Medical Association* 295 (2006): 2374–2384.

CHAPTER 5. UNDERSTANDING RISK

1. Guy R. Newell and Victor G. Vogel, "Personal Risk Factors: What Do They Mean?," *Cancer* 62, no. S1 (October 1988): 1695–1701.

2. A. B. Miller, "Epidemiology and Prevention," in *Breast Diseases*, ed. Jay R. Harris, Samuel Hellman, I. Craig Henderson, and David W. Kinne (Philadelphia: Lippincott, 1987).

3. M. Terris and M. C. Oalmann, "Carcinoma of the Cervix: An Epidemiological Study," *Journal of the American Medical Association* 174, no. 14 (1960): 1847–1851.

4. Herbert Seidman, Steven D. Stellman, and Margaret H. Mushinski, "A Different Perspective on Breast Cancer Risk Factors: Some Implications of the Nonattributable Risk," *Cancer Journal for Clinicians* 32 (1982): 301.

5. W. C. Willett, M. J. Stampfer, G. A. Colditz, et al., "Moderate Alcohol Consumption and the Risk of Breast Cancer," *New England Journal of Medicine* 316, no. 19 (1980): 1174–1180.

6. W. Yue, R. J. Santen, J. P. Wang, et al., "Genotoxic Metabolites of Estradiol in Breast: Potential Mechanism of Estradiol-Induced Carcinogenesis," *Journal of Steroid Biochemistry and Molecular Biology* 86, nos. 3–5 (2003): 477–486.

7. W. F. Anderson, P. S. Rosenberg, A. Prat, et al., "How Many Etiological Subtypes of Breast Cancer—Two, Three, Four, or More?," *Journal of the National Cancer Institute* 106, no. 8 (2014): dju165.

8. M. D. Althuis, J. M. Dozier, W. F. Anderson, et al., "Global Trends in Breast Cancer Incidence and Mortality, 1973—1997," *International Journal of Epidemiology* 34, no. 2 (2005): 405–412.

9. Tessa J. Murray, Maricel V. Maffini, Angelo A. Ucci, et al., "Induction of Mammary Gland Ductal Hyperplasias and Carcinoma In Situ Following Fetal Bisphenol A Exposure," *Reproductive Toxicology* 23, no. 3 (2007): 383–390.

10. Julie R. Palmer, Elizabeth E. Hatch, Carol Rosenberg, et al., "Risk of Breast Cancer in Women Exposed to Diethylstilbestrol In Utero: Preliminary Results (United States)," *Cancer Causes and Control* 13, no. 8 (2002): 753–758.

11. K. B. Michels, D. Trichopoulos, J. M. Robins, et al., "Birthweight as a Risk Factor for Breast Cancer," *Lancet* 348, no. 9041 (1996): 1542–1546.

12. Nancy Potischman and Rebecca Troisi, "In Utero and Early Life Exposures in Relation to Risk of Breast Cancer," *Cancer Causes and Control* 10, no. 6 (1999): 561–573; Mona Okasha, Peter McCarron, David Gunnell, et al., "Exposures in Childhood, Adolescence, and Early Adulthood and Breast Cancer Risk: A Systematic Review of the Literature," *Breast Cancer Research and Treatment* 78, no. 2 (2003): 223–276.

13. D. Trichopoulos, "Hypothesis: Does Breast Cancer Originate In Utero?," *Lancet* 335, no. 8695 (1990): 939–940.

14. B. MacMahon, P. Cole, and J. Brown, "Etiology of Human Breast Cancer: A Review," *Journal of the National Cancer Institute* 50, no. 1 (1973): 21–42.

15. W. H. Parker, M. S. Broder, E. Chang, et al., "Ovarian Conservation at the Time of Hysterectomy and Long-Term Health Outcomes in the Nurses' Health Study," *Obstetrics and Gynecology* 113, no. 5 (May 2009): 1027–1037.

16. M. C. Pike, M. D. Krailo, B. E. Henderson, et al., "'Hormonal' Risk Factors, 'Breast Tissue Age' and the Age-Incidence of Breast Cancer," *Nature* 303, no. 5920 (1983): 767–770; B. Rosner, G. A. Colditz, and W. C. Willett, "Reproductive Risk Factors in a Prospective Study of Breast Cancer: The Nurses' Health Study," *American Journal of Epidemiology* 139, no. 8 (1994): 819–835.

17. Traci R. Lyons, Pepper J. Schedin, and Virginia F. Borges, "Pregnancy and Breast Cancer: When They Collide," *Journal of Mammary Gland Biology and Neoplasia* 14, no. 2 (June 2009): 87–98.

18. M. Melbye, "Induced Abortion and the Risk of Breast Cancer," *New England Journal of Medicine* 336, no. 2 (1997): 81–85; Z. Ye, D. L. Gao, Q. Qin, et al., "Breast Cancer in Relation to Induced Abortions in a Cohort of Chinese Women," *British Journal of Cancer* 87, no. 9 (2002): 977–981; N. Hamajima, Katarina Kosmelj, Maja Primic-Zakelj, et al., "Breast Cancer and Abortion: Collaborative Reanalysis of Data of 53 Epidemiological Studies, Including 83,000 Women with Breast Cancer from 16 Countries," *Lancet* 363 (2004): 1007–1016.

19. Collaborative Group on Hormonal Factors in Breast Cancer, "Breast Cancer and Breastfeeding: Collaborative Reanalysis of Individual Data from 47 Epidemiological Studies in 30 Countries, Including 50,302 Women with Breast Cancer and 96,973 Women Without the Disease," *Lancet* 360, no. 9328 (2002): 187–195.

20. T. J. Key, P. N. Appleby, G. K. Reeves, et al., "Circulating Sex Hormones and Breast Cancer Risk Factors in Postmenopausal Women: Reanalysis of 13 Studies," *British Journal of Cancer* 105, no. 5 (2011): 709–722.

21. E. Folkerd and M. Dowsett, "Sex Hormones and Breast Cancer Risk and Prognosis," *The Breast* 22 (2013): S38–S43.

22. Hironobu Sasano, Yasuhiro Miki, Shuji Nagasaki, et al., "In Situ Estrogen Production and Its Regulation in Human Breast Carcinoma: From Endocrinology to Intracrinology," *Pathology International* 59, no. 11 (November 2009): 777–789.

23. W. R. Miller, P. Mullen, P. Sourdaine, et al., "Regulation of Aromatase Activity Within the Breast," *Journal of Steroid Biochemistry and Molecular Biology* 61, nos. 3–6 (1997): 193–202.

24. S. S. Tworoger and S. E. Hankinson, "Prolactin and Breast Cancer Etiology: An Epidemiologic Perspective," *Journal of Mammary Gland Biology and Neoplasia* 13, no. 1 (March 2008): 41–53.

25. E. Folkerd and M. Dowsett, "Sex Hormones and Breast Cancer Risk in Premenopausal Women: Collaborative Reanalysis of Seven Prospective Studies," *Lancet Oncology* 14, no. 10 (2013): 1009–1019; E. Folkerd and M. Dowsett, "Sex Hormones and Breast Cancer Risk and Prognosis," *The Breast* 22 (2013): 538–543.

26. Debra L. Monticciolo, MD, Sharp F. Malak, MD, MPH, Sarah M. Friedewald, MD, et al., "Breast Cancer Screening Recommendations Inclusive of All Women at Average Risk: Update from the ACR and Society of Breast Imaging," *Journal of the American College of Radiology* 18, no. 9 (September 2021): 1280–1288.

27. Dejan Nikolić et al., "Breast Cancer and Its Impact in Male Transsexuals," *Breast Cancer Research and Treatment* 171, no. 3 (2018): 565–569, doi:10.1007/s10549-018-4875; Dejan Nikolić et al., "Breast Cancer Risk and Prognosis," *The Breast* 22 (2013): 538–543.

28. Endogenous Hormones and Breast Cancer Collaborative Group, "Sex Hormones and Breast Cancer Risk in Premenopausal Women: Collaborative Reanalysis of Seven Prospective Studies," *Lancet Oncology* 14, no. 10 (2013): 1009–1019; E. Folkerd and M. Dowsett, "Sex Hormones and Breast Cancer Risk and Prognosis," *The Breast* 22 (2013): 538–543.

29. V. A. McCormack and Silva I. dos Santos, "Breast Density and Parenchymal Patterns as Markers of Breast Cancer Risk: A Meta-Analysis," *Cancer Epidemiology, Biomarkers and Prevention* 15, no. 6 (2006): 1159–1169.

30. K. Kerlikowske, W. Zhu, A. N. Tosteson, et al., "Identifying Women with Dense Breasts at High Risk for Interval Cancer: A Cohort Study," *Annals of Internal Medicine* 162, no. 10 (2015): 673–681.

31. K. Kerlikowske, L. Ichikawa, D. L. Miglioretti, et al., "National Institutes of Health Breast Cancer Surveillance Consortium: Longitudinal Measurement of Clinical Mammographic Breast Density to Improve Estimation of Breast Cancer Risk," *Journal of the National Cancer Institute* 99 (2007): 386–395; M. E. Work, L. L. Reimers, A. S. Quante, et al., "Changes in Mammographic Density over Time in Breast Cancer Cases and Women at High Risk for Breast Cancer," *International Journal of Cancer* 135 (2014): 1740–1744.

32. L. C. Hartmann, T. A. Sellers, M. H. Frost, et al., "Benign Breast Disease and the Risk of Breast Cancer," *New England Journal of Medicine* 353, no. 3 (2005): 229–237.

33. A. Gayet, J. Esteve, B. Seradour, et al., "Does Hormone Replacement Therapy Increase the Frequency of Breast Atypical Hyperplasia in Postmenopausal Women? Results from the Bouches du Rhone District Screening Campaign," *European Journal of Cancer* 39, no. 12 (2003): 1738–1745.

34. W. D. Dupont and D. L. Page, "Risk Factors for Breast Cancer in Women with Proliferative Breast Disease," *New England Journal of Medicine* 312, no. 3 (1985): 146–151.

35. A. C. Degnim, D. W. Visscher, T. L. Hoskin, et al., "Histologic Findings in Normal Breast Tissues: Comparison to Reduction Mammoplasty and Benign Breast Disease Tissues," *Breast Cancer Research and Treatment* 133, no. 1 (May 2012): 169–177.

36. E. Rubin, D. W. Visscher, R. W. Alexander, et al., "Proliferative Disease and Atypia in Biopsies Performed for Nonpalpable Lesions Detected Mammographically," *Cancer* 61 (1988): 2077–2082.

37. B. Fisher, J. P. Costantino, D. L. Wickerham, et al., "Tamoxifen for Prevention of Breast Cancer: Report of the National Surgical Adjuvant Breast and Bowel Project P–1 study," *Journal of the National Cancer Institute* 90, no. 18 (1998): 1371–1388.

38. D. C. Radisky and I. C. Hartmann, "Mammary Involution and Breast Cancer Risk: Transgenic Models and Clinical Studies," *Journal of Mammary Gland Biology and Neoplasia* 14, no. 2 (June 2009): 181–191.

39. J. D. Figueroa, R. M. Pfeiffer, D. A. Patel, et al., "Terminal Duct Lobular Unit Involution of the Normal Breast: Implications for Breast Cancer Etiology," *Journal of the National Cancer Institute* 106, no. 10 (October 2014).

40. R. Leborgne, "Intraductal Biopsy of Certain Pathologic Processes of the Breast," *Surgery* 19 (1946): 47–54.

41. G. N. Papanicolaou, D. G. Holmquist, G. M. Bader, et al., "Exfoliative Cytology of the Human Mammary Gland and Its Value in the Diagnosis of Cancer and the Diseases of the Breast," *Cancer* 2, no. 2 (1958): 377–409.

42. G. C. Buehring, "Screening for Breast Atypias Using Exfoliative Cytology," *Cancer* 43, no. 5 (1979): 1788–1799; O. W. Sartorius, H. S. Smith, P. Morris, et al., "Cytologic Evaluation of Breast Fluid in the Detection of Breast Disease," *Journal of the National Cancer Institute* 67 (1977): 277–284; M. R. Wrensch, N. L. Petrakis, E. B. King, et al., "Breast Cancer Incidence in Women with Abnormal Cytology in Nipple Aspirates of Breast Fluid," *American Journal of Epidemiology* 135 (1992): 130–141.

43. Gertrude C. Buehring, Amy Letscher, Kathleen M. McGirr, et al., "Presence of Epithelial Cells in Nipple Aspirate Fluid Is Associated with Subsequent Breast Cancer: A 25-Year Prospective Study," *Breast Cancer Research and Treatment* 98, no. 1 (March 2007): 63–70.

44. Kimberly A. Baltzell, Michelle Moghadassi, Terri Rice, et al., "Epithelial Cells in Nipple Aspirate Fluid and Subsequent Breast Cancer Risk: A Historic Prospective Study," *BioMed Central Cancer* 8, no. 1 (March 2008): 1–6.

45. E. Sauter, E. Ross, M. Daly, et al., "Nipple Aspirate Fluid: A Promising Non-Invasive Method to Identify Cellular Markers of Breast Cancer Risk," *British Journal of Cancer* 76, no. 4 (1997): 494–501.

46. John Hornberger, Shu-Chih Chen, Qianyi Li, et al., "Proliferative Epithelial Disease Identified in Nipple Aspirate Fluid and Risk of Developing Breast Cancer: A Systematic Review," *Current Medical Research and Opinion* 31, no. 2 (February 2015): 253–262.

47. W. C. Dooley, B. Ljung, U. Veronesi, et al., "Ductal Lavage for Detection of Cellular Atypia in Women at High Risk for Breast Cancer," *Journal of the National Cancer Institute* 93, no. 21 (2001): 1624–1632.

48. B. L. King, G. M. Crisi, S. Tsai, et al., "Immunocytochemical Analysis of Breast Cells Obtained by Ductal Lavage," *Cancer Cytopathology* 96 (2002): 244–249.

49. D. Yamamoto and K. Tanaka, "A Review of Mammary Ductoscopy in Breast Cancer," *Breast Journal* 10, no. 4 (2004): 295–297.

50. C. Fabian, C. Zalles, S. Kamel, et al., "Correlation of Breast Tissue Biomarkers with Hyperplasia and Dysplasia in Fine-Needle Aspirates (FNAs) of Women at High and Low Risk for Breast Cancer," *Proceedings of Annual Meeting of American Association of Cancer Researchers* 35, no. A1703 (1994): 153–160.

51. M. H. Gail, J. P. Costantino, D. Pee, et al., "Projecting Individualized Absolute Invasive Breast Cancer Risk in African American Women," *Journal of the National Cancer Institute* 99, no. 23 (December 2007): 1782–1792.

52. Julie R. Palmer et al., "A Validated Risk Prediction Model for Breast Cancer in US Black Women," *Journal of Clinical Oncology* 39, no. 34 (2021): 3866–3877, doi:10.1200/JCO.21.01236.

53. J. A. Tice, S. R. Cummings, R. Smith-Bindman, et al., "Using Clinical Factors and Mammographic Breast Density to Estimate Breast Cancer Risk: Development and Validation of a New Predictive Model," *Annals of Internal Medicine* 148, no. 5 (March 2008): 337–347; summary for patients in *Annals of Internal Medicine* 148, no. 5 (March 2008): 134.

54. Adam R. Brentnall et al., "Mammographic Density Adds Accuracy to Both the Tyrer-Cuzick and Gail Breast Cancer Risk Models in a Prospective UK Screening Cohort," *Breast Cancer Research* 17, no. 1 (December 2015): 147, doi:10.1186/s13058-015-0653-5; Bolette Mikela Vilmun et al., "Impact of Adding Breast Density to Breast Cancer Risk Models: A Systematic Review," *European Journal of Radiology* 127 (2020): 109019, doi:10.1016/j.ejrad.2020.109019.

55. Jonathan Tyrer, Stephen W. Duffy, and Jack Cuzick, "A Breast Cancer Prediction Model Incorporating Familial and Personal Risk Factors," *Statistics in Medicine* 23, no. 7 (April 2004): 1111–1130; erratum in *Statistics in Medicine* 24, no. 1 (January 2005): 156.

56. E. Mazzola, J. Chipman, S. C. Cheng, et al., "Recent BRCAPRO Upgrades Significantly Improve Calibration," *Cancer Epidemiology, Biomarkers and Prevention* 23, no. 8 (August 2014): 1689–1695.

CHAPTER 6. PREVENTION AND RISK REDUCTION

1. K. L. Campbell, K. E. Foster-Schubert, C. M. Alfano, et al., "Reduced-Calorie Dietary Weight Loss, Exercise, and Sex Hormones in Postmenopausal Women: Randomized Controlled Trial," *Journal of Clinical Oncology* 30, no. 19 (2012): 2314–2326.

2. A. M. Stuebe, W. C. Willett, F. Xue, et al., "Lactation and Incidence of Premenopausal Breast Cancer: Longitudinal Study," *Archives of Internal Medicine* 169, no. 15 (August 2009): 1364–1371.

3. A. Harding, "Could Half of All Breast Cancers Be Prevented?," Reuters Health News, March 26, 2014, https://www.reuters.com/article/us-breast-cancers/could-half-of-all-breast-cancers-be-prevented-idUKBREA2P12E20140326.

4. C. H. Van Gils, P. H. Peeters, H. B. Bueno-de-Mesquita, et al., "Consumption of Vegetables and Fruits and Risk of Breast Cancer," *Journal of the American Medical Association* 293 (2005): 183–193.

5. S. Jung, D. Spiegelman, L. Baglietto, et al., "Fruit and Vegetable Intake and Risk of Breast Cancer by Hormone Receptor Status," *Journal of the National Cancer Institute* 105, no. 3 (February 2013): 219–236.

6. R. L. Prentice, B. Caan, R. T. Chlebowski, et al., "Low-Fat Dietary Pattern and Risk of Invasive Breast Cancer: The Women's Health Initiative Randomized Controlled

Dietary Modification Trial," *Journal of the American Medical Association* 295, no. 6 (February 2006): 629–642.

7. A. H. Wu, P. Wan, J. Hankin, et al., "Adolescent and Adult Soy Intake and Risk of Breast Cancer in Asian Americans," *Carcinogenesis* 23, no. 9 (2002): 1491–1496.

8. S. A. Lee, X. O. Shu, H. Li, et al., "Adolescent and Adult Soy Food Intake and Breast Cancer Risk: Results from the Shanghai Women's Health Study," *American Journal of Clinical Nutrition* 89, no. 6 (June 2009): 1920–1926.

9. M. Messina and A. H. Wu, "Perspectives on the Soy-Breast Cancer Relations," *American Journal of Clinical Nutrition* 89, no. 5 (May 2009): 1673S–1679S.

10. L. A. Korde, A. H. Wu, T. Fears, et al., "Childhood Soy Intake and Breast Cancer Risk in Asian American Women," *Cancer Epidemiology, Biomarkers and Prevention* 18, no. 4 (April 2009): 1050–1059.

11. V. Rosolowich, E. Saettler, B. Szuck, et al., "Mastalgia," *Journal of Obstetrics and Gynaecology Canada* 28, no. 1 (2006): 49–71; P. E. Goss, T. Li, M. Theriault, et al., "Effects of Dietary Flaxseed in Women with Cyclical Mastalgia," *Breast Cancer Research and Treatment* 64 (2000): 49.

12. L. U. Thompson, J. M. Chen, T. Li, et al., "Dietary Flaxseed Alters Tumor Biological Markers in Postmenopausal Breast Cancer," *Clinical Cancer Research* 11, no. 10 (2005): 3828–3835.

13. Carol J. Fabian, Seema A. Khan, Judy E. Garber, et al., "Randomized Phase IIB Trial of the Lignan Secoisolariciresinol Diglucoside in Premenopausal Women at Increased Risk for Development of Breast Cancer," *Cancer Prevention Research* 13, no. 7 (July 1, 2020): 623–634, doi:10.1158/1940-6207.CAPR-20-0050.

14. A. H. Wu, G. Ursin, W. P. Koh, et al., "Green Tea, Soy, and Mammographic Density in Singapore Chinese Women," *Cancer Epidemiology, Biomarkers and Prevention* 17, no. 12 (December 2008): 3358–3365.

15. Nathalie Druesne-Pecollo, Paule Latino-Martel, Teresa Norat, et al., "Beta-Carotene Supplementation and Cancer Risk: A Systematic Review and Meta-Analysis of Randomized Controlled Trials," *International Journal of Cancer* 127, no. 1 (July 2010): 172–184.

16. M. L. Morton and C. L. Thompson, "Decreasing 25-Hydroxy-Vitamin D Levels Account for Portion of the Effect of Increasing Body Mass Index on Breast Cancer Mortality," *Molecular Nutrition and Food Research* 57, no. 2 (2013): 260–266.

17. J. M. Lappe, D. Travers-Gustafson, K. M. Davies, et al., "Vitamin D and Calcium Supplementation Reduces Cancer Risk: Results of a Randomized Trial," *American Journal of Clinical Nutrition* 85 (2007): 1586–1591.

18. R. Chlebowski, K. C. Johnson, C. Kooperberg, et al., "Calcium Plus Vitamin D Supplementation and the Risk of Breast Cancer," *Journal of the National Cancer Institute* 100 (November 2008): 1581–1591.

19. C. F. Garland, E. D. Gorham, S. B. Mohr, et al., "Vitamin D and Prevention of Breast Cancer: Pooled Analysis," *Journal of Steroid Biochemistry and Molecular Biology* 103 (2007): 708–711.

20. Rowan T. Chlebowski, Karen C. Johnson, Charles Kooperberg, et al., "Calcium plus Vitamin D Supplementation and the Risk of Breast Cancer," *Journal of the National Cancer Institute* 100, no. 22 (November 2008): 1581–1591.

21. JoAnn E. Manson et al., "Vitamin D Supplements and Prevention of Cancer and Cardiovascular Disease," *New England Journal of Medicine* 380, no. 1 (2019):

33–44; JoAnn E. Manson et al., "Marine n-3 Fatty Acids and Prevention of Cardiovascular Disease and Cancer," *New England Journal of Medicine* 380, no. 1 (2019): 23–32.

22. M. F. Holick, "Vitamin D Deficiency," *New England Journal of Medicine* 357 (2007): 266–281.

23. M. D. Holmes and W. C. Willet, "Does Diet Affect Breast Cancer Risk?," *Breast Cancer Research* 6 (2004): 170–178.

24. P. Toniolo, A. L. Van Kappel, A. Akhmedkhanov, et al., "Serum Carotenoids and Breast Cancer," *American Journal of Epidemiology* 153 (2001): 1142–1147; R. Sato, K. J. Helzlsouer, A. J. Alberg, et al., "Prospective Study of Carotenoids, Tocopherols, and Retinoid Concentrations and the Risk of Breast Cancer," *Cancer Epidemiology, Biomarkers and Prevention* 11 (2002): 451–457.

25. Kimberly Kline, Karla A. Lawson, Weiping Yu, et al., "Vitamin E and Breast Cancer Prevention: Current Status and Future Potential," *Journal of Mammary Gland Biology and Neoplasia* 8, no. 1 (2003).

26. M. L. Neuhouser, S. Wassertheil-Smoller, C. Thomson, et al., "Multivitamin Use and Risk of Cancer and Cardiovascular Disease in the Women's Health Initiative Cohorts," *Archives of Internal Medicine* 169, no. 3 (2009): 294–304.

27. L. Bernstein, B. E. Henderson, R. Hansich, et al., "Physical Exercise Activity and Reduced Risk of Breast Cancer in Young Women," *Journal of the National Cancer Institute* 86, no. 18 (September 1994): 1403–1408.

28. C. M. Dallal, J. Sullivan-Halley, R. K. Ross, et al., "Long-Term Recreational Physical Activity and Risk of Invasive and In Situ Breast Cancer," *Archives of Internal Medicine* 167 (2007): 408–415.

29. L. Bernstein, R. K. Ross, R. A. Lovo, et al., "The Effects of Moderate Physical Activity on Menstrual Cycle Patterns in Adolescence: Implications for Breast Cancer Prevention," *British Journal of Cancer* 55, no. 6 (1987): 681–685.

30. A. J. Smith, W. R. Phipps, W. Thomas, et al., "The Effects of Aerobic Exercise on Estrogen Metabolism in Healthy Premenopausal Women," *Cancer Epidemiology, Biomarkers and Prevention* 22, no. 5 (2013): 756–764.

31. R. E. Frisch, G. Wyshak, N. L. Albright, et al., "Lower Lifetime Occurrence of Breast Cancer and Cancer of the Reproductive System Among Former College Athletes," *American Journal of Clinical Nutrition* 45, no. 1 (1987): 328–335.

32. D. V. Spicer, M. C. Pike, A. Pike, et al., "Pilot Trial of a Gonadotropin Hormone Agonist with Replacement Hormones as a Prototype Contraceptive to Prevent Breast Cancer," *Contraception* 47 (1993): 427–444.

33. D. V. Spicer, G. Ursin, Y. R. Parisky, et al., "Changes in Mammographic Densities Induced by a Hormonal Contraceptive Designed to Reduce Breast Cancer Risk," *Journal of the National Cancer Institute* 86, no. 6 (1994): 431–436.

34. L. Bernstein, R. Hanisch, J. Sullivan-Halley, et al., "Treatment with Human Chorionic Gonadotropin (HCG) and Risk of Breast Cancer," *Cancer Epidemiology, Biomarkers and Prevention* 4, no. 5 (1995): 437–440.

35. J. Cuzick, I. Sestak, B. Bonanni, et al., "Selective Oestrogen Receptor Modulators in Prevention of Breast Cancer: An Updated Meta-Analysis of Individual Participant Data," *Lancet* 38, no. 9880 (2013): 1827–1834.

36. P. E. Goss, J. N. Ingle, J. E. Ales-Martinez, et al., "Exemestane for Breast-Cancer Prevention in Postmenopausal Women," *New England Journal of Medicine* 364, no. 25 (2011): 2381–2391.

37. Tara Hyder et al., "Aromatase Inhibitor-Associated Musculoskeletal Syndrome: Understanding Mechanisms and Management," *Frontiers in Endocrinology* (2021): 914.

38. J. Cuzick, I. Sestak, J. F. Forbes, et al., "Anastrozole for Prevention of Breast Cancer in High-Risk Postmenopausal Women (IBIS-II): An International, Double-Blind, Randomized Placebo-Controlled Trial," *Lancet* 383 (2014): 1041–1048.

39. Jack Cuzick et al., "Use of Anastrozole for Breast Cancer Prevention (IBIS-II): Long-Term Results of a Randomised Controlled Trial," *Lancet* 395, no. 10218 (2020): 117–122, doi:10.1016/S0140-6736(19)32955.

40. Kala Visvanathan, Carol J. Fabian, Elissa Bantug, et al., "Use of Endocrine Therapy for Breast Cancer Risk Reduction: ASCO Clinical Practice Guideline Update," *Journal of Clinical Oncology* 37, no. 33 (2019): 3152–3165.

41. Jasenca Piljac Zegarac, PhD, "ASCO Updates Breast Cancer Risk Reduction Guideline to Include Anastrozole," *ASCO Post*, November 25, 2019, https://ascopost.com/issues/november-25-2019/asco-updates-breast-cancer-risk-reduction-guideline-to-include-anastrozole/.

42. X. Zhang, S. A. Smith-Warner, L. C. Collins, et al., "Use of Aspirin, Other Nonsteroidal Anti-Inflammatory Drugs, and Acetaminophen and Postmenopausal Breast Cancer Incidence," *Journal of Clinical Oncology* 30 (2012): 3468–3477.

43. C. Duggin, C. Y. Wang, L. Xiao, et al., "Aspirin and Serum Estrogens in Postmenopausal Women: A Randomized Controlled Clinical Trial," *Cancer Prevention Research* 7, no. 9 (2014): 906–912.

44. J. D. Potter, "Aspirin and Cancer Prevention and Treatment: Are We There Yet?," *Cancer Epidemiology, Biomarkers and Prevention* 21, no. 9 (2012): 1439–1440.

45. Michelle Holmes and Wendy Chen, "A Cancer Treatment in Your Medicine Cabinet?," *New York Times*, May 19, 2014, https://www.nytimes.com/2014/05/20/opinion/a-cancer-treatment-in-your-medicine-cabinet.html?_r=0.

46. A. Decensi, M. Puntoni, P. Goodwin, et al., "Metformin and Cancer Risk in Diabetic Patients: A Systemic Review and Meta-Analysis," *Cancer Prevention Research* 3, no. 11 (2010): 1451–1461.

47. S. Gandini, M. Puntoni, E. Ospedali Galliera, et al., "Metformin and Cancer Risk and Mortality: A Systematic Review and Meta-Analysis Taking into Account Biases and Confounders," *Cancer Prevention Research* 7, no. 9 (2014): 867–885.

48. Katsuya Nakai et al., "A Perspective on Anti-EGFR Therapies Targeting Triple-Negative Breast Cancer," *American Journal of Cancer Research* 6, no. 8 (August 1, 2016): 1609–1623; Renaud Sabatier et al., "High Response to Cetuximab in a Patient with EGFR-Amplified Heavily Pretreated Metastatic Triple-Negative Breast Cancer," *JCO Precision Oncology* 3 (2019): 1–8, doi:10.1200/PO.18.00310.

49. M. Fracol, S. Xu, R. Mick, et al., "Response to HER-2 Pulsed DC1 Vaccines Is Predicted by Both HER-2 and Estrogen Receptor Expression in DCIS," *Annals of Surgical Oncology* 10 (2013): 3233–3239.

50. V. Tiriveehdi, N. Tucker, J. Herndon, et al., "Safety and Preliminary Evidence of Biologic Efficacy of a Mammaglobin—a DNA Vaccine in Patients with Stable Metastatic Breast Cancer," *Clinical Cancer Research* 20, no. 23 (2014): 5964–5975.

51. W. J. Temple, R. L. Lindsay, E. Magi, et al., "Technical Considerations for Prophylactic Mastectomy in Patients at High Risk for Breast Cancer," *American Journal of Surgery* 161, no. 4 (1991): 413.

52. Rajini Katipamula, Amy C. Degnim, Tanya Hoskin, et al., "Trends in Mastectomy Rates at the Mayo Clinic, Rochester: Effect of Surgical Year and Preoperative Magnetic Resonance," *Journal of Clinical Oncology* 27, no. 25 (September 2009): 4082–4088.

53. W. H. Parker, M. S. Broder, E. Chang, et al., "Ovarian Conservation at the Time of Hysterectomy and Long-Term Health Outcomes in the Nurses' Health Study," *Obstetrics and Gynecology* 113, no. 5 (May 2009): 1027–1037.

54. T. B. Rebbeck, T. Friebel, H. T. Lynch, et al., "Bilateral Prophylactic Mastectomy Reduces Breast Cancer Risk in BRCA 1 and BRCA 2 Mutation Carriers: The PROSE Study Group," *Journal of Clinical Oncology* 22 (2004): 1055–1062.

55. B. A. Heemskerk-Gerritsen, C. T. Brekelmans, M. B. Menke-Pluymers, et al., "Prophylactic Mastectomy in BRCA 1/2 Mutation Carriers and Women at Risk of Hereditary Breast Cancer: Long-Term Experiences at the Rotterdam Family Cancer Clinic," *Annals of Surgical Oncology* 14 (2007): 3335–3344.

56. O. I. Olopade and G. Artioli, "Efficacy of Risk-Reducing Salpingo-Oophorectomy in Women with BRCA-1 and BRCA-2 Mutations," *Breast Journal* 10, supp. 1 (January–February 2004): S5–S9.

57. M. Steven Piver, Mohannad F. Jishi, Yoshiaki Tsukada, et al., "Primary Peritoneal Carcinoma After Prophylactic Oophorectomy in Women with a Family History of Ovarian Cancer," *Cancer* 71, no. 9 (1993): 2751–2755.

58. T. R. Rebbeck, H. T. Lynch, S. L. Neuhausen, et al., "Prophylactic Oophorectomy in Carriers of BRCA 1 or BRCA 2 Mutations," *New England Journal of Medicine* 346 (2002): 1616–1622.

59. A. W. Kurian, B. M. Sigal, and S. K. Plevritis, "Survival Analysis of Cancer Risk Reduction Strategies for BRCA 1/2 Mutation Carriers," *Journal of Clinical Oncology* 28 (2009): 222–231.

60. S. A. Narod, "Modifiers of Risk of Hereditary Breast Cancer," *Oncogene* 25 (2006): 5832–5836.

61. S. Murata, S. L. Kominsky, M. Vali, et al., "Ductal Access for Prevention and Therapy of Mammary Tumors," *Cancer Research* 66, no. 2 (January 2006): 638–645.

CHAPTER 7. SCREENING

1. N. B. Biller-Andorno and P. Juni, "Abolishing Mammography Screening Programs? A View from the Swiss Medical Board," *New England Journal of Medicine* 370, no. 21 (2014): 1965–1967; R. A. Smith, "The Value of Modern Mammography Screening in the Control of Breast Cancer: Understanding the Underpinnings of the Current Debates," *Cancer Epidemiology, Biomarkers and Prevention* 23 (2014): 1139–1146.

2. American College of Radiology, "New Breast Cancer Screening Guidelines Address Heightened Risk for LGBTQ Persons and Black Women," June 22, 2021, https://www.acr.org/Media-Center/ACR-News-Releases/2021/New-Breast -Cáncer-Screening-Guidelines-Address-Heightened-Risk-for-LGBTQ-Persons-and -Black-Women; Debra Monticciolo et al., "Breast Cancer Screening Recommendations Inclusive of All Women of Average Risk: Update from the ACR and Society of Breast Imaging," *Journal of the American College of Radiology* 18, no. 9 (2021): 1280–1288, doi:10.1016/j.jacr.2021.04.021.

3. L. M. Schwartz, S. Wolloshin, H. C. Sox, et al., "US Women's Attitudes to False Positive Mammography Results and Detection of Ductal Carcinoma In Situ: Cross Sectional Survey," *British Medical Journal* 320 (2000): 1635–1640.

4. L. E. Pace and N. L. Keating, "A Systematic Assessment of Benefits and Risks to Guide Breast Cancer Screening Decisions," *Journal of the American Medical Association* 311, no. 13 (2014): 1327–1335.

5. A. Bleyer and H. G. Welch, "Effect of Three Decades of Screening Mammography on Breast Cancer Incidence," *New England Journal of Medicine* 367 (2012): 1998–2005.

6. J. S. Mandelbatt, K. A. Cronin, S. Bailey, et al., "Effects of Mammography Screening Under Different Screening Schedules: Model Estimates of Potential Benefits and Harms," *Annals of Internal Medicine* 151 (2009): 738–747.

7. L. E. Pace and N. L. Keating, "A Systematic Assessment of Benefits and Risks to Guide Breast Cancer Screening Decisions," *Journal of the American Medical Association* 311, no. 13 (2014): 1327–1335.

8. M. J. Yaffe and J. G. Mainprize, "Risk of Radiation-Induced Breast Cancer from Mammographic Screening," *Radiology* 258, no. 1 (January 2011): 98–105.

9. D. L. Miglioretti, J. Lange, J. J. van den Broek, et al., "Radiation–Induced Breast Cancer Incidence and Mortality from Digital Mammography Screening: A Modeling Study," *Annals of Internal Medicine* 164, no. 4 (February 16, 2016): 205–214, doi:10.7326/M15-1241.

10. A. Coldman, N. Phillips, C. Wilson, et al., "Pan-Canadian Study of Mammography Screening and Mortality from Breast Cancer," *Journal of the National Cancer Institute* 106, no. 11 (2014): 261.

11. Stacey Wolfson, Eric Kim, Anastasia Plaunova, et al., "Axillary Adenopathy After COVID-19 Vaccine: No Reason to Delay Screening Mammogram," *Radiology* 303, no. 2 (2022): 297–299.

12. Ana I. Velazquez et al., "Trends in Breast Cancer Screening in a Safety-Net Hospital During the COVID-19 Pandemic," *JAMA Network Open* 4, no. 8 (August 2, 2021): e2119929, doi:10.1001/jamanetworkopen.2021.19929.

13. American Psychological Association, "Stress in America 2021: One Year Later, A New Wave of Pandemic Health Concerns," APA.org, March 11, 2021, https://www.apa.org/news/press/releases/stress/2021/one-year-pandemic-stress.

14. Manisha Bahl, Sarah Mercaldo, Anne Marie McCarthy, et al., "Imaging Surveillance of Breast Cancer Survivors with Digital Mammography Versus Digital Breast Tomosynthesis," *Radiology* 298, no. 2 (2021): 308–316; Regina Hooley and Reni Butler, "Digital Breast Tomosynthesis May Not Provide Optimal Surveillance of Breast Cancer Survivors," *Radiology* 298, no. 2 (2021): 317–318.

15. C. K. Kuhl, S. Schrading, K. Strobel, et al., "Abbreviated Breast Magnetic Resonance Imaging (MRI): First Postcontrast Subtracted Images and Maximum-Intensity Projection—a Novel Approach to Breast Cancer Screening with MRI," *Journal of Clinical Oncology* 32 (2014): 2304–2310.

16. Min Sun Bae, Janice Sung, Wonshik Han, et al., "Survival Outcomes of Screening with Breast MRI in High-Risk Women," *Journal of Clinical Oncology* 35, no. 15 suppl. (May 20, 2017): 1508–1508.

17. Hayley Virgil, "Earlier MRI Screenings Could Significantly Cut Breast Cancer Mortality for Certain Pathogenic Variants," Cancer Network, May 19, 2022, https://cancernetwork.com/view/earlier-mri-screenings-could-significantly-cut-breast-cancer-mortality-for-certain-pathogenic-variants; Kathryn P. Lowry et al., "Breast Cancer Screening Strategies for Women with ATM, CHEK2, and PALB2 Pathogenic Variants: A Comparative Modeling Analysis," *JAMA Oncology* 8, no. 4 (2022): 587–596, doi:10.1001/jamaoncol.2021.6204.

18. Mieke Kriege, Cecile T. M. Brekelmans, Carla Boetes, et al., "Efficacy of MRI and Mammography for Breast Cancer Screening in Women with a Familial or Genetic Predisposition," *New England Journal of Medicine* 351 (2004): 427–437.

19. E. Warner, K. Hill, P. Causer, et al., "Prospective Study of Breast Cancer Incidence in Women with a BRCA1 or BRCA2 Mutation Under Surveillance with and Without Magnetic Resonance Imaging," *Journal of Clinical Oncology* 29 (2011): 1664–1669.

20. E. A. M. Heijinsdijik, E. Warner, F. J. Gilbert, et al., "Differences in Natural History Between Breast Cancers in BRCA 1 and BRCA 2 Mutation Carriers and Effects of MRI Screening—MRISC, MARIBS and Canadian Studies Combined," *Cancer Epidemiology, Biomarkers and Prevention* 21 (2012): 1458–1468.

21. W. A. Berg, Z. Zhang, D. Lehrer, et al., "Detection of Breast Cancer with Addition of Annual Screening Ultrasound or a Single Screening MRI to Mammography in Women with Elevated Breast Cancer Risk," *Journal of the American Medical Association* 307, no. 17 (2012): 1394–1404.

22. Min Sun Bae et al., "Survival Outcomes of Screening with Breast MRI in Women at Elevated Risk of Breast Cancer," *Journal of Breast Imaging* 2, no. 1 (2020): 29–35, doi:10.1093/jbi/wbz083.

23. W. A. Berg, J. D. Blume, A. M. Adams, et al., "Reasons Women at Elevated Risk of Breast Cancer Refuse Breast MRI Screening: ACRIN 6666," *Radiology* 254, no. 1 (January 2010): 79–87.

24. W. A. Berg, Z. Zhang, D. Lehrer, et al., "Detection of Breast Cancer with Addition of Annual Screening Ultrasound or a Single Screening MRI to Mammography in Women with Elevated Breast Cancer Risk," *Journal of the American Medical Association* 307, no. 17 (2012): 1394–1404.

25. V. Corsetti, N. Houssami, M. Ghirardi, et al., "Evidence of the Effect of Adjunct Ultrasound Screening in Women with Mammography-Negative Dense Breasts: Interval Breast Cancers at 1-Year Follow-up," *European Journal of Cancer* 47, no. 7 (2011): 1021–1026.

26. W. A. Berg and E. B. Mendelson, "Technologist-Performed Handheld Screening Breast US Imaging: How Is It Performed and What Are the Outcomes to Date?," *Radiology* 272 (2014): 12–27.

27. R. F. Brem, L. Tabar, S. W. Duffy, et al., "Assessing Improvement in Detection of Breast Cancer with Three-Dimensional Automated Breast US in Women with Dense Breast Tissue: The SomoInsight Study," *Radiology* 274, no. 3 (2015): 663–673.

28. D. B. Thomas, D. L. Gao, S. G. Self, et al., "Randomized Trial of Breast Self-Examination in Shanghai: Methodology and Preliminary Results," *Journal of the National Cancer Institute* 89 (1997): 355–365.

29. U.S. Preventive Services Task Force, "Guidelines Screening for Breast Cancer: U.S. Preventive Services Task Force Recommendation Statement," *Annals of Internal Medicine* 151 (2009): 716–726.

30. T. S. Menes, D. Coster, D. Coster, et al., "Contribution of Clinical Breast Exam to Cancer Detection in Women Participating in a Modern Screening Program," *BMC Women's Health* 21, no. 1 (October 19, 2021): 368.

31. W. H. Goodson, T. K. Hunt, J. N. Plotnik, et al., "Optimization of Clinical Breast Examination," *American Journal of Medicine* 123, no. 4 (2010): 329–334.

32. Centers for Disease Control and Prevention, "Breast Cancer Screening Guidelines for Women," CDC.gov, September 22, 2020, https://www.cdc.gov/cancer/breast/pdf/breast-cancer-screening-guidelines-508.pdf.

33. Debbie Saslow, Carla Boetes, Wylie Burke, et al., "American Cancer Society Guidelines for Breast Screening with MRI as an Adjunct to Mammography," *CA: A Cancer Journal for Clinicians* 57, no. 2 (2007): 75–89.

34. Stephen W. Duffy, László Tabár, Amy Ming-Fang Yen, et al., "Beneficial Effect of Consecutive Screening Mammography Examinations on Mortality from Breast Cancer: A Prospective Study," *Radiology* 299, no. 3 (March 2, 2021): 541–547.

35. Lisa Rosenbaum, "Invisible Risks, Emotional Choices—Mammography and Medical Decision Making," *New England Journal of Medicine* 371 (2014): 1549–1552.

CHAPTER 8. DIAGNOSIS

1. H. I. Vargas, M. P. Vargas, K. Eldrageely, et al., "Outcomes of Surgical and Sonographic Assessment of Breast Masses in Women Younger Than 30," *American Surgeon* 71, no. 9 (2005): 716–719.

2. M. Morrow, S. Wong, and L. Venta, "The Evaluation of Breast Masses in Women Younger Than Forty Years of Age," *Surgery* 124, no. 4 (1998): 634–640.

3. S. V. Hilton, G. R. Leopold, L. K. lson, et al., "Real-Time Breast Sonography: Application in 300 Consecutive Patients," *American Journal of Roentgenology* 147, no. 3 (1986): 479–486.

4. B. L. Sprague, R. E. Gangnon, V. Burt, et al., "Prevalence of Mammographically Dense Breasts in the United States," *Journal of the National Cancer Institute* 106, no. 10 (2014).

5. M. A. Roubidoux, "Invasive Cancers Detected After Breast Cancer Screening Yielded a Negative Result: Relationship of Mammographic Density to Tumor Prognostic Factors," *Radiology* 230, no. 1 (January 2004): 42–48.

6. M. J. Homer, "Nonpalpable Breast Microcalcifications: Frequency, Management, and Results of Incisional Biopsy," *Radiology* 185 (1992): 411–413.

7. M. E. Berend, D. C. Sullivan, P. J. Kornguth, et al., "The Natural History of Mammographic Calcifications Subjected to Interval Follow-Up," *Archives of Surgery* 127, no. 11 (November 1992): 1309–1313.

8. D. Gur, J. H. Sumkin, H. E. Rockette, et al., "Changes in Breast Cancer Detection and Mammography Recall Rates After the Introduction of a Computer Aided Detection System," *Journal of the National Cancer Institute* 96, no. 3 (February 2004): 185–190; J. G. Elmore and P. Carney, "Computer-Aided Detection of Breast Cancer: Has Promise Outstripped Performance?," *Journal of the National Cancer Institute* 96, no. 3 (2004): 162–163.

9. Julie Sogani et al., "Contrast-Enhanced Mammography: Past, Present and Future," *Clinical Imaging* 69 (2021): 269–279, doi:10.1016/j.clinimag.2020.09.003.

10. S. H. Parker, J. D. Lovin, W. E. Jobe, et al., "Stereotactic Breast Biopsy with a Biopsy Gun," *Radiology* 176, no. 3 (September 1990): 741–747.

11. R. F. Brem, L. Tabar, S. W. Duffy, et al., "Assessing Improvement in Detection of Breast Cancer with Three-Dimensional Automated Breast US in Women with Dense Breast Tissue: The SomoInsight Study," *Radiology* 274, no. 3 (March 2015): 663–673.

12. J. P. Delille, P. J. Slanetz, E. D. Yeh, et al., "Physiologic Changes in Breast Magnetic Resonance Imaging During the Menstrual Cycle: Perfusion Imaging, Signal

Enhancement, and Influence of the T1 Relaxation Time of Breast Tissue," *Breast Journal* 11 (2006): 236–241.

13. E. Warner, D. B. Plewes, R. S. Shumak, et al., "Comparison of Breast Magnetic Resonance Imaging, Mammography, and Ultrasound for Surveillance of Women at High Risk for Hereditary Breast Cancer," *Journal of Clinical Oncology* 19, no. 15 (August 2001): 3524–3531.

14. Debra L. Monticciolo et al., "Breast Cancer Screening in Women at Higher-Than-Average Risk: Recommendations from the ACR," *Journal of the American College of Radiology* 15, no. 3, pt. A (2018): 408–414, doi:10.1016/j.jacr.2017.11.034.

15. J. E. Kalinyak, W. A. Berg, K. Schilling, et al., "Breast Cancer Detection Using High-Resolution Breast PET Compared to Whole-Body or PET/CT," *European Journal of Nuclear Medicine and Molecular Imaging* 41, no. 2 (February 2014): 260–275.

16. FDA Consumer Updates, "Breast Cancer Screening: Thermogram No Substitute for Mammogram," FDA.gov, January 13, 2021, https://www.fda.gov/consumers/consumer-updates/breast-cancer-screening-thermogram-no-substitute-mammogram.

17. G. Martelli, S. Pilotti, G. C. De Yoldi, et al., "Diagnostic Efficacy of Physical Examination, Mammography, Fine Needle Aspiration, Cytology (Triple-Test) in Solid Breast Lumps: An Analysis of 1708 Consecutive Cases," *Tumori* 76, no. 5 (October 1990): 476–479.

CHAPTER 9. COPING WITH A BREAST CANCER DIAGNOSIS

1. Rose Kushner, *Alternatives* (Cambridge, MA: Kensington, 1984).

2. H. Peters-Golden, "Breast Cancer: Varied Perceptions of Social Support in the Illness Experience," *Social Science Medicine* 16, no. 4 (1982): 483–491.

3. Ann Kaspar, personal communication.

4. D. K. Wellisch, E. R. Gritz, W. Schain, et al., "Psychological Functioning of Daughters of Breast Cancer Patients: Part II: Characterizing the Distressed Daughter of the Breast Cancer Patient," *Psychosomatics* 33, no. 2 (Spring 1992): 171–179.

5. Rosemary R. Lichtman, Shelley E. Taylor, Joanne V. Wood, et al., "Relations with Children After Breast Cancer: The Mother-Daughter Relationship at Risk," *Journal of Psychosocial Oncology* 2, no. 3–4 (1985): 1–19.

6. Michael Singer, "Advocating for Men with Breast Cancer—My Advocacy Story," Cancer.net, November 17, 2017, https://www.cancer.net/blog/2017-11/advocating-men-with-breast-cancer.

7. Naama Levin-Dagan and Nehami Baum, "Passing as Normal: Negotiating Boundaries and Coping with Male Breast Cancer," *Social Science and Medicine* 284 (September 2021): 114239, doi:10.1016/j.socscimed.2021.114239; Weber Rainer, Johannes C. Ehrenthal, Evamarie Brock-Midding, et al., "Defense Mechanisms and Repressive Coping Among Male Breast Cancer Patients," *Frontiers in Psychiatry* 12 (2021): 718076, doi:10.3389/fpsyt.2021.718076.

CHAPTER 10. WHAT KIND OF BREAST CANCER DO I HAVE?

1. J. M. Dixon, T. J. Anderson, D. L. Page, et al., "Infiltrating Lobular Carcinoma of the Breast: An Evaluation of the Incidence and Consequence of Bilateral Disease," *British Journal of Surgery* 70, no. 9 (September 1983): 513–516.

2. M. S. Moran, S. J. Schnitt, A. E. Giuliano, et al., "Society of Surgical Oncology—American Society for Radiation Oncology Consensus Guideline on Margins for Breast-Conserving Surgery with Whole Breast Irradiation in Stages I

and II Invasive Breast Cancer," *Journal of Clinical Oncology* 32, no. 14 (May 2014): 1507–1515.

3. J. L. Mansi, H. Gogas, J. M. Bliss, et al., "Outcome of Primary Breast Cancer Patients with Micrometastases: A Long-Term Follow-Up Study," *Lancet* 354, no. 9174 (July 1999): 197–202.

4. Marianne Gotteland, Evelyne May, Francoise May-Levin, et al., "Estrogen Receptors (ER) in Human Breast Cancer," *Cancer* 74, no. 3 (August 1994): 864–871.

5. D. Slamon, W. Godolphin, L. Jones, et al., "Studies of the HER-2/neu Proto-Oncogene in Human Breast and Ovarian Cancer," *Science* 244, no. 4905 (1989): 707–712.

6. B. Dybdal, G. Leiberman, S. Anderson, et al., "Determination of HER2 Gene Amplification by Fluorescence In Situ Hybridization and Concordance with the Clinical Trials Immunohistochemical Assay in Women with Metastatic Breast Cancer Evaluated for Treatment with Trastuzumab," *Breast Cancer Research and Treatment* 93, no. 1 (2005): 3–11.

7. Daniel Eiger et al., "The Exciting New Field of HER2-Low Breast Cancer Treatment," *Cancers* 13, no. 5 (March 1, 2021): 1015, doi:10.3390/cancers13051015.

8. S. Modi, W. Jacot, T. Yamashita, et al., "Trastuzumab Deruxtecan in Previously Treated HER2-Low Advanced Breast Cancer," *New England Journal of Medicine* 387, no. 1 (July 7, 2022): 9–20, doi:10.1056/NEJMoa2203690.

9. M. Van Bockstal, K. Lambein, H. Denys, et al., "Histopathological Characterization of Ductal Carcinoma In Situ (DCIS) of the Breast According to HER-2 Amplification Status and Molecular Subtype," *Virchows Archiv* 465, no. 3 (September 2014): 275–289.

10. C. M. Perou, T. Sorlie, M. B. Eisen, et al., "Molecular Portraits of Human Breast Tumors," *Nature* 406 (2000): 747–752.

11. W. Y. Chen and G. A. Colditz, "Risk Factors and Hormone-Receptor Status: Epidemiology Risk-Prediction Models and Treatment Implications for Breast Cancer," *National Clinical Practice: Oncology* 4, no. 7 (July 2007): 415–423.

12. C. Sotiriou, S. Y. Neo, L. M. McShane, et al., "Breast Cancer Classification and Prognosis Based on Gene Expression Profiles from a Population-Based Study," *Proceedings of the National Academy of Sciences of the USA* 100, no. 18 (September 2003): 10393–10398.

13. William D. Foulkes, Ingunn M. Stefansson, Pierre O. Chappuis, et al., "Germline BRCA 1 Mutations and a Basal Epithelial Phenotype in Breast Cancer," *Journal of the National Cancer Institute* 95 (2003): 1482–1485.

14. R. Rouzier, C. M. Perou, W. F. Symmans, et al., "Breast Cancer Molecular Subtypes Respond Differently to Preoperative Chemotherapy," *Clinical Cancer Research* 11, no. 16 (August 2005): 5678–5685.

15. F. Bertucci, P. Finetti, N. Cervera, et al., "How Basal Are Triple Negative Breast Cancers?," *International Journal of Cancer* 123 (2008): 236–240.

16. S. Paik, S. Shak, G. Tang, et al., "A Multigene Assay to Predict Recurrence of Tamoxifen-Treated, Node-Negative Breast Cancer," *New England Journal of Medicine* 351, no. 27 (2004): 2817–2865.

17. G. Tang, S. Shak, S. Paik, et al., "Comparison of the Prognostic and Predictive Utilities of the 21-Gene Recurrence Score Assay and Adjuvant! for Women with Node-Negative, ER-Positive Breast Cancer: Results from NSABP B-14 and NSABP B-20," *Breast Cancer Research and Treatment* 127, no. 1 (May 2011): 133–142.

18. K. Albain, Breast Cancer Intergroup of North America, W. E. Barlow, et al., "Prognostic and Predictive Value of the 21 Gene Recurrence Score Assay in Postmenopausal Node-Positive Estrogen-Receptor-Positive Breast Cancer on Chemotherapy: A Retrospective Analysis of a Randomized Trial," *Lancet Oncology* 11, no. 1 (January 2010): 55–65.

19. Joseph A. Sparano et al., "Adjuvant Chemotherapy Guided by a 21-Gene Expression Assay in Breast Cancer," *New England Journal of Medicine* 379, no. 2 (2018): 111–121, doi:10.1056/ NEJMoa1804710.

20. C. A. Drukker, J. M. Bueno-de-Mesquita, V. P. Retèl, et al., "A Prospective Evaluation of a Breast Cancer Prognosis Signature in the Observational RASTER Study," *International Journal of Cancer* 133, no. 4 (August 2013): 929–936.

21. Martine Piccart et al., "70-Gene Signature as an Aid for Treatment Decisions in Early Breast Cancer: Updated Results of the Phase 3 Randomised MINDACT Trial with an Exploratory Analysis by Age," *Lancet Oncology* 22, no. 4 (2021): 476–488, doi:10.1016/S1470-2045(21)00007-3.

22. E. Schaafsma, B. Zhang, M. Schaafsma, et al., "Impact of Oncotype DX Testing on ER+ Breast Cancer Treatment and Survival in the First Decade of Use," *Breast Cancer Research* 23, no. 1 (July 17, 2021): 74, doi:10.1186/s13058-021-01453-4.

23. S. B. Edge, D. R. Byrd, C. C. Compton, et al., "Breast," in *AJCC Cancer Staging Manual*, 7th ed., ed. Frederick L. Greene, David L. Page, Irvin D. Fleming, April G. Fritz, Charles M. Balch, Daniel G. Haller, and Monica Morrow, 347–376 (New York: Springer, 2010).

24. Jenni S. Likanen et al., "Prognostic Value of Isolated Tumor Cells in Sentinel Lymph Nodes in Early-Stage Breast Cancer: A Prospective Study," *British Journal of Cancer* 118, no. 11 (2018): 1529–1535, doi:10.1038/s41416-018-0052-7; Yijun Li, Huimin Zhang, Wei Zhang, et al., "A Competing Risk Analysis Model to Determine the Prognostic Value of Isolated Tumor Cells in Axillary Lymph Nodes for T1N0M0 Breast Cancer Patients Based on the Surveillance, Epidemiology, and End Results Database," *Frontiers in Oncology* 10 (September 18, 2020): 572316, doi:10.3389/fonc.2020572316; Gilles Houvenaeghel, Jean-Marc Classe, Jean Rémy Garbay, et al., "Prognostic Value of Isolated Tumor Cells and Micrometastases of Lymph Nodes in Early Stage Breast Cancer: A French Sentinel Node Multicenter Cohort Study," *The Breast* 23, no. 5 (October 2014): 561–566.

25. C. Paoletti, J. Smerage, and D. F. Hayes, "Circulating Tumor Cells as a Marker of Prognosis," *Principles and Practice of Oncology* 26, no. 2 (2012): 1–8; A. Matikas, A. Kotsakis, S. Apostolaki, et al., "Detection of Circulating Tumour Cells Before and Following Adjuvant Chemotherapy and Long-Term Prognosis of Early Breast Cancer," *British Journal of Cancer* 126 (2022): 1563–1569, doi:10.1038/s41416-022-01699-5.

26. Daniel Fernandez-Garcia et al., "Plasma Cell-Free DNA (cfDNA) as a Predictive and Prognostic Marker in Patients with Metastatic Breast Cancer," *Breast Cancer Research* 21, no. 1 (December 19, 2019): 149, doi:10.1186/s13058-019-1235-8.

CHAPTER 11. DECISIONS ABOUT TREATMENT

1. Maria Ekholm et al., "Effects of Adjuvant Tamoxifen over Three Decades on Breast Cancer-Free and Distant Recurrence-Free Interval Among Premenopausal Women with Oestrogen Receptor-Positive Breast Cancer Randomised in the Swedish SBII:2pre Trial," *European Journal of Cancer* 110 (2019): 53–61, doi:10.1016/j.ejca.2018.12.034.

2. B. Fisher, S. Anderson, J. Bryant, et al., "Twenty-Year Follow-Up of a Randomized Trial Comparing Total Mastectomy, Lumpectomy, and Lumpectomy Plus Irradiation for the Treatment of Breast Cancer," *New England Journal of Medicine* 347 (2002): 1233–1241.

3. U. Veronesi, N. Cascinelli, L. Mariani, et al., "Twenty-Year Follow-Up of a Randomized Study Comparing Breast-Conserving Surgery with Radical Mastectomy for Early Breast Cancer," *New England Journal of Medicine* 347 (2002): 1227–1232.

4. S. Agarwal, L. Pappas, L. Neumayer, et al., "Effect of Breast Conservation Therapy vs Mastectomy on Disease-Specific Survival for Early Stage Breast Cancer," *JAMA Surgery* 149, no. 3 (January 2014): 267–274.

5. E. S. Hwang, D. Y. Lichtenszatajin, S. L. Gomez, et al., "Survival After Lumpectomy and Mastectomy for Early Stage Invasive Breast Cancer: The Effect of Age and Hormone Receptor Status," *Cancer* 119, no. 7 (April 2013): 1402–1411.

6. A. K. Bajaj, P. S. Kon, K. C. Oberg, et al., "Aesthetic Outcomes in Patients Undergoing Breast Conservation Therapy for the Treatment of Localized Breast Cancer," *Plastic and Reconstructive Surgery* 114, no. 6 (November 2004): 1442–1449; K. L. Kummerow, L. Du, D. F. Penson, et al., "Nationwide Trends in Mastectomy for Early-Stage Breast Cancer," *JAMA Surgery* 150, no. 1 (January 2015): 9–16.

7. E. S. Hwang, S. J. Nyante, Y. Yi Chen, et al., "Clonality of Lobular Carcinoma In Situ and Synchronous Invasive Lobular Carcinoma," *JAMA* 150, no. 1 (January 2015): 9–16.

8. A. J. Lowery, M. R. Kell, R. W. Glynn, et al., "Locoregional Recurrence After Breast Cancer Surgery: A Systematic Review by Receptor Phenotype," *Breast Cancer Research and Treatment* 133 (2012): 831–841; Zachary S. Zumsteg, Monica Morrow, Brittany Arnold, et al., "Breast-Conserving Therapy Achieves Locoregional Outcomes Comparable to Mastectomy in Women with T1-2N0 Triple-Negative Breast Cancer," *Annals of Surgical Oncology* 20, no. 11 (October 2013): 3469–3476.

9. S. J. Schnitt, A. Abner, R. Gelman, et al., "The Relationship Between Microscopic Margins of Resection and the Risk of Local Recurrence in Patients with Breast Cancer Treated with Breast Conserving Surgery and Radiotherapy," *Cancer* 74, no. 6 (September 1994): 1746–1751.

10. R. Holland, S. Veling, M. Mravunac, et al., "Histological Multifocality of Tis, T1-2 Breast Carcinomas: Implications for Clinical Trials of Breast-Conserving Treatment," *Cancer* 56, no. 5 (September 1985): 979–990.

11. L. W. Turnbull, S. R. Brown, C. Olivier, et al., "Multicentre Randomized Controlled Trial Examining the Cost-Effectiveness of Contrast- Enhanced High Yield Magnetic Resonance Imaging in Women with Primary Breast Cancer Scheduled for Wide Local Excision (CMICE)," *Health Technology Assessment* 14, no. 1 (January 2010): 1–182; L. J. Solin, S. G. Orel, W. T. Hwang, et al., "Relationship of Breast Magnetic Resonance Imaging to Outcome After Breast Conservation Treatment with Radiation for Women with Early-Stage Invasive Breast Carcinoma or Ductal Carcinoma In Situ," *Journal of Clinical Oncology* 26, no. 3 (January 2008): 386–391; R. J. Bleicher, R. M. Ciocca, B. L. Egleston, et al., "Association of Routine Pretreatment Magnetic Resonance Imaging with Time to Surgery, Mastectomy Rate, and Margin Status," *Journal of the American College of Surgeons* 209, no. 2 (August 2009): 180–187.

12. American Society of Breast Surgeons, "Consensus Guideline on Diagnostic and Screening Magnetic Resonance Imaging of the Breast," ASBrS Forums, June 22, 2017, https://www.breastsurgeons.org/docs/statements/Consensus

-Guideline-on-Diagnostic-and-Screening-Magnetic-Resonance-Imaging-of-the
-Breast.pdf.

13. A. M. Munhoz, E. Montag, and R. Gemperli, "Oncoplastic Breast Surgery: Indications, Techniques and Perspectives," *Gland Surgery* 2, no. 3 (August 2013): 143–157.

14. B. S. Abdulkarim, J. Cuartero, J. Hansen, et al., "Increased Risk of Locoregional Recurrence for Women with T1-2N0 Triple-Negative Breast Cancer Treated with Modified Radical Mastectomy Without Adjuvant Radiation Therapy with Breast-Conserving Therapy," *Journal of Clinical Oncology* 29, no. 21 (2011): 2852–2858; F. C. Adkins, A. M. Gonzalez-Angulo, X. Lei, et al., "Triple Negative Breast Cancer Is Not a Contraindication for Breast Conservation," *Annals of Surgical Oncology* 18, no. 11 (2011): 3164–3173; A. Y. Ho, G. Gupta, T. A. King, et al., "Favorable Prognosis in Patients with T1a/T1bn0 Triple Negative Breast Cancers Treated with Multimodality Therapy," *Cancer* 118, no. 20 (2012): 4944–4952.

15. M. Chadha, H. Yoon, S. Feldman, et al., "Partial Breast Brachytherapy as the Primary Treatment for Breast Cancer Diagnosed After Mantle Radiation Therapy for Hodgkin's Disease," *American Journal of Clinical Oncology* 32, no. 2 (2009): 132–136.

16. S. S. Kroll, M. A. Schusterman, G. P. Reece, et al., "Breast Reconstruction with Myocutaneous Flaps in Previously Irradiated Patients," *Plastic and Reconstructive Surgery* 93, no. 3 (March 1994): 460–469.

17. Icro Meattini et al., "Accelerated Partial-Breast Irradiation Compared with Whole-Breast Irradiation for Early Breast Cancer: Long-Term Results of the Randomized Phase III APBI-IMRT-Florence Trial," *Journal of Clinical Oncology* 38, no. 35 (2020): 4175–4183, doi:10.1200/JCO.20.00650; Frank A. Vicini et al., "Long-Term Primary Results of Accelerated Partial Breast Irradiation After Breast-Conserving Surgery for Early-Stage Breast Cancer: A Randomised, Phase 3, Equivalence Trial," *Lancet* 394, no. 10215 (2019): 2155–2164, doi:10.1016/S0140-6736(19)32514-0.

18. Candace Correa et al., "Accelerated Partial Breast Irradiation: Executive Summary for the Update of an ASTRO Evidence-Based Consensus Statement," *Practical Radiation Oncology* 7, no. 2 (2017): 73–79, doi:10.1016/j.prro.2016.09.007.

19. T. J. Whelan, J. P. Pignol, M. Levine, et al., "Long-Term Results of Hypofractionated Radiation Therapy for Breast Cancer," *New England Journal of Medicine* 362, no. 6 (2010): 513–520.

20. Adrian Murray Brunt et al., "Hypofractionated Breast Radiotherapy for 1 Week Versus 3 Weeks (FAST-Forward): 5-Year Efficacy and Late Normal Tissue Effects Results from a Multicentre, Non-Inferiority, Randomised, Phase 3 Trial," *Lancet* 395, no. 10237 (2020): 1613–1626, doi:10.1016/S0140-6736(20)30932-6.

21. Abram Recht et al., "Postmastectomy Radiotherapy: An American Society of Clinical Oncology, American Society for Radiation Oncology, and Society of Surgical Oncology Focused Guideline Update," *Practical Radiation Oncology* 6, no. 6 (2016): e219–e234, doi:10.1016/j.prro.2016.08.009.

22. EBCTCG (Early Breast Cancer Trialists' Collaborative Group) et al., "Effect of Radiotherapy After Mastectomy and Axillary Surgery on 10-Year Recurrence and 20-Year Breast Cancer Mortality: Meta-Analysis of Individual Patient Data for 8135 Women in 22 Randomised Trials," *Lancet* 383, no. 9935 (2014): 2127–2135, doi:10.1016/S0140-6736(14)60488-8.

23. Jill Remick and Neha P. Amin, "Postmastectomy Breast Cancer Radiation Therapy," *StatPearls*, January 4, 2022.

24. S. H. Giordano, Y. F. Kuo, J. L. Freeman, et al., "Risk of Cardiac Death After Adjuvant Radiotherapy for Breast Cancer," *Journal of the National Cancer Institute* 97, no. 6 (2005): 416–424.

25. M. Deutsch, S. R. Land, M. Begovic, et al., "The Incidence of Lung Carcinoma After Surgery for Breast Carcinoma with and Without Postoperative Radiotherapy: Results of National Surgical Adjuvant Breast and Bowel Project (NSABP) Clinical Trials B-04 and B-06," *Cancer* 98 (2003): 1362–1368; L. B. Zablotska and A. I. Neugut, "Lung Carcinoma After Radiation Therapy in Women Treated with Lumpectomy or Mastectomy for Primary Breast Carcinoma," *Cancer* 97 (2003): 1404–1411.

26. S. C. Formenti, J. K. Dewyngaert, G. Jozsef, et al., "Prone vs. Supine Positioning for Breast Cancer Radiotherapy," *Journal of the American Medical Association* 308, no. 9 (September 2012): 861–863; S. C. Formenti and J. K. DeWyngaert, "Positioning During Radiotherapy for Breast Cancer—Reply," *Journal of the American Medical Association* 309, no. 2 (January 2013): 137, erratum in *Journal of the American Medical Association* 309, no. 11 (March 2013): 1112; D. J. Brenner, I. Shuryak, G. Jozsef, et al., "Risk and Risk Reduction of Major Coronary Events Associated with Contemporary Breast Radiotherapy," *JAMA Internal Medicine* 174, no. 1 (January 2014): 15–60.

27. A. E. Giuliano, R. C. Jones, M. Brennan, et al., "Sentinel Lymphadenectomy in Breast Cancer," *Journal of Clinical Oncology* 5 (1997): 2345–2350.

28. A. E. Guiliano, K. K. Hunt, K. V. Ballman, et al., "Axillary Dissection vs No Axillary Dissection in Women with Invasive Breast Cancer and Sentinel Node Metastasis: A Randomized Clinical Trial," *Journal of the American Medical Association* 305, no. 6 (2011): 569–575.

29. M. Donker, G. Van Tienhoven, M. E. Straver, et al., "Radiotherapy or Surgery of the Axilla After a Positive Sentinel Node in Breast Cancer (EORTC 10981-22023 AMAROS): A Randomised, Multicentre, Open-Label, Phase 3 Non-Inferiority Trial," *Lancet Oncology* 15, no. 12 (November 2014): 1303–1310.

30. Abigail S. Caudle et al., "Improved Axillary Evaluation Following Neoadjuvant Therapy for Patients with Node-Positive Breast Cancer Using Selective Evaluation of Clipped Nodes: Implementation of Targeted Axillary Dissection," *Journal of Clinical Oncology* 34, no. 10 (2016): 1072–1078, doi:10.1200/JCO.2015.64.0094; Kavitha Kanesalingam et al., "Targeted Axillary Dissection After Neoadjuvant Systemic Therapy in Patients with Node-Positive Breast Cancer," *ANZ Journal of Surgery* 90, no. 3 (2020): 332–338, doi:10.1111/ans.15604.

31. A. B. Gropper, K. Z. Calvillo, L. Dominici, et al., "Sentinel Lymph Node Biopsy in Pregnant Women with Breast Cancer," *Annals of Surgical Oncology* 21, no. 8 (August 2014): 2506–2511.

32. S. M. Love, K. A. McGuigan, and L. Chap, "The Revlon/UCLA Breast Center Practice Guidelines for the Treatment of Breast Disease," *Cancer Journal from Scientific American* 2, no. 1 (1996): 2–15.

33. P. P. Rosen, S. Groshen, D. W. Kinne, et al., "Contralateral Breast Carcinoma: An Assessment of Risk and Prognosis in Stage I (TIN0M0) and Stage II (T1N1M0) Patients with 20-Year Follow-Up," *Surgery* 106, no. 5 (1989): 904–910; T. G. Hislop, J. M. Elwood, A. J. Coldman, et al., "Second Primary Cancers of the Breast: Incidence and Risk Factors," *British Journal of Cancer* 49, no. 1 (January 1984): 79–85.

34. L. J. Herrington, W. E. Barlow, O. Yu, et al., "Efficacy of Prophylactic Mastectomy in Women with Unilateral Breast Cancer: A Cancer Research Network Project," *Journal of Clinical Oncology* 23, no. 19 (July 2005): 4275–4286.

35. Early Breast Cancer Collaborative Trialists' Group, "Polychemotherapy for Early Breast Cancer: An Overview of the Randomized Trials," *Lancet* 352 (September 1998): 930–942.

36. S. Rajagopal, P. J. Goodman, and I. F. Tannock, "Adjuvant Chemotherapy for Breast Cancer: Discordance Between Physicians' Perception of Benefit and the Results of Clinical Trials," *Journal of Clinical Oncology* 12, no. 6 (1994): 1296–1304.

37. G. Von Minckwitz, M. Untch, J. U. Clohmer, et al., "Definition and Impact of Pathologic Complete Response on Prognosis After Neoadjuvant Chemotherapy in Various Intrinsic Breast Cancer Subtypes," *Journal of Clinical Oncology* 30, no. 15 (May 2012): 1796–1804.

38. Laura M. Spring et al., "Pathologic Complete Response After Neoadjuvant Chemotherapy and Impact on Breast Cancer Recurrence and Survival: A Comprehensive Meta-Analysis," *Clinical Cancer Research* 26, no. 12 (2020): 2838–2848, doi:10.1158/1078-0432.CCR-19-3492.

39. Gunter von Minckwitz et al., "Trastuzumab Emtansine for Residual Invasive HER2-Positive Breast Cancer," *New England Journal of Medicine* 380, no. 7 (2019): 617–628, doi:10.1056/NEJMoa1814017.

40. Shanu Modi et al., "Trastuzumab Deruxtecan in Previously Treated HER2-Positive Breast Cancer," *New England Journal of Medicine* 382, no. 7 (2020): 610–621, doi:10.1056/NEJMoa1914510.

41. Norikazu Masuda et al., "Adjuvant Capecitabine for Breast Cancer After Preoperative Chemotherapy," *New England Journal of Medicine* 376, no. 22 (2017): 2147–2159, doi:10.1056/NEJMoa1612645.

42. D. B. Y. Fontein, A. Charehbili, J. W. R. Nortier, et al., "Efficacy of Six Month Neoadjuvant Endocrine Therapy in Postmenopausal, Hormone Receptor-Positive Breast Cancer Patients—a Phase II Trial," *European Journal of Cancer* 50, no. 13 (September 2014): 2190–2200.

43. Early Breast Cancer Trialists' Cooperative Group, "Effects of Chemotherapy and Hormonal Therapy for Early Breast Cancer on Recurrence and 15-Year Survival: An Overview of the Randomized Trials," *Lancet* 365, no. 9472 (2005): 1687–1717.

44. W. H. Parker, M. S. Broder, E. Chang, et al., "Ovarian Conservation at the Time of Hysterectomy and Long-Term Health Outcomes in the Nurses' Health Study," *Obstetrics and Gynecology* 113, no. 5 (May 2009): 1027–1037.

45. Andrea DeCensi et al., "Randomized Placebo Controlled Trial of Low-Dose Tamoxifen to Prevent Local and Contralateral Recurrence in Breast Intraepithelial Neoplasia," *Journal of Clinical Oncology* 37, no. 19 (2019): 1629–1637, doi:10.1200/JCO.18.01779.

46. Mikael Eriksson et al., "Low-Dose Tamoxifen for Mammographic Density Reduction: A Randomized Controlled Trial," *Journal of Clinical Oncology* 39, no. 17 (2021): 1899–1908, doi:10.1200/JCO.20.02598.

47. C. W. Taylor, S. Green, W. S. Dalton, et al., "Multicenter Randomized Clinical Trial of Goserelin Versus Surgical Ovariectomy in Premenopausal Patients with Receptor-Positive Metastatic Breast Cancer: An Intergroup Study," *Journal of Clinical Oncology* 16, no. 3 (March 1998): 994–999.

48. M. Kaufmann, W. Jonat, R. Blamey, et al., "Survival Analyses from the ZEBRA Study: Goserelin (Zoladex) Versus CMF in Premenopausal Women with Node-Positive Breast Cancer," *European Journal of Cancer* 39 (2003): 1711–1717.

49. R. Jakesz, H. Hausmaninger, E. Kubista, et al., "Randomized Adjuvant Trial of Tamoxifen and Goserelin Versus Cyclophosphamide Methotrexate and Fluorouracil: Evidence for the Superiority of Treatment with Endocrine Blockade in Premenopausal Patients with Hormone-Responsive Breast Cancer—Austrian Breast and Colorectal Cancer Study Group Trial 5," *Journal of Clinical Oncology* 20, no. 24 (December 2002): 4621–4627.

50. S. J. Santner, R. J. Pauley, L. Tait, et al., "Aromatase Activity and Expression in Breast Cancer and Benign Breast Tissue Stromal Cells," *Journal of Clinical Endocrinology and Metabolism* 82, no. 1 (January 1997): 200–208.

51. Michael Gnant, Brigitte Mlineritsch, Walter Schippinger, et al., "Endocrine Therapy plus Zolendronic Acid in Premenopausal Breast Cancer," *New England Journal of Medicine* 360, no. 7 (February 2009): 679–691.

52. O. Pagani, M. M. Regan, B. A. Walley, et al., "Adjuvant Exemestane with Ovarian Suppression in Premenopausal Breast Cancer," *New England Journal of Medicine* 371, no. 2 (July 2014): 107–118.

53. P. A. Francis, SOFT Investigators, International Breast Cancer Study Group, et al., "Adjuvant Ovarian Suppression in Premenopausal Breast Cancer," *New England Journal of Medicine* 372, no. 5 (January 2015): 436–446.

54. O. Pagani, M. M. Regan, G. F. Fleming, et al., "Abstract GS4-02: Randomized Comparison of Adjuvant Aromatase Inhibitor Exemestane (E) plus Ovarian Function Suppression (OFS) vs Tamoxifen (T) plus OFS in Premenopausal Women with Hormone Receptor Positive (HR+) Early Breast Cancer (BC): Update of the Combined TEXT and SOFT Trials," *Cancer Research* 78, no. 4_suppl. (February 15, 2018): GS4–02, doi:10.1158/1538-7445.SABCS17-GS4-02.

55. Early Breast Cancer Trialists' Collaborative Group (EBCTCG), "Aromatase Inhibitors Versus Tamoxifen in Premenopausal Women with Oestrogen Receptor-Positive Early-Stage Breast Cancer Treated with Ovarian Suppression: A Patient-Level Meta-Analysis of 7030 Women from Four Randomised Trials," *Lancet Oncology* 23, no. 3 (2022): 382–392, doi:10.1016/S1470-2045(21)00758-0.

56. M. A. Cobleigh, C. L. Vogel, D. Tripathy, et al., "Multinational Study of the Efficacy and Safety of Humanized Anti-HER2 Monoclonal Antibody in Women Who Have HER2-Overexpressing Metastatic Breast Cancer," *Journal of Clinical Oncology* 17 (1999): 2639–2648; C. L. Vogel, M. A. Cobleigh, D. Tripathy, et al., "Efficacy and Safety of Trastuzumab as a Single Agent in First-Line Treatment of HER2-Overexpressing Metastatic Breast Cancer," *Journal of Clinical Oncology* 20 (2002): 719–772.

57. J. Baselga, E. A. Perez, T. Pienkowski, et al., "Adjuvant Trastuzumab: A Milestone in the Treatment of HER-2 Positive Early Breast Cancer," *Oncologist* 11, suppl. 1 (2006): 4–12.

58. A. M. Gonzalez-Angulo, J. K. Litton, K. R. Brogilo, et al., "High Risk of Recurrence for Patients with Breast Cancer Who Have Human Epidermal Growth Factor Receptor 2–Positive, Node-Negative Tumors 1 cm or Smaller," *Journal of Clinical Oncology* 27, no. 34 (December 2009): 5700–5706.

59. Arlene Chan et al., "Final Efficacy Results of Neratinib in HER2-Positive Hormone Receptor-Positive Early-Stage Breast Cancer From the Phase III ExteNET Trial," *Clinical Breast Cancer* 21, no. 1 (2021): 80–91.e7, doi:10.1016/j.clbc.2020.09.014.

60. Gunter von Minckwitz et al., "Adjuvant Pertuzumab and Trastuzumab in Early HER2-Positive Breast Cancer," *New England Journal of Medicine* 377, no. 2 (2017): 122–131, doi:10.1056/NEJMoa1703643.

61. Sandra M. Swain et al., "Pertuzumab, Trastuzumab, and Docetaxel in HER2-Positive Metastatic Breast Cancer," *New England Journal of Medicine* 372, no. 8 (2015): 724–734, doi:10.1056/NEJMoa1413513.

62. Julie R. Gralow et al., "Phase III Randomized Trial of Bisphosphonates as Adjuvant Therapy in Breast Cancer: S0307," *Journal of the National Cancer Institute* 112, no. 7 (2020): 698–707, doi:10.1093/jnci/djz215.

63. R. E. Coleman, H. Marshall, D. Cameron, et al., "Breast-Cancer Adjuvant Treatment with Zoledronic Acid," *New England Journal of Medicine* 365 (2011): 1396–1405; A. H. Paterson, S. J. Anderson, B. C. Lembersky, et al., "Oral Clodronate for Adjuvant Treatment of Operable Breast Cancer (National Surgical Adjuvant Breast and Bowel Project Protocol B-34): A Multicentre, Placebo-Controlled, Randomized Trial," *Lancet Oncology* 13, no. 7 (2012): 734–742.

64. Peter Schmid et al., "Pembrolizumab for Early Triple-Negative Breast Cancer," *New England Journal of Medicine* 382, no. 9 (2020): 810–821, doi:10.1056/NEJMoa1910549.

65. Javier Cortes et al., "Pembrolizumab plus Chemotherapy in Advanced Triple-Negative Breast Cancer," *New England Journal of Medicine* 387, no. 3 (2022): 217–226, doi:10.1056/NEJMoa2202809.

66. Nikolaos Zacharakis et al., "Breast Cancers Are Immunogenic: Immunologic Analyses and a Phase II Pilot Clinical Trial Using Mutation-Reactive Autologous Lymphocytes," *Journal of Clinical Oncology* 40, no. 16 (June 1, 2022): 1741–1754, doi:10.1200/JCO.21.02170.

67. Gregory M. Cresswell et al., "Folate Receptor Beta Designates Immunosuppressive Tumor-Associated Myeloid Cells That Can Be Reprogrammed with Folate-Targeted Drugs," *Cancer Research* 81, no. 3 (2021): 671–684, doi:10.1158/0008-5472.CAN-20-1414.

68. Chiara Corti et al., "Therapeutic Vaccines for Breast Cancer: Has the Time Finally Come?," *European Journal of Cancer* 160 (January 2022): 150–174, doi:10.1016/j.ejca.(2021).10.027.

69. U. Wiedermann, A. B. Davis, and C. C. Zielinski, "Vaccination for the Prevention and Treatment of Breast Cancer with Special Focus on HER-2/Neu Peptide Vaccines," *Breast Cancer Research and Treatment* 138, no. 1 (February 2013): 1–12; J. Tobias et al., "Vaccination Against Her-2/neu, with Focus on Peptide-Based Vaccines," *ESMO Open* 7, no. 1 (February 2022): 100361, doi:10.1016/j.esmoop.2021.100361.

70. V. Tiriveedhi, N. Tucker, J. Herndon, et al., "Safety and Preliminary Evidence of Biologic Efficacy of a Mammaglobin-A DNA Vaccine in Patients with Stable Metastatic Breast Cancer," *Clinical Cancer Research* 20, no. 23 (December 2014): 5964–5675.

71. N. J. Chu, T. D. Armstrong, and E. M. Jaffee, "Nonviral Oncogenic Antigens and the Inflammatory Signals Driving Early Cancer Development as Targets for Cancer Immunoprevention," *Clinical Cancer Research* 21, no. 7 (2015): 1–9; You Liu et al., "Synthetic MUC1 Breast Cancer Vaccine Containing a Toll-Like Receptor 7 Agonist Exerts Antitumor Effects," *Oncology Letters* 20, no. 3 (2020): 2369–2377, doi:10.3892/ol.2020.11762.

72. Si-Yuan Zhu and Ke-Da Yu, "Breast Cancer Vaccines: Disappointing or Promising?," *Frontiers in Immunology* 13 (January 28, 2022): 828386, doi:10.3389/fimmu.2022.828386.

73. B. Majed, T. Moreau, K. Senouci, et al., "Is Obesity an Independent Prognosis Factor in Woman Breast Cancer?," *Breast Cancer Research and Treatment* 111, no. 2 (September 2008): 329–342.

74. R. Cheblowski, G. L. Blackburn, M. K. Hoy, et al., "Survival Analyses from the Women's Intervention Nutrition Study (WINS) Evaluating Dietary Fat Reduction and Breast Cancer Outcome," *Journal of Clinical Oncology* 26, no. 15_suppl. (May 20, 2008): 522–522.

75. D. S. Chan, A. R. Vieira, D. Aune, et al., "Body Mass Index and Survival in Women with Breast Cancer—Systematic Literature Review and Meta-Analysis of 82 Follow-Up Studies," *Annals of Oncology* 25, no. 10 (October 2014): 1901–1914.

76. Charlotte Debras et al., "Glycaemic Index, Glycaemic Load and Cancer Risk: Results from the Prospective NutriNet-Santé Cohort," *International Journal of Epidemiology* 51, no. 1 (2022): 250–264, doi:10.1093/ije/dyab169.

77. Christine B. Ambrosone et al., "Dietary Supplement Use During Chemotherapy and Survival Outcomes of Patients with Breast Cancer Enrolled in a Cooperative Group Clinical Trial (SWOG S0221)," *Journal of Clinical Oncology* 38, no. 8 (2020): 804–814, doi:10.1200/JCO.19.01203.

78. U. Veronesi, "Randomized Trials Comparing Conservative Techniques with Conventional Surgery: An Overview," in *Primary Management of Breast Cancer: Alternatives to Mastectomy, Management of Malignant Diseases Series*, ed. Jeffrey S. Tobias and Michael J. Peckham, 131–152 (London: Arnold, 1985).

79. W. P. Peters, M. Ross, J. J. Vredenburgh, et al., "High-Dose Chemotherapy and Autologous Bone Marrow Support as Consolidation After Standard-Dose Adjuvant Therapy for High-Risk Primary Breast Cancer," *Journal of Clinical Oncology* 11, no. 6 (June 1993): 1132–1143.

80. M. S. Tallman, R. Gray, N. J. Robert, et al., "Conventional Adjuvant Chemotherapy with or Without High-Dose Chemotherapy and Autologous Stem Cell Transplantation in High-Risk Breast Cancer," *New England Journal of Medicine* 349, no. 1 (July 2003): 17–26.

81. R. Garcia-Carbonero, M. Hidalgo, L. Paz-Ares, et al., "Patient Selection in High-Dose Chemotherapy Trials: Relevance in High-Risk Breast Cancer," *Journal of Clinical Oncology* 15, no. 10 (October 1997): 3178–3184.

82. Early Breast Cancer Trialists' Cooperative Group, "Effects of Chemotherapy and Hormonal Therapy for Early Breast Cancer on Recurrence and 15-Year Survival: An Overview of the Randomized Trials," *Lancet* 365, no. 9472 (May 2005): 1687–1717.

83. Audre Lorde, *A Burst of Light: Essays* (New York: Firebrand, 1988).

CHAPTER 12. SPECIAL SITUATIONS AND POPULATIONS

1. M. A. Lopez-Garcia, F. C. Geyer, M. Lacroix-Triki, et al., "Breast Cancer Precursors Revisited: Molecular Features and Progression Pathways," *Histopathology* 57, no. 2 (August 2010): 171–192.

2. R. M. Tamimi, H. J. Baer, J. Marotti, et al., "Comparison of Molecular Phenotypes of Ductal Carcinoma In Situ and Invasive Breast Cancer," *Breast Cancer Research* 10, no. 4 (August 2008): R67.

3. D. C. Allred, Y. Wu, S. Mao, et al., "Ductal Carcinoma In Situ and the Emergence of Diversity During Breast Cancer Evolution," *Clinical Cancer Research* 14, no. 2 (January 2008): 370–378.

4. T. To, Institute for Clinical Evaluative Sciences, C. Wall, et al., "Is Carcinoma In Situ a Precursor Lesion of Invasive Breast Cancer?," *International Journal of Cancer* 135, no. 7 (October 2014): 1646–1652; E. Rakovitch, S. Nofech-Mozes, W.

Hanna, et al., "A Population-Based Validation Study of the DCIS Score Predicting Recurrence Risk in Individuals Treated by Breast-Conserving Surgery Alone," *Breast Cancer Research and Treatment* 152, no. 2 (July 2015): 389–398, doi:10.1007/s10549-015-3464-6.

5. K. Kerlikowske, A. Molinaro, I. Cha, et al., "Characteristics Associated with Recurrence Among Women with Ductal Carcinoma In Situ Treated by Lumpectomy," *Journal of the National Cancer Institute* 95 (2003): 1692–1702; Lawrence J. Solin, Alain Fourquet, Frank A. Vicini, et al., "Long-Term Outcome After Breast-Conservation Treatment with Radiation for Mammographically Detected Ductal Carcinoma In Situ of the Breast," *Cancer* 103, no. 6 (2005): 1137–1146; J. B. Wilkinson, F. A. Vicini, C. Shah, et al., "Twenty-Year Outcomes After Breast-Conserving Surgery and Definitive Radiotherapy for Mammographically Detected Ductal Carcinoma In Situ," *Annals of Surgical Oncology* 19 (2012): 3785–3791; Anthony B. Miller, Claus Wall, Cornelia J. Baines, et al., "Twenty-Five-Year Follow-Up for Breast Cancer Incidence and Mortality of the Canadian National Breast Screening Study: A Randomised Screening Trial," *British Medical Journal* 348 (2014): G366.

6. E. R. Fisher, S. R. Land, B. Fisher, et al., "Pathological Findings from the National Surgical Adjuvant Breast and Bowel Project: Twelve-Year Observations Concerning Lobular Carcinoma In Situ," *Cancer* 100 (2004): 238–244.

7. E. S. Hwang, S. J. Nyante, Y. Y. Chen, et al., "Clonality of Lobular Carcinoma In Situ and Synchronous Invasive Lobular Carcinoma," *Cancer* 100 (2004): 2562–2572.

8. U. Raju, L. Mei, S. Seema, et al., "Molecular Classification of Breast Carcinoma In Situ," *Current Genomics* 7, no. 8 (November 2006): 523–532.

9. Tari A. King et al., "Lobular Carcinoma In Situ: A 29-Year Longitudinal Experience Evaluating Clinicopathologic Features and Breast Cancer Risk," *Journal of Clinical Oncology* 33, no. 33 (2015): 3945–3952, doi:10.1200/JCO.2015.61.4743.

10. T. A. King, S. Muhsen, S. Patil, et al., "Is There a Role for Routine Screening MRI in Women with LCIS?," *Breast Cancer Research and Treatment* 142, no. 2 (November 2013): 445–453.

11. Patient and Caregiver Resources, National Comprehensive Cancer Network (NCCN), http://www.nccn.org/patients.

12. M. Moran and B. G. Haffty, "Lobular Carcinoma In Situ as a Component of Breast Cancer: The Long-Term Outcome in Patients Treated with Breast Conservation Therapy," *International Journal of Radiation, Oncology, Biology and Physics* 40 (1998): 353–358; A. L. Abner, J. L. Connolly, A. Recht, et al., "The Relation Between the Presence and Extent of Lobular Carcinoma In Situ and the Risk of Local Recurrence for Patients with Infiltrating Carcinoma of the Breast Treated with Conservative Surgery and Radiation Therapy," *Cancer* 88 (2000): 1072–1077; A. R. Sasson, B. Fowble, A. L. Hanlon, et al., "Lobular Carcinoma In Situ Increases the Risk of Local Recurrence in Selected Patients with Stages I and II Breast Carcinoma Treated with Conservative Surgery and Radiation," *Cancer* 91 (2001): 1862–1869; K. A. Carolin, S. Tekyi-Mensah, and H. A. Pass, "Lobular Carcinoma In Situ and Invasive Cancer: The Contralateral Breast Controversy," *Breast Journal* 8 (2002): 263–268.

13. C. E. Alpers and S. R. Wellings, "The Prevalence of Carcinoma In Situ in Normal and Cancer-Associated Breasts," *Human Pathology* 16 (1985): 796–807; M. Nielsen, J. Jensen, and J. Andersen, "Non-Invasive Cancerous and Cancerous Breast Lesions During Lifetime and at Autopsy," *Cancer* 54 (1984): 612–615.

14. W. L. Betsill, P. P. Rosen, P. H. Lieberman, et al., "Intraductal Carcinoma: Long-Term Follow-Up After Treatment by Biopsy Alone," *Journal of the American Medical Association* 239 (1978): 1863–1867; D. L. Page and W. D. Dupont, "Intraductal Carcinoma of the Breast," *Cancer* 49, no. 4 (February 1982): 751–758.

15. T. To, "The Theory of the Sick Breast Lobe and the Possible Consequences," *International Journal of Surgical Pathology* 15, no. 4 (2007): 369–375.

16. M. Morrow, C. Bucci, and A. Rademaker, "Medical Contraindications Are Not a Major Factor in the Underutilization of Breast Conserving Therapy," *Journal of the American College of Surgeons* 186, no. 3 (March 1998): 269–274.

17. L. J. Solin, S. G. Orel, W. T. Hwang, et al., "Relationship of Breast Magnetic Resonance Imaging to Outcome After Breast Conservation Treatment with Radiation for Women with Early-Stage Invasive Breast Carcinoma or Ductal Carcinoma In Situ," *Journal of Clinical Oncology* 26, no. 3 (January 2008): 386–391; A. S. Kumar, D. F. Chen, A. Au, et al., "Biologic Significance of False-Positive Magnetic Resonance Imaging Enhancement in the Setting of Ductal Carcinoma In Situ," *American Journal of Surgery* 192, no. 4 (October 2006): 520–524.

18. N. Bijker, P. Meijnen, J. L. Peterse, et al., "Breast-Conserving Treatment with or Without Radiotherapy in Ductal Carcinoma-In-Situ: Ten-Year Results of European Organization for Research and Treatment of Cancer Randomized Phase III Trial 10853—a Study by the EORTC Breast Cancer Cooperative Group and EORTC Radiotherapy Group," *Journal of Clinical Oncology* 24, no. 21 (July 2006): 3381–3387; S. O. Emdin, B. Granstrand, A. Ringberg, et al., "SWEDCIS: Radiotherapy After Sector Resection for Ductal Carcinoma In Situ of the Breast: Results of a Randomised Trial in a Population Offered Mammography Screening," *Acta Oncologica* 45, no. 5 (2006): 536–543; B. Fisher, S. Land, E. Mamounas, et al., "Prevention of Invasive Breast Cancer in Women with Ductal Carcinoma In Situ: An Update of the National Surgical Adjuvant Breast and Bowel Project Experience," *Seminars in Oncology* 28, no. 4 (2001): 400–418; J. Houghton, W. D. George, J. Cuzick, et al., "Radiotherapy and Tamoxifen in Women with Completely Excised Ductal Carcinoma In Situ of the Breast in the UK, Australia, and New Zealand: Randomized Controlled Trial," *Lancet* 362, no. 9378 (2003): 95–102.

19. "Oncotype DX DCIS Score Predicts Recurrence," *Cancer Discovery* 5, no. 2 (February 2015): F3.

20. M. Silverstein, J. Waisman, P. Gamagami, et al., "Intraductal Carcinoma of the Breast (208 Cases): Clinical Factors Influencing Treatment Choice," *Cancer* 66, no. 1 (July 1990): 102–108.

21. L. A. Habel, N. S. Achacoso, R. Haque, et al., "Declining Recurrence Among Ductal Carcinoma In Situ Patients Treated with Breast-Conserving Surgery in the Community Setting," *Breast Cancer Research* 11, no. 6 (November 2009): R85.

22. S. D. Finkelstein, R. Sayegh, and W. R. Thompson, "Late Recurrence of Ductal Carcinoma In Situ at the Cutaneous End of Surgical Drainage Following Total Mastectomy," *American Surgeon* 59 (July 1993): 410–414; D. E. Fisher, S. J. Schnitt, R. Christian, et al., "Chest Wall Recurrence of Ductal Carcinoma In Situ of the Breast After Mastectomy," *Cancer* 71, no. 10 (1993): 3025–3028.

23. E. Shelley Hwang et al., "Phase II Single-Arm Study of Preoperative Letrozole for Estrogen Receptor-Positive Postmenopausal Ductal Carcinoma In Situ: CALGB 40903 (Alliance)," *Journal of Clinical Oncology* 38, no. 12 (2020): 1284–1292, doi:10.1200/JCO.19.00510.

24. E. Shelley Hwang and Lawrence Solin, "De-Escalation of Locoregional Therapy in Low-Risk Disease for DCIS and Early-Stage Invasive Cancer," *Journal of Clinical Oncology* 38, no. 20 (2020): 2230–2239, doi:10.1200/JCO.19.02888.

25. A. U. Budzar, S. E. Singletary, D. J. Booser, et al., "Combined Modality Treatment of Stage III and Inflammatory Breast Cancer: MD Anderson Cancer Center Experience," *Surgical Oncology Clinics of North America* 4, no. 4 (1995): 715–734.

26. R. Mehra and B. Burtness, "Antibody Therapy for Early-Stage Breast Cancer: Trastuzumab Adjuvant and Neoadjuvant Trials," *Expert Opinion on Biological Therapy* 6, no. 9 (2006): 951–962.

27. C. Liedtke, C. Hatzis, W. F. Symmans, et al., "Genomic Grade Index Is Associated with Response to Chemotherapy in Patients with Breast Cancer," *Journal of Clinical Oncology* 27, no. 19 (2009): 3185–3191.

28. A. M. Chen, F. Meric-Bernstam, K. K. Hunt, et al., "Breast Conservation After Neoadjuvant Chemotherapy," *Cancer* 103, no. 4 (2005): 689–695; S. D. M. Merajver, B. L. Weber, R. Cody, et al., "Breast Conservation and Prolonged Chemotherapy for Locally Advanced Breast Cancer: The University of Michigan Experience," *Journal of Clinical Oncology* 15, no. 8 (1997): 2873–2881.

29. Flávia L. C. Faldoni et al., "Inflammatory Breast Cancer: Clinical Implications of Genomic Alterations and Mutational Profiling," *Cancers* 12, no. 10 (September 20, 2020): 2816, doi:10.3390/cancer12102816.

30. S. L. Liauw, R. K. Benda, C. G. Morris, et al., "Inflammatory Breast Carcinoma: Outcomes with Trimodality Therapy for Nonmetastatic Disease," *Cancer* 1000, no. 5 (2004): 920–928.

31. A. Fourquet, A. de la Rochefordiere, and F. Campana, "Occult Primary Cancer with Axillary Metastases," in *Diseases of the Breast*, 3rd ed., ed. J. R. Harris, M. E. Lippman, M. Morrow, and C. K. Osborne, 802–896 (Philadelphia: Lippincott Raven, 1996).

32. B. Van Ooijen, M. Bontenbal, S. C. Henzen-Logmans, et al., "Axillary Nodal Metastases from an Occult Primary Consistent with Breast Carcinoma," *British Journal of Surgery* 80, no. 10 (1993): 1299–1300.

33. Harvey Graham, *The Story of Surgery* (New York: Doubleday, Doran, 1939).

34. W. S. Wood and C. Hegedus, "Mammary Paget's Disease and Intraductal Carcinoma: Histologic, Histochemical and Immunocytochemical Comparison," *American Journal of Dermapathology* 10 (1988): 183–188.

35. W. Fu, V. K. Mittel, and S. C. Young, "Paget Disease of the Breast: Analysis of 41 Patients," *American Journal of Clinical Oncology* 24 (2001): 397–400.

36. C. Kaelin, "Paget's Disease," in *Diseases of the Breast*, 3rd ed., ed. J. R. Harris, M. E. Lippman, M. Morrow, and C. K. Osborne, 1007–1013 (Philadelphia: Lippincott Raven, 1996).

37. J. K. Marshall, K. A. Griffith, B. G. Haffty, et al., "Conservative Management of Paget Disease of the Breast with Radiotherapy: 10–15 Year Results," *Cancer* 97 (2003): 2142–2149.

38. M. D. Lagios, P. R. Westdahl, M. R. Rose, et al., "Paget's Disease of the Nipple," *Cancer* 54 (1984): 545–551.

39. S. J. Kister and C. D. Haagensen, "Paget's Disease of the Breast," *American Journal of Surgery* 119 (1970): 606–609; G. Malak and L. Tapolcsanyi, "Characteristics of Paget's Carcinoma of the Nipple and Problems of Its Negligence," *Oncology* 30 (1974): 278–293.

40. M. A. Guerrero, B. R. Ballard, and A. M. Grau, "Malignant Phyllodes Tumor of the Breast: Review of the Literature and Case Report of Stromal Overgrowth," *Surgical Oncology* 12 (2003): 27–37; A. W. Chaney, A. Pollack, M. D. McNeese, et al., "Primary Treatment of Cystosarcoma Phyllodes of the Breast," *Cancer* 89, no. 7 (2000): 1502–1511.

41. M. Intra, N. Rotmensz, G. Viale, et al., "Clinicopathologic Characteristics of 143 Patients with Synchronous Bilateral Invasive Breast Carcinomas Treated in a Single Institution," *Cancer* 101 (2004): 905–912.

42. Carey K. Anders, Rebecca Johnson, Jennifer Litton, et al., "Breast Cancer Before Age 40 Years," *Seminars in Oncology* 36, no. 3 (June 2009): 237–249.

43. S. R. Young, Robert T. Pilarski, Talia Donenberg, et al., "The Prevalence of BRCA1 Mutations Among Young Women with Triple-Negative Breast Cancer," *BMC Cancer* 9 (March 19, 2009): 86; Solene De Talhouet et al., "Clinical Outcome of Breast Cancer in Carriers of BRCA1 and BRCA2 Mutations According to Molecular Subtypes," *Scientific Reports* 10, no. 1 (April 27, 2020): 7073, doi:10.1038/s41598-020-63759-1.

44. H. A. Azim Jr., S. Michiels, P. L. Bedard, et al., "Elucidating Prognosis and Biology of Breast Cancer Arising in Young Women Using Gene Expression Profiling," *Clinical Cancer Research* 18 (2012): 1341–1351; Hatem A. Azim Jr. and Ann H. Patridge, "Biology of Breast Cancer in Young Women," *Breast Cancer Research* 16 (2014): 427.

45. J. Kotsopoulos, J. Lubinski, L. Salmena, et al., "Breastfeeding and the Risk of Breast Cancer in BRCA1 and BRCA2 Mutation Carriers," *Breast Cancer Research* 14, no. 2 (March 2012): R42.

46. Huiyan Ma et al., "Reproductive Factors and the Risk of Triple-Negative Breast Cancer in White Women and African-American Women: A Pooled Analysis," *Breast Cancer Research* 19, no. 1 (January 13, 2017): 6, doi:10.1186/s13058-016-0799-9.

47. H. Bartelink, J. C. Horiot, P. M Poortmans, et al., "Impact of Higher Radiation Dose on Local Control and Survival in Breast Conserving Therapy of Early Breast Cancer: 10-Year Result of the Randomized Boost Versus No Boost ERTC 22881-10882 Trial," *Journal of Clinical Oncology* 25, no. 22 (August 2007): 3259–3265.

48. S. Aebi, S. Gelber, M. Castiglione-Gertsch, et al., "Is Chemotherapy Alone Adequate for Young Women with Estrogen-Receptor-Positive Breast Cancer?," *Lancet* 355, no. 9218 (2000): 1869–1874.

49. A. Goldhirsch, R. D. Gelber, and M. Castiglione, "The Magnitude of Endocrine Effects of Adjuvant Chemotherapy for Premenopausal Breast Cancer Patients: The International Breast Cancer Study Group," *Annals of Oncology* 1, no. 3 (1990): 183–188; O. Pagani, A. O'Neill, M. Castiglione, et al., "Prognostic Impact of Amenorrhoea After Adjuvant Chemotherapy in Premenopausal Breast Cancer Patients with Axillary Node Involvement: Results of the International Breast Cancer Study Group (IBCSG) Trial VI," *European Journal of Cancer* 34, no. 5 (1998): 632–640; J. N. M. Walshe, N. Denduluri, and S. M. Swain, "Amenorrhea in Premenopausal Women After Adjuvant Chemotherapy for Breast Cancer," *Journal of Clinical Oncology* 24, no. 36 (2006): 5769–5779.

50. Prudence A. Francis, Meredith M. Regan, Gini F. Fleming, et al., "Adjuvant Ovarian Suppression in Premenopausal Breast Cancer," *New England Journal of Medicine* 372 (2015): 436–446.

51. Joseph A. Sparano et al., "Clinical and Genomic Risk to Guide the Use of Adjuvant Therapy for Breast Cancer," *New England Journal of Medicine* 380, no. 25 (2019): 2395–2405, doi:10.1056/NEJMoa1904819.

52. Kevin Kalinsky et al., "21-Gene Assay to Inform Chemotherapy Benefit in Node-Positive Breast Cancer," *New England Journal of Medicine* 385, no. 25 (2021): 2336–2347, doi:10.1056/NEJMoa2108873.

53. Joseph A. Sparano et al., "Adjuvant Chemotherapy Guided by a 21-Gene Expression Assay in Breast Cancer," *New England Journal of Medicine* 379, no. 2 (2018): 111–121, doi:10.1056/NEJMoa1804710.

54. M. Lambertini, H. Moore, R. Leonard, et al., "Gonadotropin-Releasing Hormone Agonists During Chemotherapy for Preservation of Ovarian Function and Fertility in Premenopausal Patients with Early Breast Cancer: A Systematic Review and Meta-Analysis of Individual Patient-Level Data," *Journal of Clinical Oncology* 36, no. 19 (July 1, 2018): 1981–1990, doi.org/10.1200/JCO.2018.78.0858.

55. K. Okaty, E. Buyuk, N. Libertella, et al., "Fertility Preservation in Breast Cancer Patients: A Prospective Controlled Comparison of Ovarian Stimulation with Tamoxifen and Letrozole for Embryo Cryopreservation," *Journal of Clinical Oncology* 23 (2005): 4347–4353; A. A. Azim, M. Costantini-Ferrando, and Kutluk Oktay, "Safety of Fertility Preservation by Ovarian Stimulation with Letrozole and Gonadotropins in Patients with Breast Cancer: A Prospective Controlled Study," *Journal of Clinical Oncology* 26 (2008): 2630–2635.

56. A. H. Partridge and K. J. Ruddy, "Fertility and Adjuvant Treatment in Young Women with Breast Cancer," *Breast* 16, suppl. 2 (2007): S175–S181; Anna Marklund et al., "Reproductive Outcomes After Breast Cancer in Women with vs Without Fertility Preservation," *JAMA Oncology* 7, no. 1 (2021): 86–91, doi:10.1001/jamaoncol.2020.5957.

57. Hatem A. Azim. Jr., Luigi Santoro, William Russell-Edu, et al., "Prognosis of Pregnancy-Associated Breast Cancer: A Meta-Analysis of 30 Studies," *Cancer Treatment Reviews* 38 (2012): 834–842.

58. M. Lambertini, E. Blondeaux, M. Bruzzone, et al., "Pregnancy After Breast Cancer: A Systematic Review and Meta-Analysis," *Journal of Clinical Oncology* 39, no. 29 (October 10, 2021): 3293–3305, doi:10.1200/JCO.21.00535.

59. L. J. Blakely, A. U. Buzdarm, J. A. Lozada, et al., "Effects of Pregnancy After Treatment for Breast Carcinoma on Survival and Risk of Recurrence," *Cancer* 100 (2004): 465–469; S. Gelber, A. Coates, A. Goldhirsch, et al., "Effect of Pregnancy on Overall Survival After the Diagnosis of Early-Stage Breast Cancer," *Journal of Clinical Oncology* 19 (2001): 1671–1675; B. A. Mueller, M. S. Simon, D. Deapen, et al., "Childbearing and Survival After Breast Carcinoma in Young Women," *Cancer* 98 (2003): 1131–1140.

60. R. A. Silliman, L. Balducci, J. S. Goodwin, et al., "Breast Cancer Care in Old Age: What We Know, Don't Know, and Do," *Journal of the National Cancer Institute* 85, no. 3 (1993): 190–199.

61. I. H. Kunkler, L. J. Williams, W. Jack, et al., "PRIME II Randomized Trial (Postoperative Radiotherapy in Minimum-Risk Elderly): Wide Local Excision and Adjuvant Hormonal Therapy Whole Breast Irradiation in Women ≥65 years with Early Invasive Cancer: 10-Year Results," paper presented at the 2020 San Antonio Breast Cancer Symposium, December 9, 2020, San Antonio, TX (virtual presentation); Y. Zhong, Y. Xu, Y. Zhou, et al., "Omitting Radiotherapy Is Safe in Breast Cancer

Patients ≥ 70 Years Old After Breast-Conserving Surgery Without Axillary Lymph Node Operation," *Scientific Reports* 10, no. 1 (November 10, 2020): 19481, doi:10.1038/s41598-020-76663-5.

62. Arti Hurria et al., "Validation of a Prediction Tool for Chemotherapy Toxicity in Older Adults with Cancer," *Journal of Clinical Oncology* 34, no. 20 (2016): 2366–2371, doi:10.1200/JCO.2015.65.4327.

63. K. S. Hughes, L. A. Schnapper, D. Berry, et al., "Lumpectomy plus Tamoxifen with or Without Irradiation in Women 70 Years of Age or Older with Early Breast Cancer," *New England Journal of Medicine* 351 (2004): 971–977.

64. M. D. Deapen, M. C. Pike, J. T. Casagrande, et al., "The Relationship Between Breast Cancer and Augmentation Mammoplasty: An Epidemiologic Study," *Plastic and Reconstructive Surgery* 77, no. 3 (March 1986): 361–368.

65. G. M. Jacobson, W. T. Sause, J. W. Thomson, et al., "Breast Irradiation Following Silicone Gel Implants," *International Journal of Radiation, Oncology, Biology and Physics* 12, no. 5 (1986): 835–838.

66. Mariana Chavez-MacGregor et al., "Male Breast Cancer According to Tumor Subtype and Race: A Population-Based Study," *Cancer* 119, no. 9 (2013): 1611–1617, doi:10.1002/cncr.27905.

67. Richard M. Schwartz, Robert B. Newell, James F. Hauch, et al., "A Study of Familial Male Breast Carcinoma and a Second Report," *Cancer* 46, no. 12 (December 1980): 2697–2701.

68. A. W. Jackson, S. Muldal, C. H. Ockey, et al., "Carcinoma of Male Breast in Association with the Klinefelter Syndrome," *British Medical Journal* 1, no. 5429 (January 1965): 223–225.

69. Elaine Ron, Takayoshi Ikeda, Dale L. Preston, et al., "Male Breast Cancer Incidence Among Atomic Bomb Survivors," *Journal of the National Cancer Institute* 97, no. 8 (April 2005): 603–605.

70. J. H. Campbell and S. D. Cummins, "Metastases Simulating Mammary Cancer in Prostatic Carcinoma Under Estrogenic Therapy," *Cancer* 4 (1951): 303–311.

71. E. R. Port, J. V. Fey, H. S. Cody III, et al., "Sentinel Lymph Node Biopsy in Patients with Male Breast Carcinoma," *Cancer* 91, no. 2 (2001): 319–323.

72. A. Chakravarthy and C. R. Kim, "Post-Mastectomy Radiation in Male Breast Cancer," *Radiotherapy and Oncology* 65, no. 2 (2002): 99–103.

73. C. J. M. de Blok, C. M. Wiepjes, N. M. Nota, et al., "Breast Cancer Risk in Transgender People Receiving Hormone Treatment: Nationwide Cohort Study in the Netherlands," *British Medical Journal* 365 (2019): l1652, doi:10.1136/bmj.l1652.

74. Ujas Parikh, Elizabeth Mausner, Chloe M. Chhor, et al., "Breast Imaging in Transgender Patients: What the Radiologist Should Know," *RadioGraphics* 40, no. 1 (2020): 13–27.

CHAPTER 13. LOCAL TREATMENT: SURGERY

1. A. K. Exadaktylos, D. J. Buggy, D. C. Moriarty, et al., "Can Anesthetic Technique for Primary Breast Cancer Surgery Affect Recurrence or Metastasis?," *Anesthesiology* 105, no. 4 (2006): 660–664.

2. Daniel I. Sessler et al., "Recurrence of Breast Cancer After Regional or General Anaesthesia: A Randomised Controlled Trial," *Lancet* 394, no. 10211 (2019): 1807–1815, doi:10.1016/S0140-6736(19)32313-X.

3. C. Boneti, S. Korourian, Z. Diaz, et al., "Scientific Impact Award: Axillary Reverse Mapping (Arm) to Identify and Protect Lymphatics Draining the Arm During Axillary Lymphadenectomy," *American Journal of Surgery* 198, no. 4 (October 2009): 482–487.

4. Siyao Liu et al., "Using the Axillary Reverse Mapping Technique to Screen Breast Cancer Patients with a High Risk of Lymphedema," *World Journal of Surgical Oncology* 18, no. 1 (June 1, 2020): 118, doi:10.1186/s12957-020-01886-9; Evan Tummel et al., "Does Axillary Reverse Mapping Prevent Lymphedema After Lymphadenectomy?," *Annals of Surgery* 265, no. 5 (2017): 987–992, doi:10.1097/SLA.0000000000001778.

5. Malcolm R. Kell, John P. Burke, Mitchel Barry, et al., "Outcome of Axillary Staging in Early Breast Cancer: A Meta-Analysis," *Breast Cancer Research and Treatment* 120, no. 2 (January 2010): 441–447.

6. A. H. Moskovitz, B. O. Anderson, R. S. Yeung, et al., "Axillary Web Syndrome After Axillary Dissection," *American Journal of Surgery* 181, no. 5 (2001): 434–439.

7. R. H. Baron, J. V. Fey, P. I. Borgen, et al., "Eighteen Sensations After Breast Cancer Surgery: A 5-Year Comparison of Sentinel Lymph Node Biopsy and Axillary Lymph Node Dissection," *Annals of Surgical Oncology* 14, no. 5 (May 2007): 1653–1661.

8. Toan T. Nguyen et al., "Breast Cancer-Related Lymphedema Risk Is Related to Multidisciplinary Treatment and Not Surgery Alone: Results from a Large Cohort Study," *Annals of Surgical Oncology* 24, no. 10 (2017): 2972–2980, doi:10.1245/s10434-017-5960-x.

9. Amparo García-Tejedor et al., "Radiofrequency Ablation Followed by Surgical Excision Versus Lumpectomy for Early Stage Breast Cancer: A Randomized Phase II Clinical Trial," *Radiology* 289, no. 2 (2018): 317–324, doi:10.1148/radiol.2018180235.

10. Wenbin Zhou et al., "Microwave Ablation Induces Th1-Type Immune Response with Activation of ICOS Pathway in Early-Stage Breast Cancer," *Journal for Immunotherapy of Cancer* 9, no. 4 (2021): e002343, doi:10.1136/jitc-2021-002343.

11. Richard E. Fine et al., "Cryoablation Without Excision for Low-Risk Early-Stage Breast Cancer: 3-Year Interim Analysis of Ipsilateral Breast Tumor Recurrence in the ICE3 Trial," *Annals of Surgical Oncology* 28, no. 10 (2021): 5525–5534, doi:10.1245/s10434-021-10501-4.

12. M. Thompson, R. Henry-Tillman, A. Margulies, et al., "Hematoma-Directed Ultrasound-Guided (Hug) Breast Lumpectomy," *Annals of Surgical Oncology* 14, no. 1 (January 2007): 148–156.

13. J. W. Jakub, R. J. Gray, A. C. Degnim, et al., "Current Status of Radioactive Seed for Localization of Non-Palpable Breast Lesions," *American Journal of Surgery* 199, no. 4 (April 2010): 522–528.

14. B. O. Anderson, R. Masetti, and M. J. Silverstein, "Oncoplastic Approaches to Partial Mastectomy: An Overview of Volume-Displacement Techniques," *Lancet Oncology* 6, no. 3 (2005): 145–157.

15. F. Bertolini, J.-Y. Petit, and M. G. Kolonin, "Stem Cells from Adipose Tissue and Breast Cancer: Hype, Risks and Hope," *British Journal of Cancer* 112 (2015): 419–423.

16. Todor Krastev et al., "Long-Term Follow-Up of Autologous Fat Transfer vs Conventional Breast Reconstruction and Association with Cancer Relapse in Patients with Breast Cancer," *JAMA Surgery* 154, no. 1 (2019): 56–63, doi:10.1001/jamasurg.2018.3744.

17. Rafaella Genova and Robert F. Garza, "Breast Fat Necrosis," StatPearls, August 11, 2021.

18. S. Paepke, R. Schmid, S. Fleckner, et al., "Subcutaneous Mastectomy with Conservation of the Nipple-Areola Skin: Broadening the Indications," *Annals of Surgery* 250, no. 2 (August 2009): 288–292.

19. Audre Lorde, *The Cancer Journals* (New York: Spinsters, 1980), 44.

20. Rose Kushner, *Why Me?* (Cambridge, MA: Kensington, 1982).

21. Ana M. Fernández-Frias, Jose Aguilar, Juan A. Sánchez, et al., "Immediate Reconstruction After Mastectomy for Breast Cancer: Which Factors Affect Its Course and Final Outcome?," *Journal of the American College of Surgeons* 208, no. 1 (January 2009): 126–133.

22. B. A. Pockaj, A. C. Degnim, J. C. Boughey, et al., "Quality of Life After Breast Cancer Surgery: What Have We Learned and Where Should We Go Next?," *Journal of Surgical Oncology* 99 (2009): 447–455.

23. M. H. Frost, J. M. Slzak, N. V. Tran, et al., "Satisfaction After Contralateral Prophylactic Mastectomy: The Significance of Mastectomy Type, Reconstructive Complications, and Body Appearance," *Journal of Clinical Oncology* 23 (2005): 7849–7856.

24. M. B. El-Tamer, B. M. Ward, T. Schifftner, et al., "Morbidity and Mortality Following Breast Cancer Surgery in Women: National Benchmarks for Standards of Care," *Annals of Surgery* 245 (2007): 665–671.

25. American Society of Plastic Surgeons, "Plastic Surgery Statistics Report 2020," Plasticsurgery.org, https://www.plasticsurgery.org/documents/News/Statistics/2020/plastic-surgery-statistics-full-report-2020.pdf.

26. National Breast Implant Registry, "National Breast Implant Registry Annual Report 2020," Plastic Surgery Foundation, 2020, https://www.thepsf.org/documents/Research/Registries/NBIR/NBIR-Annual-Report-2020.pdf.

27. U.S. Food and Drug Administration, "What to Know About Breast Implants," FDA.gov, September 8, 2022, https://www.fda.gov/consumers/consumer-updates/what-know-about-breast-implants.

28. Mark Lee, et al., "Breast Implant Illness: A Biofilm Hypothesis," *Plastic and Reconstructive Surgery. Global Open* 8, no. 4 (April 30, 2020): e2755, doi:10.1097/GOX.0000000000002755.

29. Deena Metzger, *Tree and the Woman Who Slept with Men to Take the War out of Them* (Oakland, CA: Wingbow, 1983).

CHAPTER 14. LOCAL TREATMENT: RADIATION THERAPY

1. Icro Meattini et al., "Accelerated Partial-Breast Irradiation Compared with Whole-Breast Irradiation for Early Breast Cancer: Long-Term Results of the Randomized Phase III APBI-IMRT-Florence Trial," *Journal of Clinical Oncology* 38, no. 35 (2020): 4175–4183, doi:10.1200/JCO.20.00650.

2. T. Whelan, R. Mackenzie, Jim Julian, et al., "Randomized Trial of Breast Irradiation Schedules After Lumpectomy for Women with Lymph Node-Negative Breast Cancer," *Journal of the National Cancer Institute* 94, no. 15 (August 2002): 1143–1150.

3. F. M. Dirbas, S. S. Jeffrey, and D. R. Goffinet, "The Evolution of Accelerated, Partial-Breast Irradiation as a Potential Treatment Option for Women with Newly Diagnosed Breast Cancer Considering Breast Conservation," *Cancer Biotherapy and Radiopharmaceuticals* 19, no. 6 (2004): 673–705.

4. F. A. Vicini, K. L. Baglan, L. L. Kestin, et al., "Accelerated Treatment of Breast Cancer," *Journal of Clinical Oncology* 19 (2001): 1993–2001.

5. Jayant S. Vaidya et al., "Long-Term Survival and Local Control Outcomes from Single Dose Targeted Intraoperative Radiotherapy During Lumpectomy (TARGIT-IORT) for Early Breast Cancer: TARGIT-A Randomised Clinical Trial," *British Medical Journal* 370 (August 19, 2020): m2836, doi:10.1136/bmj.m2836.

6. J. M. Kurtz, R. Amalric, H. Brandone, et al., "Contralateral Breast Cancer and Other Second Malignancies in Patients Treated by Breast-Conserving Therapy with Radiation," *International Journal of Radiation, Oncology, Biology and Physics* 15 (1987): 277–284.

CHAPTER 15. SYSTEMIC THERAPY: CHEMOTHERAPY, HORMONES, TARGETED THERAPIES, AND IMMUNOTHERAPY

1. G. Bonadonna, V. E. Valagussa, A. Rossi, et al., "Ten-Year Experience with CMF-Based Adjuvant Chemotherapy in Resectable Breast Cancer," *Breast Cancer Research and Treatment* 5 (1985): 95–115.

2. American Society of Clinical Oncology, "American Society of Clinical Oncology Recommendations for the Use of Hematopoetic Colony Stimulating Factors: Evidence-Based Clinical Practice Guidelines," *Journal of Clinical Oncology* 12 (1994): 2471–2508.

3. Gregory S. Calip et al., "Myelodysplastic Syndrome and Acute Myeloid Leukemia Following Adjuvant Chemotherapy with and Without Granulocyte Colony-Stimulating Factors for Breast Cancer," *Breast Cancer Research and Treatment* 154, no. 1 (2015): 133–143, doi:10.1007/s10549-015-3590-1.

4. National Comprehensive Cancer Network, "NCCN Practice Guidelines in Oncology 2004, Vol. 1: High Emetic Risk, Chemotherapy-Emesis Prevention," https://www.nccn.org/professionals/physician_gls/pdf/breast.pdf.

5. L. N. Chaudhary, S. Wen, J. Xiao, et al., "Weight Change Associated with Third-Generation Adjuvant Chemotherapy in Breast Cancer Patients," *Journal of Community Support Oncology* 12, no. 10 (October 2014): 355–360.

6. C. Printz, "Obesity Associated with Higher Mortality in Women with ER-Positive Breast Cancer," *Cancer* 120, no. 21 (November 2014): 3267.

7. R. M. Speck, A. Demichele, J. T. Farrar, et al., "Taste Alteration in Breast Cancer Patients Treated with Taxane Chemotherapy: Experience, Effect and Coping Strategies Support Care," *Cancer* 21, no. 2 (2013): 549–555.

8. I. IJpma, R. J. Renken, G. J. Ter Horst, et al., "Metallic Taste in Cancer Patients Treated with Chemotherapy," *Cancer Treatment Reviews* 41, no. 2 (February 2015): 179–186.

9. Renate Haidinger and Ingo Bauerfeind, "Long-Term Side Effects of Adjuvant Therapy in Primary Breast Cancer Patients: Results of a Web-Based Survey," *Breast Care* 14, no. 4 (2019): 111–116, doi:10.1159/000497233.

10. P. J. Goodwin, M. Ennis, K. I. Pritchard, et al., "Risk of Menopause During the First Year After Breast Cancer Diagnosis," *Journal of Clinical Oncology* 17, no. 8 (1999): 2365–2370; J. Bines, D. M. Oleske, and M. A. Cobleigh, "Ovarian Function in Premenopausal Women Treated with Adjuvant Chemotherapy for Breast Cancer," *Journal of Clinical Oncology* 14, no. 5 (1996): 1718–1729.

11. M. A. Cobleigh, J. Bines, D. Harris, et al., "Amenorrhea Following Adjuvant Chemotherapy for Breast Cancer," *Proceedings of the American Society of Clinical Oncology*

14 (1995): 115; C. J. Bryce, T. Shenkier, K. Gelmon, et al., "Menstrual Disruption in Premenopausal Breast Cancer Patients Receiving CMF (V) vs AC Adjuvant Chemotherapy," *Breast Cancer Research and Treatment* 50, no. 3 (1998): 336.

12. H. C. F. Moore, J. M. Unger, K. A. Phillips, et al., "Goserelin for Ovarian Protection During Breast-Cancer Adjuvant Chemotherapy," *New England Journal of Medicine* 372 (2015): 923–932.

13. Joachim Chan et al., "Permanent Hair Loss Associated with Taxane Chemotherapy Use in Breast Cancer: A Retrospective Survey at Two Tertiary UK Cancer Centres," *European Journal of Cancer Care* 30, no. 3 (2021): e13395, doi:10.1111/ecc.13395.

14. D. Irvine, L. Vincent, J. E. Graydon, et al., "The Prevalence and Correlates of Fatigue in Patients Receiving Treatment with Chemotherapy and Radiotherapy: Comparison with the Fatigue Experienced by Healthy Individuals," *Cancer Nursing* 17, no. 5 (1994): 367–378.

15. J. F. Meneses-Echávez, E. González-Jiménez, and R. Ramírez-Vélez, "Effects of Supervised Exercise on Cancer-Related Fatigue in Breast Cancer Survivors: A Systematic Review and Meta-Analysis," *BMC Cancer* 15, no. 1 (2015): 77.

16. Arti Hurris, George Somlo, and Tim Ahles, "Renaming 'Chemobrain,'" *Cancer Investigation* 25, no. 6 (2007): 373–377; N. Biglia, V. E. Bounous, A. Malabaila, et al., "Objective and Self-Reported Cognitive Dysfunction in Breast Cancer Women Treated with Chemotherapy: A Prospective Study," *European Journal of Cancer Care* 21, no. 4 (2012): 485–492; J. S. Wefel, A. K. Saleeba, A. U. Buzdar, et al., "Acute and Late Onset Cognitive Dysfunction Associated with Chemotherapy in Women with Breast Cancer," *Cancer* 116 (2010): 3348–3356.

17. R. E. Smith, J. Bryant, A. Decillis, et al., "Acute Myeloid Leukemia and Myelodysplastic Syndrome After Doxorubicin-Cyclophosphamide Adjuvant Therapy for Operable Breast Cancer: The National Surgical Breast and Bowel Project Experience," *Journal of Clinical Oncology* 21 (2003): 1195–1204.

18. S. M. Swain, F. S. Whatley, and M. S. Ewer, "Congestive Heart Failure in Patients Treated with Doxorubicin: A Retrospective Analysis of Three Trials," *Cancer* 97 (2003): 2869–2879.

19. E. Rivera and M. Cianfrocca, "Overview of Neuropathy Associated with Taxanes for the Treatment of Metastatic Breast Cancer," *Cancer Chemotherapy and Pharmacology* 75, no. 4 (April 2015): 659–670.

20. Bernie S. Siegel, *Love, Medicine and Miracles: Lessons Learned About Self-Healing from a Surgeon's Experience with Exceptional Patients* (New York: Harper & Row, 1986).

21. C. L. Loprinski, J. Dugler, J. A. Sloan, et al., "Venlafaxine Alleviates Hot Flashes: An NCCTG Trial," *Proceedings of the American Society of Clinical Oncology* 19 (2000), abstract 4.

22. T. Saphner, D. C. Tormey, and R. Gray, "Venous and Arterial Thrombosis in Patients Who Received Adjuvant Therapy for Breast Cancer," *Journal of Clinical Oncology* 9, no. 2 (1991): 286–294.

23. B. Fisher, J. P. Costantino, D. L. Wickerham, et al., "Tamoxifen for the Prevention of Breast Cancer: Current Status of the National Surgical Adjuvant Breast and Bowel Project P-1 Study," *Journal of the National Cancer Institute* 97, no. 22 (November 16, 2005): 1652–1662, doi:10.1093/jnci/dji372.

24. E. Chalas, J. P. Costantino, D. L. Wickerham, et al., "Benign Gynecological Conditions Among Participants in the Breast Cancer Prevention Trial," *American Journal of Obstetrics and Gynecology* 192, no. 4 (2005): 1230–1237.

25. M. Caleffi, I. S. Fentiman, G. M. Clark, et al., "Effect of Tamoxifen on Oestrogen Binding, Lipid and Lipoprotein Concentrations and Blood Clotting Parameters in Premenopausal Women with Breast Pain," *Journal of Endocrinology* 119, no. 2 (1988): 335–339.

26. B. Kristensen, B. Ejlertsen, P. Dalgaard, et al., "Tamoxifen and Bone Metabolism in Postmenopausal Low-Risk Breast Cancer Patients: A Randomized Study," *Journal of Clinical Oncology* 12, no. 5 (1994): 992–997.

27. C. Davies, H. Pan, J. Godwin, et al., "Adjuvant Tamoxifen: Longer Against Shorter (ATLAS) Collaborative Group. Long-Term Effects of Continuing Adjuvant Tamoxifen to 10 Years Versus Stopping at 5 Years After Diagnosis of Oestrogen Receptor-Positive Breast Cancer: ATLAS, A Randomised Trial," *Lancet* 381, no. 9869 (March 9, 2013): 805–816, doi:10.1016/S0140-6736(12)61963-1; Erratum in *Lancet* 381, no. 9869 (March 9, 2013): 804; Erratum in *Lancet* 389, no. 10082 (May 13, 2017): 1884.

28. A. U. Budzar, C. Marcus, F. Holmes, et al., "Phase II Evaluation of Ly156758 in Metastatic Breast Cancer," *Oncology* 45, no. 5 (1988): 344–345.

29. W. J. Gradishar, J. E. Glusman, C. L. Vogel, et al., "Raloxifene HCL: A New Endocrine Agent Is Active in Estrogen-Receptor-Positive Metastatic Breast Cancer," *Breast Cancer Research and Treatment* 46, no. 53 (1997), abstract no. 209.

30. K. Strasser-Weippl, T. Badovinac-Crnjevic, L. Fan, et al., "Extended Adjuvant Endocrine Therapy in Hormone-Receptor-Positive Breast Cancer," *Breast* 22, suppl. 2 (August 2013): S171–S175.

31. Olivia Pagani et al., "Absolute Improvements in Freedom from Distant Recurrence to Tailor Adjuvant Endocrine Therapies for Premenopausal Women: Results from TEXT and SOFT," *Journal of Clinical Oncology* 38, no. 12 (2020): 1293–1303, doi:10.1200/JCO.18.01967.

32. Michael Gnant, Florian Fitzal, Gabriel Rinnerthaler, et al., "Duration of Adjuvant Aromatase-Inhibitor Therapy in Postmenopausal Breast Cancer," *New England Journal of Medicine* 385 (July 2021): 395–405, doi:10.1056/NEJMoa2104162.

33. A. U. Buzdar and the ATAC Trialists' Group, "Clinical Features of Joint Symptoms Observed in the 'Arimidex,' Tamoxifen Alone or in Combination (ATAC) Trial," *Journal of Clinical Oncology* 24, no. 18S (2006): 551.

34. K. Briot, M. Tubiana-Hulin, L. Bastit, et al., "Effect of a Switch of Aromatase Inhibitors on Musculoskeletal Symptoms in Postmenopausal Women with Hormone-Receptor-Positive Breast Cancer: The Atoll (Articular Tolerance of Letrozole) Study," *Breast Cancer Research and Treatment* 120, no. 1 (February 2010): 127–134.

35. D. L. Hersman, "Perfecting Breast Cancer Treatment—Incremental Gains and Musculoskeletal Pains," *New England Journal of Medicine* 372 (January 2015): 477–478.

36. L. E. Geisler, P. E. Lonning, L. Krag, et al., "Changes in Bone and Lipid Metabolism in Postmenopausal Women with Early Breast Cancer After Terminating 2-Year Treatment with Exemestane: A Randomized, Placebo-Controlled Study," *European Journal of Cancer* 42, no. 17 (November 2006): 2968–2975.

37. S. Hines, J. A. Sloan, P. J. Atherton, et al., "Zoledronic Acid for Treatment of Osteopenia and Osteoporosis in Women with Primary Breast Cancer Undergoing Adjuvant Aromatase Inhibitor Therapy," *Breast* 19, no. 2 (April 2010): 92–96.

38. S. G. Ahn, S. H. Kim, H. M. Lee, et al., "Survival Benefit of Zolendronic Acid in Postmenopausal Breast Cancer Patients Receiving Aromatase Inhibitors," *Journal of Breast Cancer* 17, no. 4 (December 2014): 350–355.

39. Shanu Modi et al., "Trastuzumab Deruxtecan in Previously Treated HER2-Positive Breast Cancer," *New England Journal of Medicine* 382, no. 7 (2020): 610–621, doi:10.1056/NEJMoa1914510.

40. Daniel Eiger et al., "The Exciting New Field of HER2-Low Breast Cancer Treatment," *Cancers* 13, no. 5 (March 1, 2021): 1015, doi:10.3390/cancers13051015.

41. S. Modi, W. Jacot, T. Yamashita, et al., "Trastuzumab Deruxtecan in Previously Treated HER2-Low Advanced Breast Cancer," *New England Journal of Medicine* 387, no. 1 (July 7, 2022): 9–20, doi:10.1056/NEJMoa2203690.

42. Arlene Chan et al., "Neratinib After Trastuzumab-Based Adjuvant Therapy in Patients with HER2-Positive Breast Cancer (ExteNET): A Multicentre, Randomised, Double-Blind, Placebo-Controlled, Phase 3 Trial," *Lancet Oncology* 17, no. 3 (2016): 367–377, doi:10.1016/S1470-2045(15)00551-3.

43. Komal Jhaveri, Haeseong Park, James Waisman, et al., "Abstract GS4-10: Neratinib + Fulvestrant + Trastuzumab for Hormone Receptor-Positive, HER2-Mutant Metastatic Breast Cancer and Neratinib + Trastuzumab for Triple-Negative Disease: Latest Updates from the SUMMIT Trial," *Cancer Research* 82, 4_suppl. (February 15, 2022): GS4–GS10, doi:10.1158/1538-7445.SABCS21-GS4-10.

44. Javier Cortés et al., "Trastuzumab Deruxtecan Versus Trastuzumab Emtansine for Breast Cancer," *New England Journal of Medicine* 386, no. 12 (2022): 1143–1154, doi:10.1056/NEJMoa2115022.

45. G. Curigliano et al., "Tucatinib Versus Placebo Added to Trastuzumab and Capecitabine for Patients with Pretreated HER2+ Metastatic Breast Cancer with and Without Brain Metastases (HER2CLIMB): Final Overall Survival Analysis," *Annals of Oncology* 33, no. 3 (2022): 321–329, doi:10.1016/j.annonc. 2021.12.005; Rashmi K. Murthy et al., "Tucatinib, Trastuzumab, and Capecitabine for HER2-Positive Metastatic Breast Cancer," *New England Journal of Medicine* 382, no. 7 (2020): 597–609, doi:10.1056/NEJMoa1914609.

46. So Yi Lam, Wing Sze Liu, Chung-Shien Lee, et al., "A Review of CDK4/6 Inhibitors," U.S. Pharmacist, May 15, 2020, https://www.uspharmacist.com /article/a-review-of-cdk4-6-inhibitors; Ryohei Ogata et al., "Resistance to Cyclin-Dependent Kinase (CDK) 4/6 Inhibitors Confers Cross-Resistance to Other CDK Inhibitors but Not to Chemotherapeutic Agents in Breast Cancer Cells," *Breast Cancer* 28, no. 1 (2021): 206–215, doi:10.1007/s12282-020-01150-8.

47. Stephen R. D. Johnston et al., "Abemaciclib Combined with Endocrine Therapy for the Adjuvant Treatment of HR+, HER2-, Node-Positive, High-Risk, Early Breast Cancer (monarchE)," *Journal of Clinical Oncology* 38, no. 34 (2020): 3987–3998, doi:10.1200/JCO.20.02514.

48. Michael Gnant et al., "Adjuvant Palbociclib for Early Breast Cancer: The PALLAS Trial Results (ABCSG-42/AFT-05/BIG-14-03)," *Journal of Clinical Oncology* 40, no. 3 (2022): 282–293, doi:10.1200/JCO.21.02554.

49. Mitch Dowsett et al., "Biomarkers of Response and Resistance to Palbociclib plus Letrozole in Patients with ER+/HER2- Breast Cancer," *Clinical Cancer Research* 28, no. 1 (2022): 163–174, doi:10.1158/1078-0432.CCR-21-1628.

50. D. E. Dolan and S. Gupta, "Pd-1 Pathway Inhibitors: Changing the Landscape of Cancer Immunotherapy," *Cancer Control* 21, no. 3 (2014): 231–237.

51. Ren Xin-yu, Song Yu, Wang Jing, et al., "Mismatch Repair Deficiency and Microsatellite Instability in Triple-Negative Breast Cancer: A Retrospective Study of 440 Patients," *Frontiers in Oncology* 11 (March 4, 2021), doi:10.3389/fonc.2021.570623.

52. M. Fracol, S. Xu, R. Mick, et al., "Response to Her-2 Pulsed Dc1 Vaccines Is Predicted by Both Her-S and Estrogen Receptor Expression in DCIS," *Annals of Surgical Oncology* 20, no. 10 (October 2013): 3233–3239.

53. S. E. Stanton and M. L. Disis, "Designing Vaccines to Prevent Breast Cancer Recurrence or Invasive Disease," *Immunotherapy* 7, no. 2 (February 2015): 69–72.

54. You Liu et al., "Synthetic MUC1 Breast Cancer Vaccine Containing a Toll-Like Receptor 7 Agonist Exerts Antitumor Effects," *Oncology Letters* 20, no. 3 (2020): 2369–2377, doi:10.3892/ol.2020.11762; Du Jing-Jing, Zhou Shi-Hao, Cheng Zi-Ru, et al., "Specific Immune Responses Enhanced by Coadministration of Liposomal DDA/ MPLA and Lipoglycopeptide," *Frontiers in Chemistry* 10 (February 4, 2022), doi:10.3389 /fchem.2022.814880.

55. Lerner Research Institute News, "Researchers Open Clinical Trial for Triple-Negative Breast Cancer Vaccine," Cleveland Clinic, October 26, 2021, https://www.lerner.ccf.org/news/article/index.php?id=84d7f977cfef00657df60ce 0bf4d30b1389b5d90.

56. Si-Yuan Zhu and Ke-Da Yu. "Breast Cancer Vaccines: Disappointing or Promising?," *Frontiers in Immunology* 13 (January 28, 2022): 828386, doi:10.3389 /fimmu.2022.828386.

CHAPTER 16. SYSTEMIC THERAPY: LIFESTYLE CHANGES AND COMPLEMENTARY TREATMENTS

1. A. M. Lorincz and S. Sukumar, "Molecular Links Between Obesity and Breast Cancer," *Endocrine-Related Cancer* 13, no. 2 (2006): 279–292.

2. P. J. Goodwin, M. Ennis, M. Bahl, et al., "High Insulin Levels in Newly Diagnosed Breast Cancer Patients Reflect Underlying Insulin Resistance and Are Associated with Components of the Insulin Resistance Syndrome," *Breast Cancer Research and Treatment* 114, no. 3 (2009): 517–525; P. J. Goodwin, M. Ennis, K. I. Pritchard, et al., "Fasting Insulin and Outcome in Early-Stage Breast Cancer: Results of a Prospective Cohort Study," *Journal of Clinical Oncology* 20 (2001): 42–51.

3. P. J. Goodwin, R. J. O. Dowling, M. Ennis, et al., "Effect of Metformin Versus Placebo on Metabolic Factors in the MA.32 Randomized Breast Cancer Trial," *npj Breast Cancer* 7, no. 74 (2021), doi:10.1038/s41523-021-00275-z.

4. B. I. Pierce, R. Ballard-Barbash, L. Bernstein, et al., "Elevated Biomarkers of Inflammation Are Associated with Reduced Survival Among Breast Cancer Patients," *Journal of Clinical Oncology* 27 (2009): 3437–3444.

5. R. T. Chlebowski, E. Aiello, and A. McTiernan, "Weight Loss in Breast Cancer Patient Management," *Journal of Clinical Oncology* 20, no. 4 (February 2002): 1128–1143; L. H. Kushi, M. L. Kwan, M. M. Lee, et al., "Lifestyle Factors and Survival in Women with Breast Cancer," *Journal of Nutrition* 137 (2007): 236S–242S; M. D. Holmes, W. Y. Chen, D. Feskanich, et al., "Physical Activity and Survival After Breast Cancer Diagnosis," *Journal of the American Medical Association* 293, no. 20 (2005): 2479–2486.

6. G. Berclaz, S. Li, K. N. Price, et al., "Body Mass Index as a Prognostic Feature in Operable Breast Cancer: The International Breast Cancer Study Group Experience," *Annals of Oncology* 15, no. 6 (June 2004): 875–884; M. Portani, M. Coory, and J. H. Martin, "Effect of Obesity on Survival of Women with Breast Cancer: Systematic Review and Meta-Analysis," *Breast Cancer Research and Treatment* 123 (2010): 627–635.

7. E. De Azambuja, W. Mccaskill-Stevens, P. Francis, et al., "The Effect of Body Mass Index on Overall and Disease-Free Survival in Node-Positive Breast Cancer

Patients Treated with Docetaxel and Doxorubicin-Containing Adjuvant Chemotherapy: The Experience of the BIG 02-98 Trial," *Breast Cancer Research and Treatment* 119 (2010): 145–153.

8. C. H. Kroenke, W. Y. Chen, B. Rosner, et al., "Weight, Weight Gain and Survival After Breast Cancer Diagnosis," *Journal of Clinical Oncology* 23, no. 7 (2005): 1370–1378.

9. P. Goodwin, M. J. Esplen, K. Butler, et al., "Multidisciplinary Weight Management in Locoregional Breast Cancer: Results of a Phase II Study," *Breast Cancer Research and Treatment* 48, no. 1 (March 1998): 53–64; Z. Dujuric, N. M. Dilaura, I. Jenkins, et al., "Combining Weight-Loss Counseling with the Weight Watchers Plan for Obese Breast Cancer Survivors," *Obesity Research* 10, no. 7 (July 2002): 657–665.

10. R. Ballard-Barbash, C. M. Friedenreich, K. S. Courneya, et al., "Physical Activity, Biomarkers and Disease Outcomes in Cancer Survivors: A Systematic Review," *Journal of the National Cancer Institute* 104, no. 11 (2012): 815–840.

11. C. N. Holick, P. A. Newcomb, A. Trentham-Dietz, et al., "Physical Activity and Survival After Diagnosis of Invasive Breast Cancer," *Cancer Epidemiology, Biomarkers and Prevention* 17, no. 2 (February 2008): 379–386.

12. R. Segal, W. Evans, D. Johnson, et al., "Structured Exercise Improves Physical Functioning in Women with Stages I and II Breast Cancer Results of a Randomized Controlled Trial," *Journal of Clinical Oncology* 19, no. 3 (February 2001): 657–665; V. Mock, C. Frangakis, and N. E. Davidson, "Exercise Manages Fatigue During Breast Cancer Treatment: A Randomized Controlled Trial," *Psycho-Oncology* 14, no. 6 (June 2005): 464–477; M. L. McNeely, K. L. Campbell, B. H. Rowe, et al., "Effects of Exercise on Breast Cancer Patients and Survivors: A Systematic Review and Meta-Analysis," *Canadian Medical Association Journal* 175, no. 1 (July 2006): 34–41.

13. B. K. Pedersen, "The Diseasome of Physical Inactivity—and the Role of Myokines in Muscle-Fat Cross Talk," *Journal of Physiology* 587, no. 23 (2009): 5559–5568.

14. J. Weuve, J. H. Kand, J. E. Manson, et al., "Physical Activity, Including Walking, and Cognitive Function in Older Women," *Journal of the American Medical Association* 292 (2004): 1454–1461.

15. G. L. Blackburn and K. A. Wang, "Dietary Fat Reduction and Breast Cancer Outcome: Results from the Women's Intervention Nutrition Study (WINS)," *American Journal of Clinical Nutrition* 86, no. 3 (September 2007): S878–S881.

16. J. P. Pierce, I. Natarajan, B. J. Caan, et al., "Influence of a Diet Very High in Vegetables, Fruit and Fiber and Low in Fat on Prognosis Following Treatment for Breast Cancer: The Women's Healthy Eating and Living (WHEL) Randomized Trial," *Journal of the American Medical Association* 98 (2007): 289–298.

17. Rowan T. Chlebowski et al., "Association of Low-Fat Dietary Pattern with Breast Cancer Overall Survival: A Secondary Analysis of the Women's Health Initiative Randomized Clinical Trial," *JAMA Oncology* 4, no. 10 (2018): e181212, doi:10.1001/jamaoncol.2018.1212.

18. J. P. Pierce, M. L. Stefanick, S. W. Flatt, et al., "Greater Survival After Breast Cancer in Physically Active Women with High Vegetable-Fruit Intake Regardless of Obesity," *Journal of Clinical Oncology* 25 (2007): 2345–2351.

19. Tengteng Wang et al., "Diabetes Risk Reduction Diet and Survival After Breast Cancer Diagnosis," *Cancer Research* 81, no. 15 (2021): 4155–4162, doi:10.1158/0008-5472.CAN-21-0256.

20. Kim T. Knoops, Lisette C. P. G. M. De Groot, Daan Kromhout, et al., "Mediterranean Diet, Lifestyle Factors, and 10-Year Mortality in Elderly European Men and Women," *Journal of the American Medical Association* 292 (2004): 1433–1439; M. J. Stampfer, F. B. Hu, M. J. Manson, et al., "Primary Prevention of Coronary Heart Disease in Women Through Diet and Lifestyle," *New England Journal of Medicine* 343 (2000): 16–22.

21. Noelle K. LoConte et al., "Alcohol and Cancer: A Statement of the American Society of Clinical Oncology," *Journal of Clinical Oncology* 36, no. 1 (2018): 83–93, doi:10.1200/JCO.2017.76.1155.

22. Alexandra J. White et al., "Lifetime Alcohol Intake, Binge Drinking Behaviors, and Breast Cancer Risk," *American Journal of Epidemiology* 186, no. 5 (2017): 541–549, doi:10.1093/aje/kwx118.

23. Harriet Rumgay et al., "Global Burden of Cancer in 2020 Attributable to Alcohol Consumption: A Population-Based Study," *Lancet Oncology* 22, no. 8 (July 13, 2021): 1071–1080, doi:10.1016/S1470-2045(21)00279-5.

24. N. Hamajima, K. Hirose, K. Tajima, et al., "Alcohol, Tobacco and Breast Cancer—Collaborative Reanalysis of Individual Data from 53 Epidemiological Studies, Including 58,515 Women with Breast Cancer and 95,067 Women Without the Disease," *British Journal of Cancer* 87, no. 11 (2002): 1234–1245.

25. H. Greenlee, M. DuPont-Reyes, L. G. Balneaves, et al., "Clinical Practice Guidelines on the Use of Integrative Therapies as Supportive Care in Patients Treated for Breast Cancer," *American Cancer Society Journal* 67 (April 2017): 194–232, doi:10.3322/caac.21397.

26. Norman Cousins, *Anatomy of an Illness as Perceived by the Patient: Reflections on Healing and Regeneration* (New York: Bantam Books, 1979).

27. G. Chvetzoff and I. F. Tannock, "Placebo Effects in Oncology," *Journal of the National Cancer Institute* 95 (2003): 19–29.

28. D. Spiegel, "Effects of Psychotherapy on Cancer Survival," *Nature Reviews Cancer* 2 (2002): 383–388.

29. P. J. Goodwin, M. L. Lezcz, and M. Ennis, "The Effect of Group Psychosocial Support on Survival in Metastatic Breast Cancer," *New England Journal of Medicine* 345 (2001): 1719–1726.

30. B. L. Andersen, L. M. Thornton, C. L. Shapiro, et al., "Biobehavioral, Immune, and Health Benefits Following Recurrence for Psychological Intervention Participants," *Clinical Cancer Research* 16, no. 12 (2010): 3270–3278.

31. P. Duckro and P. R. Magaletta, "The Effect of Prayer on Physical Health: Experimental Evidence," *Journal of Health and Religion* 33, no. 3 (September 1994): 211–219; Larry Dossey, *Healing Words: The Healing Power of Prayer* (San Francisco: Harper, 1993).

32. H. Benson, J. A. Dusek, J. B. Sherwood, et al., "Study of the Therapeutic Effects of Intercessory Prayer (STEP) in Cardiac Bypass Patients: A Multicenter Randomized Trial of Uncertainty and Certainty of Receiving Intercessory Prayer," *American Heart Journal* 151, no. 4 (2006): 934–942.

33. Carl Simonton, Stephanie Simonton, and James L. Creighton, *Getting Well Again: A Step-by-Step, Self-Help Guide to Overcoming Cancer for Patients and Their Families* (New York: Bantam Books, 1992).

34. M. J. Ott, R. L. Norris, and S. M. Bauer-Wu, "Mindfulness Meditation for Oncology Patients: A Discussion and Critical Review," *Integrative Cancer Therapies* 2 (June 2006): 98–108.

35. H. Wurtzen, S. O. Dalton, J. Christensen, et al., "Effect of Mindfulness-Based Stress Reduction on Somatic Symptoms, Distress, Mindfulness and Spiritual Wellbeing in Women with Breast Cancer: Results of a Randomized Controlled Trial," *Acta Oncologica* 54, no. 5 (May 2015): 712–719.

36. L. E. Carlson, R. Tamagawa, J. Stephine, et al., "Tailoring Mind-Body Therapies to Individual Needs: Patients' Program Preference and Psychological Traits as Moderators of the Effects of Mindfulness-Based Cancer Recovery and Supportive-Expressive Therapy in Distressed Breast Cancer Survivors," *Journal of the National Cancer Institute Monographs* 2014, no. 50 (November 2014): 308–314.

37. Norman Cousins, *Anatomy of an Illness* (New York: Norton, 1985).

38. M. A. Navo, J. Phan, C. Vaughan, et al., "An Assessment of the Utilization of Complementary and Alternative Medication in Women with Gynecologic or Breast Malignancies," *Journal of Clinical Oncology* 22, no. 4 (February 2004): 671–677.

39. Pius S. Fasinu and Gloria K. Rapp, "Herbal Interaction with Chemotherapeutic Drugs—a Focus on Clinically Significant Findings," *Frontiers in Oncology* 9 (December 3, 2019): 1356, doi:10.3389/fonc.2019.01356.

40. Christine B. Ambrosone et al., "Dietary Supplement Use During Chemotherapy and Survival Outcomes of Patients with Breast Cancer Enrolled in a Cooperative Group Clinical Trial (SWOG S0221)," *Journal of Clinical Oncology* 38, no. 8 (2020): 804–814, doi:10.1200/JCO.19.01203.

41. Jenna Tucker et al., "Unapproved Pharmaceutical Ingredients Included in Dietary Supplements Associated with US Food and Drug Administration Warnings," *JAMA Network Open* 1, no. 6 (October 5, 2018): e183337, doi:10.1001/jamanetworkopen.2018.3337.

42. S. Leggett, B. Koczwara, and M. Miller, "The Impact of Complementary and Alternative Medicines on Cancer Symptoms, Treatment Disease Effects, Quality of Life, and Survival in Women with Breast Cancer: A Systematic Review," *Nutrition and Cancer* 26 (March 2015): 1–19.

43. M. Zhang, X. Liu, J. Li, et al., "Chinese Medicinal Herbs to Treat the Side-Effects of Chemotherapy in Breast Cancer Patients," *Cochrane Database of Systematic Reviews* no. 2 (April 18, 2007): CD004921.

44. P. Pommier, F. Gomez, M. P. Sunyach, et al., "Phase III Randomized Trial of Calendula Officinalis Compared with Trolamine for the Prevention of Acute Dermatitis During Irradiation for Breast Cancer," *Journal of Clinical Oncology* 22, no. 8 (April 2004): 1447–1453.

45. M. Oberbaum, "A Randomized Controlled Clinical Trial of the Homeopathic Medication TRAUMEEL S in the Treatment of Chemotherapy-Induced Stomatitis in Children Undergoing Stem Cell Transplantation," *Cancer* 92, no. 3 (August 2001): 664–690.

46. J. Jacobs, P. Herman, K. Heron, et al., "Homeopathy for Menopausal Symptoms in Breast Cancer Survivors: A Preliminary Randomized Controlled Trial," *Journal of Alternative and Complementary Medicine* 11, no. 1 (February 2005): 21–27.

47. E. A. Thompson and D. Reilly, "The Homeopathic Approach to the Treatment of Symptoms of Oestrogen Withdrawal in Breast Cancer Patients: A Prospective Observational Study," *Homeopathy* 92, no. 3 (July 2003): 131–134.

48. M. A. Horneber, G. Bueschel, R. Huber, et al., "Mistletoe Therapy in Oncology," *Cochrane Database of Systematic Reviews* no. 2 (April 16, 2008): CD003297.

49. S. Milazzo, S. Lejeune, and E. Ernst, "Laetrile for Cancer: A Systematic Review of the Clinical Evidence," *Supportive Care in Cancer* 15, no. 6 (June 2007): 583–595.

50. Donald Kennedy, "Laetrile Warning," U.S. Food and Drug Administration, n.d., http://resource.nlm.nih.gov/101438443.

51. S. R. Burzynski and E. Kubove, "Initial Clinical Study with Antineoplaston A2 Injections in Cancer Patients with Five Years' Follow-Up," *Drugs Under Experimental and Clinical Research* 13, suppl. 1 (1987): 1–11; S. Green, "Antineoplastons: An Unproven Cancer Therapy," *Journal of the American Medical Association* 267 (1992): 2924–2928; S. R. Burzynski, "The Present State of Antineoplaston Research," *Integrated Cancer Therapy* 3, no. 1 (2004): 47–58.

52. D. R. Miller, G. T. Anderson, J. J. Stark, et al., "Phase I/II Trial of the Safety and Efficacy of Shark Cartilage in the Treatment of Advanced Cancer," *Journal of Clinical Oncology* 16 (1998): 3649–3655.

53. Louise B. Trull, *The CanCell Controversy: Why Is a Possible Cure for Cancer Being Suppressed?* (Norfolk, VA: Hampton Roads, 1993).

54. S. M. Zick, A. Sen, Y. Feng, et al., "Trial of Essiac to Ascertain Its Effect in Women with Breast Cancer (TEA-BC)," *Journal of Alternative and Complementary Medicine* 12, no. 10 (2006): 971–980.

55. L. M. Bennett, J. L. Montgomery, S. M. Steinberg, et al., "Flor-Essence Herbal Tonic Does Not Inhibit Mammary Tumor Development in Sprague Dawley Rats," *Breast Cancer Research and Treatment* 88, no. 1 (2004): 87–93.

CHAPTER 17. FOLLOW-UP

1. Carolyn D. Runowicz, Corinne R. Leach, N. Lynn Henry, et al., "Breast Cancer Survivorship Care Guideline," *Journal of Clinical Oncology* 34, no. 6 (2016): 611–635, doi:10.1200/jco.2015.64.3809.

2. E. Joseph, M. Hyacinthe, G. H. Lyman, et al., "Evaluation of an Intensive Strategy for Follow-Up and Surveillance of Primary Breast Cancer," *Annals of Surgical Oncology* 5 (1998): 552–528.

3. P. A. Ganz, K. A. Desmond, B. Leedham, et al., "Quality of Life in Long-Term, Disease-Free Survivors of Breast Cancer: A Follow-Up Study," *Journal of the National Cancer Institute* 94 (2002): 39–49.

4. Guy F. Robbins and John W. Berg, "Bilateral Primary Breast Cancers: A Prospective Clinical Pathological Study," *Cancer* 17 (1964): 1501–1527.

5. C. D. Haagensen, N. Lane, and C. Bodian, "Coexisting Lobular Neoplasia and Carcinoma of the Breast," *Cancer* 51 (1983): 1468–1482.

6. E. Grunfeld, D. Mant, P. Yudkin, et al., "Routine Follow-Up of Breast Cancer in Primary Care: Randomised Trial," *British Medical Journal* 313 (1996): 665–669.

7. R. J. Cossetti, S. K. Tyldesley, C. H. Speers, et al., "Comparison of Breast Cancer Recurrence and Outcome Patterns Between Patients Treated from 1986 to 1992 and from 2004 to 2008," *Journal of Clinical Oncology* 33, no. 1 (January 2015): 65–73.

CHAPTER 18. AFTER BREAST CANCER TREATMENT: LIVING WITH COLLATERAL DAMAGE

1. N. Vadivelu, M. Schreck, J. Lopez, et al., "Pain After Mastectomy and Breast Reconstruction," *American Surgeon* 74, no. 4 (2008): 285–296.

2. J. S. Crawford, J. Simpson, and P. Crawford, "Myofascial Release Provides Symptomatic Relief from Chest Wall Tenderness Occasionally Seen Following Lumpectomy

and Radiation in Breast Cancer Patients," *International Journal of Radiation, Oncology, Biology and Physics* 34, no. 5 (1996): 1188–1189.

3. M. Teshome, "Lymphedema Lingers Long After Sentinel Lymph Node Dissection for Early Breast Cancer," *Society of Surgical Oncology Cancer Symposium* (2014), abstract 3.

4. J. A. Petrek, R. T. Senie, M. Peters, et al., "Lymphedema in a Cohort of Breast Carcinoma Survivors 20 Years After Diagnosis," *Cancer* 92 (2001): 1368–1377.

5. K. H. Schmitz, R. L. Ahmed, A. B. Troxel, et al., "Weight Lifting for Women at Risk for Breast Cancer-Related Lymphedema: A Randomized Trial," *Journal of the American Medical Association* 304, no. 24 (2010): 2699–2705.

6. P. H. Graham, "Compression Prophylaxis May Increase the Potential for Flight-Associated Lymphoedema After Breast Cancer Treatment," *The Breast* 11, no. 1 (2002): 66–71.

7. S. L. Showalter, J. C. Brown, A. L. Cheville, et al., "Lifestyle Risk Factors Associated with Arm Swelling Among Women with Breast Cancer," *Annals of Surgical Oncology* 20, no. 3 (2013): 842–849.

8. M. L. Kwan, J. C. Cohn, J. M. Armer, et al., "Exercise in Patients with Lymphedema: A Systematic Review of the Contemporary Literature," *Journal of Cancer Survivorship* 5, no. 4 (2011): 320–336.

9. S. Vignes, R. Porcher, M. Arrault, et al., "Long-Term Management of Breast Cancer-Related Lymphedema After Intensive Decongestive Physiotherapy," *Breast Cancer Research and Treatment* 101, no. 3 (2007): 285–290.

10. S. O. Gurdal, A. Kostanoglu, I. Cavdar, et al., "Comparison of Intermittent Pneumatic Compression with Manual Lymphatic Drainage for Treatment of Breast Cancer-Related Lymphedema," *Lymphatic Research and Biology* 10, no. 3 (2012): 129–135.

11. Claire Ketterer, "Surgical Options for Lymphedema Following Breast Cancer Treatment," *Plastic Surgical Nursing* 34, no. 2 (April–June 2014): 82–85.

12. M. T. Omar, A. A. Shaheen, and H. Zafar, "A Systematic Review of the Effect of Low-Level Laser Therapy in the Management of Breast Cancer- Related Lymphedema," *Supportive Care in Cancer* 20, no. 11 (2012): 2977–2984.

13. Li Wang et al., "Predictors of Persistent Pain After Breast Cancer Surgery: A Systematic Review and Meta-Analysis of Observational Studies," *Canadian Medical Association Journal* 188, no. 14 (2016): E352–E361, doi.10.1503/cmaj.151276.

14. T. Meretoja, M. H. K. Leidenius, T. Tasmuth, et al., "Pain at 12 Months After Surgery for Breast Cancer," *Journal of the American Medical Association* 311 (2014): 90–92.

15. W. M. Yeung, S. M. McPhail, and S. S. Kuys, "A Systematic Review of Axillary Web Syndrome," *Journal of Cancer Survivorship* 9, no. 4 (December 2015): 576–598.

16. J. S. Crawford, J. Simpson, and P. Crawford, "Myofascial Release Provides Symptomatic Relief from Chest Wall Tenderness Occasionally Seen Following Lumpectomy and Radiation in Breast Cancer Patients," *International Journal of Radiation, Oncology, Biology and Physics* 34, no. 5 (1996): 1188–1189.

17. K. Eija, T. Tiina, and N. J. Pertti, "Amitriptyline Effectively Relieves Neuropathic Pain Following Treatment of Breast Cancer," *Pain* 64, no. 2 (1996): 293–302.

18. T. Grantzau, M. S. Thomsen, M. Vaeth, et al., "Risk of Second Primary Lung Cancer in Women After Radiotherapy for Breast Cancer," *Radiotherapy and Oncology* 111, no. 3 (2014): 366–373.

19. R. Jagsi, K. A. Griffin, T. Koelling, et al., "Rates of Myocardial Infarction and Coronary Artery Disease and Risk Factors in Patients Treated with Radiation Therapy for Early Stage Breast Cancer," *Cancer* 109 (2007): 650–657.

20. S. C. Darby, M. Ewertz, P. McGale, et al., "Risk of Ischemic Heart Disease in Women After Radiotherapy for Breast Cancer," *New England Journal of Medicine* 368, no. 11 (2013): 987–998.

21. E. O. Osa, K. Dewyngaert, D. Roses, et al., "Prone Breast Intensity Modulated Radiation Therapy: 5-Year Results," *International Journal of Radiation, Oncology, Biology and Physics* 89, no. 4 (July 2014): 899–906.

22. T. A. Ahles, A. J. Saykin, B. C. McDonald, et al., "Cognitive Function in Breast Cancer Patients Prior to Adjuvant Treatment," *Breast Cancer Research and Treatment* 110 (2008): 143–152.

23. P. A. Ganz, J. E. Bower, L. Kwan, et al., "Does Tumor Necrosis Factor-Alpha (TNF-Alpha) Play a Role in Post-Chemotherapy Cerebral Dysfunction?," *Brain, Behavior, and Immunity* 30 (2013): S99–S108.

24. M. G. Falleti, A. Sanfilippo, P. Maruff, et al., "The Nature and Severity of Cognitive Impairment Associated with Adjuvant Chemotherapy in Women with Breast Cancer: A Meta-Analysis of the Current Literature," *Brain and Cognition* 59 (2005): 60–70.

25. T. A. Ahles, J. C. Root, and E. L. Ryan, "Cancer- and Cancer Treatment–Associated Cognitive Change: An Update on the State of the Science," *Journal of Clinical Oncology* 30 (2012): 3675–3686.

26. M. Simo, X. Rifa-Ros, A. Rodrigues-Fornells, et al., "Chemobrain: A Systematic Review of Structural and Functional Neuroimaging Studies," *Neuroscience and Biobehavioral Reviews* 37 (2013): 1311–1321.

27. B. C. McDonald, S. K. Conroy, T. A. Ahles, et al., "Alterations in Brain Activation During Working Memory Processing Associated with Breast Cancer and Treatment: A Prospective Functional Magnetic Resonance Imaging Study," *Journal of Clinical Oncology* 30 (June 2012): 2500–2508; R. A. Lopez Sunini, C. Scherling, N. Wallis, et al., "Differences in Verbal Memory Retrieval in Breast Cancer Chemotherapy Patients Compared to Healthy Controls: A Prospective fmRI Study," *Brain Imaging and Behavior* 7, no. 4 (January 2013): 460–477.

28. M. M. Stouten-Kemperman, M. B. de Ruiter, W. Boogerd, et al., "Very Late Treatment-Related Alterations in Brain Function of Breast Cancer Survivors," *Journal of the International Neuropsychological Society* 21 (2015): 50–61.

29. V. Koppelmans, M. M. Breteler, W. Boogerd, et al., "Neuropsychological Performance in Survivors of Breast Cancer More Than 20 Years After Adjuvant Chemotherapy," *Journal of Clinical Oncology* 30, no. 10 (April 2012): 1080–1086.

30. V. Koppelmans, M. de Groot, M. B. de Ruiter, et al., "Global and Focal White Matter Integrity in Breast Cancer Survivors 20 Years After Adjuvant Chemotherapy," *Human Brain Mapping* 35, no. 3 (March 2014): 889–899.

31. X. Chen, J. Li, J. Chen, et al., "Decision-Making Impairments in Breast Cancer Patients Treated with Tamoxifen," *Hormones and Behavior* 66 (2014): 449–456.

32. P. A. Ganz, L. Petersen, S. A. Castellon, et al., "Cognitive Function After the Initiation of Adjuvant Endocrine Therapy in Early Stage Breast Cancer: An Observational Cohort Study," *Journal of Clinical Oncology* 32, no. 31 (November 2014): 3559–3567.

33. S. Kesler, S. M. Hadi Hosseini, C. Heckler, et al., "Cognitive Training for Improving Executive Function in Chemotherapy Treated Breast Cancer Survivors," *Clinical Breast Cancer* 13, no. 4 (2013): 299–306.

34. K. A. Biegler, M. A. Chaoul, and L. Cohen, "Cancer, Cognitive Impairment, and Meditation," *Acta Oncologica* 48, no. 1 (2009): 18–26; R. J. Ferguson, T. A. Ahles, A. J. Saykin, et al., "Cognitive-Behavioral Management of Chemotherapy-Related Cognitive Change," *Psycho-Oncology* 16, no. 8 (2007): 772–777; J. J. Ratey and E. S. Hagerman, *The Revolutionary New Science of Exercise and the Brain* (New York: Little, Brown, 2008); S. N. Culos-Reed, L. E. Carlson, L. M. Daroux, et al., "A Pilot Study of Yoga for Breast Cancer Survivors: Physical and Psychological Benefits," *Psycho-Oncology* 15, no. 10 (2006): 891–897.

35. L. M. Ercoli, L. Petersen, A. M. Hunter, et al., "Cognitive Rehabilitation Group Intervention for Breast Cancer Survivors: Results of a Randomized Clinical Trial," *Psycho-Oncology* (March 2015).

36. S. Kohli, S. G. Fisher, Y. Tra, et al., "The Effect of Modafinil on Cognitive Function in Breast Cancer Survivors," *Cancer* 115 (2009): 2605–2616.

37. Laxmi S. Mehta et al., "Cardiovascular Disease and Breast Cancer: Where These Entities Intersect: A Scientific Statement from the American Heart Association," *Circulation* 137, no. 8 (2018): e30–e66, doi:10.1161/CIR.0000000000000556.

38. Ann Banke et al., "Long-Term Risk of Heart Failure in Breast Cancer Patients After Adjuvant Chemotherapy with or Without Trastuzumab," *JACC Heart Failure* 7, no. 3 (2019): 217–224, doi:10.1016/j.jchf.2018.09.001.

39. Muhammad Mustafa Alhussein et al., "Pertuzumab Cardiotoxicity in Patients with HER2-Positive Cancer: A Systematic Review and Meta-Analysis," *CJC Open* 3, no. 11 (July 14, 2021): 1372–1382, doi:10.1016/j.cjco.2021.06.019.

40. D. A. Patt, Z. Duan, S. Fang, et al., "Acute Myeloid Leukemia After Adjuvant Breast Cancer Therapy in Older Women: Understanding Risk," *Journal of Clinical Oncology* 25 (2007): 3871–3876.

41. Gregory S. Calip et al., "Myelodysplastic Syndrome and Acute Myeloid Leukemia Following Adjuvant Chemotherapy with and Without Granulocyte Colony-Stimulating Factors for Breast Cancer," *Breast Cancer Research and Treatment* 154, no. 1 (2015): 133–143, doi:10.1007/s10549-015-3590-1.

42. H. G. Kaplan, J. A. Malmgren, and M. K. Atwood, "Increased Incidence of Myelodysplastic Syndrome and Acute Myeloid Leukemia Following Breast Cancer Treatment with Radiation Alone or Combined with Chemotherapy: A Registry Cohort Analysis, 1990–2005," *BMC Cancer* 11 (2011): 260.

43. A. J. Swerdlow, M. E. Jones, and British Tamoxifen Second Cancer Study Group, "Tamoxifen Treatment for Breast Cancer and Risk of Endometrial Cancer: A Case-Control Study," *Journal of the National Cancer Institute* 97 (2005): 375–384.

44. G. A. Curt, W. Breitbart, D. Cella, et al., "Impact of Cancer-Related Fatigue on the Lives of Patients: New Findings from the Fatigue Coalition," *Oncologist* 5 (2000): 353–360.

45. J. E. Bower, P. A. Ganz, K. A. Desmond, et al., "Fatigue in Breast Cancer Survivors: Occurrence Correlates and Impact on Quality of Life," *Journal of Clinical Oncology* 18 (2000): 743–753.

46. L. M. Nail, "Fatigue in Patients with Cancer," *Oncology Nursing Forum* 29 (2002): 537–544; K. Meeske, A. W. Smith, C. M. Alfano, et al., "Fatigue in Breast Cancer

Survivors Two to Five Years Post Diagnosis: A HEAL Study Report," *Quality of Life Research* 16 (2007): 947–960.

47. J. E. Bower, P. A. Ganz, M. L. Tao, et al., "Inflammatory Biomarkers and Fatigue During Radiation Therapy for Breast and Prostate Cancer," *Clinical Cancer Research* 15, no. 17 (2009): 5534–5540.

48. Julienne E. Bower, Patricia A. Ganz, Najib Aziz, et al., "Inflammatory Responses to Psychological Stress in Fatigued Breast Cancer Survivors: Relationship to Glucocorticoids," *Brain, Behavior, and Immunity* 3 (2007): 251–258.

49. J. E. Bower, P. A. Ganz, M. R. Irwain, et al., "Cytokine Genetic Variations and Fatigue Among Patients with Breast Cancer," *Journal of Clinical Oncology* 31 (2013): 1–7.

50. R. R. Spence, K. C. Heesch, and W. J. Brown, "Exercise and Cancer Rehabilitation: A Systematic Review," *Cancer Treatment Reviews* 36, no. 2 (2009): 185–194.

51. J. Finnegan-John, A. Molassiotis, A. Richardson, et al., "A Systematic Review of Complementary and Alternative Medicine Interventions for the Management of Cancer-Related Fatigue," *Integrative Cancer Therapies* 12, no. 4 (July 2013): 276–290.

52. C. J. Hoffman, S. J. Ersser, J. B. Hopkinson, et al., "Effectiveness of Mindfulness-Based Stress Reduction in Mood, Breast- and Endocrine-Related Quality of Life, and Well-Being in Stage 0 to III Breast Cancer: A Randomized, Controlled Trial," *Journal of Clinical Oncology* 30, no. 12 (April 2012): 1335–1342.

53. A. Molassiotis, J. Bardy, J. Finnegan-John, et al., "Acupuncture for Cancer-Related Fatigue in Patients with Breast Cancer: A Pragmatic Randomized Controlled Trial," *Journal of Clinical Oncology* 30, no. 36 (December 2012): 4470–4476.

54. J. E. Bower, D. Garet, B. Sternlieb, et al., "Yoga for Persistent Fatigue in Breast Cancer Survivors: A Randomized Controlled Trial," *Cancer* 118 (2012): 3766–3775.

55. P. Jean-Pierre, G. R. Morrow, J. A. Roscoe, et al., "A Phase 3 Randomized, Placebo-Controlled, Double-Blind, Clinical Trial of the Effect of Modafinil on Cancer-Related Fatigue Among 631 Patients Receiving Chemotherapy: A University of Rochester Cancer Center Community Clinical Oncology Program Research Base Study," *Cancer* 116, no. 14 (July 2010): 3513–3520.

56. J. C. Fehrenbacher, "Chemotherapy-Induced Peripheral Neuropathy," *Progress in Molecular Biology and Translational Science* 131 (2015): 471–508.

57. J. H. Kim, P. M. Dougherty, and S. Abdi, "Basic Science and Clinical Management of Painful and Non-Painful Chemotherapy-Related Neuropathy," *Gynecologic Oncology* 1336 (2015): 453–459.

58. Palliative Doctors, http://www.palliativedoctors.org.

59. K. D. Crew, H. Greenlee, J. Capodice, et al., "Prevalence of Joint Symptoms in Postmenopausal Women Taking Aromatase Inhibitors for Early-Stage Breast Cancer," *Journal of Clinical Oncology* 19 (2001): 3685–3691.

60. Melinda L. Irwin, Brenda Cartmel, Cary Gross, et al., "Randomized Exercise Trial of Aromatase Inhibitor-Induced Arthralgia in Breast Cancer Survivors," *Journal of Clinical Oncology* 33, no. 10 (April 2015): 1104–1111.

61. J. K. Dixon, D. A. Moritz, and F. L. Baker, "Breast Cancer and Weight Gain: An Unexpected Finding," *Oncology Nursing Forum* 5 (1978): 5–7.

62. P. J. Goodwin, "Weight Gain in Early-Stage Breast Cancer: Where Do We Go From Here?," *Journal of Clinical Oncology* 19 (2001): 2367–2369.

63. S. R. Cummings, D. M. Black, E. D. Thompson, et al., "Effect of Alendronate on Risk of Fracture in Women with Low Bone Density but Without Vertebral

Fractures: Results from the Fracture Intervention Trial," *Journal of the American Medical Association* 280 (1998): 2077–2082.

64. P. J. Goodwin, M. Ennis, K. I. Pritchard, et al., "Prognostic Effects of 25-Hydroxyvitamin D Levels in Early Breast Cancer," *Journal of Clinical Oncology* 27 (2009): 3757–3763.

65. R. Coleman, R. de Boer, H. Eidtmann, et al., "Zoledronic Acid (Zoledronate) for Postmenopausal Women with Early Breast Cancer Receiving Adjuvant Letrozole (Z-FAST Study): Final 60-Month Results," *Annals of Oncology* 24, no. 2 (February 2013): 398–405.

66. C. Domschke and F. Schuetz, "Side Effects of Bone-Targeted Therapies in Advanced Breast Cancer," *Breast Care* 9, no. 5 (October 2014): 332–336; F. Borumandi, T. Aghaloo, L. Cascarinil, et al., "Anti-Resorptive Drugs and Their Impact on Maxillofacial Bone Among Cancer Patients," *Anticancer Agents in Medicinal Chemistry* 15, no. 6 (March 2015): 736–743.

67. Andrea Eisen, Mark R. Somerfield, Melissa K. Accordino, et al., "Use of Adjuvant Bisphosphonates and Other Bone-Modifying Agents in Breast Cancer: ASCO-OH (CCO) Guideline Update," *Journal of Clinical Oncology* 40, no. 7 (2022): 787–800, doi:10.1200/JCO.21.02647.

68. Nobuyuki Hamajima et al., "Type and Timing of Menopausal Hormone Therapy and Breast Cancer Risk: Individual Participant Meta-Analysis of the Worldwide Epidemiological Evidence," *Lancet* 394 (2019): 1159–1168.

69. L. Holmberg, H. Anderson, and HABITS Steering and Data-Monitoring Committees, "HABITS (Hormonal Replacement Therapy After Breast Cancer): Is It Safe?: A Randomized Comparison: Trial Stopped," *Lancet* 363, no. 9407 (2004): 453–455.

70. Nobuyuki Hamajima et al., "Type and Timing of Menopausal Hormone Therapy and Breast Cancer Risk: Individual Participant Meta-Analysis of the Worldwide Epidemiological Evidence," *Lancet* 394 (2019): 1159–1168.

71. M. Morrow, R. T. Chatterton Jr., A. W. Rademaker, et al., "A Prospective Study of Variability in Mammographic Density During the Menstrual Cycle," *Breast Cancer Research and Treatment* 121, no. 3 (June 2010): 565–574.

72. The Writing Group for the PEPI Trial, "Effects of Estrogen or Estrogen/Progestin Regimens on Heart Disease Risk Factors in Postmenopausal Women: The Postmenopausal Estrogen/Progestin Interventions (PEPI) Trial," *Journal of the American Medical Association* 273, no. 3 (1995): 199–208.

73. A. R. Cialli and A. Fugh-Berman, "Is Estriol Safe?," *Alternative Therapies in Women's Health* 14, no. 10 (2002): 73–74.

74. Rogerio A. Lobo et al., "A 17β-Estradiol-Progesterone Oral Capsule for Vasomotor Symptoms in Postmenopausal Women: A Randomized Controlled Trial," *Obstetrics and Gynecology* 132, no. 1 (2018): 161–170, doi:10.1097/AOG.00000000 00002645.

75. USPSTF Bulletin, "Task Force Issues Draft Recommendation Statement on Hormone Therapy for Preventing Chronic Conditions in Postmenopausal People," U.S. Preventative Services Task Force, May 2022, https://www.uspreventiveservicestaskforce.org/uspstf/sites/default/files/file/supporting_documents/hormone-therapy-postmenopause-draft-rec-bulletin.pdf.

76. V. Beral and Million Women Study Coordinators, "Breast Cancer and Hormone Replacement Therapy in the Million Women Study," *Lancet* 362, no. 9390 (2003): 419–427; Million Women Study Collaborators, "Endometrial Cancer and

Hormone-Replacement Therapy in the Million Women Study," *Lancet* 365 (2005): 1543–1545.

77. P. Kenemans, "Safety and Efficacy of Tibolone in Breast-Cancer Patients with Vasomotor Symptoms: A Double Blind, Randomized, Non-Inferiority Trial," *Lancet Oncology* 10, no. 2 (2009): 135–146.

78. D. L. Barton, C. L. Loprinzi, S. K. Quella, et al., "Prospective Evaluation of Vitamin E for Hot Flashes in Breast Cancer Survivors," *Journal of Clinical Oncology* 16 (1998): 495–500.

79. C. L. Loprinzi, D. L. Barron, J. A. Sloan, et al., "Mayo Clinic and North Central Cancer Treatment Group Hot Flash Studies: A 20-Year Experience," *Menopause* 15, no. 4, pt. 1 (July–August 2008): 655–660.

80. H. D. Nelson, K. K. Vesco, E. Haney, et al., "Nonhormonal Therapies for Menopausal Hot Flashes: Systematic Review and Meta-Analysis," *Journal of the American Medical Association* 295 (2006): 2057–2071.

81. Roberto A. Leon-Ferre et al., "Oxybutynin vs Placebo for Hot Flashes in Women with or Without Breast Cancer: A Randomized, Double-Blind Clinical Trial (ACCRU SC-1603)," *JNCI Cancer Spectrum* 4, no. 1 (October 21, 2019): pkz088, doi:10.1093/jncics/pkz088.

82. D. L. Barton, D. B. Wender, J. A. Sloan, et al., "Randomized Controlled Trial to Evaluate Transdermal Testosterone in Female Cancer Survivors with Decreased Libido; North Central Cancer Treatment Group Protocol No.2C3," *Journal of the National Cancer Institute* 99 (2007): 672–679.

83. Debra L. Barton et al., "Systemic and Local Effects of Vaginal Dehydroepi-androsterone (DHEA): NCCTG N10C1 (Alliance)," *Supportive Care in Cancer* 26, no. 4 (2018): 1335–1343, doi:10.1007/s00520-017-3960-9.

84. P. A. Ganz and G. A. Greendale, "Female Sexual Desire—Beyond Testosterone," *Journal of the National Cancer Institute* 99, no. 9 (2007): 659–661.

85. P. A. Ganz, J. H. Rowland, K. Desmond, et al., "Life After Breast Cancer: Understanding Women's Health-Related Quality of Life and Sexual Functioning," *Journal of Clinical Oncology* 16, no. 2 (1998): 501–514; C. L. Thors, J. A. Broeckel, and P. B. Jacobsen, "Sexual Functioning in Breast Cancer Survivors," *Cancer Control* 8, no. 5 (2001): 442–448.

86. S. Kitzinger, *Woman's Experience of Sex* (New York: Putnam, 1983).

87. D. K. Wellisch, K. R. Jamison, and R. O. Pasnau, "Psychosocial Aspects of Mastectomy: II. The Man's Perspective," *American Journal of Psychiatry* 135 (1978): 543–546.

88. L. Baider and A. Kaplan-Denour, "Couples' Reactions and Adjustments to Mastectomy: A Preliminary Report," *International Journal of Psychiatry and Medicine* 14 (1984): 265–276.

89. P. A. Ganz, J. H. Rowland, K. Desmond, et al., "Life After Breast Cancer: Understanding Women's Health-Related Quality of Life and Sexual Functioning," *Journal of Clinical Oncology* 16, no. 2 (1998): 501–514.

90. J. H. Rowland, B. E. Meyerowitz, C. M. Crespi, et al., "Addressing Intimacy and Partner Communication After Breast Cancer: A Randomized Controlled Group Intervention," *Breast Cancer Research and Treatment* 118, no. 1 (2009): 99–111.

91. Matteo Lambertini, Eva Blondeaux, Marco Bruzzone, et al., "Pregnancy After Breast Cancer: A Systematic Review and Meta-Analysis," *Journal of Clinical Oncology* 39, no. 29 (October 10, 2021): 3293–3305, doi: 10.1200/JCO.21.00535.

92. R. L. Whitney, J. Bell, S. Reed, et al., "Work and Financial Disparities Among Adult Cancer Survivors in the United States," *Journal of Clinical Oncology* 32, suppl. 31 (2014): abstract 238.

93. S. Y. Zafar, J. M. Peppercorn, D. Schrag, et al., "The Financial Toxicity of Cancer Treatment: A Pilot Study Assessing Out-of-Pocket Expenses and the Insured Cancer Patient's Experience," *Oncologist* 18 (2013): 381–390.

94. R. Jagsi, S. T. Hawley, P. Abrahamse, et al., "Impact of Adjuvant Chemotherapy on Long-Term Employment of Survivors of Early-Stage Breast Cancer," *Cancer* 120, no. 12 (June 2014): 1854–1862.

CHAPTER 19. WHEN CANCER COMES BACK

1. Theodoros Foukakis, Tommy Fornander, Tobias Lekberg, et al., "Age-Specific Trends of Survival in Metastatic Breast Cancer: 26 Years Longitudinal Data from a Population-Based Cancer Registry in Stockholm," *Sweden Breast Cancer Research and Treatment* 130, no. 2 (2011) 130: 553–560.

2. L. J. Solin, E. E. R. Harris, S. P. Weinstein, et al., "Local-Regional Recurrence After Breast Conservation Treatment of Mastectomy," in *Diseases of the Breast*, 4th ed., ed. Jay R. Harris, Marc E. Lippman, Monica Morrow, and C. Kent Osborne, 844–847 (Philadelphia: Lippincott Williams & Wilkins, 2010).

3. E. Rutgers, E. Van Slooten, and H. Kluck, "Follow-Up After Treatment of Primary Breast Cancer," *British Journal of Surgery* 76 (1989): 187–190; John Kurtz, Jean-Maurice Spitalier, Robert Amalric, et al., "The Prognostic Significance of Late Local Recurrence After Breast Conserving Therapy," *International Journal of Radiation Oncology, Biology and Physics* 18 (1990): 87–93.

4. Douglas W. Arthur et al., "Effectiveness of Breast-Conserving Surgery and 3-Dimensional Conformal Partial Breast Reirradiation for Recurrence of Breast Cancer in the Ipsilateral Breast: The NRG Oncology/RTOG 1014 Phase 2 Clinical Trial," *JAMA Oncology* 6, no. 1 (2020): 75–82, doi:10.1001/jamaoncol .2019.4320.

5. L. J. Solin, E. E. R. Harris, S. P. Weinstein, et al., "Local-Regional Recurrence After Breast Conservation Treatment of Mastectomy," in *Diseases of the Breast*, 4th ed., ed. Jay R. Harris, Marc E. Lippman, Monica Morrow, and C. Kent Osborne, 844–847 (Philadelphia: Lippincott Williams & Wilkins, 2010).

6. A. C. Voogd, G. Tienhoven, H. L. Peterse, et al., "Local Recurrence After Breast Conservation Therapy for Early Stage Breast Carcinoma: Detection, Treatment and Outcome in 266 Patients: Dutch Study Group on Local Recurrence After Breast Conservation (BORST)," *Cancer* 85, no. 2 (January 1999): 437–446; S. Galper, E. Blood, R. Gelman, et al., "Prognosis After Local Recurrence After Conservative Surgery and Radiation Therapy for Early-Stage Breast Cancer," *International Journal of Radiation, Oncology, Biology and Physics* 61 (2005): 348–357.

7. M. D. Gilliland, R. M. Barton, and E. M. Copeland, "The Implications of Local Recurrence of Breast Cancer as the First Site of Therapeutic Failure," *Annals of Surgery* 197 (1983): 284–287.

8. S. A. Slavin, S. M. Love, and R. M. Goldwyn, "Recurrent Breast Cancer Following Immediate Reconstruction with Myocutaneous Flaps," *Plastic and Reconstructive Surgery* 93, no. 6 (May 1994): 1191–1204.

9. S. K. Childs, Y. H. Chen, M. M. Duggan, et al., "Surgical Margins and the Risk of Local-Regional Recurrence After Mastectomy Without Radiation Therapy,"

International Journal of Radiation, Oncology, Biology and Physics 84, no. 5 (December 2012): 1133–1138.

10. M. Borner, A. Bacchi, A. Goldhirsch, et al., "First Isolated Locoregional Recurrence Following Mastectomy for Breast Cancer: Results of a Phase III Multicenter Study Comparing Systemic Treatment with Observation After Excision and Radiation," *Journal of Clinical Oncology* 12 (1994): 2071–2077; G. Hortobagyi, "Can We Cure Limited Metastatic Breast Cancer?," *Journal of Clinical Oncology* 20, no. 3 (2001): 620–623.

11. A. Recht, S. Pierce, A. Abner, et al., "Regional Nodal Failure After Conservative Surgery and Radiotherapy for Early-Stage Breast Carcinoma," *Journal of Clinical Oncology* 9 (1991): 988–986.

12. A. Wells, L. Griffith, J. Z. Wells, et al., "The Dormancy Dilemma: Quiescence Versus Balanced Proliferation," *Cancer Research* 73, no. 13 (July 2013): 3811–3816.

13. J. A. Aguirre-Ghiso, P. Bragado, and M. S. Sosa, "Targeting Dormant Cancer," *Nature Medicine* 19, no. 3 (March 2013): 276–277.

14. E. Young, "Written in Blood: DNA Circulating in the Bloodstream Could Guide Cancer Treatment—If Researchers Can Work Out How Best to Use It," *Nature* 511 (July 31, 2014): 524–526.

15. D. A. Haber and V. E. Velculescu, "Blood-Based Analysis of Cancer: Circulating Tumor Cells and Circulating Tumor DNA," *Cancer Discovery* 4, no. 6 (June 2014): 650–661.

16. C. Fedele, R. W. Tothill, and G. A. McArthur, "Navigating the Challenge of Tumor Heterogeneity in Cancer Therapy," *Cancer Discovery* 4, no. 2 (2014): 146–148.

17. A. D. Seidman, "Sequential Single-Agent Chemotherapy for Metastatic Breast Cancer: Therapeutic Nihilism or Realism?," *Journal of Clinical Oncology* 21, no. 4 (2003): 577–579.

18. L. Gerratana, V. Fanotto, M. Bonotto, et al., "Pattern of Metastasis and Outcome in Patients with Breast Cancer," *Clinical and Experimental Metastasis* 32 (2015): 125–133.

19. Hai Wang, C. Yu, X. Gao, et al., "The Osteogenic Niche Promotes Early-Stage Bone Colonization of Disseminated Breast Cancer Cells," *Cancer Cell* 27 (May 2015): 2–28.

20. G. N. Hortobagyi, "Can We Cure Limited Metastatic Breast Cancer?," *Journal of Clinical Oncology* 20 (2002): 620–623.

21. S. M. Parker, J. M. Clayton, K. Hancock, et al., "A Systematic Review of Prognostic/End-of-Life Communication with Adults in the Advanced Stages of a Life-Limiting Illness: Patient/Caregiver Preferences for the Content, Style and Timing of Information," *Journal of Pain and Symptom Management* 34, no. 1 (2007): 81–93.

22. T. Hamaoka, J. E. Madewell, D. A. Podoloff, et al., "Bone Imaging in Metastatic Breast Cancer," *Journal of Clinical Oncology* 22 (2004): 2942–2953.

23. B. E. Hillner, J. N. Ingle, R. T. Chlebowski, et al., "Update on the Role of Bisphosphonates and Bone Health Issues in Women with Breast Cancer," *Journal of Clinical Oncology* 21 (2003): 4042–4057.

24. N. U. Lin, A. Vanderokas, M. E. Hughes, et al., "Clinicopathologic Features, Patterns of Recurrence and Survival Among Women with Triple-Negative Breast Cancer in the National Comprehensive Cancer Network," *Cancer* 118, no. 22 (2012): 5463–5472.

25. A. M. Brufsky, M. Mayer, H. S. Rugo, et al., "Central Nervous System Metastases in Patients with HER2-Positive Metastatic Breast Cancer: Incidence, Treatment,

and Survival in Patients from RegistHER," *Clinical Cancer Research* 17, no. 14 (July 2011): 4834–4843.

26. Masaaki Yamamoto et al., "A Multi-Institutional Prospective Observational Study of Stereotactic Radiosurgery for Patients with Multiple Brain Metastases (JLGK0901 Study Update): Irradiation-Related Complications and Long-Term Maintenance of Mini-Mental State Examination Scores," *International Journal of Radiation, Oncology, Biology and Physics* 99, no. 1 (2017): 31–40, doi:10.1016/j.ijrobp.2017.04.037.

CHAPTER 20. LIVING WITH RECURRENCE

1. NCI SEER 2015–2019 Statistics, "Cancer Stat Facts: Female Breast Cancer Subtypes," Cancer.gov, National Cancer Institute Surveillance, Epidemiology and End Results, May 10, 2022, https://seer.cancer.gov/statfacts/html/breast-subtypes.html.

2. Junjie Li, Zhonghua Wang, and Zhimin Shao, "Fulvestrant in the Treatment of Hormone Receptor-Positive/Human Epidermal Growth Factor Receptor 2-Negative Advanced Breast Cancer: A Review," *Cancer Medicine* 8 (2019): 1943–1957.

3. Rashmi K. Murthy et al., "Tucatinib, Trastuzumab, and Capecitabine for HER2-Positive Metastatic Breast Cancer," *New England Journal of Medicine* 382, no. 7 (2020): 597–609, doi:10.1056/NEJMoa1914609.

4. Javier Cortés et al., "Trastuzumab Deruxtecan Versus Trastuzumab Emtansine for Breast Cancer," *New England Journal of Medicine* 386, no. 12 (2022): 1143–1154, doi:10.1056/NEJMoa2115022.

5. Javier Cortes et al., "Pembrolizumab plus Chemotherapy Versus Placebo plus Chemotherapy for Previously Untreated Locally Recurrent Inoperable or Metastatic Triple-Negative Breast Cancer (KEYNOTE-355): A Randomised, Placebo-Controlled, Double-Blind, Phase 3 Clinical Trial," *Lancet* 396, no. 10265 (2020): 1817–1828, doi:10.1016/S0140-6736(20)32531-9.

6. D. J. Slamon, B. Leyland-Jones, S. Shak, et al., "Use of Chemotherapy plus a Monoclonal Antibody Against HER2 for Metastatic Breast Cancer That Overexpresses HER 2," *New England Journal of Medicine* 334, no. 11 (March 2001): 783–792.

7. A. Howell, J. F. R. Robertson, P. Abram, et al., "Comparison of Fulvestrant Versus Tamoxifen for the Treatment of Advanced Breast Cancer in Postmenopausal Women Previously Untreated with Endocrine Therapy: A Multinational Double-Blind, Randomized Trial," *Journal of Clinical Oncology* 22, no. 9 (2004): 1605–1613; J. F. Robertson, C. K. Osborne, A. Howell, et al., "Fulvestrant Versus Anastrozole for the Treatment of Advanced Breast Carcinoma in Postmenopausal Women: A Prospective Combined Analysis of Two Multicenter Trials," *Cancer* 98, no. 2 (2003): 229–238; C. K. Osborne, J. Pippen, S. E. Jones, et al., "Double-Blind, Randomized Trial Comparing the Efficacy and Tolerability of Fulvestrant Versus Anastrozole in Postmenopausal Women with Advanced Breast Cancer Progressing on Prior Endocrine Therapy: Results of a North American Trial," *Journal of Clinical Oncology* 16 (2002): 3386–3395.

8. M. J. Ellis, F. Gao, F. Dehdashti, et al., "Lower-Dose vs High-Dose Oral Estradiol Therapy of Hormone Receptor-Positive Aromatase Inhibitor Resistant Advanced Breast Cancer: A Phase 2 Randomized Study," *Journal of the American Medical Association* 302, no. 7 (2009): 774–780.

9. Rita S. Mehta et al., "Overall Survival with Fulvestrant plus Anastrozole in Metastatic Breast Cancer," *New England Journal of Medicine* 380, no. 13 (2019): 1226–1234, doi:10.1056/NEJMoa1811714.

10. I. C. Henderson, *Breast Cancer* (New York: Oxford University Press, 2015).

11. Massimo Cristofanilli, G. Thomas Budd, Matthew J. Ellis, et al., "Circulating Tumor Cells, Disease Progression and Survival in Metastatic Breast Cancer," *New England Journal of Medicine* 351 (2004): 781–791.

12. Francois-Clement Bidard et al., "Circulating Tumor Cells in Breast Cancer," *Molecular Oncology* 10, no. 3 (2016): 418–430.

13. C. Farquhar, J. Marjoribanks, R. Basser, et al., "High Dose Chemotherapy and Autologous Bone Marrow or Stem Cell Transplantation Versus Conventional Chemotherapy for Women with Metastatic Breast Cancer," *Cochrane Database of Systematic Reviews* 20, no. 3 (July 2005): CD003142.

14. Dennis J. Slamon, Brian Leyland-Jones, Steven Shak, et al., "Use of Chemotherapy plus a Monoclonal Antibody Against HER2 for Metastatic Breast Cancer That Over-Expresses HER2," *New England Journal of Medicine* 344, no. 11 (2001): 783–792.

15. J. Baselga, K. A. Gelmon, S. Verna, et al., "Phase II Trial of Pertusumab and Trastuzumab in Patients with Human Epidermal Growth Factor Receptor 2 Positive Metastatic Breast Cancer That Progressed During Prior Trastuzumab Therapy," *Journal of Clinical Oncology* 28, no. 7 (2010): 1138–1144.

16. G. Von Minckwitz, A. Du Bois, M. Schmidt, et al., "Trastuzumab Beyond Progression in Human Epidermal Growth Factor Receptor 2-Positive Advanced Breast Cancer: A German Breast Group 26/Breast International Group 03-05 Study," *Journal of Clinical Oncology* 27, no. 12 (April 2009): 1999–2006.

17. G. Mustacchi, L. Biganzoli, P. Pronzato, et al., "HER2-Positive Metastatic Breast Cancer: A Changing Scenario," *Critical Reviews in Oncology/Hematology* 95, no. 1 (February 2015): 78–87, doi:10.1016/j.critrevonco.2015 .02.002.

18. C. Bighin, P. Pronzato, and L. Del Mastro, "Trastuzumab Emtansine in the Treatment of HER-2-Positive Metastatic Breast Cancer Patients," *Future Oncology* 9, no. 7 (July 2013): 955–957.

19. R. S. Finn, J. P. Crown, I. Lang, et al., "The Cyclin-Dependent Kinase 4/6 Inhibitor Palbociclib in Combination with Letrozole Versus Letrozole Alone as First-Line Treatment of Oestrogen Receptor Positive, Her2-Negative, Advanced Breast Cancer (Paloma_1trio-18): A Randomized Phase 2 Study," *Lancet Oncology* 16, no. 1 (January 2015): 25–35.

20. Javier Cortes et al., "Pembrolizumab plus Chemotherapy Versus Placebo plus Chemotherapy for Previously Untreated Locally Recurrent Inoperable or Metastatic Triple-Negative Breast Cancer (KEYNOTE-355): A Randomised, Placebo-Controlled, Double-Blind, Phase 3 Clinical Trial," *Lancet* 396, no. 10265 (2020): 1817–1828, doi:10.1016/S0140-6736(20)32531-9.

21. A. Milani, D. Sangiolo, M. Aglietta, et al., "Recent Advances in the Development of Breast Cancer Vaccines," *Breast Cancer* 6 (October 2014): 159–168.

22. A. Lipton, R. L. Theriault, G. N. Hortobagyi, et al., "Pamidronate Prevents Skeletal Complications and Is Effective Palliative Treatment in Women with Breast Carcinoma and Osteolytic Bone Metastases: Long-Term Follow-Up of Two Randomized, Placebo-Controlled Trials," *Cancer* 88, no. 5 (2000): 1082–1090; B. E. Hillner, J. N. Ingle, R. T. Chlebowski, et al., "American Society of Clinical Oncology 2003 Update on the Role of Bisphosphonates and Bone Health Issues in Women with Breast Cancer," *Journal of Clinical Oncology* 21, no. 21 (November 2003): 4042–4057.

23. A. T. Stopeck, A. Lipton, J. J. Brody, et al., "Denosumab Compared with Zoledronic Acid for the Treatment of Bone Metastases in Patients with Advanced Breast

Cancer: A Randomized Double Blind Study," *Journal of Clinical Oncology* 28 (2010): 5132–5139.

24. Kelly Shanahan (@stage4kelly), "We should not limit #clinicaltrial enrollment to the cancer olympians—trials need to reflect the population who will eventually be using the drugs, comorbidities, brain mets, and all. #WhatFriendsDoes," Twitter, April 9, 2021, 10:48 a.m., https://twitter.com/stage4kelly/status/1380578405272281089.

25. David Spiegel, *Living Beyond Limits: New Hope and Help for Facing Life-Threatening Illness* (New York: Times Books, 1993).

26. Atul Gawande, *Being Mortal: Medicine and What Matters in the End* (New York: Henry Holt, 2014); David Spiegel, *Living Beyond Limits: New Hope and Help for Facing Life-Threatening Illness* (New York: Times Books, 1993).

27. Atul Gawande, *Being Mortal: Medicine and What Matters in the End* (New York: Henry Holt, 2014).

28. Daniel R. Tobin, with Karen Lindsey, *Peaceful Dying: The Step-by-Step Guide to Preserving Your Dignity, Your Choice, and Your Inner Peace at the End of Life* (Reading, MA: Perseus Books, 1999).

Glossary

abscess: Infection that has formed a pocket of pus.

adenine: Nucleotide base that pairs with thymine in forming DNA.

adenocarcinoma: Cancer arising in gland forming tissue. Breast cancer is a type of adenocarcinoma.

adjuvant chemotherapy: Anticancer drugs used in combination with surgery and/or radiation as an initial treatment before there is detectable spread, to prevent or delay recurrence.

adrenal gland: Small gland found above each kidney that secretes cortisone, adrenaline, aldosterone, and many other important hormones.

alopecia: Hair loss, a common side effect of chemotherapy.

amenorrhea: Absence or stoppage of menstrual period.

amino acid: The building block of proteins.

androgen: Hormone that produces male characteristics.

angiogenesis (angiogenic): Stimulates new blood vessels to be formed.

anorexia: Loss of appetite.

apoptosis: Cell suicide.

areola: Area of pigment around the nipple.

aromatase inhibitors: A class of drugs that block an enzyme called aromatase, thereby reducing estrogen levels in the breast tissue.

arthralgia: Pain in joints.

aspiration: Putting a hypodermic needle into a tissue and drawing back on the syringe to obtain fluid or cells.

asymmetrical: Not matching.

ataxia telangectasia: Disease of the nervous system; carriers of the gene are more sensitive to radiation and have a higher risk of cancer.

atypical cell: Mild to moderately abnormal cell.

atypical hyperplasia: Cells that are not only abnormal but increased in number.

augmented: Added to, such as an augmented breast: one that has had a silicone implant added to it.

autologous: From the same person. An autologous blood transfusion is blood removed and then transfused back to the same person at a later date.

axilla: Armpit.

axillary lymph node dissection: Surgical removal of lymph nodes found in the armpit region.

axillary lymph nodes: Lymph nodes found in the armpit area.

balloon catheter: Method for delivering radiation to the site of a lumpectomy.

basal type: Triple-negative or ER-negative, PR-negative and HER2/neu-negative.

base pairs: Two nucleic acids that bind together in DNA and RNA.

benign: Not cancerous.

bilateral: Involving both sides, such as both breasts.

biological response modifier: Usually natural substances such as colony-stimulating factor that stimulates the bone marrow to make blood cells that alter the body's natural response.

biomarker: Measurable biological property that can be used to identify people at risk.

biopsy: Removal of tissue. This term does not indicate how *much* tissue will be removed.

bone marrow: The soft inner part of large bones that produces blood cells.

bone scan: Test to determine if there is any sign of cancer in the bones.

brachial plexus: Bundle of nerves in the armpit that go on to supply the arm.

breast reconstruction: Creation of an artificial breast after mastectomy by a plastic surgeon.

bromocriptine: Drug used to block the hormone prolactin.

calcifications: Small calcium deposits in the breast tissue that can be seen by mammography.

carcinoembryonic antigen (CEA): Nonspecific (not specific to cancer) blood test used to follow women with metastatic breast cancer to help determine if the treatment is working.

carcinogen: Substance that can cause cancer.

carcinoma: Cancer arising in the epithelial tissue (skin, glands, and lining of internal organs). Most cancers are carcinomas.

cell cycle: The steps a cell goes through in order to reproduce itself.

cellulitis: Infection of the soft tissues.

centigray: Measurement of radiation absorbed dose; same as a *rad*.

cfDNA: The remnants and DNA of dead tumor cells found in the bloodstream. An analysis of cfDNA can help diagnose a tumor and guide treatment.

checkpoint: Point in the cell cycle where the cell's DNA is checked for mutations before it is allowed to move forward.

chemo brain: Experience of having one's brain not function as well in attention and memory after receiving a course of chemotherapy.

chemotherapy: Treatment of disease with certain chemicals. The term usually refers to *cytotoxic* drugs given for cancer treatment.

chromosome: Genes are strung together in a chromosome.

cohort study: Study of a group of people who have something in common when they are first assembled and who are then observed for a period of time to see what happens to them.

colostrum: Liquid produced by the breast before the milk comes in: pre-milk.

comedo: Type of DCIS where the cells filling the duct are more aggressive-looking.

comedon: Whitehead pimple.

complete response: Term used in clinical trials to indicate no evidence of cancer after treatment.

contracture: Formation of a thick scar tissue; in the breast a contracture can form around an implant.

core biopsy: Type of needle biopsy where a small core of tissue is removed from a lump without surgery.

corpus luteum: Ovarian follicle after ovulation.

cortisol: Hormone produced by the adrenal gland.

costochondritis: Inflammation of the connection between ribs and breast bone, a type of arthritis.

cribriform: Type of DCIS where the cells filling the duct have punched out areas.

cyclical: In a cycle like the menstrual period, which is every twenty-eight days, or chemotherapy treatment, which is periodic.

cyst: Fluid-filled sac.

cystosarcoma phyllodes: Unusual type of breast tumor.

cytologist: One who specializes in studying cells.

cytology: Study of cells.

cytosine: Nucleotide base that pairs with guanine in DNA.

cytotoxic: Causing the death of cells. The term usually refers to drugs used in chemotherapy.

dense breasts: Breasts with less fat and more glandular and fibrous tissue, making it more difficult to spot any suspicious masses on a mammogram.

diethylstilbesterol (DES): Synthetic estrogen once used to prevent miscarriages, now shown to cause vaginal cancer in the daughters of the women who took it. DES is sometimes used to treat metastatic breast cancer.

DNA: Deoxyriboneucleic acid, the genetic code.

DNA microarray analysis: Way of analyzing the many mutations in many tumors at the same time.

dose dense: Chemotherapy where the interval between two courses is shortened while the dose of each course may be increased, decreased, or made equivalent to a standard dose so that the dose per unit of time is higher.

double helix: Structure of DNA that allows it to be easily replicated.

doubling time: Time it takes the cell population to double in number.

ductal carcinoma in situ (DCIS): Ductal cancer cells that have not grown outside their site of origin, sometimes referred to as precancer.

ductoscope: Tiny endoscope that is threaded through the nipple into a duct.

eczema: Skin irritation characterized by redness and open weeping.

edema: Swelling caused by a collection of fluid in the soft tissues.

electrocautery: Instrument used in surgery to cut, coagulate, or destroy tissue by heating it with an electric current.

embolus: Plug or clot of tumor cells within a blood vessel.

engorgement: Swelling with fluid, as in a breast engorged with milk.

epidermal growth factor: Protein that stimulates growth of certain cells.

epigenetic: Changes in DNA that can be reversible as opposed to permanent mutations; similar to taping the light switch so that it cannot be turned off rather than permanently damaging it.

erbB-2: Another name for the HER2/neu oncogene.

esophagus (esophageal): Organ carrying food from the mouth to the stomach.

estrogen: Female sex hormones produced by the ovaries, adrenal glands, placenta, and fat.

estrogen receptor: Protein found on some cells to which estrogen molecules will attach. If a tumor is positive for estrogen receptors, it is sensitive to hormones.

excisional biopsy: Taking the whole lump out.

extracellular matrix: Material that surrounds the cells.

fat necrosis: Area of dead fat usually following some form of trauma or surgery, a cause of lumps.

fibroadenoma: Benign fibrous tumor of the breast most common in young people.

fibrocystic disease: Much-misused term for any benign condition of the breast.

fibroid: Benign fibrous tumor of the uterus (not in the breast).

flow cytometry: Test that measures DNA content in tumors.

fluoroscopy: Use of an X-ray machine to examine parts of the body directly rather than taking a picture and developing it as in conventional X-rays. Fluoroscopy uses more radiation than a single X-ray.

follicle-stimulating hormone (FSH): Hormone from the pituitary gland that stimulates the ovary.

follicles: In the ovaries, eggs encased in their developmental sacs.

free flap: Flap or island of tissue where the blood supply has been cut and then is reconnected to a vessel at a new site.

frozen section: Freezing and slicing tissue to make a slide immediately for diagnosis.

frozen shoulder: Stiffness of the shoulder, which is painful and makes it hard to lift the arm over your head.

galactocele: Milk cyst sometimes found in a nursing mother's breast.

GCSF (granulocyte-stimulating factor): Drug that stimulates the bone marrow to recover faster from chemotherapy.

gene: Linear sequence of DNA that is required to produce a protein.

genetic: Relating to genes or inherited characteristics.

genome: All the chromosomes that together form the genetic map.

germ line: Cells that are involved in reproduction: sperm and eggs.

ghostectomy: Removal of breast tissue in the area where there was a previous lump.

GnRH agonist: A drug that blocks the pituitary production of hormones that stimulate the ovaries.

guanine: One of the base pairs that form DNA; pairs with cytosine.

gynecomastia: Swollen breast tissue in a man or boy.

hemangioma: Birthmark consisting of overgrowth of blood vessels.

hematoma: Collection of blood in the tissues. Hematomas may occur in the breast after surgery.

hemorrhage: Bleeding.

HER2/neu: Oncogene that, when overexpressed, leads to more cell growth.

heterogeneous: Composed of many different elements. In relation to breast cancer, "heterogeneous" refers to the fact that there are many different types of breast cancer cells within one tumor.

homeopathy: System of therapy using very small doses of drugs, which can produce in healthy people symptoms similar to those of the disease being treated. These are believed to stimulate the immune system.

hormone: Chemical substance produced by glands in the body that enters the bloodstream and causes effects in other tissues.

hot flashes: Sudden sensations of heat and swelling associated with menopause.

HRT: Hormone replacement therapy.

human chorionic gonadotropin (HCG): Hormone produced by the *corpus luteum*.

hyperplasia: Excessive growth of cells.

hypothalamus: Area at the base of the brain that controls various functions including hormone production in the pituitary.

hysterectomy: Removal of the uterus. Hysterectomy does not necessarily mean the removal of ovaries (*oophorectomy*).

immune system: Complex system by which the body is able to protect itself from foreign invaders.

immunocytochemistry: Study of the chemistry of cells using techniques that employ immune mechanisms.

immunotherapy: Therapy that takes advantage of the immune system to treat a cancer.

incisional biopsy: Taking a piece of the lump out.

infiltrating cancer: Cancer that can grow beyond its site of origin into neighboring tissue. "Infiltrating" does not imply that the cancer has already spread outside the breast. "Infiltrating" has the same meaning as *invasive*.

informed consent: Process in which the patient is fully informed of all risks and complications of a planned procedure and agrees to proceed.

in situ: In the site of. In regard to cancer, "in situ" refers to tumors that haven't grown beyond their site of origin and invaded neighboring tissue.

interstitial brachytherapy: Partial-breast irradiation through tubes loaded with radioactive seeds.

intracavitary brachytherapy: Partial-breast irradiation through a balloon filling the biopsy cavity.

intraductal: Within the duct. "Intraductal" can describe a benign or malignant process.

intraductal papilloma: Benign tumor that projects like a finger from the lining of the duct.

intraoperative limited radiation therapy: Irradiation applied in the operating room to the bed of the tumor.

invasive cancer: Cancers that are capable of growing beyond their site of origin and invading neighboring tissue. "Invasive" does not imply that the cancer is aggressive or has already spread.

lactation: Production of milk from the breast.

latissimus flap: Flap of skin and muscle taken from the back used for reconstruction after mastectomy or partial mastectomy.

lidocaine: Drug most commonly used for local anesthesia.

liquid biopsy: Test done on a sample of blood or breast fluid to find circulating cancer cells or tumor cell DNA.

lobular: Having to do with the lobules of the breast.

lobular carcinoma in situ: Abnormal cells within the lobule that don't form lumps. They can serve as a marker of future cancer risk.

lobules: Parts of the breast capable of making milk.

local treatment of cancer: Treatment of the tumor only.

Luminal A and B: Molecular types of breast cancer that are positive for estrogen receptors.

lumpectomy: Surgery to remove a lump with a small rim of normal tissue around it.

luteinizing hormone: Hormone produced by the pituitary, which helps control the menstrual cycle.

lymphatic vessels: Vessels that carry lymph (tissue fluid) to and from lymph nodes.

lymphedema: Milk arm. This swelling of the arm can follow surgery to the lymph nodes under the arm. It can be temporary or permanent and occur immediately or any time later.

lymph nodes: Glands found throughout the body that help defend against foreign invaders such as bacteria. Lymph nodes can be a location of cancer spread.

macrophages: Blood cells that are part of the immune system.

malignant: Cancerous.

mastalgia: Pain in the breast.

mastitis: Infection of the breast. "Mastitis" is sometimes used loosely to refer to any benign process in the breast.

mastodynia: Pain in the breast.

mastopexy: Uplift of the breast through plastic surgery.

MBI: Injection of technetium that can be detected by a nuclear medicine scanner.

menarche: First menstrual period.

metastasis: Spread of cancer to another organ, usually through the bloodstream.

metastasizing: Spreading to a distant site.

methylxanthine: Chemical group to which caffeine belongs.

microarray: Grid of DNA segments of known sequence that is used to test and map DNA fragments, antibodies, or proteins.

microcalcifications: Tiny calcifications in the breast tissue usually seen only on a mammogram. When clustered, they can be a sign of ductal carcinoma in situ.

micrometastasis: Microscopic and as yet undetectable but presumed spread of tumor cells to other organs.

micropapillary: Type of DCIS where the cells filling the duct take the form of "finger" projections into the center.

mitosis: Cell division.

mutation: Alteration of the genetic code.

myocutaneous flap: Flap of skin and muscle and fat taken from one part of the body to fill in an empty space.

myoepithelial cells: Cells that surround the ductal lining cells and may serve to contain the cells.

necrosis: Dead tissue.

neoadjuvant therapy: Steps taken to shrink the tumor prior to the main treatment of a cancer.

neuropathy: Disease of a nerve, often used to describe pain caused by nerve damage as with chemotherapy.

nodular: Forming little nodules.

nuclear magnetic resonance (NMR or MRI): Imaging technique using a magnet and electrical coil to transmit radio waves through the body.

nucleotide: One of the base pairs forming DNA.

observational study: Study in which a factor is observed in a group of people.

oncogenes: Altered DNA that can lead to cancerous growth.

oncology: Study of cancer.

oncoplastic surgery: Surgery on the breast using plastic surgery techniques to improve the cosmetic results.

oophorectomy: Removal of the ovaries.

osteoporosis: Softening of the bones, and bone loss, that occurs with age in some people.

ovarian ablation: Destroying the tissue in the ovary that makes estrogen through surgery, radiation therapy, or drugs.

ovarian suppression: Treatment that reduces or suspends the production of estrogen by the ovaries that can be reversed.

oxytocin: Hormone produced by the pituitary gland, involved in lactation.

p53: Tumor suppressor gene.

palliation: Act of relieving a symptom without curing the cause.

partial-breast irradiation: Radiation just to the bed of the tumor rather than to the whole breast.

pathologist: Doctor who specializes in examining tissue and diagnosing disease.

pectoralis major: Muscle that lies under the breast.

perforator flap: Flap of tissue where the vessel supplying the blood is a perforator through the muscle.

phlebitis: Irritation of a vein.

pituitary gland: Gland located in the brain that secretes many hormones to regulate other glands in the body: the master gland.

placebo: Inert treatment used in a clinical trial for comparison when there is no treatment standard.

Poland syndrome: Congenital condition in which there is no breast development on one side of the chest.

polychemotherapy: Chemotherapy with more than one drug at a time.

polygenic: Relating to more than one gene.

polymastia: Literally many breasts. Existence of an extra breast or breasts.

postmenopausal: After menopause has occurred.

Premarin (conjugated estrogen): Estrogen from pregnant horses' urine that is sometimes given to women after menopause.

progesterone: Hormone produced by the ovary involved in the normal menstrual cycle.

prognosis: Expected or probable outcome.

prolactin: Hormone produced by the pituitary that stimulates progesterone production by the ovaries and lactation.

prophylactic subcutaneous mastectomy: Removal of all breast tissue beneath the skin and nipple, to prevent future breast cancer risk.

prosthesis: Artificial substitute for an absent part of the body, as in breast prosthesis.

protein: Formed from amino acids, this is the building block of life.

protocol: Research designed to answer a hypothesis. Protocols often involve testing a specific new treatment under controlled conditions.

proto-oncogene: Normal gene controlling cell growth or turnover.

Provera (medroxyprogesterone acetate): Progesterone that is sometimes given to women in combination with Premarin after menopause.

pseudolump: Breast tissue that feels like a lump but when removed proves to be normal.

ptosis: Drooping, as in breasts that hang down.

punch biopsy: Biopsy of skin that just punches a small hole out of the skin.

quadrantectomy: Removal of a quarter of the breast.

rad: Radiation absorbed dose; same as a *centigray*. One chest X-ray equals 1/10 of a rad.

radial scar: Benign lesion where glands are trapped in fibrous tissue; often difficult to distinguish from cancer.

randomized: Chosen at random. In regard to a research study it means choosing the subjects to be given a particular treatment by means of a computer programmed to choose names at random.

randomized controlled study: Study in which the participants are randomized to one treatment or another.

recurrence: Return of cancer after its apparent complete disappearance.

recurrence score: Score developed from analyzing different mutations and predicting the risk of recurrence with tamoxifen or chemotherapy.

remission: Disappearance of detectable disease.

repair endonucleases: Enzymes that can repair mutations.

RNA: Ribonucleic acid; carries the message from the DNA into the cell to make proteins.

sarcoma: Cancer arising in the connective tissue.

scleroderma: Autoimmune disease that involves thickening of the skin and difficulty swallowing, among other symptoms.

scoliosis: Deformity of the spine that causes a person to bend to one side or the other.

sebaceous: Oily, cheesy material secreted by glands in the skin.

selenium: Metallic element found in food.

sentinel node: First lymph node to which cancer is likely to spread from a tumor in the breast.

SERM: Selective estrogen receptor modulator; a compound that is estrogenic in some organs and antiestrogenic in others.

seroma: Collection of tissue fluid.

side effect: Unintentional or undesirable secondary effect of treatment.

silicone: Synthetic material used in breast implants because of its flexibility, resilience, and durability.

SNP (pronounced "snip"): Single nucleotide polymorphism; occurs when there is a variation at a single position in a DNA sequence among individuals.

somatic: Cell that forms the organs of the body but is not involved in reproduction.

S phase fraction: Measure of how many cells are dividing at a time; if it is high it is thought to indicate an aggressive tumor.

stem cell: Primitive cell that is self-renewing as well as capable of giving rise to daughter cells.

stroma: Tissue and cells forming the support structure of an organ or gland; many include fat cells, fibrous cells, white blood cells, blood vessels, and nerves.

subareolar abscess: Infection of the glands under the nipple.

subcutaneous tissue: Tissue under the skin.

systemic treatment: Treatment involving the whole body, usually using drugs.

T cells: Type of immune cell that recognizes threats and foreign substances and fights them.

tamoxifen: Estrogen blocker used in treating breast cancer.

targeted therapy: Antibody directed to a specific molecular target, for example, Herceptin.

telomerase: Enzyme that reattaches the end of a chromosome when it divides.

telomere: End of a chromosome, a bit of which is clipped off every time a cell divides.

thoracic: Concerning the chest (thorax).

thoracic nerves: Nerves in the chest area.

thoracoepigastric vein: Vein that starts under the arm and passes along the side of the breast and then down into the abdomen.

thymine: Nucleotide base that pairs with adenine in DNA formation.

TILs: Tumor-infiltrating lymphocytes; white blood cells that recognize and penetrate cancer tumors. They can be extracted from tumors, multiplied in labs, and returned to patients to fight cancer.

titration: System of balancing. In chemotherapy, "titration" means using the largest amount of a drug possible while keeping the side effects from becoming intolerable.

tomosynthesis: Creation of a 3D image of part of the body by digital processing of multiple X-rays.

trauma: Wound or injury.

triglyceride: Form in which fat is stored in the body, consisting of glycerol and three fatty acids.

tru-cut biopsy: Type of core needle biopsy where a small core of tissue is removed from a lump without surgery.

tumor: Abnormal mass of tissue. Strictly speaking, a tumor can be benign or malignant.

tumor dormancy: Tumors that are present in a stable state.

tumor suppressor gene: Gene that prevents cells from growing if they have a mutation.

vegf: Vascular epidermal growth factor; a protein that stimulates new blood vessels to grow.

virginal hypertrophy: Inappropriately large breasts in a young woman.

xeroradiography: Type of mammogram taken on a Xerox plate and transferred to paper rather than X-ray film.

Index

abbreviated MRI (AB-MRI), 175

abdomen, flaps from, 378–381, 379 (fig.), 383 (fig.), 384–385

abemaciclib (Verzenio), 443, 543, 554

ablation
breast, 350, 542
ovarian (*see* ovarian ablation)

Abraxane. *See* nab-paclitaxel

abscess, 40–42, 41 (fig.)

absolute risk, 97, 98 (fig.), 100–101

AC (Adriamycin and cyclophosphamide), 310, 426

accelerated partial-breast irradiation (APBI), 395, 400, 403–405

accelerated radiation, 246–248, 395, 400, 403–405

accelerated whole-breast irradiation (AWBI), 395

acetyl-L-carnitine, 453

acupuncture, 35, 424, 437, 453, 458–459, 481, 491

acute myeloid leukemia (AML), 418–419, 490

adaptive immune system, 70, 71–72, 71 (fig.)

adenocarcinoma, 209

ADH. *See* atypical ductal hyperplasia

adjuvant therapy, 259–262, 412
chemotherapy, 258–262, 416–422
definition of, 259, 412
first randomized trial of, 260
hormone, 432–443
See also specific therapies

adrenal glands, 10, 14 (fig.), 269, 435, 495, 544

Adriamycin. *See* doxorubicin

Adrucil. *See* 5-fluorouracil

advance directives, 566–567

affirmations, 456

Afinitor. *See* everolimus

afterloader, 404

age
at first period, 82, 102, 108, 309
at first pregnancy, 124–125, 130, 132
in screening guidelines, 149–150, 157–159
See also elderly women; young women

age-specific risks, 101, 102 (table)

Ahles, Timothy, 487

AIs. *See* aromatase inhibitors

Alaskan natives, risk of female breast cancer in, 101 (fig.)

alcohol consumption, 124–125, 446, 452–453

alendronate (Fosamax), 272–273, 439

ALH. *See* atypical lobular hyperplasia

alkylating agents, 263

Allen, Robert, 382

Allison, James, 73

Allred, Craig, 295

aloe, 407

alopecia (hair loss), 426–428, 550–551

Aloxi. *See* palonosetron

alpelisib (Piqray), 555

alpha-carotene, 457

alternative treatments, 203, 447, 460–462

amastia, 19

amenorrhea, 48

American Cancer Society
BI-RADS categories, 163 (table)
breast cancer risk, 102 (table)
on complementary therapies, 462
factors that increase risk, 103 (table)
on follow-up, 468–469
political activism of, 572

About the Authors

Susan Love, MD, MBA, was an author, surgeon, researcher, entrepreneur, and mother. She was the chief visionary officer of the Dr. Susan Love Foundation for Breast Cancer Research, and a founder and director of the National Breast Cancer Coalition. Dr. Love was responsible for the Love Research Army, formerly known as the Army of Women, a pioneering online approach to linking those who are willing to participate in breast cancer studies and the scientists who need them. This has developed into a vital resource for fast-tracking research on the disease. Dr. Love passed away with recurrent leukemia in July of 2023.

Elizabeth Love is a journalist, researcher, and translator who has worked for various publications while living in Latin America, South Africa, and Egypt. She currently lives in California.